# Sudden Death

Haiyan Zhu
Editor

# Sudden Death

## Advances in Diagnosis and Treatment

Springer

*Editor*
Haiyan Zhu
Emergency Department
The First Medical Center of Chinese PLA General Hospital
Beijing, China

Emergency Department
Hainan hospital of Chinese PLA General Hospital
Haitangwan Bay, Sanya City
Hainan Province, China

ISBN 978-981-15-7001-8 ISBN 978-981-15-7002-5 (eBook)
https://doi.org/10.1007/978-981-15-7002-5



This Springer imprint is published by the registered company Springer Nature Singapore Pte Ltd.
The registered company address is: 152 Beach Road, #21-01/04 Gateway East, Singapore 189721, Singapore

# Foreword I

For humankind, sudden death is considered an unexpected event as well as a tragedy. For thousands of years, people have been pursuing the skill of bringing back the dead to life. From ancient fables to modern resuscitation techniques, all of them place great hopes on life. With the development of modern recovery science and technology, more and more medical or public welfare personnel are engaged in the research and promotion of saving lives and preventing sudden death.

Sudden death usually refers to the sudden and unexpected nonviolent death of a seemingly healthy person due to an underlying disease or body dysfunction, especially sudden cardiac death, which usually occurs within an hour from the onset of clinical symptoms. According to statistics, there are about three million sudden deaths in the world every year, about 450,000 in the United States, 400,000 in Europe, and 540,000 in China, while the survival rate is less than 5%. With the development of urbanization and industrialization, the number of patients suffering from cardiovascular and cerebrovascular diseases increases year by year in China. The occurrence of sudden death also shows a gradually increasing trend, and what's more, sudden cardiac death takes the first place. According to domestic reports, men from 55 to 60 years of age and women from 65 to 70 years of age are at high risk of sudden death, and the incidence of out-of-hospital sudden death is up to 75–80%. Therefore, the prevention and treatment of sudden death caused by heart diseases are early identification of the signs of sudden death and timely and effective treatment, which is vital to medical professionals as well as the public.

For nearly more than half a century, scholars have been committed to research about the physiological and pathological mechanism of sudden death and effective cardiopulmonary cerebral resuscitation technology. However, the core problem is still about how to improve the success rate of patient recovery after sudden death, related problems after recovery of organ dysfunction, the survival rate, and the recovery degree of neurological function. With the use of advanced technology, people had further understood the pathogenesis of sudden death, accumulated basic theory and clinical experience, and formed updated academic consensus and application, such as high-quality heart compressions standard, suitable pressure ventilation, early application of electric defibrillation method, and low temperature method after the recovery, which had played a promoting role in cardiac arrest treatment. Still, the basic cure for sudden death remains elusive and the key to resuscitation is the beginning time of rescue. It is difficult to control the process from recognizing symptoms to cardiac arrest. To use a Chinese idiom—prepare for the rainy day; it is important to shift the focus of dealing with sudden death from rescue to prevention.

This book discusses the etiology of sudden cardiac death from the perspective of pathological physiology and elaborates the mechanism of brain injury and death, research on the injury of important organs caused by ischemia-reperfusion, and the progress in the diagnosis of sudden death. It also explains problems such as chronic fatigue and stress that lead to sudden cardiac death and pays particular attention to sudden death of female patients, young adults, and infants. In the progress of treatment technology and methods of sudden death, something remains to be resolved, that is how to prevent the occurrence of sudden death, early warning of many factors which would induce sudden death, and the genomic differences leading to population prone to sudden death.

This is a great book written mainly by Chinese scholars exploring sudden death. Haiyan Zhu, editor in chief and professor, has been engaged in the clinical diagnosis and treatment of cardiovascular diseases and related basic research for more than 20 years. She accumulated relatively rich experience and knowledge. She has devoted herself to this area for a long time because of her strong sense of identity with traditional Chinese culture. More than 1800 years ago, in the Eastern Han Dynasty of China, the great physician Zhongjing Zhang expatiated the procedure of CPR in his book named *Synopsis of the Golden Chamber*, the same as today's steps A, B, C. Coincidently, the place of cardiac compression recommended by modern resuscitation guide, the midpoint of the connection between two nipples, happens to be on the "shan zhong point" described in *Lingshu Meridian*, treating chest pain, palpitation, and other diseases mainly. In our existing experimental studies of the use of electrical stimulation of "shan zhong point" alone after 4 min of cardiac arrest in rats, the success rate of resuscitation is higher than 24%, compared with the control group without any resuscitation of rats. The combined CPR technique is twice as successful as CPR alone. Although the study is preliminary, the extent of its effect is obvious.

Another problem in cardiac arrest is about epinephrine application which is controversial in academic circle. Epinephrine can effectively increase the pressure in the aorta and improve the recovery of autonomic circulation. It is difficult to achieve a satisfactory success rate of resuscitation. One of the reasons is that epinephrine destroys the microcirculation of myocardial tissue when arterial pressure is raised, resulting in eventual ischemic damage. According to an experiment in the 1960s, they used high dose of anisodamine extracted from an endemic plant to China and extensive clinical experience in the treatment of septic shock with vasopressors. We also organized and carried out a series of experimental studies on the recovery of epinephrine combined with anisodamine, which significantly improved the success rate of recovery, and discussed the mechanism of its effect at the level of pathophysiology and molecular biology, further verifying its effectiveness in human clinical trials.

All in all, breakthroughs in the treatment of sudden death needs to pay attention to the possible occurrence of sudden death's early prevention or warning. There are many ways to prevent sudden death. The artificial intelligence used in wearables could help gain health data of a person to mine beneficial and potential risk information of sudden death. Take timely and necessary preventive measures at an earlier stage.

Hong Shen, MD, MM
The General Hospital of People's Liberation Army
28 fuxing road, Haidian district
Beijing, China

# Foreword II

It is a great pleasure to recommend the book host edited by Professor Haiyan Zhu. *Sudden Death: Advances in Diagnosis and Treatment* is a book full of awe for life and death. In recent years, there is a lot of news about the sudden death of doctors, nurses, academic masters, and corporate executives. Do we still feel that sudden death is far away from us? Modern medicine has gradually changed from "medical treatment as the center" to "prevention as the center," from "Cure before you get sick" to "prevent before you get sick." The core of our health maintenance is to prevent before you get sick, rather than just do what needs to mend. Therefore, to master the characteristics of etiology, pathogenesis, and clinical expression of sudden death is of particular importance. I believe that *Sudden Death: Advances in Diagnosis and Treatment* should be rooted in everyone's mind as a kind of consciousness of health management. It is a fantastic book suitable for emergency doctors, general practitioners, cardiologists, and practitioners in related disciplines as well as medical students.


Yucheng Guo
Chinese Health Association
General Hospital of Chinese People's Liberation Army
Beijing, China

# Preface

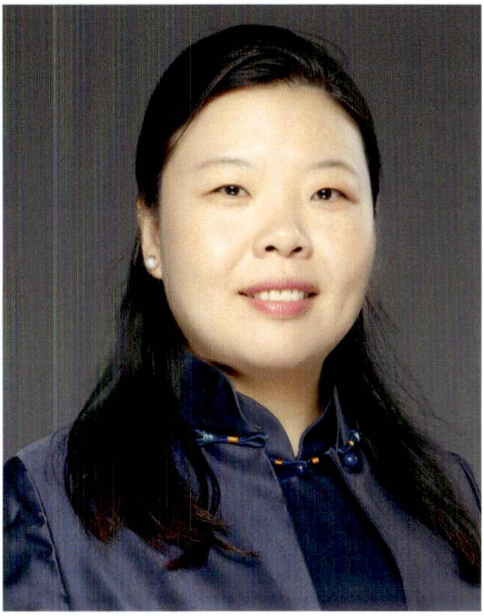

Ladies and gentlemen:

I am a Chinese clinician who has been engaged in cardiovascular medicine, emergency medicine, and critical medicine for about 20 years. In my career, I have seen a lot of sickness and death. What I regret most is sudden death. I have seen the youngest patient with myocardial infarction who was 18 years old, the youngest patient with aortic dissection who was 28 years old, and the youngest patient with explosive myocarditis who was only 1 year old. These patients all suffered suddenly and deteriorated quickly, with sudden cardiac arrest or respiratory arrest within a short period. Besides, my colleagues died of sudden asphyxiation due to hemoptysis at 34, the 48-year-old academic leader died of sudden myocardial infarction, and the 56-year-old academician candidate died of sudden myocardial infarction. The sudden departure of one life after another shocked me, which made me have a very intuitive understanding of sudden death and accumulate a lot of treatment experience in clinical work. Prevention is the most effective way to avoid sudden death. As an old Chinese saying goes, "if we know ourselves and the enemy, we can fight a hundred battles without danger." Nowadays, the success rate for resuscitation in China is less than 1%.

Therefore, I would like to dedicate this book to all those involved in the prevention and treatment of patients such as cardiopulmonary doctors, peers, and researchers, including high-risk patients. I hope everyone through this book can understand sudden death and its epidemiology, pathologic physiology, clinical manifestation, diagnosis, treatment, and prevention. The editors of this book have not only finished a great deal of literature reading but also put their own experience of clinical work into the text and spent a great deal of effort. I, as chief editor of the book, chair of the emergency branch of China Medical Women's Association, would like to recommend this book to everyone. The chapters covering chronic fatigue stress and sudden death, sudden death in women, sudden death in the young, extracorporeal membrane oxygenation therapy, as well as the hot spots of diagnosis and treatment of sudden death largely resonate with readers.

I would like to thank all those who have helped me in constructing and editing the book including the director of my department, the teachers, students, colleagues, editors, as well as my family. The book was written during the China's tough period battling the new virus causing "COVID-19" outbreak. Many writers were devoted to the treatment of the epidemic. Your courage, professionalism, and wisdom cure the patients with "COVID-19," defend the takeoff of China, and embody the spirit of the book and the core essence—salvage as much as possible as we can.

Knowledge is limitless; I will continue to update the content of this book and continue to work hard!

Beijing, China
Sanya, Hainan, China
March 16, 2020

Haiyan Zhu

# Contents

## Part V Chinese Medicine to Prevent Sudden Death

# 1 Introduction of Sudden Death

Haiyan Zhu and Guoxin Han

**Abstract**

Sudden death is unpredictable; it is the most serious disease of human beings. With the development of economy and society, people's pace of work and life is accelerating, which results in long-term physical fatigue, excessive mental burden, and the accompanying bad emotions, such as depression and irritability. Due to the bad influence, the number of sudden deaths is increasing, which has brought huge disaster to the whole society and family. This chapter introduces the connotation, epidemiology, and classification of sudden death in detail.

**Keywords**

Sudden death · Connotation · Epidemiology · Classification

H. Zhu (✉)
Emergency Department, The First Medical Center of Chinese PLA General Hospital, Beijing, China

Emergency Department, Hainan Hospital of Chinese PLA General Hospital, Haitangwan Bay, Sanya City, Hainan Province, China

G. Han
Emergency Department of Strategic Support Force Special Medical Center, Chaoyang, Beijing, China



H. Zhu (ed.), *Sudden Death*, https://doi.org/10.1007/978-981-15-7002-5_1

# 1.1 Introduction

## 1.1.1 Evolution of the Concept of Sudden Death

### 1.1.1.1 Death

It is generally known that all lives will die. From ancient to modern times, many philosophers, writers, medical scientists, and other scholars have profoundly studied the facts of death from different angles. When people live in the world, they will eventually face death, which is judged by nature. No one can get rid of the control of fate. The deaths in life are happening at any time and in just different ways such as death, natural death, or accidental death. Death is the last link that constitutes the complete life process of people. Hegel believes that the moment of the birth of life has already buried the seeds of death, and in the process of human growth, all activities are cultivating this seed and continue to advance the process of death. The meaning and value of death is based on the existence of life, and it ensures the integrity of life. Whether the life of a person lacks life or does not achieve death, the meaning and value as well as the integrity and finiteness of life cannot be judged.

Death is originally interpreted in myth. Primitive religion is the main form of primitive culture. It often needs to be expressed by means of mythology, rituals, etc., all of which are trying to interpret death. Humans have studied the original myths of death around the world and found that the most primitive tribes refuse to recognize the fact that "death is inevitable." With the further development of scientific practice and modern medicine, traditional death standards no longer pose a threat to death because of the wide application of heart transplants and respirators. In addition, effective techniques such as cardiac pacing, intracardiac injection, and cardiopulmonary resuscitation help some people recover their heartbeat and breathing, thus gaining new life. Medical experts have therefore explored new standards of death. The standard of modern medical death is brain death, also known as whole brain death, including irreversible death of the brain, midbrain, cerebellum, and brainstem. The concept of brain death was first proposed by French medical practitioners in 1959, and they first used the term "excessive coma." Because the probability of a patient waking up in this state tends to zero, it can be expressed as "brain death." The criteria for brain death in 1968 were formally proposed, that is, "the irreversibility loss of brain function." This criterion has been recognized by many medical scientists all over the world. Today, more than 80 countries worldwide use brain death as criteria for determining death, and based on this, many European countries and the United States have established special laws and regulations for brain death criteria.

### 1.1.1.2 Sudden Death

Sudden death (SD), as a special type of death, is the most serious disease of human beings. It was known to people thousand years ago. In the ancient Egypt, about more than 4000 years ago, the ancient Abbots medical book stated that the patient may die if there is pain in chest, shoulder, and back. Different literatures have different definitions of sudden death. It is scientifically defined by World Health

Organization (WHO) as an unexpected death which occurs within minutes from disease for those who are healthy and seemingly healthy people.

At present, there is no uniform standard to decide how long exactly can be considered as sudden death from onset to death. For example, the World Health Organization (WHO) in 1970 and the International Heart Association in 1979 defined the sudden death as the immediate accidental death or 24 h after acute symptoms occur. The time from onset to death was within 1 h, 6 h, 12 h, and 24 h, and it was considered to include deaths within 48 h. Most of the deaths within 1 h were sudden cardiac death.

#### 1.1.1.3 The Elements of Sudden Death

The definition "sudden death due to illness" refines the three elements of them sudden death:

- Element 1: The patient has died. If the patient is not dead, he cannot be considered as sudden death. Sudden death is a final diagnosis and a conclusion. Therefore, sudden death is a disease that can only be prevented and cannot be treated. Any situation that can be treated or even cured or successfully recovered cannot be called sudden death.
- Element 2: The patient belongs to natural death, that is, death due to his own disease, and death is caused by internal factors of the patient's body instead of the external factors or unnatural causes such as drowning, electric shock, self-destruction, poisoning, low temperature, high temperature, violence, blood loss, trauma, anesthesia, and surgery.
- Element 3: Sudden death occurs suddenly. The time of its occurrence is unpredictable. The patient does not have signs of imminent death. No one thinks that the patient will die, but death has occurred. Therefore, all expected deaths are not sudden death. The most common clinical patients are end-stage diseases, such as advanced cancer and late stage of various diseases, the patient's life is gradually coming to an end, and the clinical manifestations are obvious to all. Once the patient leaves, this death is not sudden death.

### 1.1.2 Epidemiology of Sudden Death

#### 1.1.2.1 Cardiac Sudden Death

##### Incidence Rate

About two thirds of the sudden deaths result from diseases of circulatory system. The sudden death caused by the heart is also called "Cardiac Sudden Death" [1]. Death often occurs within 1 h after the symptoms appear. If the main cause of sudden death outside the hospital is sudden cardiac death, the incidence of sudden cardiac death in the United States is between 300,000 and 450,000, but this may overestimate the incidence of sudden cardiac death [2]. If cardiac death is strictly defined as death within 1 h of symptom onset, the case of no witnesses is not included, thus underestimating the incidence of cardiac death. So to get a true rate of sudden cardiac death, you need to collect information from multiple sources.

Two prospective studies using multiple sources of information found that the incidence of sudden cardiac death was lower than previously reported, and a data-based study from first responders showed an incidence of sudden cardiac death is 40–90 per 100,000 people. The incidence of sudden death from the center of residents aged 20–75 years in Maastricht, the Netherlands, is 100 per 100,000 people. Research in Ireland shows that the annual rate of sudden death in the country is between 40 and 50 per 100,000 people [3]. The Framingham Heart Study showed that the incidence of sudden cardiac death was 6.8% of the 5000 people included in the study after more than 50 years of follow-up. A prospective study in Paris showed that the incidence of sudden cardiac death in 7000 people enrolled in the study over a 23-year period was 4.4% [4]. If we conclude from these data, the incidence of sudden death in the United States should be between 180,000 and 250,000 per year. With the advancement of primary prevention and secondary prevention of coronary heart disease in recent decades, deaths from coronary heart disease have decreased significantly. The incidence of corresponding sudden cardiac death is also decreasing. In China, through a 1-year monitoring of rural and urban residents selected in Beijing, Guangzhou and Xinjiang, according to the incidence and population of 1.3 billion, the number of sudden cardiac deaths in China is 550,000/year [5]. However, when China's 1.3 billion population is further calculated, the total number of sudden cardiac deaths in China is 544,000, ranking first in the world. The total number of people killed in the United States is 300,000 per year, that is, one person per minute will have sudden cardiac death, and the total number of sudden deaths in China is twice that of the United States, which means that two people will have sudden cardiac death every minute. The data also suggest that with the further aging of the Chinese population, and the increase in the incidence of coronary heart disease as well as the cardiovascular disease the total number of sudden cardiac deaths in China will further increase.

Whether there are differences in epidemiology among different ethnic groups is not yet fully understood. The available data show that the proportion of sudden deaths among the black Americans is higher than that of the white Americans [6], and the rate of discharge after cardiac arrest and survival after cardiopulmonary resuscitation are lower than the white people. At present, the sudden death and risk factors of various people's heart are still unknown.

### Age and Gender Distribution

In the reported epidemiological studies, the incidence of adolescents and young people (<35 years old) ranged from 0.5 to 8/100,000 per year, and the incidence of those who are under 35 years old was lower. The average is 4.5/ten million and 1.4/ten million in London of the United Kingdom and the Veneto area of Italy, respectively. The risk of sudden death of adults increases with age and coronary heart disease. Middle-aged men are four times more likely to have sudden cardiac death than women of the same age. However, this gap decreases with age and may be associated with postmenopausal women who are also susceptible to coronary heart disease. A Chinese study showed that the incidence of sudden cardiac death in middle-aged men was significantly increased, and most cases occurred in people aged 65 years or older. The annual incidence of SCD in 80-year-old males is about 7 times that of 40-year-old males; the distribution of sudden cardiac death in women is more extreme with age: the incidence in those who are over 70-year-old women is more than 40 times that in women aged 45 years or younger. Foreign studies have shown that the incidence of male SCD is 2–3 times that of women; Chinese Hua and other studies have shown that the incidence of males in rural areas is twice that of urban males, about three times that of females. The overall incidence rates of male and female in China were 44.6/100,000 and 39.0/100,000, respectively, and the difference was not statistically significant. In the young population, SCD is predominantly male, with a gender ratio of 1.5 to 3.6:1; the risk of SCD in middle-aged men is four times that of women of the same age, but the difference decreases with age, which may be due to women. The prevalence of postmenopausal CHD is gradually increasing, while CHD is the primary risk factor for SCD.

### 1.1.3 Classification of Sudden Death

#### 1.1.3.1 Cardiac Death

Sudden death due to heart disease is the most common cause.

1. Acute coronary syndrome (ACS). Acute coronary syndrome (ACS) includes plaque rupture, vascular endothelial damage, various inflammatory factors platelet aggregation, and thrombosis after coronary atherosclerosis, causing coronary artery stenosis or even obstruction [7]. With the occurrence of clinical syndrome of insufficient blood supply, subsequent myocardial hypoxic necrosis, the most dangerous type of CHD may occur. In recent years, its morbidity, lethality, and disability rate have been increasing year by year, and it is often accompanied by risks such as malignant arrhythmia, heart failure, sudden cardiac death, and sudden cardiac arrest. In clinical work, it is the most common reason for death. ACS mainly includes ST segment elevation myocardial infarction (STEMI), non-ST segment elevation myocardial infarction (NSTEMI), and unstable angina pectoris (UAP). The first two are collectively called acute myocardial infarction (AMI) [8]. ACS, a serious acute cardiovascular disease, has the characteristics of rapid onset, rapid change of condition, and high mortality. It threatens human health and survival. The Global Acute Coronary Artery Events Registry (GRACE) shows that the mortality rate of ACS patients is about 15% after 1 year and that the cumulative mortality rate is about 20% after 5 years. Bougouin and his team reported the 5-year follow-up results of 3670 patients with acute myocardial infarction. The hospital mortality rate was 5.6%, and the all-cause mortality rate of surviving patients within 5 years was 25.6% [9]. Since 2004, cardiovascular disease (CVD) deaths have been the leading cause of death for urban and rural residents in China and are higher than tumors and other diseases, accounting for more than 40% of deaths from residents. According to the "2017 Chinese

Cardiovascular Disease Report," the number of AMI patients in China is about 2.5 million, and the mortality rate of AMI generally shows an upward trend. The Taiwan ACS full-spectrum registration form shows that among the 183 ACS patients registered, STEMI, NSTEMI, and UAP mortality rates after 1 year were 6.1%, 10.1%, and 6.2%, respectively. Such a high fatality rate not only causes a heavy financial burden on patients, families, and society, but also significantly reduces the quality of life of patients, which shows the urgency and importance of prevention and treatment of ACS.

2. Stress and sudden death. Patients can induce myocardial ischemia under mental and psychological stress, which is different from myocardial ischemia caused by exercise and drug load as inducing factors. This is called mental stress–induced myocardial ischemia (MSIM) [10]. It is closely related to characters and weight. People in a more obvious state of anger and personality traits are more likely to have myocardial ischemia. A rise in weight index leads to increased risk of MSIMI in patients with coronary heart disease, which can be used as an independent risk factor for myocardial ischemia under mental stress. This may have nothing to do with coronary artery stenosis and coronary artery calcification, and may be related to patients' depression and anxiety [11]. Mental stress is different from exercise/drug stress–induced myocardial ischemia. Mental stress mainly increases diastolic blood pressure, the symptoms are concealed, and there are fewer changes in electrocardiogram; while exercise/drug stress increases systolic blood pressure and heart rate. ECG changes. However, this is not conclusive. A study included 34 patients with coronary heart disease and heart failure. The stress test and the drug adenosine test were used to evaluate the myocardial ischemia of the patients by PET examination. The results showed that the stress test and adenosine have the same effect on myocardial ischemia [12].

   Most research results on gender and MSIMI show that MSIMI has gender differences. The incidence of MSIMI in young women after myocardial infarction is twice that of men. There is no clear relationship between the gender differences of MSIMI and psychosocial factors and clinical risk factors. Peripheral arterial tension (PAT) index and reactive hyperemia index cannot explain this difference, but can be used as a predictor of MSIMI in women. Female patients with angina symptoms have a higher incidence of MSIMI, and young women are more likely to develop MSIMI than men and older women. For every 10 years of decline in female age, the total reversibility severity score under mental stress increased by 9.6 points, and the incidence of MSIMI in women was 82.6% higher than that in men [13]. However, York et al. included 154 patients with coronary heart disease, including 61 women and 93 men. Myocardial ischemia was used to diagnose myocardial ischemia. There was no gender difference in the incidence of MSIMI, and there was no difference in hemodynamics and myocardial perfusion.

   A meta-analysis included five clinical studies, a total of 555 patients with coronary heart disease (85% of the patients were male), a follow-up period of 35 days to 8.8 years and a total of 117 events [14]. A comprehensive analysis showed that MSIMI makes the end point (event or total mortality), and the risk of occurrence increases by a factor of 2. Indicators that reflect cardiac function, such as ventricular wall motor function, LVEF, mitral annulus movement, and hemodynamic indicators, can help predict the relationship between MSIMI and cardiac adverse events. The REMIT study has different results for the study of LVEF. The study shows that the continuous variables of mental stress–induced LVEF changes are significantly related to the end events. For every 5% decrease in LVEF caused by mental stress, patients have significant adverse cardiovascular during the average follow-up period. The probability of occurrence increased by 5%, and after 6 years of follow-up, a significant adverse cardiovascular event increased by 20%. Babyak et al. found that changes in LVEF during mental stress were related to clinical events through 5.9 years of follow-up [15]. For every 4% decrease in LVEF during the stress test compared to resting, the risk of clinical events increased by 1.7 times.

Changes in myocardial valve ring motion caused by mental stress are independent predictors of the prognosis of adverse cardiovascular events in patients with stable coronary heart disease. Changes in myocardial valve ring motion caused by mental stress in early diastole and systole are important predictors of major adverse cardiovascular events, while late diastolic changes are marginal. Cardiac annulus motion measurement relationship model shows that early diastolic and/or systolic phases are significantly reduced, and major adverse cardiovascular events are more likely to occur. Late diastolic changes and marginal adverse cardiovascular events are marginal, but have the same trend.

Mental stress increases myocardial oxygen consumption requirements. Physiological responses to mental stress include increased heart rate, peripheral vasoconstrictor response, and increased left ventricular afterload. Mental pressure has an effect on cardiac output and is related to a decrease in LVEF. There is a clear relationship between the changes of neurohormones and the mechanism of MSIMI when coping with mental stress. The heart has its own endocrine function, which affects microcirculation and endothelial signal changes. At the same time, it activates the hypothalamic–pituitary–adrenal axis, promotes the release of cortisol and corticotropin-releasing hormone, and has a systemic effect on inflammation, cardiac function, microcirculation, platelet function, and hemodynamics.

3. Cardiomyopathy (dilated, hypertrophic) is another important disease contributing to ventricular arrhythmia and sudden death. Sustained or induced sustained ventricular tachycardia, mean signal electrocardiogram positive, and right heart involvement are risky patients of sudden death [16–18]. Right ventricular cardiomyopathy can contribute to right ventricular tachycardia and sudden death [19–21]. Myocarditis intrigued by virus leads to the sudden death in children and young people.
4. Congenital heart disease. In patients with Faure's quadruple syndrome, the incidence of sudden death after repair was 6%. Two flap prolapses with complicated ventricular tachyarrhythmia, high-risk patients with sudden death, family history of sudden death, syncope history, and prolonged Q-T interval. Aortic stenosis, regurgitation, and pulmonary stenosis can also occur sudden death [22–24].

5. Arrhythmia. Long Q-T interval prolongation syndrome includes congenital and acquired two major categories. Congenital Q-T interval prolongation syndrome, corrected Q-T interval over 500 ms, and the risk of sudden death in families with sudden death [25, 26]. Pre-excitation syndrome combined with short-term refractory forward conduction has a rapid ventricular rate of atrial fibrillation, which has a certain risk of sudden death. Brugada syndrome refers to "idiopathic" ventricular fibrillation (IVF) in the absence of structural heart disease [27, 28], electrocardiogram with right bundle branch block, V1 to V3 lead ST segment elevation, and sudden death with a group of symptoms [29].
6. Atrial myxoma [30–33]. A benign tumor originating from the endocardial primitive interstitial cells grows to a certain extent. Under the influence of blood flow, it can block the position of the mitral valve. In severe cases, it may cause sudden death. It should be detected early and operated as soon as possible.
7. Viral myocarditis [34, 35]. Many viruses can cause myocarditis, leading to myocardial interstitial hyperplasia, edema, and congestion. The clinical manifestations vary greatly in severity and can be completely symptom-free or sudden death.
8. Heart shock sudden death syndrome [36]. Refers to the heart area in front of a healthy chest, suddenly hit by some reason and drowned.

### 1.1.3.2 Non-cardiac Sudden Death

#### Arrhythmia Drugs and Cardiotoxic Drugs

It can cause severe arrhythmia and sudden cardiac death. Certain drugs and serum preparations may cause cardiac arrest due to severe allergic reactions.

#### Drowning

Drowning refers to the fact that people are drowning in the water, often due to accidents when they fall into the water or swim. Because the respiratory tract is blocked by water, sludge, algae, etc. (90% of wet sudden death) or by the reflex spasm of the head of the throat and trachea (dry drowning accounts for 10%), it causes suffocation and hypoxia and even causes the stop of breathing and heartbeat, even death. The drowning process is very fast, which can cause death if the rescue does not take place in 4–6 min. The study pointed out that the drowning person's 6–9 min mortality rate reached 65%. It can cause serious sequelae and even death if the rescue does not take place in 25 min. However, if the rescue is obtained within 1–2 min, the success rate of salvage can reach 100%. Therefore, weak water first aid must be obtained in time. The early death in drowning is mainly caused by water, sludge, algae, etc. entering the mouth, nose, trachea, and lungs which obstructs the respiratory tract. The death can also be caused by obstruction of throat, trachea, and bronchospasm due to inhaling water, panic, cold, etc. Dilution of blood in fresh water, hemolysis, and ventricular fibrillation can cause elevated blood potassium and cardiac arrest. Electrolyte imbalance of seawater sputum and acute pulmonary edema lead to heart failure and death. When diving, head impact or wood piles can cause craniocerebral trauma, coma, and death in the water. The basic pathological changes of sputum are brain and heart function damage caused by asphyxia and hypoxia, myocardial hypoxia, degeneration and necrosis, and circulatory failure. Pulmonary dysfunction caused by hydronephrosis in the lungs and hypoxia in the body can lead to metabolic acidosis. The environment and duration of drowning determine the severity of the illness after asphyxia. Generally, respiratory arrest occurs first, followed by cardiac arrest.

### Electric Shock

Electric shock refers to the local and systemic injury or dysfunction caused by a certain amount of current passing through the human body. In severe cases, cardiac arrest and respiratory arrest can occur. Whether it is current or static current, it can cause electric shock. It is mostly due to a lack of attention to the safety regulations of the electric industry, especially in rural areas. People are lacking in knowledge of safe electricity use and install wire without permit or rescue electric shockers directly by hand. When people work in high-temperature, high-humidity workplaces or corrosive chemical workshops, especially in the rainy season, their electrical insulation performance is reduced, and the body's resistance to skin contact points is significantly reduced due to sweating and skin moisture, causing injury through the human body. At low voltage (220–380 V) electric shock, current through the heart can cause ion disturbance in the myocardial cells and cause fatal ventricular fibrillation, which is life-threatening. At high voltage >1 kV electric shock, the most common is severe electrical burns, or respiratory numbness caused by high-voltage electric injury in the respiratory center, respiratory muscle tonic contraction caused by apnea and asphyxia, secondary cardiac arrest, or ventricular fibrillation. Muscles contract strongly during an electric shock, causing limb fractures or joint dislocation. Especially falling from high altitude can cause serious combined injuries, such as craniocerebral trauma, chest and abdominal visceral rupture, and so on.

### Obstetric Death

Obstetric death accounts for about 5% of diagnosed deaths [37–39]. Sudden death during pregnancy is mainly caused by sudden deterioration of the original disease, more common heart disease combined with pregnancy, or sudden changes in pregnancy complications, such as eclampsia died of asphyxia, cerebrovascular accident, HELLP syndrome, and DIC. During childbirth, sudden accidents are common, such as amniotic fluid embolism and postpartum hemorrhage. During the puerperium period, the original disease is aggravated during the puerperium, such as pulmonary embolism, dielectric disorder, and puerperal infection.

### Sudden Death of the Respiratory System

1. Acute laryngeal embolism. Acute tonsillitis (occlusion of airway, acute asphyxia, septic shock); posterior pharyngeal abscess (compression obstruction of the throat, pus into the airway, acute asphyxia); acute laryngitis with glottic edema (laryngeal obstruction, suffocation death); glottic fistula, edema (inflammation, allergies, infectious diseases, etc.); throat tumors (polyps, papilloma, fibroids, cancer, obstructive asphyxia, etc.); inhalation injury (hot air, liquid, toxic or irritant gas inhalation).

2. Bronchial asthma [40]. Pulmonary allergic disease, characterized by bronchospasm, is considered a special type of chronic obstructive bronchitis. Bronchial asthma causes asphyxia (occlusion, spasm, spontaneous pneumothorax, respiratory failure) and right heart failure (severe ventilatory disorders, myocardial hypoxia, increased resistance to pulmonary circulation) causing sudden death.
3. Pneumonia [41]. Pneumonia is a frequently occurring disease of the respiratory system. Most people do not die, and some types of pneumonia or those who are infirm can die suddenly.
4. Pulmonary embolism [42]. Pulmonary embolism is a pathological process in which a loose thrombus or other substance blocks the pulmonary artery or its branches. It is often a complication. A patient with pulmonary tissue necrosis after vascular occlusion is called a pulmonary infarction. Clinical symptoms include dyspnea, severe chest pain, hemoptysis, and fever. Acute pulmonary embolism is a clinical and pathophysiological syndrome caused by endogenous or exogenous emboli to block pulmonary circulatory trunk or branch. Its morbidity is second only to coronary heart disease and hypertension. Pulmonary artery trunk or large branch embolization can cause pulmonary artery resistance to suddenly increase, pressure rise, leading to acute right heart failure and sudden death, while pulmonary embolism can cause pulmonary artery, coronary artery, and bronchial artery spasm through lung-heart vagus nerve reflex, or 5-serotonin is released in large amounts, causing pulmonary vasospasm to cause acute heart failure and sudden death.

### Sudden Death Due to Digestive System Disease

1. Acute gastrointestinal bleeding [43–45]. Stomach and duodenal ulcer complicated by massive hemorrhage, cirrhosis complicated with esophageal varices bleeding, acute gastric mucosal hemorrhagic erosion and ulcer, hemorrhage of longitudinal mucosal laceration in the lower esophagus or gastric cardia. Mechanism—hemorrhagic shock.
2. Acute diffuse peritonitis [46]. Appendicitis, gastroduodenal ulcer, enteric typhoid, ulcerative colitis, intestinal tuberculosis, intestinal amebiasis and other perforations, liver abscess, and pancreatic abscess rupture. Sudden death mechanism—ulcer perforation (toxic shock, neurological shock).
3. Acute necrotizing pancreatitis [47–49]. Acute hemorrhagic necrotic pancreatitis is a type of acute pancreatitis that is caused by the continued development of acute edematous pancreatitis, which include pancreatic acinar, fat, large blood vessels necrosis, pancreatic tissue edema, volume increase, extensive hemorrhage, and necrosis. A large amount of bloody exudate in the retroperitoneal space. The omentum and mesangial tissue are digested by the exuded trypsin. This type of pancreatitis is a serious condition with many complications, and high mortality. Pancreatic juice stimulates peritoneal plexus-induced neurogenic shock; massive exudation of sputum, decreased body fluid caused by vomiting, hypovolemia caused by insufficient circulating blood volume; pancreatic tissue necrosis, increased absorption of inflammation and protein breakdown products,

toxic shock; pancreatic juice stimulation, abdominal plexus, nerve reflex caused by sudden cardiac arrest and sudden death.

**Brain Hernia**

When there is a space-occupying lesion in a certain cavity in the skull, the pressure of the sub-chamber is greater than the pressure of the adjacent sub-chamber, and the brain tissue is displaced from the high-pressure area to the low-pressure area, resulting in a series of serious clinical signs and symptoms when sometimes squeezed into the interdural space or in the diverticulum, which is called brain hernia. Various intracranial hematoma is caused by common cause damage, such as acute epidural hematoma, subdural hematoma, and intracerebral hematoma; various intracranial tumors, especially tumors located in one side of the cerebral hemisphere and posterior fossa tumor; intracranial abscess; intracranial parasitic diseases and various other chronic granulomas; congenital factors such as cerebellar tonsil malformation. In addition, if the intracranial pressure is increased, lumbar puncture releases too much cerebrospinal fluid, which leads to an increase in the pressure difference between the intracranial segments, which can promote the formation of cerebral palsy. It can be divided into cerebellar incision, occipital foramen, and cerebral palsy. Among them, the cerebellum incision is the most serious manifestation of changes in blood pressure, pulse, respiration, and body temperature. In severe cases, the blood pressure is high and low, the breathing is fast and slow, sometimes the face is flushed, sweating, sometimes turning pale, and sweaty, the body temperature can be as high as 41 °C or higher, but can be as low as 35 °C or less, and finally breath and blood pressure drop, causing heart arrest and death.

**Other Causes of Sudden Death**

1. Cardiac catheterization and treatment, bronchoscopy, anesthesia, etc. lead to autonomic nervous instability and arrhythmia caused by cardiac arrest.
2. Sudden death from sports [50–52]: Athletes and those who do physical exercise with or without symptoms accidentally die within or after 24 h of exercise. It is mainly due to sudden loss of consciousness, the disappearance of aorta beat, and the breathing stops after 20–30 s of sigh-like breathing. Chest pain and shortness of breath may occur before sudden death, and they may occur suddenly without any warning. The ratio of male to female sports death is 7.2:1, which may be due to the low incidence of ischemic heart disease in women with low exercise load, and difficulty in tolerating fatigue or other excessive overload. The study reported that the average age of sudden death in sports was 30.8 ± 17.9 years old. The data suggest that sudden death may also be affected by the time, but it is not clear. There are a wide range of people involved in sports death, including athletes, coaches, physical education teachers, teachers, cadres, workers, and middle school students aged from 9 to 67 years. Studies have shown that sudden death in sports occurs in projects with high intensity or competition, but some projects with smaller intensity also account for a considerable proportion. Common causes of sudden death in sports are coronary heart disease (SCD is the most common, accounting for 73%–95%, the most common cause of people aged

over 40 years), Marfan syndrome (the most common cause of people under 40 years), hypertrophic cardiomyopathy, coronary artery malformation, idiopathic left ventricular hypertrophy, myocarditis, pre-excitation syndrome, QT syndrome, concussion, and Brugada syndrome.

## References


1. Basso C, Aguilera B, Banner J, et al. Guidelines for autopsy investigation of sudden cardiac death: 2017 update from the Association for European Cardiovascular Pathology. Virchows Arch. 2017;471:691–705.
2. Hayashi M, Shimizu W, Albert CM. The spectrum of epidemiology underlying sudden cardiac death. Circ Res. 2015;116:1887–906.
3. Boudoulas KD, Borer JS, Boudoulas H. Etiology of valvular heart disease in the 21st century. Cardiology. 2013;126:139–52.
4. Adabag AS, Luepker RV, Roger VL, Gersh BJ. Sudden cardiac death: epidemiology and risk factors. Nat Rev Cardiol. 2010;7:216–25.
5. Shao F, Li CS, Liang LR, Li D, Ma SK. Outcome of out-of-hospital cardiac arrests in Beijing, China. Resuscitation. 2014;85:1411–7.
6. Kong MH, Fonarow GC, Peterson ED, et al. Systematic review of the incidence of sudden cardiac death in the United States. J Am Coll Cardiol. 2011;57:794–801.
7. Fox KA, Carruthers KF, Dunbar DR, et al. Underestimated and under-recognized: the late consequences of acute coronary syndrome (GRACE UK-Belgian study). Eur Heart J. 2010;31:2755–64.
8. Benjamin EJ, Blaha MJ, Chiuve SE, et al. Heart disease and stroke Statistics-2017 update: a report from the American Heart Association. Circulation. 2017;135:e146–603.
9. Behnes M, Mashayekhi K, Weiß C, et al. Prognostic impact of acute myocardial infarction in patients presenting with ventricular Tachyarrhythmias and aborted cardiac arrest. J Am Heart Assoc. 2018;7:e10004.
10. Esler M. Mental stress and human cardiovascular disease. Neurosci Biobehav Rev. 2017;74:269–76.
11. Williams RB. Anger and mental stress-induced myocardial ischemia: mechanisms and clinical implications. Am Heart J. 2015;169:4–5.
12. Soufer R, Fernandez AB, Meadows J, Collins D, Burg MM. Body mass index and risk for mental stress induced ischemia in coronary artery disease. Mol Med. 2016;22:286–91.
13. Vaccarino V, Sullivan S, Hammadah M, et al. Mental stress-induced-myocardial ischemia in young patients with recent myocardial infarction: sex differences and mechanisms. Circulation. 2018;137:794–805.
14. Wei J, Rooks C, Ramadan R, et al. Meta-analysis of mental stress-induced myocardial ischemia and subsequent cardiac events in patients with coronary artery disease. Am J Cardiol. 2014;114:187–92.
15. Babyak MA, Blumenthal JA, Hinderliter A, et al. Prognosis after change in left ventricular ejection fraction during mental stress testing in patients with stable coronary artery disease. Am J Cardiol. 2010;105:25–8.
16. Nappi G, Dialetto G, De Feo M, et al. Apico-aortic conduit for severe hypertrophic cardiomyopathy: sudden death despite conduit patency 31 years postoperatively. Ann Thorac Cardiovasc Surg. 2013;19:63–6.
17. Beggs S, Jhund PS, Jackson CE, McMurray J, Gardner RS. Non-ischaemic cardiomyopathy, sudden death and implantable defibrillators: a review and meta-analysis. Heart. 2018;104:144–50.
18. Wald DS, Law M. Hypertrophic cardiomyopathy. Sudden death is rare in young people with hypertrophic cardiomyopathy. BMJ. 2006;333:96–7.

19. Bunck AC, Baessler B, Ritter C, et al. Structured reporting in cross-sectional imaging of the heart: reporting templates for CMR imaging of cardiomyopathies (myocarditis, dilated cardiomyopathy, hypertrophic cardiomyopathy, Arrhythmogenic right ventricular cardiomyopathy and Siderosis). Rofo. 2020;192(1):27–37.
20. James CA, Calkins H. Arrhythmogenic right ventricular cardiomyopathy: evidence for progression increases. Eur Heart J. 2020;41(14):1411–3.
21. Padron-Barthe L, Villalba-Orero M, Gomez-Salinero JM, et al. Severe cardiac dysfunction and death caused by Arrhythmogenic right ventricular cardiomyopathy type 5 are improved by inhibition of glycogen synthase kinase-3beta. Circulation. 2019;140:1188–204.
22. Quality of life in congenital heart disease. J Paediatr Child Health. 2019;55:1286.
23. Cedars A, Burchill L, Roche SL, et al. Impact of durable ventricular assist devices on post-transplant outcomes in adults with congenital heart disease. Congenit Heart Dis. 2019;14(6):958–62.
24. Sigmon ER, Kelleman M, Susi A, Nylund CM, Oster ME. Congenital heart disease and autism: a case-control study. Pediatrics. 2019;144(5):e20184114.
25. Pignata C, Farina V, Andria G, et al. Prolonged Q-T interval syndrome presenting as idiopathic epilepsy. Neuropediatrics. 1983;14:235–6.
26. Bassan J. Hereditary prolonged Q-T interval syndrome: Romano-Ward type. Rev Med Panama. 1988;13:153–9.
27. Batra AS, Watson R, McCanta AC. Exercise-induced syncope and Brugada syndrome. Ann Pediatr Cardiol. 2019;12:292–4.
28. Letsas KP, Bazoukis G, Efremidis M, et al. Clinical characteristics and long-term clinical course of patients with Brugada syndrome without previous cardiac arrest: a multiparametric risk stratification approach. Europace. 2019:euz288.
29. Waldmann V, Khairy P. Ventricular arrhythmias and sudden death in patients with Ebstein anomaly: insights from a retrospective cohort study. J Thorac Dis. 2018;10:S2172–5.
30. Cervetti MR, Camporrotondo M, Clusa NM, Navia D. Advanced calcification of a left atrial myxoma. Eur J Cardiothorac Surg. 2019;57(1):196.
31. Mathew R, Agrawal N, Aggarwal P, Jamshed N. Atrial Myxoma presenting as acute bilateral limb ischemia. J Emerg Med. 2019;57:710.
32. Lalla S, Kawall J, Seecheran R, et al. Atrial myxoma presenting as a non-ST-segment elevation myocardial infarction. Int Med Case Rep J. 2019;12:179–83.
33. Yi SY, Han MJ, Kong YH, Joo CU, Kim SJ. Acute blindness as a presenting sign of left atrial myxoma in a pediatric patient: a case report and literature review. Medicine (Baltimore). 2019;98:e17250.
34. Zhao L, Fu Z. Roles of host immunity in viral myocarditis and dilated cardiomyopathy. J Immunol Res. 2018;2018:5301548.
35. Jois A, Zannino D, Curtis N, et al. Arterial structure and function following viral myocarditis. Pediatr Cardiol. 2019;40:133–7.
36. Yang CP, Guillan RA. Sudden death syndrome. Reports of 16 patients on high doses of phenothiazine. J Kans Med Soc. 1979;80:547–9, 563.
37. STEIN Z, SUSSER M. A study of obstetric results in an under-developed community. III. The role of the hospital in the prevention of obstetric death. J Obstet Gynaecol Br Emp. 1959;66:62–7.
38. Primrose T. Maternal mortality: the non-obstetric death. Clin Obstet Gynecol. 1963;30:893–9.
39. Kaiser IH. The obstetric death of Mary Wollstonecraft. Am J Obstet Gynecol. 1976;125:1–2.
40. Perskvist N, Edston E. Differential accumulation of pulmonary and cardiac mast cell-subsets and eosinophils between fatal anaphylaxis and asthma death: a postmortem comparative study. Forensic Sci Int. 2007;169:43–9.
41. Manabe K, Tanji F, Tomata Y, Zhang S, Tsuji I. Preventive effect of oral self-care on pneumonia death among the elderly with tooth loss: the Ohsaki cohort 2006 study. Tohoku J Exp Med. 2019;247:251–7.

42. Khan A, Kiryluk S, Fordyce MJ. Fatal pulmonary embolism, death rates and standardised mortality ratios after primary total hip replacement in a joint replacement centre. Hip Int. 2007;17:59–63.
43. Ogawa Y, Asayama N, Nagata S. Acute gastrointestinal bleeding from appendiceal diverticulitis diagnosed preoperatively by combined short-interval computed tomography and colonoscopy: a case report. Dig Endosc. 2018;30:392–4.
44. Soyer P, Fohlen A, Dohan A. Acute gastrointestinal bleeding: a slowly changing paradigm. Diagn Interv Imaging. 2017;98:451–3.
45. Hudacko R, Siegel L. Acute gastrointestinal bleeding in Olmesartan-associated collagenous gastroduodenitis: a potential endoscopic complication. Case Rep Gastrointest Med. 2018;2018:3295204.
46. Deceanu D, Cazacu M, Tudose M, et al. Acute diffuse peritonitis of a rare cause. Chirurgia (Bucur). 2004;99:177–80.
47. Soulaidopoulos S, Chalevas P, Cholongitas E. Acute necrotizing pancreatitis after chemoembolization for hepatocellular. Hippokratia. 2016;20:95.
48. Jamaluddin MA, Kataria K. Management of Acute Necrotizing Pancreatitis. Indian J Surg. 2016;78:168–9.
49. Hajimaghsoudi M, Zeinali F, Mansouri M, Dehghani MH. Acute necrotizing pancreatitis following coronary artery angiography: a case report. ARYA Atheroscler. 2017;13:156–8.
50. Lippi G, Favaloro EJ, Sanchis-Gomar F. Sudden cardiac and noncardiac death in sports: epidemiology, causes, pathogenesis, and prevention. Semin Thromb Hemost. 2018;44:780–6.
51. Endres BD, Kerr ZY, Stearns RL, et al. Epidemiology of sudden death in organized youth sports in the United States, 2007–2015. J Athl Train. 2019;54:349–55.
52. Karam N, Marijon E, Jouven X. Cardiac arrest during competitive sports. N Engl J Med. 2018;378:1463.

# Part I

# Sudden Cardiac Death: Pathophysiological Mechanism

# Etiology of Sudden Death

2

Chunyuan Wang and Jing Wang

**Abstract**

Sudden death is defined as unexpected, nontraumatic death occurring within 1 h of the onset of new or worsening symptoms (witnessed arrest) or, if unwitnessed, within 24 h of last being seen alive (Zipes et al., J Am Coll Cardiol 27(17):2099–2140, 2006). It is a main cause of mortality among the general population. Consequently, sudden death is an important public health problem, which constitutes a clinical challenge. There are many sorts of sudden death arranged from cardiac sudden death to noncardiac-derived sudden death. The most common pre-manifestations of sudden cardiac death include palpitation, chest tightness, chest pain, dyspnea, and syncope. The purpose of this chapter is to summarize and elaborate different types of sudden death and its risk factors, describe the pathophysiological mechanism of sudden death caused by different diseases, which could guide us to acquire a better understanding to deal with the patients suffered from sudden death.

**Keywords**

Sudden death · Risk factors · Cardiac sudden death · Noncardiac-derived sudden death · Risk prediction

## 2.1 Introduction

Sudden death is an extremely important cause of death in both China and abroad, that make a big challenge to the global public health system [1–5]. It includes cardiac sudden death and noncardiac sudden death, during which sudden cardiac death

C. Wang · J. Wang (✉)
Emergency Department, Xuanwu Hospital, Capital Medical University, Beijing, China
e-mail: wwwangchunyuan@xwhosp.org; wj139113@xwhosp.org



H. Zhu (ed.), *Sudden Death*, https://doi.org/10.1007/978-981-15-7002-5_2

accounts for a major proportion. With the rapid development of China's economy and the improvement of people's life, the disease spectrum of China's population has gradually changed, leading to the subsequent change of cause of death. At present, cardiovascular and cerebrovascular diseases are the main causes of sudden death in China. The purpose of this chapter is to elaborate the cause of death in different aspects such as risk factors, etiology classification, and risk stratification.

## 2.2 Risk Factors

Many patients do not suffer from serious heart disease or significantly reduced ejection fraction before sudden death, or even diagnosis of heart disease [2]. Therefore, it is very important to identify the common risk factors of sudden death, especially sudden cardiac death. Age and gender are the first concerned risk factors of sudden death. It is well known that the occurrence of sudden death is higher in elder people than that in young which shows that the incidence of sudden death increases with age. In addition, the morbidity and severity of cardiovascular and cerebrovascular diseases are quite different between men and women during the same age group. For example, the morbidity of cardiovascular and cerebrovascular diseases in premenopausal women is lower than that in men.

The risk factors also include genetic, regional, and ethnic factors. The incidence of sudden death varies from different regions and ethnic groups. For example, the risk of sudden cardiac death in African Americans is higher than that in whites and Hispanics [6]. Furthermore, most of the sudden cardiac death in young is related to genetic defects, with a certain tendency of family aggregation.

Other risk factors include smoking, obesity, hyperlipidemia, hypertension, coronary heart disease, diabetes, and so on [7]. Continuous high-intensity exercise increases the risk of sudden death, while regular physical exercise can reduce the incidence of sudden death [8, 9]. Long-term heavy drinking also increased the risk of sudden cardiac death [10]. Other studies have shown that the level of plasma polyunsaturated fatty acids and C-reactive protein are also related to the occurrence of sudden death [11, 12].

## 2.3 Etiology and Classification

Broad categories of cardiac sudden death range from vast cardiac disease to noncardiac disease. Cardiac sudden death accounts for the main reason of sudden death. Generally, ischemic heart disease is the most common contributor to cardiac sudden death, such as acute myocardial infarction in coronary heart disease. Other cardiac diseases range from structural heart disease, valve membranous heart disease, and congenital heart disease to hereditary ion channel disease [5]. Besides, there are many cardiogenic disease such as cerebral hemorrhage, epilepsy, aortic dissection, pulmonary embolism, chronic lung disease, malignant tumor, electrolyte disorder, metabolic disorder, acid–base balance disorder, etc. The most common direct cause of sudden death is malignant arrhythmia during both cardiogenic and noncardiogenic disease, especially the occurrence of ventricular fibrillation.

## 2.3.1 Cardiac Disease and Sudden Death

### 2.3.1.1 Ischemic Heart Disease

Coronary heart disease is the main cause of sudden cardiac death in ischemic heart disease. Acute coronary occlusion can lead to myocardial hypoxia, myocardial necrosis, myocardium dysfunction, adjacent cell edema, and subsequent electrophysiological disorder, which eventually lead to ventricular fibrillation or cardiac arrest. Meanwhile, excessive catecholamine substances increase the risk of malignant arrhythmia and sudden cardiac death due to the increase of adrenergic and cholinergic activities and autonomic nervous regulation disorder after myocardial infarction [13].

Owing to the changes of ion channels and action potentials in the process of myocardial remodeling after myocardial infarction, the remolded myocardium is more sensitive to hypokalemia and more likely to develop malignant arrhythmias than normal people [14]. Studies have shown that magnesium and spironolactone can reduce the incidence of sudden cardiac death by countering the effects of low potassium ion in patients during the period of myocardial remodeling after myocardial infarction [15, 16]. Another research indicates that mutation of ion channel caused by genetic factors also increases the risk of sudden cardiac death in patients with ischemic cardiomyopathy [17].

### 2.3.1.2 Structure Heart Disease

#### Valvular Heart Disease and Cardiac Sudden Death

Various valvular heart diseases lead to the change of heart structure, ventricular dilation, cardiac myasthenia, and electrical activity disorder, which is easy to cause cardiac sudden death. The management depending on the current clinical guidelines is still confronting great challenge [18]. In addition, many patients with valvular heart diseases also have suffered from ischemic heart disease, which aggravates the occurrence of malignant arrhythmia.

Studies have shown that aortic valve stenosis carries one of the highest risk of cardiac sudden death. As the left ventricle contracts, the blood in the left ventricle enters the aorta through the aortic valve and supplies oxygen to organs and tissues of the whole body. Severe stenosis of the aortic valve can cause significant reduce of blood flow from ventricle to aorta, thus leading to severely reduced myocardial blood supply, which can eventually induce malignant arrhythmia and cardiac sudden death.

Severe mitral stenosis is another considerable disease related to cardiac sudden death. Owing to seriously narrowed mitral valve, the filling of the left ventricle was obviously restricted, leading to the sharp reduction of blood filling during the next cardiac cycle. In some special cases, the reduction of blood supply can be further aggravated, which increase the risk of sudden cardiac attack. Other valvular heart diseases include myxomatous mitral valve prolapse and Ebstein's anomaly, etc. Ebstein's anomaly is known as tricuspid valve downward movement deformity. This kind of patients may be suffered from multiple bypass involved preexcitation syndrome, which may cause the occurrence of malignant arrhythmias, leading to cardiac sudden death [19, 20].

### Congenital Heart Disease and Cardiac Sudden Death

Congenital heart disease (CHD) is a sort of relatively common cardiovascular disease, ranging from tetralogy of Fallot to patent ductus arteriosus (PDA). The patient suffered from congenital heart disease is often manifested as chest pain, wheezing, cyanosis, crouching after activity, clubbing fingers, pulmonary hypertension, erythrocytosis, heart failure, etc. The risk of sudden death in such patients is significantly increased because of its congenital anatomical abnormalities, hemodynamic abnormalities, and electrical activity disorders. Patients with severe congenital heart disease often die during childhood, while others with mild condition can survive to adulthood, but still with a high risk of sudden death. With the improvement of diagnosis and surgical operation method, the survival time and quality of life of patients with congenital heart disease are significantly improved. However, many patients with congenital heart disease cannot be completely cured; therefore, there is still a potential risk of sudden death even if the operation is carried out. At the present research, ventricular fibrillation or hemodynamic unstable ventricular tachycardia are still a significant cause of sudden death in patients of congenital heart disease. For example, after the repair of tetralogy of Fallot, the incidence rate of ventricular fibrillation or ventricular tachycardia is 3%–14%, and the *occurrence* of sudden cardiac death is 2%–5% every 10 years [21, 22].

At present, the main method to improve the survival rate and reduce the risk of sudden death of patients with congenital heart disease is surgical treatment, including pulmonary arterioplasty, percutaneous balloon aortic valvuloplasty, occlusion of atrial/ventricular septum defect, occlusion of patent ductus arteriosus, etc. Study shows that the incidence of sudden death is higher in patients with abnormal origin of coronary artery, especially in patients with left coronary artery originating from right coronary artery cusp, and surgical treatment should be considered in priority [23, 24]. Patients with tetralogy of Fallot, prolonged QRS duration, palliative shunt, or ventricular dysfunction who have a tendency to develop ventricular fibrillation are recommended to take implantable cardioverter defibrillator (ICD) which has been proved to be effective in preventing sudden cardiac death. Catheter ablation is considered as the main treatment for patients with single, stable, slow ventricular tachycardia [21]. As congenital heart disease is a constant challenge to human health, more research is needed to improve the diagnose and treatment in order to decrease its high risk of sudden death.

## Cardiomyopathy and Cardiac Sudden Death

### Hypertrophic Cardiomyopathy

Dilated cardiomyopathy (DCM) is a kind of primary cardiomyopathy with unknown reason. It is characterized by enlargement of the left or right ventricles or both, with decreased systolic function of the ventricles and congestive heart failure. The main clinical manifestation in the later stage include wheezing after activity and paroxysmal dyspnea at night. Patients suffered from DCM may present with various malignant arrhythmias, which can cause syncope and A-S syndrome, leading to sudden cardiac death [25–27]. As one of the most common cardiomyopathy, DCM accounts for 1/400 of incidence in the United States and has a high mortality rate at any period of the disease [28]. It is well-known that gene mutation, virus infection, and cellular immune response are the main important causes of this kind of disease.

The pathological changes include nonspecific hypertrophy, degenerative change, and interstitial fibrosis. Studies have shown that there are both alternative fibrosis and interstitial fibrosis in myocardial tissue. The swelling of mitochondria, rupture or disappearance of cristae, and disappearance of myofibrils can also be observed from electron microscopy, besides hypertrophy, degeneration, apoptosis, and fibrosis of cardiomyocytes [29, 30]. It is reported that myocardial fibrosis is closely related to delayed conduction and conduction block, which is the basic reason of malignant arrhythmia [31, 32].

In the cases of DCM, the cardiac contractility wakened with expanding cardiac cavity, leading to decreased output of stroke volume. In the early stage, the decrease of output can be compensated by the acceleration of heart rate. With increase of end diastolic pressure of left ventricle, it gradually lead to congestive left heart failure. In the later period, the pressure of left atrium and pulmonary artery increased and finally right heart failure occurred. In addition, due to the increased tension of the ventricular wall and heart rate, myocardial oxygen consumption increased simultaneously, resulting in the aggravation of myocardial ischemia and cardiomyocyte apoptosis. Moreover, myocardial lesions have influence on all parts of myocardial tissue including sinoatrial node and conduction system that can cause various arrhythmias such as ventricular tachycardia, ventricular fibrillation, and high atrioventricular block. As most of sudden cardiac death in patients with dilated cardiomyopathy is difficult to anticipate, it is consequently quite harmful to the suffered individuals. Therefore, ICD implantation is the main means to prevent sudden cardiac death which can quickly identify and treat ventricular arrhythmias [33–37].

### Restrictive Cardiomyopathy

Restricted cardiomyopathy (RCM) is a kind of relatively rare cardiomyopathy characterized by restrictive filling disorder. The typical pathological changes are progressive fibrosis of the endocardium and subendocardium of the ventricle, which lead to decreased compliance of the ventricular wall and ventricular volume. The limitation occurs in either the left ventricle or both, while ventricular systolic function and wall thickness are in nearly normal condition. Restrictive cardiomyopathy is rare among the unexplained cardiomyopathy with regional differences [38]. The main clinical manifestations of RCM are fatigue and decreased exercise endurance. In severe cases, patients of RCM may present with orthopnea, oliguria, and systemic congestion.

RCM can be idiopathic, hereditary, or secondary changes of various systemic diseases. It can be divided into two categories: cardiomyopathy and endocardial cardiomyopathy. There are mainly three types of cardiomyopathy depicted as follows: (1) non-infiltrative cardiomyopathy (idiopathic and familial cardiomyopathy, etc.), (2) infiltrative cardiomyopathy (amyloidosis, sarcoidosis [39, 40], etc.), (3) storage cardiomyopathy (hemochromatosis [41], Fabry's disease, etc.).

Myocardial fibrosis, myocardial infiltration, and endocardial scarring are the main causes of restrictive filling disorder. According to the different stages of endocardial cardiomyopathy, there are three pathological changes including necrosis, thrombosis, and fibrosis, during which the ventricular compliance and end-diastolic volume decreased gradually, finally leading to the decreased cardiac output and returned blood volume. Meanwhile, because of the inflammatory reaction of cardiomyocyte, the damage of the capillary in the myocardium and the formation of scars, the cardiac nervous system is damaged, leading to various arrhythmias or sudden cardiac death. Clinically, the usual appropriate use of diuretics and anticoagulants can relieve the symptoms and reduce the occurrence of complications. Surgical removal of fibrotic and thickened endocardium can significantly improve cardiac function and reduce the incidence of sudden death.

#### Arrhythmogenic RV Cardiomyopathy

Arrhythmogenic right ventricular cardiomyopathy (ARVC) is other kind of relatively rare cardiomyopathy characterized by degenerative myocardium of right ventricle replaced by fat or fibrofatty tissue. Without certain cause, the degenerative changes of ARVC mainly involve the right ventricle, occasionally involving the left ventricle in a few cases [42]. It is known as a type of autosomal dominant genetic disease. The mutant gene produces defective cell adhesion protein, which leads to dysfunction of desmosomes, loss of electrical coupling between cardiomyocytes, and subsequent degenerative change of right ventricle.

The pathological changes mainly occurred in the infundibulum of the right ventricular anterior wall, the apex and the posterior inferior wall which gradually resulting in thinning of the ventricular wall and global ventricular dilatation, even may be accompanied by the formation of ventricular aneurysm in some cases. The suffered intrinsic nerve system and conduction system of the heart then act as the original pathological reason for the occurrence of various arrhythmias in such kind of patients [43].

Clinically, recurrent arrhythmia of persistent or non-persistent ventricular tachycardia is the typical electrocardiogram of this kind of patients. Ventricular fibrillation may occur in severe cases. Patients always present with palpitation, chest distress, chest pain, and syncope [44]. Usually, the inducing factors of ventricular tachycardia include excessive emotional excitement or fatigue and may lead to sudden cardiac death in severe cases especially in young.

For clinicians, antiarrhythmic drugs are the first considered measures selected to control arrhythmia. Studies show that β receptor blocker can reduce the risk of sudden death and improve its prognosis. Surgical treatment of radiofrequency catheter ablation and ICD implantation can reliably prevent the occurrence of fatal arrhythmias [45]. Heart transplantation should be considered for patients with refractory ventricular tachycardia and heart failure.

#### 2.3.1.3 Electrical Abnormalities and Cardiac Sudden Death

##### Primary Electrical Abnormalities and Cardiac Sudden Death

Tachycardias

Wolff–Parkinson–White syndrome (W-P-W syndrome), also known as preexcitation syndrome, is a kind of ventricular preexcitation caused by the atrioventricular conduction pathway in the heart, which leads to the earlier arrival of excitation at the ventricle. Therefore, the ORS wave in ECG of WPW is actually a kind of ventricular fusion wave. The typical ECG manifestations are: (1) P-R interval shortened to less than 0.12 s; (2) QRS duration prolonged to more than 0.11 s, and δ wave at the beginning of QRS wave [46].

The congenital atrioventricular bypass outside normal atrioventricular conduction system is the main cause of preexcitation. Some organic heart diseases such as hypertrophic obstructive cardiomyopathy can also lead to W-P-W syndrome. The arrhythmias related to preexcitation syndrome mainly include atrioventricular reentrant tachycardia, atrial flutter, and atrial fibrillation. Supraventricular tachycardia is often accompanied by palpitation, which is similar to the common supraventricular tachycardia. In patients of W-P-W syndrome with atrial flutter or atrial fibrillation, the ventricular rate rises as fast as 200 times/min, which may cause hemodynamic abnormalities, even serious conditions such as hypotension and heart failure. Although with rare occurrence, ventricular fibrillation may be induced by the stimulation of excessive rapid heart rhythm when the minimum interval of δ wave is less than 250 ms, which may be the mechanism of sudden cardiac death. Considering that cardiac sudden death often occurs in young, clinicians should pay more attention to it, although the risk is quite small [47].

Usually the preexcitation does not need any special treatment. Propafenone and amiodarone are often used to slow down the conduction of the bypass and restore sinus rhythm when patients suffer from supraventricular tachycardia, atrial flutter, or fibrillation. While the ventricular rate is excessive rapid, the hemodynamics of circulation become unstable, and synchronous cardioversion should be used as soon as possible. If drugs are ineffective, the patients should receive surgical method such as catheter ablation.

Long-QT Syndrome

Long-QT syndrome (LQTS) is characterized by the prolongation of ventricular repolarization, which is prone to cause torsade de pointe and ventricular fibrillation, resulting in sudden cardiac death. LQTS can be caused by congenital channel disease and can also be a secondary disease. Congenital LQTS is prone to cause sudden cardiac death during childhood [48, 49]. Acquired LQTS is often caused by improper use of antiarrhythmic drugs, electrolytes, or metabolic disorders, such as hypokalemia, hypomagnesemia, hypothyroidism, and hypothermia, and is more likely to occur on the basis of organic heart disease. The electrocardiographic characteristics of LQTS are described as follows: Q-T interval prolongation (female QTc > 480 ms; male QTc > 470 ms); interval is likely to cause torsade de pointe, ventricular fibrillation, or cardiac arrest accompanied by clinical manifestations syncope and sudden death.

Drug therapy for LQTS includes (1) congenital types: β-blocker, potassium and magnesium supplement, and prevention of risk factors and (2) acquired types: magnesium sulfate, isoprenaline, lidocaine, atropine, etc.

Non-drug therapy included ICD implantation, permanent dual chamber pacemaker and left cervical thoracic sympathectomy.

#### Brugada Syndrome

Brugada syndrome is a type of autosomal dominant disease with ion channel disorder in the heart. The electrocardiogram expressions include ST segment elevation in the right precordial lead (V1–V3) in the form of covered type or saddleback type [50], sometimes accompanied by right bundle branch block. In most cases, patients' heart structure is normal, but repeatedly suffer from polymorphous ventricular tachycardia or ventricular fibrillation [51]. The occurrence of Brugada syndrome is usually at night or during rest while rarely related to exercise. Most of the victims are male and often suffer from unexplained syncope or sudden cardiac death.

It has been shown that the abnormalities of gene loci encoding for *sodium channel* current *(INa)*, transient outward current (ITO), ATP-sensitive potassium current (IKATP), or Na/Ca exchange current channel may be related to the incidence of the kind of disease [52]. Depending on the present research, the relationship of SCN5A mutation and Brugada syndrome has been conformed. The abnormality of this gene shortens the duration of action potential in cardiomyocytes, leading to further heterogeneity of action potential durations both across layers and within the ventricular epicardium, which increases the susceptibility to malignant arrhythmias [53].

Quinidine is known as a sort of effective drug been proved to inhibit Ito current, prolonging action potential and decreasing electrical heterogeneity [51]. Besides, ICD implantation has been described to be the most effective surgical measure at present. Other studies have shown that radiofrequency ablation and pacemaker therapy also have certain therapeutic effects, but these treatments lack further affirmation in large-scale clinical trials, which efficacy needs to be further assessed.

#### Short-QT Syndrome

Short QT interval syndrome (SQTS) includes idiopathic SQTS and secondary SQTS. Idiopathic SQTS is an autosomal dominant disease, which belongs to a kind of rare ion channel disease [54]. It is characterized by persistent shortened QT interval with unknown reason from normal test. Most of the patients with this kind of disease tend to recurrent syncope or sudden cardiac death during childhood.

Secondary SQTS is transient and reversible, usually caused by high fever, hypoxemia, hyperkalemia, hypercalcemia, sympathetic excitation, etc. [55]. From the detailed clinical examination, we may find no organic heart disease but abnormal ECG: QT interval was significantly shortened (generally $\leq$300 ms); Tall, symmetrically peaked T wave in precordial lead; T wave is always upright and the T peak-T end interval was not prolonged; Coexistence of multiple arrhythmias including paroxysmal atrial fibrillation, ventricular tachycardia, or ventricular fibrillation.

Three types of coding genes have been proved related to short QT syndrome up to now. The mutation of gene loci encoding the corresponding ion channel disturbs its normal operation, decreases the inflow of Na + and $Ca^{2+}$ and increases the outflow of K+, resulting in accelerated cell repolarization and shortened QT interval, which make patients prone to malignant arrhythmia.

Clinically, mild patients only have occasional palpitations, dizziness, or no symptoms; severe patients have recurrent syncope or sudden death. The demonstrated effective prevention of sudden death is ICD implantation. Drug therapy refers to sodium channel blockers such as flecainide and quinidine.

#### Catecholaminergic Polymorphic VT

Catecholamine-sensitive polymorphic ventricular tachycardia (CPVT) is a malignant familial cardiac arrhythmia with a very low incidence rate (1:10,000), that usually occurs during childhood. Patients with CPVT may have no clinical manifestation in general state. Thus, it is difficult to be identified from routine examination, although the mortality rate is high. CPVT is characterized by the induced polymorphic ventricular tachycardia or ventricular fibrillation by exercise or emotional stress.

The pathogenesis of CPVT is not completely clear so far. Studies have shown that the pathogenesis of CPVT is related to gene mutations of RyR2 (autosomal dominant inheritance) and CASQ2 (autosomal recessive inheritance) [56]. Patients of CPVT usually have normal cardiac structure and mechanical contraction, and their electrocardiogram shows normal QTc interval, atrioventricular conduction and intraventricular conduction while at rest. With the increase of exercise intensity, premature ventricular beat will be induced as the heart rate accelerating to 120–130 bpm. Biphasic or polymorphic ventricular tachycardia may occur when the heart rate continues to increase [57–59]. The arrhythmias can sometimes be terminated automatically, but also prone to malignant arrhythmia that leads to sudden death.

It is suggested that patients with CPVT should not take part in strenuous sports or competitive competitions. At present, β-blocker is the first choice of drug treatment described to inhibit the occurrence of polymorphous ventricular tachycardia. Other studies have shown that the application of verapamil or fluconanil may be beneficial [59, 60]. Immediate electric cardioversion is necessary if the patients suffer from ventricular tachycardia with hemodynamic instability or ventricular fibrillation. ICD implantation is the main surgical measure to prevent sudden cardiac death and should be combined with β-blocker application.

### Early Repolarization Syndrome and Idiopathic VF

Early repolarization (ER) is also a kind of hereditary ion channel disease characterized by a type of common benign ECG variation. When patients with early repolarization ECG experienced malignant arrhythmia or sudden death, it is called early repolarization syndrome (ERS). ER is more common in young and men than elderly or women with a relatively high incidence (2%–9%) and low mortality [61].

The typical ECG manifestations of early repolarization are: (1) ST segment oblique uplift, usually in leads v2–v5 and leads II, III and AVF without corresponding lead ST segment depression; T wave is generally vertical and asymmetry; usually shortened a QT interval and QRS interval. (2) J-wave can be observed at junction of QRS wave and ST segment, which would be more obvious as the vagus nerve tension increases. (3) Sinus bradycardia. (4) ST segment elevation can last for several years, with dynamic changes, and may decrease gradually along with aging. The exact ion channel disorder (mainly involving Na+, $Ca^{2+}$, and K+ channels) related to mutation of corresponding gene locus is still unclear [62–64].

Patients of ER usually have no obvious clinical symptoms, while a few have feelings of atypical palpitation, dizziness, and fatigue. Some patients present with chest tightness and chest pain, similar to variant angina, myocardial infarction or acute pericarditis, which need to be identified carefully. Malignant arrhythmia related to ERS usually occurs during rest or sleep. ER is a type of benign ECG variation, which does not need special treatment [51]. Intravenous injection of isoproterenol is recommended while patients suffer from an ERS attack [65, 66]. ICD implantation and quinidine taken simultaneously are also effective methods recommended from guidelines to prevent recurrence of malignant arrhythmia.

### Commotio Cordis

Commotio cordis refers to the malignant arrhythmia and sudden death caused by the rapid impact of blunt objects. This disease often occurs in young athletes, whose chest have been severely impacted during the process of exercise leading to sudden cardiac death. The mortality of commotio cordis is high owing to its pathogenesis [67, 68]. Report of commotio cordis increased year by year in pace with the gradually recognition of this type disease.

It can be found from the autopsy that the suffered victims died of commotio cordis did not have a structural damage on the chest, which suggested that there may exist deeper factors for the occurrence of death. Further research shows that there is a special short period of the electrocardiographic activity during which ventricular fibrillation is induced after chest been impacted. The specific pathophysiological mechanism is described below: When the stimulation of impact occurs, left ventricular pressure increases instantaneously, leading to the sharp ascending of tension in cardiomyocyte, which activates the corresponding ion channels (such as K+ ATP channels) in the myocardial tissue. During this period, the inward current abnormally occurs leading to the heterogeneous activation and repolarization, and finally induces ventricular fibrillation [69, 70]. In addition, the study also shows that impact area, speed, and strength of blunt impact are also related to the induction of ventricular fibrillation.

In recent years, the significantly improved survival of commotio cordis is considered to be related to the further understanding of its mechanisms, the upgrade of emergency equipment and popularization of first-aid skills from general public to medical staff [71, 72]. In view of the high risk of mortality caused by this disease, it is necessary to further strengthen the protective measures of athletes, reinforce their awareness of self-protection and regularly training of medical staff and general public.

#### Bradycardias

Bradycardia, a common type of arrhythmia, refers to the low hear rate (<60/min) caused by sinus node dysfunction or atrioventricular conduction system block due to various reasons, which has a low risk of mortality. Usually patients of bradycardia are present with mild fatigue, palpitation, or no symptoms. While the heart rate drops to less than 40 times per minute, patients may have symptoms of chest tightness, amaurosis, or syncope. Once bradycardia occurs, ventricular rate slows down, and/or ventricular ejection function decreases, which can reduces the cardiac output, resulting in the involved symptoms above. In rare cases, patients may suffer from sudden cardiac death.

Bradyarrhythmia includes sinus bradycardia, sinoatrial block, sinus arrest, atrioventricular block, etc. [73] Studies have shown that when atrioventricular block occurs, if the inferior ectopic excitation worked effectively, patients will be less prone to encounter serious adverse cardiac events. However, sudden cardiac death may occur in patients with high degree conduction block near the His-bundle or below [74]. Three branch block and alternating bundle branch block should be regarded as the high-risk group of sudden death. In addition, bradycardia related to sudden cardiac death, often accompanied by organic heart disease, or combined with drug overdose (digoxin), poisoning (organic phosphorus), or electrolyte abnormality (high potassium), etc. Sometimes, patients may suffer from rapid arrhythmia on the basis of original bradycardia or sick sinus syndrome. For example, patients with bradycardia and long QT interval are prone to develop into torsade de pointes, which is harmful to patients.

Cardiac pacemaker implantation is an effective treatment for bradycardia which can relieve the patient's condition and improve their qualities of life [75]. ICD implantation should be considered for patients with severe left ventricular dysfunction.

### Secondary Abnormalities and Cardiac Sudden Death

Many drugs can cause arrhythmias, including antiarrhythmic drugs, diuretics, antibiotics, narcotic drugs (cocaine), and so on, which affect the ion channels of cardiomyocyte directly or indirectly, causing the disorder of cardiac electrical activity. Drug-induced sudden cardiac death is mainly related to tachyarrhythmias especially torsade de pointes. It usually happens on the basis of electrolyte abnormalities, structural heart disease, ion channel disease, acute myocardial infarction, hypothermia, and so on.

Cocaine is known to have sympathomimetic effects, such as producing positive inotropic effect, increasing heart rate and blood pressure. High dose of cocaine can cause ventricular tachycardia/fibrillation, acute myocardial infarction or cerebral hemorrhage leading to sudden death [76]. Moreover, the application of antiarrhythmia drugs in patients also has the risk of proarrhythmic effect. Class III antiarrhythmic drugs (amiodarone) are potassium channel blockers, which can prolong QT interval and increase the risk of torsade de pointes. Single or combined use of class I (sodium channel blocker), class II (β- blocker), and class IV (calcium channel blocker) antiarrhythmic drugs is also related to the occurrence of malignant arrhythmia [77]. Therefore, clinicians should closely detect the level of electrolyte (especially the level of blood potassium and magnesium), change of electrocardiogram and renal function in order to reduce the occurrence of adverse events [78].

Other causes of cardiac sudden death include acute pericardial tamponade, myocarditis, rupture of ventricular aneurysm, and so on.

### 2.3.2 Noncardiac-Derived Sudden Death

#### 2.3.2.1 Neurologic Disorders

A large number of researches about brain-derived sudden death were published in recent years. There are complex interactions between brain and cardiovascular system depending on the research. Many kinds of brain diseases, such as epilepsy, [79] ischemia, hemorrhage, trauma, [80] infection, and even psychological stress, can cause sympathetic or parasympathetic dysfunction. The abnormal changes subsequently have effects on the heart with arrhythmia, hemodynamic disorder, neurogenic myocardial stunning, heart failure, and even sudden death. The pathophysiological mechanism of brain-derived sudden death has not been fully understood, and may include the descriptions as follows: (1) The damage of high-level nerve centers such as prefrontal cortex and limbic system can cause disconnection and dysfunction of sympathetic and parasympathetic nerve system, which brings the abnormal release of neurotransmitters from nerve endings disrupting the cardiac nervous system and myocardial contraction. (2) Cerebral disease also has an impact on neuroendocrine pathway regulation. The over activation of adrenal medulla and massive release of catecholamine into circulatory system lead to hyperactivity of cardiac nervous system characterized by myocardial over contraction and coronary ischemia. (3) Over activation of central and peripheral immune systems after brain injury results in inflammatory cascade and further tissues damage including the heart. All these factors above are prone to cause various malignant arrhythmias, myocardial stunning, and even sudden death.

#### 2.3.2.2 Acute Aortic Syndromes

Acute aortic syndrome (AAS) is a group of cardiovascular disease syndrome based on the pathological characteristics of the aorta described as follows:

Aortic dissection (AD): The pathological change of AD is the degeneration of the collagen and elastic fiber in the middle layer of aorta. When the intima of aorta is damaged, blood flow penetrates into the middle layer continuously, inducing occurrence of aortic dissection. The dissection develops continuously under the impact of blood flow with high pressure and sometimes developed into dissecting aneurysm, which could result in aneurysm rupture and sudden death. When the dissected pseudolumen is formed, the true lumen of aorta is compressed and narrowed, resulting in corresponding organ ischemia.

Intramural aortic hematoma (IMH): The pathological mechanism of IMH is that the rupture of nutrient vessels leads to the internal hematoma of the adventitia of aorta without the tear of the intima.

Penetrating atherosclerotic aortic ulcer (PAU): PAU refers to the ulcer of the aortic intima that penetrates into the internal elastic layer and forms a hematoma in the middle layer of aorta. The hematoma formed from ulcer is generally limited based on the atherosclerosis of aorta, which occasionally may develop to IMH or AD.

The cause factors of AAS include age, hypertension, atherosclerosis, and genetic factors (Marfan syndrome, Ehlers-Danlos syndrome, Turner syndrome, congenital aortic valve malformation, and coarctation of aorta). In addition, some special diseases such as syphilis can also cause inflammation of aortic wall and induce AAS.

The most common clinical manifestations are persistent severe pain in the chest and back. AAS may cause hypotension, and syncope the pericardium is involved. When the hematoma compression happens in superior vena cava, patients may present with superior vena cava syndrome, while happens in recurrent laryngeal nerve, patients may present with hoarseness. Angina and myocardial infarction may occur if the dissection involves coronary artery. Patients may also present with hemiplegia, coma, abdominal pain, anuria, and hematochezia if the dissection involves different arterial branches such as brachiocephalic trunk, common carotid artery, or branches of abdominal aorta.

Treatment: β-receptor blocker and vasodilator are recommended to control blood pressure and decrease the risk of sudden death. Generally, patients with type A should be treated with surgery method immediately, while the type B could be treated conservatively, if progresses, be treated surgically at once [81].

#### 2.3.2.3 Electrolyte, Metabolic, Endocrine Disorder, and Other Causes

Cardiomyocyte have the abilities of excitation, automaticity, conduction, and contraction, which is based on the bioelectric activity of cardiomyocyte membrane. Therefore, these abilities are closely related to the concentration of various ions inside and outside the cardiomyocyte. Any electrolyte abnormalities, especially the level of blood potassium, magnesium and calcium, can cause dysregulation of ion channels on the cardiomyocyte membrane, thus affecting the resting potential, action potential threshold, depolarization, and repolarization. For example, electrolyte disturbance with hyperkalemia, hypermagnesemia, and hypercalcemia can decrease the automaticity, excitability and conductivity of cardiomyocytes, causing high-degree atrioventricular block and prolonged QT interval. Conversely, hypokalemia, hypocalcemia, and hypocalcemia can increase the automaticity, excitability, and conductivity of cardiomyocytes, causing tachyarrhythmia such as ventricular tachycardia and ventricular fibrillation. Severe hypokalemia and hypomagnesemia are known to be associated with torsade de pointes. In addition, hypermagnesemia can inhibit the release of acetylcholine from neuromuscular junction and sympathetic preganglionic fibers, which can cause respiratory failure and dropped blood pressure, which increase the risk of sudden death.

Severe acidosis (diabetic ketoacidosis, renal failure, poisoning) can cause significant changes in the concentration of hydrogen ions inside and outside the cardiomyocytes, thus further affecting the status of cardiomyocytes in different periods of action potential, leading to malignant arrhythmias, especially ventricular fibrillation [82].

Serious endocrine system disorder is also related to the occurrence of sudden death. Pituitary crisis is a type of acute neuroendocrine disease caused by sudden hemorrhage, infarction, and necrosis of pituitary tumor, mainly manifested as hyperthermia/hypothermia, hypoglycemia, circulatory failure, and water poisoning. Thyroid crisis is related to the sharp increase of thyroxine levels in the circulation, manifested as hyperthermia, sweating, tachycardia, heart failure, shock, and coma. Other types of serious endocrine disorders such as adrenal crisis and severe hypothyroidism can also disrupt the intracellular environment of myocardium from in many ways. If not handled properly, these diseases can also develop into ventricular tachycardia, ventricular fibrillation, and even sudden death.

Treatment: It is important to closely monitor the different clinical indicators of patients, manage underlying disorders. Try to prevent the occurrence of electrolyte disorder, metabolic disorder, and endocrine disorder. Once it happens effective treatment should be taken in time.

Other causes of noncardiac-derived sudden death include pulmonary embolism, tension pneumothorax, massive hemorrhage of digestive tract, rupture of ectopic pregnancy, etc., which are relatively rare.

## 2.4 Risk Prediction for Sudden Death

Sudden cardiac death has a rapid onset with serious consequences, and the suffered numbers are increasing in recent years. Therefore, the prediction for sudden death is very important. For example, a significant reduction in left ventricular ejection fraction (<35%) is a definite risk predictor of sudden cardiac death [83]. The prognosis of this group of patients can be greatly improved by ICD implanting to prevent sudden cardiac death. The risk of sudden death in patients with cardiomyopathy and coronary heart disease (especially myocardial infarction) is significantly higher. Studies have shown that if patients with cardiomyopathy have ECG manifestations of QT interval prolongation, high degree atrioventricular block, ventricular tachycardia, and ventricular fibrillation, it reveals high predictive ability for the occurrence of sudden cardiac death. Patients with broken QRS waves and significantly reduced ejection fraction after myocardial infarction, also revealed a good predictive value for sudden cardiac death [84–86]. It is reported that cMRI can reveal the functional state of myocardium in patients with cardiomyopathy, and also has a certain prediction ability. Other indicators include high resting heart rate, heart rate variability, and T wave alternation, etc. [84, 87]. At present, many related studies are still in the early stage, and more evidence is needed to improve the predictive power of sudden death.

## References


1. Stecker EC, Reinier K, Marijon E, et al. Public health burden of sudden cardiac death in the United States. Circ Arrhythm Electrophysiol. 2014;7:212–7.
2. Lippert FK, Raffay V, Georgiou M, Steen PA, Bossaert L. European resuscitation council guidelines for resuscitation 2010 section 10. The ethics of resuscitation and end-of-life decisions. Resuscitation. 2010;81:1445–51.
3. Mathers CD, Loncar D. Projections of global mortality and burden of disease from 2002 to 2030. PLoS Med. 2006;3(e442):2011–29.
4. Gillum RF. Geographic variation in sudden coronary death. Am Heart J. 1990;119:380–9.
5. Myerburg RJ, Junttila MJ. Sudden cardiac death caused by coronary heart disease. Circulation. 2012;125:1043–52.
6. Zipes DP, Camm A, Borggrefe M, et al. ACC/AHA/ESC 2006 guidelines for the management of patients with ventricular arrhythmias and the prevention of sudden cardiac death: a report of the American College Of Cardiology/American Heart Association task force and the European Society Of Cardiology Committee for practice guidelines (writing committee to develop guidelines for management of patients with ventricular arrhythmias and the prevention of sudden cardiac death). J Am Coll Cardiol. 2006;27(17):2099–140.
7. Wellens HJ, Schwartz PJ, Lindemans FW, et al. Risk stratification for sudden cardiac death: current status and challenges for the future. Eur Heart J. 2014;35:1642–51.
8. Albert CM, Mittleman MA, Chae CU, Lee IM, Hennekens CH, Manson JE. Triggering of sudden death from cardiac causes by vigorous exertion. N Engl J Med. 2000;343:1355–61.
9. Kark J, Goldman S, Epstein L. Iraqi missile attacks on Israel. The association of mortality with a life-threatening stressor. JAMA. 1995;273:1208.
10. Albert CM, Manson JE, Cook NR, Ajani UA, Gaziano JM, Hennekens CH. Moderate alcohol consumption and the risk of sudden cardiac death among US male physicians. Circulation. 1999;100:944–50.
11. Albert CM, Campos H, Stampfer MJ, et al. Blood levels of long-chain n-3 fatty acids and the risk of sudden death. N Engl J Med. 2002;346:1113–8.
12. Albert CM, Ma J, Rifai N, Stampfer MJ, Ridker PM. Prospective study of C-reactive protein, homocysteine, and plasma lipid levels as predictors of sudden cardiac death. Circulation. 2002;105:2595–9.
13. Muller JE. Circadian variation and triggering of acute coronary events. Am Heart J. 1999;137(Pt 2):51–8.
14. Huang B, Qin D, El-Sherif N. Early down-regulation of K+ channel genes and currents in the post infarction heart. J Cardiovasc Electrophysiol. 2000;11:1252–61.
15. Gyamlani G, Parikh C, Kulkani AG. Benefits of magnesium in acute myocardial infarction. Timing is crucial. Am Heart J. 2000;139(4):703.
16. Pitt B, Zannad F, Remme WJ, et al. The effect of spironolactone on morbidity and mortality in patients with severe heart failure. N Engl J Med. 1999;341:709–17.
17. Rubart M, Zipes DP. Genes and cardiac repolarization: the 428 challenge ahead. Circulation. 2005;112:1242–4.
18. Nishimura RA, Otto CM, Bonow RO, et al. 2014 AHA/ACC guideline for the management of patients with valvular heart disease: a report of the American College of Cardiology/American Heart Association task force on practice guidelines. J Thorac Cardiovasc Surg. 2014;148:e1–32.

19. Sriram CS, Syed FF, Ferguson ME, et al. Malignant bileaflet mitral valve prolapse syndrome in patients with otherwise idiopathic out-of-hospital cardiac arrest. J Am Coll Cardiol. 2013;62:222–30.
20. Kligfield P, Levy D, Devereux RB, Savage DD. Arrhythmias and sudden death in mitral valve prolapse. Am Heart J. 1987;113:1298–307.
21. Walsh EP. Interventional electrophysiology in patients with congenital heart disease. Circulation. 2007;115:3224–34.
22. Mondesert B, Khairy P. Implantable cardioverter-defibrillators in congenital heart disease. Curr Opin Cardiol. 2014;29:45–52.
23. Zeppenfeld K, Schalij MJ, Bartelings MM, et al. Catheter ablation of ventricular tachycardia after repair of congenital heart disease: electroanatomic identification of the critical right ventricular isthmus. Circulation. 2007;116:2241–52.
24. Gersony WM. Management of anomalous coronary artery from the contralateral coronary sinus. J Am Coll Cardiol. 2007;50:2083–4.
25. Pinto YM, Elliott PM, Arbustini E, Adler Y, Anastasakis A, Bohm M, Duboc D, Gimeno J, de Groote P, Imazio M, Heymans S, Klingel K, Komajda M, Limongelli G, Linhart A, Mogensen J, Moon J, Pieper PG, Seferovic PM, Schueler S, Zamorano JL, Caforio AL, Charron P. Proposal for a revised definition of dilated cardiomyopathy, hypokinetic non-dilated cardiomyopathy, and its implications for clinical practice: a position statement of the ESC working group on myocardial and pericardial diseases. Eur Heart J. 2016;37:1850–8.
26. Gorgels AP, Gijsbers C, de Vreede-Swagemakers J, Lousberg A, Wellens HJ. Out-of-hospital cardiac arrest–the relevance of heart failure. The Maastricht circulatory arrest registry. Eur Heart J. 2003;24:1204–9.
27. Stecker EC, Vickers C, Waltz J, Socoteanu C, John BT, Mariani R, McAnulty JH, Gunson K, Jui J, Chugh SS. Population-based analysis of sudden cardiac death with and without left ventricular systolic dysfunction: two-year findings from the Oregon sudden unexpected death study. J Am Coll Cardiol. 2006;47:1161–6.
28. Hershberger RE, Hedges DJ, Morales A. Dilated cardiomyopathy: the complexity of a diverse genetic architecture. Nat Rev Cardiol. 2013;10:531–47.
29. Beltrami CA, Finato N, Rocco M, Feruglio GA, Puricelli C, Cigola E, Sonnenblick EH, Olivetti G, Anversa P. The cellular basis of dilated cardiomyopathy in humans. J Mol Cell Cardiol. 1995;27:291–305.
30. Mewton N, Liu CY, Croisille P, Bluemke D, Lima JA. Assessment of myocardial fibrosis with cardiovascular magnetic resonance. J Am Coll Cardiol. 2011;57:891–903.
31. Hsia HH, Marchlinski FE. Electrophysiology studies in patients with dilated cardiomyopathies. Card Electrophysiol Rev. 2002;6:472–681.
32. Liuba I, Marchlinski FE. The substrate and ablation of ventricular tachycardia in patients with nonischemic cardiomyopathy. Circ J. 2013;77:1957–66.
33. Bansch D, Antz M, Boczor S, Volkmer M, Tebbenjohanns J, Seidl K, Block M, Gietzen F, Berger J, Kuck KH. Primary prevention of sudden cardiac death in idiopathic dilated cardiomyopathy: the cardiomyopathy trial (CAT). Circulation. 2002;105:1453–8.
34. Strickberger SA, Hummel JD, Bartlett TG, Frumin HI, Schuger CD, Beau SL, Bitar C, Morady F. Amiodarone versus implantable cardioverter-defibrillator:randomized trial in patients with nonischemic dilated cardiomyopathy and asymptomatic nonsustained ventricular tachycardia—AMIOVIRT. J Am Coll Cardiol. 2003;41:1707–12.
35. Bardy GH, Lee KL, Mark DB, Poole JE, Packer DL, Boineau R, Domanski M, Troutman C, Anderson J, Johnson G, McNulty SE, Clapp-Channing N, Davidson-Ray LD, Fraulo ES, Fishbein DP, Luceri RM, Ip JH. Amiodarone or an implantable cardioverter-defibrillator for congestive heart failure. N Engl J Med. 2005;352:225–37.
36. Kadish A, Dyer A, Daubert JP, Quigg R, Estes NA, Anderson KP, Calkins H, Hoch D, Goldberger J, Shalaby A, Sanders WE, Schaechter A, Levine JH. Prophylactic defibrillator implantation in patients with nonischemic dilated cardiomyopathy. N Engl J Med. 2004;350:2151–8.

37. Kober L, Thune JJ, Nielsen JC, Haarbo J, Videbaek L, Korup E, Jensen G, Hildebrandt P, Steffensen FH, Bruun NE, Eiskjaer H, Brandes A, Thogersen AM, Gustafsson F, Egstrup K, Videbaek R, Hassager C, Svendsen JH, Hofsten DE, Torp-Pedersen C, Pehrson S. Defibrillator implantation in patients with nonischemic systolic heart failure. N Engl J Med. 2016;375:1221–31.
38. Beaton A, Mocumbi AO. Diagnosis and Management of Endomyocardial Fibrosis. Cardiol Clin. 2017;35:87–98.
39. Baughman RP, Lower EE, du Bois RM. Sarcoidosis. Lancet. 2003;361:1111–8.
40. Martusewicz-Boros MM, Boros PW, Wiatr E, Kempisty A, Piotrowska-Kownacka D, Roszkowski-Śliż K. Cardiac sarcoidosis: is it more common in men? Lung. 2016;194:61–6.
41. Gulati V, Harikrishnan P, Palaniswamy C, Aronow WS, Jain D, Frishman WH. Cardiac involvement in hemochromatosis. Cardiol Rev. 2014;22:56–68.
42. Saguner AM, Brunckhorst C, Duru F. Arrhythmogenic ventricular cardiomyopathy: a paradigm shift from right to biventricular disease. World J Cardiol. 2014;6:154–74.
43. Azaouagh A, Churzidse S, Konorza T, Erbel R. Arrhythmogenic right ventricular cardiomyopathy/dysplasia: a review and update. Clin Res Cardiol. 2011;100:383–94.
44. Link MS, Laidlaw D, Polonsky B, et al. Ventricular arrhythmias in the north American multidisciplinary study of ARVC: predictors, characteristics, and treatment. J Am Coll Cardiol. 2014;64:119–25.
45. Marcus FI, Abidov A. Arrhythmogenic right ventricular cardiomyopathy 2012: diagnostic challenges and treatment. J Cardiovasc Electrophysiol. 2012;23:1149–53.
46. Wolff L, Parkinson J, White PD. Bundle-branch block with short P-R interval in healthy young people prone to paroxysmal tachycardia. 1930. Ann Noninvasive Electrocardiol. 2006;11:340–53.
47. Cohen MI, Triedman JK, Cannon BC, et al. PACES/HRS expert consensus statement on the management of the asymptomatic young patient with a Wolff-Parkinson-White (WPW, ventricular preexcitation) electrocardiographic pattern. Heart Rhythm. 2012;9:1006.
48. Ruan Y, Liu N, Napolitano C, Priori SG. Therapeutic strategies for long-QT syndrome: does the molecular substrate matter? Circ Arrhythm Electrophysiol. 2008;1:290–7.
49. Odening KE, Brunner M. Risk stratification in long QT syndrome: are we finally getting closer to a mutation-specific assessment of an individual patient's arrhythmo-genic risk? Heart Rhythm. 2013;10:726–7.
50. Bayes de Luna A, Brugada J, Baranchuk A, et al. Current electrocardiographic criteria for diagnosis of Brugada pattern: a consensus report. J Electrocardiol. 2012;45:433–42.
51. Priori SG, Wilde AA, Horie M, et al. HRS/EHRA/APHRS expert consensus statement on the diagnosis and management of patients with inherited primary arrhythmia syndromes: document endorsed by HRS, EHRA, and APHRS in May 2013 and by ACCF, AHA, PACES, and AEPC in June 2013. Heart Rhythm. 2013;10:1932–63.
52. Clancy CE, Kass RS. Defective cardiac ion channels: from mutations to clinical syndromes. J Clin Invest. 2002;110:1075–7.
53. Yan GX, Antzelevitch C. Cellular basis for the Brugada syndrome and other mechanisms of arrhythmogenesis associated with ST-segment elevation. Circulation. 1999;100:1660–6.
54. Gussak I, Brugada P, Brugada J, et al. Idiopathic short QT interval: a new clinical syndrome? Cardiology. 2000;94:99–102.
55. Patel U, Pavri BB. Short QT syndrome: a review. Cardiol Rev. 2009;17:300–3.
56. Priori SG, Napolitano C, Tiso N, et al. Mutations in the cardiac ryanodine receptor gene (hRyR2) underlie catecholaminergic polymorphic ventricular tachycardia. Circulation. 2001;103:196–200.
57. Hayashi M, Denjoy I, Extramiana F, et al. Incidence and risk factors of arrhythmic events in catecholaminergic polymorphic ventricular tachycardia. Circulation. 2009;119:2426–34.
58. Chapman M, Hargreaves M, Schneider H, Royle M. Bidirectional ventricular tachycardia associated with digoxin toxicity and with normal digoxin levels. Heart Rhythm. 2014;11:1222–5.

59. van der Werf C, Zwinderman AH, Wilde AA. Therapeutic approach for patients with catecholaminergic polymorphic ventricular tachycardia: state of the art and future developments. Europace. 2012;14:175–83.
60. van der Werf C, Kannankeril PJ, Sacher F, et al. Flecainide therapy reduces exercise- induced ventricular arrhythmias in patients with catecholaminergic polymorphic ventricular tachycardia. J Am Coll Cardiol. 2011;57:2244–54.
61. Obeyesekere MN, Klein GJ, Nattel S, et al. A clinical approach to early repolarization. Circulation. 2013;127:1620–9.
62. Haissaguerre M, Chatel S, Sacher F, et al. Ventricular fibrillation with prominent early repolarization associated with a rare variant of KCNJ8/KATP channel. J Cardiovasc Electrophysiol. 2009;20:93–8.
63. Burashnikov E, Pfeiffer R, Barajas-Martinez H, et al. Mutations in the cardiac L-type calcium channel associated with inherited J-wave syndromes and sudden cardiac death. Heart Rhythm. 2010;7:1872–82.
64. Li N, Wang R, Hou C, Zhang Y, Teng S, Pu J. A heterozygous missense SCN5A mutation associated with early repolarization syndrome. Int J Mol Med. 2013;32:661–7.
65. Haissaguerre M, Sacher F, Nogami A, et al. Characteristics of recurrent ventricular fibrillation associated with inferolateral early repolarization role of drug therapy. J Am Coll Cardiol. 2009;53:612–9.
66. Belhassen B, Viskin S, Fish R, Glick A, Setbon I, Eldar M. Effects of electrophysiologic-guided therapy with class IA antiarrhythmic drugs on the longterm outcome of patients with idiopathic ventricular fibrillation with or without the Brugada syndrome. J Cardiovasc Electrophysiol. 1999;10:1301–12.
67. Maron BJ, Gohman TE, Kyle SB, Estes NA 3rd, Link MS. Clinical profile and spectrum of commotio cordis. JAMA. 2002;287:1142–6.
68. Maron BJ, Doerer JJ, Haas TS, Estes NA 3rd, Link MS. Historical observation on commotio cordis. Heart Rhythm. 2006;3:605–6.
69. Link MS, Wang PJ, Pandian NG, et al. An experimental model of sudden death due to low-energy chest-wall impact (commotio cordis). N Engl J Med. 1998;338:1805–11.
70. Link MS. Commotio cordis: ventricular fibrillation triggered by chest impact induced abnormalities in repolarization. Circ Arrhythm Electrophysiol. 2012;5:425–32.
71. Maron BJ, Ahluwalia A, Haas TS, Semsarian C, Link MS, Estes NA III. Global epidemiology and demographics of commotio cordis. Heart Rhythm. 2011;8:1969–71.
72. Maron BJ, Haas TS, Ahluwalia A, Garberich RF, Estes NA III, Link MS. Increasing survival rate from commotio cordis. Heart Rhythm. 2013;10:219–23.
73. Epstein AE, Dimarco JP, Ellenbogen KA, et al. ACC/AHA/HRS 2008 guidelines for device-based therapy of cardiac rhythm abnormalities: executive summary. Heart Rhythm. 2008;5:934–55.
74. Vogler J, Breithardt G, Eckardt L. Bradyarrhythmias and conduction blocks. Rev Esp Cardiol. 2012;65:656–67.
75. Manlucu J, Tang AS. Whom should I refer in 2014 for cardiac resynchronization? Can J Cardiol. 2014;30:675–8.
76. Morentin B, Ballesteros J, Callado LF, Meana JJ. Recent cocaine use is a significant risk factor for sudden cardiovascular death in 15–49-year-old subjects: a forensic case-control study. Addiction. 2014;109(12):2071–8.
77. Echt DS, Liebson PR, Mitchell LB, et al. Mortality and morbidity in patients receiving encainide, flecainide, or placebo. The cardiac arrhythmia suppression trial. N Engl J Med. 1991;324:781–8.
78. Li EC, Esterly JS, Pohl S, Scott SD, McBride BF. Drug-induced QT-interval prolongation: considerations for clinicians. Pharmacotherapy. 2010;30:684–701.
79. Ryvlin P, Nashef L, Tomson T. Prevention of sudden unexpected death in epilepsy: a realistic goal? Epilepsia. 2013;54(suppl 2):23–8.
80. Finsterer J, Wahbi K. CNS-disease affecting the heart: brain-heart disorders. J Neurol Sci. 2014;345:8–14.

81. Bonaca MP, O'Gara PT. Diagnosis and management of acute aortic syndromes: dissection, intramural hematoma, and penetrating aortic ulcer. Curr Cardiol Rep. 2014;16:536.
82. Kanbay M, Afsar B, Goldsmith D, Covic A. Sudden death in hemodialysis: an update. Blood Purif. 2010;30:135–45.
83. Buxton AE, Lee KL, Hafley GE, et al. Relation of ejection fraction and inducible ventricular tachycardia to mode of death in patients with coronary artery disease: an analysis of patients enrolled in the multicenter unsustained tachycardia trial. Circulation. 2002;106:2466–72.
84. Zaman S, Kovoor P. Sudden cardiac death early after myocardial infarction: pathogenesis, risk stratification, and primary prevention. Circulation. 2014;129:2426–35.
85. Hohnloser SH, Kuck KH, Dorian P, et al. Prophylactic use of an implantable cardioverter-defibrillator after acute myocardial infarction. N Engl J Med. 2004;351:2481–8.
86. Das MK, Zipes DP. Fragmented QRS: a predictor of mortality and sudden cardiac death. Heart Rhythm. 2009;6:S8–14.
87. Exner DV, Kavanagh KM, Slawnych MP, et al. Noninvasive risk assessment early after a myocardial infarction the REFINE study. J Am Coll Cardiol. 2007;50:2275–84.

# 3 Etiology Mechanism of Sudden Death Derived from Brain

Chunyuan Wang and Jing Wang

**Abstract**

Along with the population aging of social structure and prolongation of life expectancy, there are more patients suffer from various acute brain diseases. Subsequently, the number of sudden death caused by brain disorders is increasing by year, which prompt a large number of researchers pay attention to the study of sudden brain-derived death. It is reported that all kinds of acute brain disorders such as ischemic stroke, intracranial bleeding, epilepsy, traumatic injury, and stress can cause heart dysfunction and at times sudden death. And its etiology mechanism has become a hot topic of research. According to the latest research, the reason for brain-derived sudden death mainly includes the following aspects: (1) Dysregulation of sympathetic and/or parasympathetic nerve after cerebral diseases results in the disorder of cardiac neural network and the abnormality of myocardial contraction. (2) Sympathetic–adrenomedullary axis hyperactivity and excessive catecholamine release into peripheral blood lead to exorbitant heart rate, blood pressure, and intense myocardial contraction. (3) The transient activation of inflammatory factors under stress increases the sensitivity of cardiomyocytes to catecholamine and other substances and the direct damage of myocardium. These etiology mechanisms alone or in combination increase the risk of heart disease in patients with cerebral disease, leading to sudden death.

**Keywords**

Sudden death · Cerebral disease · Sympathetic nerve · Parasympathetic nerve Catecholamine · Myocardium · Adrenal medulla · Inflammation

C. Wang · J. Wang (✉)
Emergency Department, Xuanwu Hospital, Capital Medical University, Beijing, China
e-mail: wwwangchunyuan@xwhosp.org; wj139113@xwhosp.org



H. Zhu (ed.), *Sudden Death*, https://doi.org/10.1007/978-981-15-7002-5_3

## 3.1 Introduction

As the main cause of natural death, sudden cardiac death (SCD) has an increasing numbers of incidence during recent years. There are different categories of SCD ranged from cardiogenic disease to brain-derived disease. Central nervous system (CNS) disorders can in many ways result in sudden death including epilepsy, ischemic stroke, intracranial bleeding, traumatic head injury, and stress-induced cardiomyopathy [1, 2]. After central nervous system injury, the involved sympathetic and parasympathetic nervous system plays in a disorder way which finally results in autonomic imbalance and severe cardiac events. It is reported that the subsequent arrhythmias (severe bradycardia or VT/VFs) originated from the brain–heart interaction after CNS injury may cause sudden death. Furthermore, the sympatho–adrenomedullary axes reaction and inflammatory waterfall after CNS injury also play an important role in the pathological process of brain–heart interaction that makes patients more predisposed to SCD.

In this chapter, we will explore the mechanism of different kinds of brain disorders such as ischemic stroke, intracranial bleeding, trauma, epilepsy, Takotsubo cardiomyopathy, neurogenic stunned myocardium, Cushing's reflex, and inflammation that lead to cardiovascular changes and sudden death.

## 3.2 The Brain–Heart Axis

In recent studies, it was well known that the cardiovascular system is regulated by both cortical and subcortical modulation. With the development of positron emission tomography and functional magnetic resonance imaging (fMRI) service, researchers built a whole network of the central autonomic nervous system consisting of prefrontal cortex, limbic system, hypothalamus, and the brainstem, which is responsible for the modulation of the central autonomic nervous system.

Catecholamine can be released from the sympathetic nervous system after stimulation-specific areas of the CNS. These special areas were defined as the "brain–cardiac axis" with a complex groups of neural pathways consisting of the prefrontal cortex, amygdala, insular cortex, the anterior cingulate cortex hypothalamus, and the brainstem which are related to the autonomic nervous system modulation [3, 4]. The acute pathologic change of any part of the axis may cause acute rise in intracranial pressure, neurogenic pulmonary edema, malignant arrhythmia, cardiac stun, and sudden death.

### 3.2.1 Cardiac Attack with Prefrontal Cortex

The prefrontal cortex has extensive neural projection connections with other cerebral cortex and subcortical structures. For example, the prefrontal cortex has an interactive fiber connection with the striate anterior visual area, temporal lobe, and parietal lobe; it has a direct or indirect fiber connection with the basal forebrain, cingulate gyrus, and hippocampus; it projects fibers to the basal ganglia; it is the only neocortex with direct projections to the hypothalamus.

Resting high-frequency HRV (HF-HRV), which can manifest vagal blocking of sympathetic activity, is an important kind of method to assess the interaction of cardiovascular changes with the nervous system. The prefrontal cortex region is a special area connective to HF-HRV, which can be proved by the impaired autonomic cardiac control that occurs following injury to the prefrontal cortex. A pathological change arrived from injury or ischemia in the prefrontal cortex can lead to parasympathetic features such as bradycardia, hypotension, and HF HRV in the ECG [5, 6].

### 3.2.2 Cardiac Attack with Limbic System Lesion

The limbic system is an important part of central autonomic network, which includes the insular cortex, hippocampal, parahippocampal gyrus and entorhinal area, dentate gyrus, cingulate gyrus, papillary body, and amygdala, is an crucial component of an internal regulation system through which the brain controls the visceromotor, neuroendocrine, heart rhythm, and blood pressure [7]. Within the central autonomic network, the insular cortex is proved to play a prominent role in limbic–autonomic integration [8]. Furthermore, the network consisting of the insular cortex, amygdala, and anterior cingulate gyrus has been involved in higher order processing of emotional information with autonomic nervous system response.

#### 3.2.2.1 Cardiac Attack with the Insular Cortex

The insular cortex, as a part of the cortex, is located at the bottom of the lateral sulcus, which is separated from the frontal, temporal, and parietal lobes with the circular sulcus around it [9, 10]. It is embedded in the deep part with the rapid development of the surrounding cortex. The insular cortex plays a vital role in controlling the sympathetic and the parasympathetic system. The insular artery from the M2 segment of the middle cerebral artery (MCA) is the main supply artery of the insular lobe. Therefore, the insular lobe tends to be exposed to a higher risk of cerebrovascular disease. In clinical studies, the insular cortex damage has been associated with arrhythmia, diurnal blood pressure (BP) variation disruption, myocardial injury, and sleep-disordered breathing, as well as higher plasma levels of brain natriuretic peptide, catecholamine, and glucose. These patients are at an elevated risk of sudden cardiovascular death. Specially, there is also lateralization of cardiac control by the insula: the right insular regions predominantly regulate the sympathetic tone, and the left insula regulates parasympathetic cardiac manifestations [11, 12]. Therefore, the left insular damage was associated with bradycardia, hypotension, and impairment of cardiac wall motion [13], while the right with more complex arrhythmias such as atrial fibrillation, atrioventricular block, premature contractions, T-wave inversion (or elevation), QT interval prolongation [14], and neurogenic stunned myocardium (NSM), which increase the risk of sudden death [15–19]. Stroke with the insular cortex involvement has also been shown to be associated with elevation of serum N-terminal B-type natriuretic peptide and troponin T levels, suggesting a relationship between the insular cortex damage and cardiac dysfunction or cardiomyopathy [20, 21].

#### 3.2.2.2 Cardiac Attack with Hippocampus Lesion

Hippocampus is located between the thalamus and the medial temporal lobe, and it is part of the limbic system. It is a component of the "brain–cardiac axis," and any pathology damage involving the hippocampus such as bleeding, infraction, or tumors could result in autonomic dysregulation such as hypertension, atrial fibrillation, myocardial infarction, and cardiac failure [22]. Hippocampal infarcts have a poor outcome as evidenced by some research, revealing an association of hippocampal damage with heart failure, severe sympathetic dysfunction, and unexpected sudden death [23].

### 3.2.3 Cardiac Attack with Hypothalamus

The hypothalamus is an integrative center for vital functions that lies above the superior, anterior aspect of the third ventricle, and below the thalamus. It sits in close apposition to central vasculature, with the mammillary bodies and infundibulum "descending through" the center of the circle of Willis [24]. It is a small but complex regulatory center of the brain with important roles in the homeostasis of energy balance, circadian rhythms, and stress responses, as well as growth and reproductive behaviors [25]. The hypothalamus is highly interconnected with other brain regions and acts as an excellent role for the automatic nerve system regulation, whose damage could contribute to the pathogenesis of sudden death.

Nervous system stimulation produces cardiac lesions that are histologically indistinguishable from those described for stress and catecholamine-induced cardiac damage. It has been known for a long time that stimulation of the hypothalamus can lead to autonomic cardiovascular disturbances [26, 27]. The damage of the lateral hypothalamus could produce hypertension and/or electrocardiographic changes ascribed to sympathetic dysregulation, and the anterior hypothalamus damage leads to bradycardia. Unilateral hypothalamic damage does not result in histological evidence of myocardial damage by light microscopy, but bilateral disruption could produce myofibrillar degeneration indistinguishable from that produced by catecholamine injections and stress [28].

### 3.2.4 Cardiac Attack with Brainstem

Brainstem is located under the brain and between the spinal cord and diencephalon. It is a small but quite essential part of the central nervous system, with irregular columnar shape. The sympathetic tone is set by a network of discrete groups of neurons located in different regions of the brainstem. These areas act as an essential regulator of cardiovascular responses to the interactive or exteroceptive environment, as well as vagal and sympathetic nerve activity [29]. It is well known that the regions including the rostral ventrolateral medulla (RVLM) and the nucleus of solitary tract (NTS) in the medulla play a vital role in the regulation of cardiac function [30, 31]. The NST receives afferents from baroreceptors and the cranial nerves, including the vagus which communicates the visceral sensorial information. The RVLM is mainly constituted by excitatory neurons, which are responsible for the initiation of the sympathetic response. Furthermore, the RVLM, along with the external lateral parabrachial nucleus of the pons, is involved in the CNS processing of excitatory cardiovascular reflexes resulting in cardiac sympathetic stimulation [32, 33]. Further advance of the ischemic front into the lower medulla oblongata can also lead to an abrupt change from bradycardia to tachycardia. Patients having brainstem lesions can present with autonomic dysfunction, ventricular arrhythmias, T-wave inversion, bradyarrhythmias, myocardial infarction (MI), and sudden cardiac death [34].

## 3.3 The Sympatho–Adrenomedullary Axes

The sympatho–adrenomedullary axis is the main biological system activated during the stress response [35, 36] that results in neuroendocrine changes, including an increase in epinephrine and norepinephrine levels.

It has been proved that the reason for cardiac attack after cerebral lesion is not only an immediate enhancement of activity in sympathetic nerve terminals with catecholamine release into the cardiac tissue [35–37] but also an indirect effect on the heart through the activation of the sympathetic–adrenomedullary axis. The adrenal medulla is located in the center of the adrenal gland. From embryological view, the medulla and sympathetic nerves, originated from the same tissue, are dominated by the preganglionic fibers of the great splanchnic nerve (belonging to sympathetic nerve), composing the sympatho–adrenomedullary axis. Adrenal medulla acts as a kind of neuroendocrine converter that transforms neural information into hormone information. Under the control of sympathetic nerve, adrenomedullin chromaffin cells can secrete catecholamine hormones such as adrenaline and noradrenaline to ensure the body complete a proper response to the outside stress. However, if suffered from serious brain diseases, such as brain trauma, acute large-area cerebral infarction, acute cerebral hemorrhage, subarachnoid hemorrhage, epilepsy, the sympatho–adrenomedullary axis will be excessively activated and will release excessive catecholamine into the blood, resulting in myocardial over contraction, malignant arrhythmia, and subsequent sudden death.

### 3.3.1 Catecholamine Storm

#### 3.3.1.1 Takotsubo Cardiomyopathy (TC)

As the well-known clinical life-threatening manifestation of brain heart interaction, Takotsubo cardiomyopathy has gradually been recognized in the acute phase of severe cerebral injury. Therefore, the occurrence of TC is mainly due to an emotional or physical stress, during this period the sympatho–adrenomedullary axis is activated resulting in a catecholamine over release. This kind of stress-related cardiomyopathy syndrome has a typical presentation with apical and mid-ventricular dysfunction which may be the causation in the pathogenesis of refractory seizures, sudden unexplained deaths in adults and sudden infant death.

#### 3.3.1.2 Neurogenic Stunned Myocardium

"Neurogenic stunned myocardium" (NSM) is another kind of stress-related cardiomyopathy, the pathophysiology of its myocardial dysfunction is attributed to the catecholamine storm which triggered by an acute neurological injury. The related areas include the caudal ventrolateral medulla, tractus solitarius, dorsal motor vagal nucleus, and posterior hypothalamus. The ischemia, bleeding, trauma, and inflammatory of these structures can result in a centrally mediated profound sympathetic release of noradrenaline which lead to a loss of vasomotor regulation, intense pulmonary vasoconstriction, and increased cardiac rate and contraction [38]. A special type of tissue lesion named as "myocardial contraction band necrosis" has been described in patients suffered from severe catecholamine storm. It is characterized by the hypercontraction of the sarcomeric myofibrils, interstitial mononuclear infiltration, and presence of eosinophilic transverse bands which results in increased extracellular matrix proteins, inflammatory cell infiltration, fibrotic changes contraction band necrosis, and cardiac attack [39, 40].

### 3.3.2 Cushing's Reflex

The sympathetic–adrenomedullar axis is also involved in the Cushing reaction which include mainly two stages. In the first stage, increased intracranial pressure (ICP) derived from severe cerebral injury consequently increases the CSF pressure accessing to the point of mean arterial pressure (MAP), which initiates the complex mechanism of the Cushing's reflex. While the ICP access to the MAP, there is diminished blood supply to the brain, resulting in cerebral ischemia. This "cerebral ischemia" can be perceived by the hypothalamus which triggers a "CNS ischemic response." The hypothalamic activation causes a sympathetic overdrive and sympatho–adrenomedullary axis hyperactivity. A large amount of catecholamine release into blood results in increased arterial blood pressure. The second stage is initiated when the resultant increased arterial blood pressure stimulates the baroreceptors in the carotid bodies resulting in decreasing of pulse and increasing of pulse pressure. In some severe case, the patient then suffers from tidal respiration, blood pressure drop, weak pulse and breathing, or finally dies of cardiac arrest [41].

## 3.4 The Brain Immune System

Inflammatory reaction also plays an important part in the pathophysiology process of brain-derived cardiac death. Stimulation of various CNS disorders can result in an inflammatory mediator-related increase in vascular permeability and tissue damage [42, 43]. It has been wildly recognized that the influence of inflammation and inflammatory cytokines contribute to the myocardial injury.

For one thing, a variety of immune cells that directly derived from spleen and lymph nodes are activated soon after cerebral disorder. As an important peripheral immune organ, the spleen was recognized as a contributor to inflammatory damage after ischemic or hemorrhagic brain injury in many studies [44–46]. The spleen can accomplish a long-distance connection with the brain through mobilizing its inside immune response when encountered a cerebral disorder. After severe central lesion, the spleen contracts, releasing pro-inflammatory immune cells and cytokines into the blood circulation [44–47]. As a result, there is a sudden increased release of immune cells such as lymphocytes, monocytes, neutrophils, and NK cells from the spleen into the peripheral circulation that then migrate into the brain and myocardium and other tissues, which promotes excessive inflammatory response and aggravate tissue damage [48]. Furthermore, the later reduction of immune cells of T lymphocytes and B lymphocytes in the spleen evokes a persistent immunosuppression and increases their susceptibility to stress and infection [49].

For another, the spleen cells activate inflammatory cytokines and chemokines, including tumor necrosis factor-α (TNF-α), interleukin-6 (IL-6), monocyte chemoattractant protein-1 (MCP-1), interferon-γ (IFN-γ), many of which has been shown to aggravate systemic myocardium damage and increase the heart's susceptibility to serious events of sympathetic disorders [50–52].

## 3.5 Conclusion

1. Sudden death derived from brain is becoming increasingly important, and the underlying etiology mechanisms become better understood in the recent years. Many research studies explore the interplay of the brain and cardiovascular systems [53, 54]. As the lesion stimulation of some areas of the brain, a sympathetic or parasympathetic response is presented as a result of a neuroendocrine release attributing to cardiac rhythm disturbances, hemodynamic perturbations, ventricular tachyarrhythmias, and in worse scenarios as neurogenic stunned myocardium, heart failure, and death [55, 56]. The reason for sudden death ranged from ischemia, hemorrhage, and trauma to psychological stress. In general, the etiology mechanism includes both direct and indirect dysregulation of sympathetic/parasympathetic nervous systems and ruins of inflammatory cytokines as the following:
   (a) The high-level nerve center dominating the heart activity is located in the prefrontal cortex, limbic system of the brain, including the insular lobe,

hypothalamus, and brain stem. After acute lesions, the neural network among these nucleus was disrupt, which lead to disconnection and maladjustment of sympathetic nerve and parasympathetic system, subsequently increase or decrease its excitability. Then the abnormal neurotransmitter release from the sympathetic nerve or parasympathetic nerve terminals disrupts the neural network of the myocardium which eventually leads to various malignant arrhythmias, overcontraction of cardiomyocytes, myocardial stunning, and finally sudden death [57].

(b) The sympatho–adrenomedullary axes are the other biological systems activated after acute brain injury that result in neuroendocrine changes, including excessive release of catecholamines from adrenal medulla into the blood. The excessive increase of peripheral blood epinephrine and norepinephrine level thus overactivate the cardiac nervous system network resulting in obviously increased blood pressure and heart rhythm, malignant arrhythmia, myocardial overcontraction, and even myocardial stunning and sudden death.

(c) The neuron cells, glial cells, and vascular endothelial cells were damaged after brain injury, which attribute to the central and peripheral immune systems overactivated as a stress response. The levels of inflammatory factors such as endothelin, thromboxane A2 and prostacyclin (TNF-$\alpha$), interleukin-6 (IL-6), monocyte chemoattractant protein-1 (MCP-1), and interferon $\gamma$ (IFN$\gamma$) in the blood are significantly increased, which cause inflammation and over immune response, affecting myocardial metabolism, and having direct toxic effect on the myocardium [58, 59].

2. Problems and Prospects:

   At present, there is still lack of further insight into the etiology mechanism of sudden death caused by different cerebral disorders at molecular level and gene level, such as the exact incidence of these interactions, the multifactorial pathogenesis, and individual susceptibility. The affective management and elaborate precautions are also needed to be further explored including new drug research and its application, further development of cryotherapy, effective application of stem cell transplantation, treatment of organ transplantation, and gene regulation.

## References

1. Finsterer J, Wahbi K. CNS-disease affecting the heart: brain-heart disorders. J Neurol Sci. 2014;345:8–14.
2. Ryvlin P, Nashef L, Tomson T. Prevention of sudden unexpected death in epilepsy: a realistic goal? Epilepsia. 2013;54(suppl 2):23–8.
3. Goldstein DS. Handbook of clinical neurology. In: Sympathetic neuroimaging, vol. 117. Amsterdam: Elsevier; 2013. p. 365–70.
4. Lizarraga KJ, Gorgulho A, Chen W, Salles AA. Molecular imaging of movement disorders. World J Radiol. 2016;8(3):226–39.
5. Nagai M, Hoshide S, Kario K. The insular cortex an cardiovascular system: a new insight into the brain-heart axis. J Am Soc Hypertens. 2010;4(4):174–82.
6. Ravindran K, Powell KL, Todaro M, O'Brien TJ. The pathophysiology of cardiac dysfunction in epilepsy. Epilepsy Res. 2016;127:19–29.

7. Benarroch EE. The central autonomic network: functional organization, dysfunction, and perspective. Mayo Clin Proc. 1993;68:988–1001.
8. Augustine JR. Circuitry and functional aspects of the insular lobe in primates including humans. Brain Res Rev. 1996;22:229–44.
9. Fink JN, Selim MH, Kumar S, Voetsch B, Fong WC, Caplan LR. Insular cortex infarction in acute middle cerebral artery territory stroke: predictor of stroke severity and vascular lesion. Arch Neurol. 2005;62:1081–5.
10. Dupont S, Bouilleret V, Hasboun D, Semah F, Baulac M. Functional anatomy of the insula: new insights from imaging. Surg Radiol Anat. 2003;25:113–9.
11. Orlandi G, Fanucchi S, Strata G, Pataleo L, Landucci PL, et al. Transient autonomic nervous system dysfunction during hyperacute stroke. Acta Neurol Scand. 2000;102(2):317–21.
12. Makovac E, Meeten F, Watson DR, Herman A, Garfinkel SN, Critchley H, et al. Alterations in amygdala-prefrontal functional connectivity account for excessive worry and autonomic dysregulation in generalized anxiety disorder. Biol Psychiatry. 2016;80(10):786–95.
13. Laowattana S, Zeger SL, Lima JA, Goodman SN, Wittstein IS, Oppenheimer SM. Left insular stroke is associated with adverse cardiac outcome. Neurology. 2006;66:477–83.
14. Eckardt M, Gerlach L, Welter FL. Prolongation of the frequency-corrected QT dispersion following cerebral strokes with involvement of the insula of Reil. Eur Neurol. 1999;42:190–3.
15. Christensen H, Boysen G, Christensen AF, Johannesen HH. Insular lesions, ECG abnormalities, and outcome in acute stroke. J Neurol Neurosurg Psychiatry. 2005;76:269–71.
16. Colivicchi F, Bassi A, Santini M, Caltagirone C. Cardiac autonomic derangement and arrhythmias in right-sided stroke with insular involvement. Stroke. 2004;35:2094–8.
17. Kothavale A, Banki NM, Kopelnik A, et al. Predictors of left ventricular regional wall motion abnormalities after subarachnoid hemorrhage. Neurocrit Care. 2006;4:199–205.
18. Abboud H, Berroir S, Labreuche J, Orjuela K, Amarenco P. GENIC Investigators. Insular involvement in brain infarction increases risk for cardiac arrhythmia and death. Ann Neurol. 2006;59:691–9.
19. Colivicchi F, Bassi A, Santini M, Caltagirone C. Prognostic implications of right-sided insular damage, cardiac autonomic derangement, and arrhythmias after ischemic stroke. Stroke. 2005;36:1710–5.
20. Iltumur K, Yavavli A, Apak I, Ariturk Z, Toprak N. Elevated plasma N-terminal pro-brain natriuretic peptide levels in acute ischemic stroke. Am Heart J. 2006;151:1115–22.
21. Ay H, Koroshetz WJ, Benner T, Vangel MG, Melinosky C, Arsava EM, et al. Neuroanatomical correlates of stroke-related myocardial injury. Neurology. 2006;66:1325–9.
22. Rauramaa T, Pikkarainen M, Englund E, Ince PG, Jellinger K, Paetau A, et al. Cardiovascular diseases and hippocampal infarcts. Hippocampus. 2011;21(3):281–7.
23. Wandschneider B, Koepp M, Scott C, Micallef C, Balestrini S, Sisodiya SM, et al. Structural imaging biomarkers of sudden unexpected death in epilepsy. Brain. 2015;138(10):2907–19.
24. Toni R, Malaguti A, Benfenati F, Martini L. The human hypothalamus: a morpho-functional perspective. J Endocrinol Invest. 2004;27(6 Suppl):73–94.
25. Burbridge S, Stewart I, Placzek M. Development of the neuroendocrine hypothalamus. Compr Physiol. 2016;6(2):623–43.
26. Zhang R, Niu H, Kang X, Ban T, Hong H, Ai J. Longterm administration of neuropeptide y in the subcutaneous infusion results in cardiac dysfunction and hypertrophy in rats. Cell Physiol Biochem. 2015;37(1):94–104.
27. Dikshit BB. The production of cardiac irregularities by excitation of the hypothalamic centres. J Physiol. 1934;81:382–94.
28. Braunwald E, Kloner RA. Myocardial reperfusion: a double-edged sword? J Clin Invest. 1985;76:13–9.
29. Cummings KJ, Commons KG, Fan KC, Li A, Nattie EE. Severe spontaneous bradycardia associated with respiratory disruptions in rat pups with fewer brain stem 5-HT neurons. Am J Physiol Regul Integr Comp Physiol. 2009;296(6):R1783–96.

30. Ardell JL, Andresen MC, Armour JA, Billman GE, Chen PS, Foreman RD, et al. Translational neurocardiology: preclinical models and cardioneural integrative aspects. J Physiol. 2016;594(14):3877–909.
31. Koppikar S, Baranchuk A, Guzmán JC, Morillo CA. Stroke and ventricular arrhythmias. Int J Cardiol. 2013;168(2):653–9.
32. Guo ZL, Longhurst JC, Tjen-A-Looi SC, Fu LW. elPBN neurons regulate rVLM activity through elPBN-rVLM projections during activation of cardiac sympathetic afferent nerves. Am J Physiol Regul Integr Comp Physiol. 2016;311(2):R410–25.
33. Constantinescu V, Matei D, Cuciureanu D, Corciova C, Ignat B, Popescu CD. Cortical modulation of cardiac autonomic activity in ischemic stroke patients. Acta Neurol Belg. 2016;116(4):473–80.
34. Oppenheimer S, Cechetto D. The insular cortex and the regulation of cardiac function. Compr Physiol. 2016;6(2):1081–133.
35. Steptoe A, Kivimaki M. Stress and cardiovascular disease. Nat Rev Cardiol. 2012;9:360–70.
36. Masuda T. Sympathetic nervous activity and myocardial damage immediately after subarachnoid hemorrhage in a unique animal model. Stroke. 2002;33:1671–6.
37. Mertes PM, Carteaux JP, Jaboin Y, et al. Estimation of myocardial interstitial norepinephrine release after brain death using cardiac microdialysis. Transplantation. 1994;57:371–7.
38. Samuels MA. The brain-heart connection. Circulation. 2007;116:77–84.
39. Lee VH, Oh JK, Mulvagh SL, Wijdicks EF. Mechanisms in neurogenic stress cardiomyopathy after aneurysmal subarachnoid hemorrhage. Neurocrit Care. 2006;5:243–9.
40. Banki NM, Zaroff JG. Neurogenic cardiac injury. Curr Treat Options Cardiovasc Med. 2003;5:451–8.
41. Heymans C. The control of heart rate consequent to changes in the cephalic blood pressure and in the intracranial pressure. Am J Physiol. 1928;85:498–505.
42. Mashaly HA, Provencio JJ. Inflammation as a link between brain injury and heart damage: the model of subarachnoid hemorrhage. Cleve Clin J Med. 2008;75(Suppl. 2):S26–30.
43. Tracey KJ. The inflammatory reflex. Nature. 2002;420:853–9.
44. Liu ZJ, Chen C, Li FW, Shen JM, Yang YY, Leak RK, et al. Splenic responses in ischemic stroke: new insights into stroke pathology. CNS Neurosci Ther. 2015;21(4):320–6.
45. Rasouli J, Lekhraj R, Ozbalik M, Lalezari P, Casper D. Brain-spleen inflammatory coupling: a literature review. Einstein J Biol Med. 2011;27(2):74–7.
46. Pennypacker KR. Targeting the peripheral inflammatory response to stroke: role of the spleen. Transl Stroke Res. 2014;5(6):635–7.
47. Seifert HA, Hall AA, Chapman CB, Collier LA, Willing AE, Pennypacker KR. A transient decrease in spleen size following stroke corresponds to splenocyte release into systemic circulation. J Neuroimmune Pharmacol. 2012;7(4):1017–24.
48. Offner H, Subramanian S, Parker SM, et al. Splenic atrophy in experimental stroke is accompanied by increased regulatory T cells and circulating macrophages. J Immunol. 2006;176:6523–31.
49. Prass K, Meisel C, Hoflich C, et al. Stroke-induced immunodeficiency promotes spontaneous bacterial infections and is mediated by sympathetic activation reversal by poststroke T helper cell type 1-like immunostimulation. J Exp Med. 2003;198:725–36.
50. Offner H, Subramanian S, Parker SM, et al. Experimental stroke induces massive, rapid activation of the peripheral immune system. J Cereb Blood Flow Metab. 2006;26:654–65.
51. Seifert HA, Leonardo CC, Hall AA, et al. The spleen contributes to stroke induced neurodegeneration through interferon gamma signaling. Metab Brain Dis. 2012;27(2):131–41.
52. Seifert HA, Collier LA, Chapman CB, et al. Pro-inflammatory interferon gamma signaling is directly associated with stroke induced neurodegeneration. J Neuroimmune Pharmacol. 2014;9:679–89.
53. Natelson BH. Neurocardiology: an interdisciplinary area for the 80s. Arch Neurol. 1985;42(2):178–84.
54. Van der Wall EE. The brain-heart connection; a round trip. Neth Heart J. 2011;19:269–70.

55. Chatterjee S. ECG changes in subarachnoid haemorrhage: a synopsis. Neth Heart J. 2011;19:31–4.
56. Kukla P, Jastrzebski M, Praefort W. J-wave-associated ventricular fibrillation in a patient with a subarachnoid haemorrhage. Europace. 2012;14:1063–4.
57. Nagai M, Hoshide S, Kario K. The insular cortex and cardiovascular system: a new insight into the brain-heart axis. J Am Soc Hypertens. 2010;4(4):174–82. https://doi.org/10.1016/j.jash.2010.05.001.
58. Mazzeo AT, Micalizzi A, Mascia L, et al. Brain-heart crosstalk: the many faces of stress-related cardiomyopathy syndromes in anaesthesia and intensive care. Br J Anaesth. 2014;112(5):803–15. https://doi.org/10.1093/bja/aeu046.
59. Chen Z, Venkat P, Seyfried D, et al. Brain-heart interaction: cardiac complications after stroke. Circ Res. 2017;121(4):451–68. https://doi.org/10.1161/CIRCRESAHA.117.311170.

# Progress in Pathophysiological Mechanism of Global Cerebral Ischemia-Reperfusion Injury

4

Jingyu He and Jing Wang

**Abstract**

Global cerebral ischemia-reperfusion injury after cardiopulmonary arrest is the majority reason for poor neurological prognosis. The pathophysiological mechanism includes endoplasmic reticulum stress (ERS), mitochondrial dysfunction, calcium overload, excessive neuro-inflammatory, platelet activation, microcirculatory thrombosis formation, delayed neurological damage, etc. All mechanisms work together to determine patients' outcomes.

**Keywords**

Mitochondrial dysfunction · Endoplasmic reticulum stress · Glutamate excitotoxicity · Cerebral edema · Oxidative stress · Ischemia-reperfusion

## 4.1 Introduction

In adults, global cerebral ischemic-reperfusion (I/R) insults typically result from cardiac arrest (CA) [1, 2]. The basic structural and functional unit of the nervous system is the neurovascular unit, which consists of neurons and their axons, astrocytes and other supporting cells, and micro-vessels [1, 3]. The neurovascular units constitute the blood–brain barrier (BBB) and have various injury mechanisms during cerebral I/R process [1, 2].

The main pathophysiology of global cerebral I/R can be separated into two dynamic stages [1, 2]: First, ischemic stage, which is a transient ischemic phase of the whole brain during cardiac arrest. There exists the supply–demand disequilibrium between metabolism and oxygen, which rapidly leads to neuronal necrosis and

J. He · J. Wang (✉)
Emergency Department, Xuanwu Hospital, Capital Medical University, Beijing, China
e-mail: hejingyu@xwhosp.org; wj139113@xwhosp.org



H. Zhu (ed.), *Sudden Death*, https://doi.org/10.1007/978-981-15-7002-5_4

vascular damage; and second, reperfusion stage. This includes the hypoperfusion stage during CRP and the hyperperfusion stage after recovery of spontaneous circulation (ROSC) [4, 5]. Both hypo- or hyperperfusions accelerate the activation of inflammatory waterfall-cascade responses which result in large release of cytokines, inflammatory mediators, and reactive oxygen species (ROS); promote the dysfunction of endothelium; facilitate the permeability of BBB; and expedite the migration and regeneration of inflammatory cell (as neutrophils), etc.

Physiopathologic mechanisms of hypo- or/and hyper- perfusion stages cotribute to delayed neuron damage, such as apoptosis or autophagy. In addition, microthrombosis, which is caused by blood stasis company with platelet activation in the microcirculation and impedes the recovery of cerebral circulation after resuscitation [4]. Early massive activation of neutrophils and ischemic injury of vascular endothelial cells also aggravate further damage to the cerebral microvascular system [4]. All of these hinder reperfusion, forming the phenomenon of "no reflow" [4] that increases CNS lesions.

After ROSC, these were regional impaired disparities because of vasoplegia [6], microcirculation collapse, immunosuppression, hypercoagulability, cells' self-tolerance, etc. [6–8]. Neurons in the CA1 region of the hippocampus, Purkinje neurons in the cerebellum, and projection neurons deep in the cerebral cortex have been observed as selective vulnerability [9, 10]. White matter, subcortical regions, and support cells are relatively resistant to short-term hypoxia-ischemia [10]. Disorders of consciousness due to progressive damage of cortical and thalamus neurons is very common among survivors of cardiopulmonary resuscitation [11]. Memory impairment due to the selective vulnerability of the hippocampus is also common in survivors with cognitive deficits [11]. Imaging examination is less sensitive to early cerebral injury after cardiopulmonary resuscitation [12, 13]; however, chronic progressive cerebral atrophy is often observed during the survivors' follow-up [14]. Selective cerebral atrophy, such as the decreased gray matter in precuneus, insular cortex, posterior hippocampus, dorsomedial thalamus, and cingulate cortex, is related to cognitive dysfunction, memory deficits, and consciousness [12, 13, 15].

The precise underlying mechanism of neuronal damage induced by I/R injury include mitochondrial dysfunction, endoplasmic reticulum stress (ERS), oxidative injury, glutamate excitotoxicity, dysregulated calcium homeostasis, and exaggerated neuroinflammation autoregulation depletion of brain circulation, etc.

The exact mechanisms are as follows:

## 4.2 Mitochondrial Dysfunction

Mitochondria is one type of intracellular double-membrane organelles. The main functions of mitochondria are to regulate cellular energy metabolism and synthesize ATP [16]. Neuronal cells are rich in mitochondria because of their high energy requirements [17]. In addition, mitochondria are involved in many other physiological processes, including regulating proliferation and metabolism of cells and participating in the transduction of the calcium pathway [18]. Under the condition of ischemia and hypoxia, mitochondria are prone to cell stress, which leads to imbalanced production of pro- and/or anti-apoptotic protein and overproduction of reactive oxygen species (ROS), and then eventually leads to cell death [19]. Keeping the dynamic balance in a certain number of mitochondrial with stable function is essential in maintaining cell homeostasis and survival.

Sophisticated quality control system, which formed by the biogenesis, clearance, dynamics, and complex interplay of mitochondria, helps to resist the pathological stress and maintain mitochondrial function [16, 20–22]. Protein folding and degradation, DNA repair, and antioxidants early help maintain cellular structure and function after mitochondrial damage. Mitochondrial biogenesis, fusion, division, and autophagy are then performed to eliminate damaged mitochondria after defense failure of first line. Mitochondrial phagocytosis may be the last guarantee for removing injured mitochondria and maintaining cellular viability before necrosis or-/and-apoptosis [23].

Mitophagy is one type of autophagy. Through isolating organelles, protein aggregates, or large cytoplasmic proteins by degradation system sequestering and dissolving by lysosomes, mitophagy eliminates injured mitochondria and maintains the structural and functional integrity of mitochondria and promote cell survival [20, 21]. Mitophagy is the targeted phagocytosis and destruction, which is the main mechanism of mitochondrial quality control.

Multiple mechanisms are involved in the regulation of mitophagy.

1. PINK1/Parkin pathway. After cerebral I/R injury, PINK1 clusters on mitochondrial outer membrane (OMM), which promotes the recruitment of parkin. Perkin ubiquitinates several OMM components. The polyubiquitin chain is then phosphorylated by PINK1 as an "eat me" signal for the autophagy. Adaptor proteins (P62, OPTN, NDP52) recognize phosphorylated polyubiquitin chains on mitochondrial proteins, and initiate the formation of autophagosome by binding to LC3. TBK1 phosphorylates OPTN, enhancing its binding affinity to the ubiquitin chain. The OPTN-TBK1 complex establishes a feedforward mechanism to promote mitochondrial clearance. Gp78, SMURF1, MUL1, SIAH1, and ARIH1 represent E3 ubiquitin ligase targeting OMM proteins prior to nucleation and phagocytosis. The pink1-parkin pathway regulates mitochondrial kinetics and locomotion through proteasomal degradation targeting MFN and Miro [24, 25].
2. The receptor-mediated pathway. The mitotic phagocytic receptors of BNIP3, NIX, and FUNDC1 were localized in OMM and directly interacted with LC3 to mediate mitochondrial clearance. After mitochondrial injury, PHB2 and cardiolipin were externalized to OMM and interacted with LC3. Different receptors guarantee the specificity of different tissues and different stimuli. NIX and BNIP3 phosphorylation enhanced their association with LC3. CK2, Sc kinase, and PGAM5 phosphatase all affect the phosphorylation state of FUNDC1 and regulate mitochondrial dynamics during hypoxia [16, 26].

The receptors-mediated pathway and PNK1/Parkin-mediated pathway share complex crosstalk mechanism. For example, PGAM5 is a well-known regulator of FUNDC1, and it was also associated with increased DRP1 translocation and PINK1/Parkin-mediated mitophagy [16, 26].

Mitophagy is also inconsistent between ischemia and reperfusion phase, for example, ALDH2 (mitochondrial isoform of aldehyde dehydrogenase) promotes autophagy through AMPK-mTOR signaling during ischemia, whereas it inhibits autophagy by Akt-mTOR signaling during reperfusion [27]. Therefore, adaptive mitophagy is protective since it helps to remove abnormal mitochondria and keep cellar homeostasis [28]; however, maladaptive autophagy is accompanied by excessive mitochondrial fragmentation and compromise mitochondrial integrity and function, especially during reperfusion, resulting in a severe reduction in ATP synthesis and a significant increase in ROS, which will seriously threaten the survival of cells [29, 30].

There are many other elements referring to mitochondrial dysfunction after I/R injury. Acute cerebral ischemia accompanies the acute decrease in the supply of oxygen and glucose, which disrupts mitochondrial function along with insufficient adenosine triphosphate (ATP) synthesis and immoderate $Ca^{2+}$ buffering impaired [28, 31, 32] and mitochondrial permeability increased with persistent patency of the mitochondrial permeability transition pore (mPTP) [33, 34]. In certain situations, overstimulation of N-methyl-D-aspartate (NMDA) receptor leads to mitochondrial calcium overload, which in turn activates protease calpain, promotes cleavage of mitofusin 2 (MFN2), leads to mitochondrial fragmentation, and results in further neuronal damage because of progressive ATP depletion [35]. In addition, the increase of intracellular $Ca^{2+}$ combined with the secondary increase of mitochondrial $Ca^{2+}$ leads to the increase of mitochondrial metabolic rate and the formation of free radicals [35–38]. Free radicals lead to excess superoxide production and apoptotic activation by inhibition of electron transport, and furthermore trigger the mitochondrial vicious cycle [35, 38]. For example, ROS induces activation of Bax/Bak, which penetrates into the mitochondrial membrane through the formed large pores and induces apoptosis [16]. ROS are also closely linked to ionic imbalance, energy loss, and excitatory toxicity [39].

Mitochondrial membrane permeabilization is another critical factor in neuronal survival. (1) The initial permeabilization antagonizes the effects of high intracellular $Ca^{2+}$ levels on mitochondrial homeostasis [39]. (2) Permeabilization of OMM facilitates displacing of pro-apoptotic substances from the intermembrane space to the cytoplasm (including inorganic ions, cytochrome c, and so on), leading to apoptosis [40]. (3) OMM permeabilization decreases mitochondrial ATP synthesis and further increases mPTP opening because of imbalance between agonists and inhibitors, specifically the increase of mPTP activators (such as $Ca^{2+}$, ROS, inorganic phosphate from ATP application), and the decrease of mPTP inhibitors (such as: ATP/ADP). Long-lasting mPTP opening, which disturbs the mitochondrial membrane potential (MMP) and uncouples the respiratory process from ATP synthase, is a point-of-no return in apoptosis [41].

All in all, dysfunctional mitochondria plays a pivotal role in the pathogenesis of I/R injury [42].

## 4.3 Endoplasmic Reticulum Stress

Endoplasmic reticulum (ER) is the main intracellular organelles for synthesis, processing and storage of protein. It participates in signal transduction because it is also the huge $Ca^{2+}$ repository. After I/R injury, intracellular accumulation of misfolded and unfolded proteins and dysregulation of calcium homeostasis induce endoplasmic reticulum stress (ERS) which is characterized by the downregulation of translation rates in specific protein, upregulation of endoplasmic reticulum chaperone expression, and degradation of misfolded proteins. The intensity and duration of ischemia determine the extent of ERS [16, 43].

ESR proceeds through the following three crosswise pathways simultaneously: (1) unfolded protein response (UPR), it is a highly conserved response. At an early stage, UPR enhances the ability to fold and process peptides by the upregulation of endoplasmic reticulum chaperone molecules and some other secreted components, helping the cells adapt to changes in the environment and restore ER function. However, when the UPR is activated for an extended time, apoptosis will be induced via post-translational modification of phosphorylation of protein kinase RNA-like endoplasmic reticulum kinase (PERK), which enhances the transcription of CCAAT-enhancer-binding protein homologous protein (CHOP) [43]. CHOP is an executive apoptotic protein, it accelerates apoptosis by reducing Bcl-2 expression and inducing successively cleavage of caspase 12 and caspase 3 [44, 45]. (2) ER-associated degradation (ERAD), it can remove excess proteins from ER. (3) Regulate the protein translation rate to reduce the load of cell. For example, posttranscriptional modification of small ubiquitin-related trim accessories (SUMO) conjugational protein influences protein stability and apoptosis [39, 46]. SUMOylation is the primary target of SUMO conjugation, inhibiting transcription of target genes [16, 39]. SUMOylation is the active form of X-box-binding protein 1 (XBP1), which upregulates reverse transport of misfolded protein transporters and UPR-related proteins, and is a key transcription factor for protein clearance [44]. Moreover, SUMO conjugation increases in response to stress-inducing stimuli, such as heat shock and high ROS production [45, 47] and coincides with neuronal apoptosis [39, 46].

ERS helps to restore homeostasis, which is an important defense mechanism in early stage, whereas prolonged or intense ESR further induces programmed cell death.

## 4.4 Cerebral Edema

There is a period of hyper-perfusion following hypoperfusion after cerebral ischemia [48, 49]. Both hyper- and hypo-perfusion exacerbate cerebral edema and obstacle cerebral recovery.

At the beginning of interruption of blood flow, ischemia-induced hypoxia in the surrounding tissue, and inorganic ions, water, proteins, or/and blood enter into the edematous extracellular space, leading to the increase in tissue pressure [50]. Cerebral tissue pressure blocks capillary inflow by over-exceeding capillary osmotic pressure and aggravates cerebral ischemia and edema. Anaerobic metabolism in the early stages of hypoxia promotes the accumulation of inorganic phosphate and lactic acid, resulting in a significant osmotic imbalance (the osmolarity increases by 50–80 mOsm) [51, 52]. Through ion channels, cation influx (such as Na+) contributes to the disequilibrium [53]. Following changes of osmotic gradient in ion flow, water further passes through BBB, resulting in cytotoxic edema and cellular excitotoxicity. Subsequently, with the recovery of blood flow and subsequently enhanced osmotic gradients between brain tissue and blood, cytotoxic edema progresses gradually into vasogenic edema, which further facilitates vascular permeability and promotes fluid extravasation [54]. Edema increases intracranial pressure that compresses the cerebral vessels and eventually attenuates the cerebral perfusion and exacerbates the initial injury [55, 56].

Aquaporin (AQPs) is a water channel protein, playing an important role in both cytotoxic and vasogenic edema [54, 57]. It is located in the astrocytic end-feet facing BBB vessels and accounts for 35% of the total membrane area [58]. Osmotic driving force that originates from ion channels, or/and cotransporters or/and accumulation of metabolites in hypoxic tissue drives water finally through AQP4 and breaks water homeostasis [57, 59]. On the contrary, AQP4-null mice (the mice that lack AQP4 by gene knockout) showed highly tolerance to cerebral edema with improved neurological prognosis in ischemic stroke model [59].

Matrix metalloproteinases (MMPs) are a large family, which are so named because they need metal ions (such as $Ca^{2+}$ and $Zn^{2+}$) as cofactors. Matrix metalloproteinase-9 (MMP-9) is an important member of MMPs. The main function of MMP-9 is to degrade and remodel the dynamic equilibrium of extracellular matrix. Under the condition of ischemia-reperfusion injury, MMP-9 plays a crucial role in modulating the permeability of the BBB [60, 61]. After stroke, significantly activated MMP-9 brought the poor prognosis by breaking the integrity of BBB and prompting the cerebral edema [62].

Finally, cerebral edema in global cerebral I/R induces high cranial pressure and low cerebral blood flow, which in turn leads to neuron death [54]. Cerebral edema has regional differences. Gray matter is more vulnerable and more sensitive to excitatory toxicity due to higher metabolic rate than white matter (GWR), and also the degree of cerebral edema in gray matter was more severe; however, GWR in basal ganglia and cerebrum changes independently [54].

## 4.5 Glutamate Excitotoxicity

Neuronal excitotoxity is another important mechanism of neuronal injury after ischemia-reperfusion. It mainly includes two aspects: numerous release of excitatory neurotransmitters suddenly and prolonged activation of excitatory receptors [1].

Glutamate excitotoxity is widely researched.

After I/R injury, insufficient ATP production and inadequate cellular energy reserves from dysfunctional mitochondria lead to an increase in glutamate release and a decrease in reabsorption, which leads to neurotoxicity and neural death [63]. By means of overstimulation or/and prolonged stimulation of excitatory receptors (such as N-methyl-D-aspartate (NMDA) receptor and AMPA/kinase receptors), excessive glutamate also leads to lethal ionic derangements, such as excessive inflow of sodium ions and calcium ions [64]. Moreover, glutamate promotes activation of catabolic enzymes. Over-activation of endonuclease leads to the breakdown of DNA and the functional failure of mitochondria. In addition, excessive-activation of phospholipase leads to rupture of cell membrane and over-synthesis release of arachidonic acid and/or oxygen free radicals [65].

Of course, there are also antagonistic factors against glutamate. Glutamine synthase (GS) is synthesized and expressed in glial cells. Under normal conditions, its main function is to reduce the excitatory toxicity of glutamate [66]. Besides, synaptic NMDA receptors composed of GluN2A subunits can prevent glutamate excitotoxicity, whereas non-synaptic NMDA receptors composed of GluN2B subunits show opposing effect with excitotoxicity [67, 68]. Therefore, selective agonists acting on synaptic NMDA receptors may be the effective neuroprotective agents.

In other words, selectively vulnerable excitotoxic injury of distinct neurons depend on the intensity of the excitatory signal input, the density of acting receptors, and the internal defense mechanisms.

## 4.6 Inflammatory Response

### 4.6.1 Neuroinflammatory Response

Although early inflammation is neuroprotective, persistent and excessive inflammatory responses further aggravate neuronal damage [69].

The resultant action of cells, cytokines, signal transduction pathways, and other factors ultimately determine neuronal prognosis as survival, necrosis, apoptosis, or autophagy [39, 70]. For example, proinflammatory cytokines (interleukin-6, 8, 1β) and inflammatory cells with chemotactic activity (such as neutrophils and monocytes) synergistically modulate the progression of neuronal damage in injured area [70]; Astroglia and microglia induce regional apoptosis through mitochondrial apoptosis pathway [70]; tumor necrosis factor-α (TNF-α) acting on tumor necrosis factor receptor 1 (TNF-R1) induces apoptosis by accelerating the release of pro-apoptotic cytochrome C and reducing the action potential of mitochondria [71]. In addition, damage-associated molecular patterns (DAMPs) released during systemic inflammation directly destroy the BBB and increase its permeability, which provokes neuronal necrosis [72], and also, circulating DAMPs acting on brain Toll-like receptors (TLRs) (specifically TLR2 and TLR4) further activate intracellular pathways and participate in pathogen identification and innate immunity [73]. Activated intracellular pathways induce the transcription of cytokines and chemokines and further accelerate apoptosis (details are given below).

On the contrary, anti-inflammatory cytokines (such as IL-4, 9, 10) act as a negative feedback system to antagonize the inflammatory response [39].

Therefore, reducing neuroinflammatory responses and improving the tolerance of inflammation are other targets for neuroprotection [39].

### 4.6.2 Oxidative Stress

Oxidative stress (OS) leads to excessive free radicals in short periods, especially in early phase of reperfusion [74]. Free radicals mainly include two categories: (1) reactive oxygen species (ROS) comprising superoxide anion free radical ($.O_2$-), hydroxyl radical (.OH), hydrogen peroxide ($.H_2O_2$), and so on. (2) Reactive nitrogen species (RNS) comprising nitric oxide (.NO), nitrogen dioxide ($.NO_2$), nitrite peroxide (.ONOO-), etc. [81.82]. Experiments demonstrate that free radicals centered oxygen and centered carbon peak within 5 min of reperfusion [75] and hydroxyl radical peaks within 15 min [76].

Overproduction of free radicals without enough scavenging is the most important characteristic of OS [77]. OS primarily destroys lipid components and protein constituents in membrane structures [1, 78] and further interferes with DNA synthesis and cells function [79] and modulates neuro-inflammation [80] and leads to necrosis and apoptosis [81–86].

Nicotinamide adenine dinucleotide phosphate oxidase, especially in neutrophils, is another main source of ROS [87–89].

There are also regional differences in cerebral OS. Compared with the striatum, OS is more prominent in the cortex due to higher energy requirements [1, 78, 86].

### 4.6.3 Nitric Oxide (NO) and Nitric Oxide Synthase (NOS)

Nitric oxide (NO) is one type of extracellular gas signaling molecule, which belongs to the first messenger responsible for information transmission between cells. NO is derived from de-guanidine of L-arginine via nitric oxide synthase (NOS) catalysis and is produced in endothelial cells, macrophages, nerve cells, and leukocyte [90, 91]. NO plays a variety of roles in the brain, including regulating CBF, conducting nerve signaling, and modulating neuroinflammation [90, 91].

Because of instability, NO study is more difficult than NOS. In reality, the functions of NO are often deduced through the studies of NOS.

Current studies have identified at least three different NOS subtypes: neural nitric oxide synthase (nNOS or NOS1), and inducible nitric oxide synthase (iNOS or NOS2) and endothelial nitric oxide synthase (eNOS or NOS3). nNOS and eNOS (also called as constructive NOS) are encoded on chromosome 12 and 7; iNOS (also called as free radical NOS) is encoded on chromosome 17 [92, 93].

nNOS are selectively distributed in the cerebral cortex, hippocampus, and brainstem [91] and play a dual role in ischemic neuropathology. On the one hand, it assists in cell signal transduction. On the other hand, it is cytotoxic. Mechanisms are as follows: (1) NO inhibits important enzyme systems (such as complexes I and II of the mitochondrial transport chain) and decreases ATP production; (2) NO combines with superoxide anion to form oxidant peroxynitrite, which is an important triggering factor of cytotoxicity, producing free radicals and promoting membrane destruction; (3) NO acts on energy-dependent activation of the DNA repair enzyme poly(ADP-ribose) polymerase, leading to consumption of ATP [94]. iNOS is activated after cell stress, which assists macrophages in the clearance of pathogens and induces delayed nerve damage, and eNOS promotes vasodilation and inhibits platelet aggregation and increases cerebral blood flow, through phosphatidylinositol-3 kinase/Akt (PI3K/Akt) pathway [1, 90–92]. The combination of these mechanisms determines the destiny of cell [1].

## 4.7 Neuronal Apoptosis

Neuronal apoptosis is one of the delayed programmed deaths associated with gene regulation. It is characterized by cell shrinkage with integrated membrane, chromatin aggregation and DNA fragmentation without injured inflammation, and formation of apoptotic bodies without surrounding tissue injured [1, 95]. It causes delayed neurological sequelae, such as: coma, delirium, neurocognitive impairment, seizures, and stroke after cerebral I/R [96].

The exact pathways of apoptosis are not yet known. The current hypothesis classifies them as mitochondrial-dependent intrinsic pathway and receptor-mediated extrinsic pathway [97, 98].

In intrinsic pathway, permeability transition pores are formed in mitochondrial inner membrane, which leads to the rupture of mitochondrial outer membrane and the release of proapoptotic substances (including endonucleases, caspases, cytochrome c, and other proteases related to interleukin-1b-converting enzyme) [97–99]. These factors ultimately lead to DNA breakage. Nuclear transcription factor, nuclear factor-b (NF-B), regulates neuronal apoptosis through mitochondrial-dependent intrinsic pathways [1, 100].

The extrinsic pathways (also called mitochondrial-independent pathways) involve several receptor families, such as Bcl-2 families and Fas families. Promoting the member actions of Bcl-2 family (such as Bcl-2, Bcl-XL, Bcl-W, Mcl-1, CED9), which control proteolytic systems, help to inhibit apoptosis, whereas other family members of bcl-2 family (such as Bax, Bcl-XL, Mcl-1) augment apoptosis by increasing translocation [1, 97–99, 101].

Protein lyase caspases are also significantly expressed in cerebral ischemia. Activated caspase-3 can instigate DNA fragmentation, whereas caspase inhibitors protect against ischemia. In addition, release of cytochrome c into the cytosol leads to the formation of apoptotic bodies [1, 101].

Mitogen-activated protein kinase (MAPK) signaling pathways are involved in the regulation of inflammation and apoptosis after cerebral ischemia-reperfusion [1]. p38 mitogen-activated protein kinase (p38MAPK), c-Jun N-terminal kinase (JNK), extracellular signal-regulated kinase (ERK 1/2), and ERK 5 are the four main elements of MAPKs [102]. The MAPK pathway plays a variety of cellular functions by regulating its downstream molecules; reversely, the downstream targets (such as: ATF2) increase the complexity of MAPKs' regulation in apoptosis, necrosis, and survival. The activation of ERK 1/2 and JNK pathways plays roles in promoting injury formation, while inhibition of them can reduce brain edema, protect cerebral function, and decrease apoptosis. Whereas, the activation of p38

MAPK pathway plays the opposite effect with a neuroprotective role. ERK 5 is an indispensable signaling protein in cell proliferation and differentiation. Phosphorylation of ERK 5 promotes the survival of nerve cells by facilitating the expression of insulin in neurons [1, 103]. Moreover, the activation of ERK 1/2 pathway is promoted by the JNK pathway and inhibited by the p38 MAPK pathway, indicating that there is mutual regulation between MAPK pathways.

## 4.8 Other Mechanisms

Brain-derived neurotrophic factor (BDNF) belongs to neurotrophin-family. After binding to tyrosine kinase B (TrkB), BDNF enhances the autophosphorylation of TrkB, stepwise activates the RAS-MAPK pathway, and finally activates transcription factor, cAMP response element-binding protein (CREB), to promote the neural survival and increase synaptic plasticity and neurogenesis [104]. BDNF participates in neuronal development and differentiation, as well as the improvement of neurological function after brain injury [105, 106]. BDNF can also active extracellular signal-regulated kinases 1/2 (ERK1/2) and induce the angiogenesis of endothelial cell [107].

Sirtuin 1 (SIRT 1) is a member of the sirtuin enzyme family [108]. It is considered to be a new target for neuroprotection after brain I/R injury [109, 110]. By deacetylating histones, SIRT 1 interacts with DNA and takes part in DNA repair, gene silencing, and metabolism [111]. The neuroprotective effects of iPoCo might be due to the activation of the SIRT 1 [112].

Micro-RNAs are often considered as regulatory factors participating in various physiological or/and pathophysiological processes, and recent studies have found that they are also involved in the regulation of mitophagy [113]. For example, the significantly upregulated micro RNA-410 in mice IR model interacts with high-mobility group box 1 protein (HMGB1), leading to the deterioration of mitochondrial function and the increase of mitophagy [16]. The overexpression of micro RNA-410 in cultured human adult cardiac myocytes (HACMs) can diminish cell viability by increasing mitophagy and decreasing energy production and also can promote cell death by promoting the release of cytochrome c and enhancing caspase-3 activity [114]; however, recent studies have found that bicarbonate may aggravate IR injury by inhibiting mitophagy [115].

Hypoxia-inducible factor 1 (HIF-1), which is a major transcriptional regulator under hypoxic conditions [116, 117], consists of constitutive-subunit and oxygen-regulated-subunit [118] and participates in apoptosis, angiogenesis, glucose metabolism, and cell survival during hypoxia [116, 117].

Acid-sensing ion channels (ASICs) are a specific type of ligand-gated channel that mediates $Ca^{2+}$ influx during activation. It protects neuron proteins and nucleic acids by eliminating toxic cell substances with low extracellular pH [119]. ASIC2a has a potential neuroprotective effect through inhibiting apoptosis and promoting regeneration [120].

Generally speaking, the mechanisms of cerebral IR injury include endoplasmic reticulum stress (ERS), mitochondrial dysfunction, calcium overload, oxidative stress, neuroinflammatory, platelet activation, and microcirculatory thrombosis formation. Targeted temperature management (TTM), cerebral ischemic postconditioning (CPOC), chinese traditional medicines, bundling therapies and etc. which were introduced below, might be beneficial.

## References


1. Li Z, Chen H, Lv J, Zhao R. The application and neuroprotective mechanisms of cerebral ischemic post-conditioning: a review. Brain Res Bull. 2017;131:39–46.
2. Koenig MA. Brain resuscitation and prognosis after cardiac arrest. Crit Care Clin. 2014;30:765–83.
3. Han D, Zhang S, Fan B, Wen LL, Sun M, Zhang H, Feng J. Ischemic postconditioning protects the neurovascular unit after focal cerebra ischemia/reperfusion injury. J Mol Neurosci. 2014;53:50–8.
4. Chalkias A, Xanthos T. Post-cardiac arrest brain injury: pathophysiology and treatment. J Neurol Sci. 2012;315:1–8.
5. Hinduja A, Gupta H, Yang JD, et al. Hypoxic ischemic brain injury following in hospital cardiac arrest—lessons from autopsy. J Forensic Leg Med. 2014;23:84–6.
6. Huynh N, Kloke J, Gu C, et al. The effect of hypothermia "dose" on vasopressor requirements and outcome after cardiac arrest. Resuscitation. 2013;84:189.
7. Neumar RW. Molecular mechanisms of ischemic neuronal injury. Ann Emerg Med. 2000;36:483–506.
8. Madder RD, Reynolds JC. Multidisciplinary management of the post–cardiac arrest patient. Cardiol Clin. 2018;36:85–101.
9. Metter RB, Rittenberger JC, Guyette FX, et al. Association between a quantitative CT scan measure of brain edema and outcome after cardiac arrest. Resuscitation. 2011;82:1180–5.
10. Fujioka M, Okuchi K, Sakaki T, et al. Specific changes in human brain following reperfusion after cardiac arrest. Stroke. 1994;25:2091–5.
11. Nolan JP, Neumar RW, Adrie C, et al. Post-cardiac arrest syndrome: epidemiology, pathophysiology, treatment, and prognostication. Resuscitation. 2008;79:350–79.
12. Arbelaez A, Castillo M, Mukherji SK. Diffusion weighted MR imaging of global cerebral anoxia. Am J Neuroradiol. 1999;20:999–1007.
13. Gutierrez LG, Rovira A, Portela LA, et al. CT and MR in non-neonatal hypoxic-ischemic encephalopathy: radiographic findings with pathophysiological correlations. Neuroradiology. 2010;52:949–76.
14. Horstmann A, Frisch S, Jentzsch RT, et al. Resuscitating the heart but losing the brain: brain atrophy in the aftermath of cardiac arrest. Neurology. 2010;74:306–12.
15. Youn CS, Park KN, Kim JY, Callaway CW, Choi SP, Rittenberger JC, Kim SH, Oh SH, Kim YM. Repeated diffusion weighted imaging in comatose cardiac arrest patients with therapeutic hypothermia. Resuscitation. 2015;96:1–8.
16. Yang M, Linn BS, Zhang Y, Ren J. Mitophagy and mitochondrial integrity in cardiac ischemia-reperfusion. Mol Basis Dis. 2019;1865:2293–302.
17. Ren J, Pulakat L, Whaley-Connell A, Sowers JR. Mitochondrial biogenesis in the metabolic syndrome and cardiovascular disease. J Mol Med (Berl). 2010;88:993–1001.
18. Rizzuto R, Bernardi P, Pozzan T. Mitochondria as all-round players of the calcium game. J Physiol. 2000;529(Pt 1):37–47.
19. Sena LA, Chandel NS. Physiological roles of mitochondrial reactive oxygen species. Mol Cell. 2012;48:158–16.

20. Ren J, Zhang Y. Targeting autophagy in aging and aging-related cardiovascular diseases. Trends Pharmacol. 2018;39:1064–76.
21. Zhang Y, Whaley-Connell AT, Sowers JR, Ren J. Autophagy as an emerging target in cardiorenal metabolic disease: from pathophysiology to management. Pharmacol Ther. 2018;191:1–22.
22. Zhou H, Wang S, Hu S, Chen Y, Ren J. ER-mitochondria microdomains in cardiac ischemia-reperfusion injury: a fresh perspective. Front Physiol. 2018;9:755.
23. Yoo SM, Jung YK. A molecular approach to mitophagy and mitochondrial dynamics. Mol Cells. 2018;41:18–26.
24. Lan R, Wu JT, Wu T, Ma YZ, Wang BQ, Zheng HZ, Li YN, Wang Y, Gu CQ, Zhang Y. Mitophagy is activated in brain damage induced by cerebral ischemia and reperfusion via the PINK1/Parkin/p62 signalling pathway. Brain Res Bull. 2018;142:63–77.
25. Feng J, Chen X, Guan B, Li C, Qiu J, Shen J. Inhibition of peroxynitrite-induced mitophagy activation attenuates cerebral ischemia-reperfusion injury. Mol Neurobiol. 2018;55:6369–86.
26. Wang Y, Lu X, Zhao P, Jiang J, Yao L. Overexpression of PPENK reduces myocardial ischemia reperfusion injury by promoting mitophagy in rats. Chin J Cell Mol Immunol. 2017;33:1335–40.
27. Ji W, Wei S, Hao P, Xing J, Yuan Q, Wang J, Xu F, Chen Y. Aldehyde dehydrogenase 2 has cardioprotective effects on myocardial ischaemia/reperfusion injury via suppressing mitophagy. Front Pharmacol. 2016;7:101.
28. Ma H, Guo R, Yu L, Zhang Y, Ren J. Aldehyde dehydrogenase 2 (ALDH2) rescues myocardial ischaemia/reperfusion injury: role of autophagy paradox and toxic aldehyde. Eur Heart J. 2011;32:1025–38.
29. Solenski NJ, di Pierro CG, Trimmer PA, Kwan AL, Helm GA. Ultrastructural changes of neuronal mitochondria after transient and permanent cerebral ischemia. Stroke. 2002;33:816–24.
30. Kumar R, Bukowski MJ, Wider JM, Reynolds CA, Calo L, Lepore B, Tousignant R, Jones M, Przyklenk K, Sanderson TH. Mitochondrial dynamics following global cerebral ischemia. Mol Cell Neurosci. 2016;76:68–75.
31. Ren J, Zhang Y. Editorial: new therapeutic approaches in the management of ischemia reperfusion injury and cardiometabolic diseases: opportunities and challenges. Curr Drug Targets. 2017;18:1687–8.
32. Murphy E, Steenbergen C. Mechanisms underlying acute protection from cardiac ischemia-reperfusion injury. Physiol Rev. 2008;88:581–609.
33. Kubli DA, Gustafsson AB. Mitochondria and mitophagy: the yin and yang of cell death control. Circ Res. 2012;111:1208–21.
34. Givvimani S, Munjal C, Tyagi N, Sen U, Metreveli N, Tyagi SC. Mitochondrial division/mitophagy inhibitor (Mdivi) ameliorates pressure overload induced heart failure. PLoS One. 2012;7:e32388.
35. Schinder AF, Olson EC, Spitzer NC, Montal M. Mitochondrial dysfunction is a primary event in glutamate neurotoxicity. J Neurosci. 1996;16(19):6125–33.
36. Loor G, Kondapalli J, Iwase H, Chandel NS, Waypa GB, Guzy RD, Vanden Hoek TL, Schumacker PT. Mitochondrial oxidant stress triggers cell death in simulated ischemia-reperfusion. Biochim Biophys Acta. 2011;1813(7):1382–94.
37. Globus MY, Busto R, Lin B, Schnippering H, Ginsberg MD. Detection of free radical activity during transient global ischemia and recirculation: effects of intra ischemic brain temperature modulation. J Neurochem. 1995;65(3):1250–6.
38. Reynolds IJ, Hastings TG. Glutamate induces the production of reactive oxygen species in cultured forebrain neurons following NMDA receptor activation. J Neurosci. 1995;15:3318–27.
39. Talma N, Kok WF, de Veij Mestdagh CF, Shanbhag NC, Bouma HR, Henning RH. Neuroprotective hypothermia—why keep your head cool during ischemia and reperfusion. Biochim Biophys Acta. 2016;1860:2521–8.
40. Kroemer G, Galluzzi L, Brenner C. Mitochondrial membrane permeabilization in cell death. Physiol Rev. 2007;87(1):99–163.

41. Gong P, Hua R, Zhang Y, Zhao H, Tang Z, Mei X, Zhang M, Cui J, Li C. Hypothermia-induced neuroprotection is associated with reduced mitochondrial membrane permeability in a swine model of cardiac arrest. J Cereb Blood Flow Metab. 2013;33(6):928–34.
42. Gazmuri RJ, Radhakrishnan J. Protecting mitochondrial bioenergetic function during resuscitation from cardiac arrest. Crit Care Clin. 2012;28:245–70.
43. Hetz C. The unfolded protein response: controlling cell fate decisions under ER stress and beyond. Nat Rev Mol Cell Biol. 2012;13:89–102.
44. Chen H, Qi L. SUMO modification regulates the transcriptional activity of XBP1. Biochem J. 2010;429(1):95–102.
45. Lee YJ, Mou Y, Klimanis D, Bernstock JD, Hallenbeck JM. Global SUMOylation is a molecular mechanism underlying hypothermia-induced ischemic tolerance. Front Cell Neurosci. 2014;8:416.
46. Wei H, Teng H, Huan W, Zhang S, Fu H, Chen F, Zhao J, et al. An upregulation of SENP3 after spinal cord injury: implications for neuronal apoptosis. Neurochem Res. 2012;37(12):2758–66.
47. Saitoh H, Hinchey J. Functional heterogeneity of small ubiquitin-related protein modifiers SUMO-1 versus SUMO-2/3. J Biol Chem. 2000;275(9):6252–8.
48. Dohmen C, Kumura E, Rosner G, Heiss WD, Graf R. Extracellular correlates of glutamate toxicity in short-term cerebral ischemia and reperfusion: a direct in vivo comparison between white and gray matter. Brain Res. 2005;1037:43–51.
49. Karapanayiotides T, Meuli R, Devuyst G, Piechowski-Jozwiak B, Dewarrat A, Ruchat P, Von Segesser L, Bogousslavsky J. Post carotid endarterectomy hyperperfusion or reperfusion syndrome. Stroke. 2005;36:21–6.
50. Ayata C, Ropper AH. Ischaemic brain oedema. J Clin Neurosci. 2002;9(2):113–24.
51. Hossmann KA. Treatment of experimental cerebral ischemia. J Cereb Blood Flow Metab. 1982;2:275–97.
52. LaManna JC. Hypoxia/ischemia and the pH paradox. Adv Exp Med Biol. 1996;388:283–92.
53. Simard JM, Sheth KN, Kimberly WT, Stern BJ, del Zoppo GJ, Jacobson S, Gerzanich V. Glibenclamide in cerebral ischemia and stroke. Neurocrit Care. 2013;20:319–33.
54. Farr GW, Hall CH, Farr SM, Wade R, Detzel JM, Adams AG, Buch JM, Beahm DL, Flask CA, Xu K, LaManna JC, McGuirk PR, Boron WF, Pelletier MF. Functionalized phenylbenzamides inhibit Aquaporin-4 reducing cerebral edema and improving outcome in two models of CNS injury. Neuroscience. 2019;404:484–98.
55. Bardutzky J, Schwab S. Antiedema therapy in ischemic stroke. Stroke. 2007;38:3084–94.
56. Marmarou A. A review of progress in understanding the pathophysiology and treatment of brain edema. Neurosurg Focus. 2007;22:E1.
57. Kozlu S, Caban S, Yerlikaya F, Fernandez-Megia E, Novoa-Carballal R, Riguera R, Yemisci M, Gursoy-Ozdemir Y, Dalkara T, Couvreur P, Capan Y. An aquaporin 4 antisense oligonucleotide loaded, brain targeted nanoparticulate system design. Pharmazie. 2014;69:340–5.
58. Papadopoulos MC, Verkman AS. Aquaporin water channels in the nervous system. Nat Rev Neurosci. 2013;14:265–77.
59. Manley GT, Fujimura M, Ma T, Noshita N, Filiz F, Bollen AW, Chan P, Verkman AS. Aquaporin-4 deletion in mice reduces brain edema after acute water intoxication and ischemic stroke. Nat Med. 2000;6:159–63.
60. Lok J, Zhao S, Leung W, Seo JH, Navaratna D, Wang X, Whalen MJ, Lo EH. Neuregulin-1 effects on endothelial and blood-brain-barrier permeability after experimental injury. Transl Stroke Res. 2012;3(Suppl. 1):S119–24.
61. Shigemori Y, Katayama Y, Mori T, Maeda T, Kawamata T. Matrixmetalloproteinase-9 is associated with blood-brain barrier opening and brain edema formation after cortical contusion in rats. Acta Neurochir Suppl. 2006;96:130–3.
62. Switzer JA, Hess DC, Ergul A, Waller JL, Machado LS, Portik-Dobos V, Pettigrew LC, Clark WM, Fagan SC. Matrix metalloproteinase-9 in anexploratory trial of intravenous minocycline for acute ischemic stroke. Stroke. 2011;42:2633–5.
63. Nishizawa Y. Glutamate release and neuronal damage in ischemia. Life. 2001;69(4):369–81.

64. Pignataro G, Cuomo O, Vinciguerra A, Sirabella R, Esposito E, Boscia F, DiRenzo G, Annunziato L. NCX as a key player in the neuroprotection exerted by ischemic preconditioning and postconditioning. Adv Exp Med Biol. 2013;961:223–40.
65. London A, Benhar I, Schwartz M. The retina as a window to the brain-from eye research to CNS disorders. Nat Rev Neurol. 2013;9(1):44–53.
66. Zhang W, Miao Y, Zhou S, Jiang J, Luo Q, Qiu Y. Neuroprotective effects of ischemic post-conditioning on global brain ischemia in rats through upregulation of hippocampal glutamine synthetase. J Clin Neurosci. 2011;18:685–9.
67. Brassai A, Suvanjeiev RG, Ban EG, Lakatos M. Role of synaptic and nonsynaptic glutamate receptors in ischaemia induced neurotoxicity. Brain Res Bull. 2015;112:1–6.
68. Vizi ES, Kisfali M, Lorincz T. Role of nonsynaptic GluN2B-containing NMDA receptors in excitotoxicity: evidence that fluoxetine selectively inhibits these receptors and may have neuroprotective effects. Brain Res Bull. 2013;93:32–8.
69. Peberdy MA, Andersen LW, Abbate A, et al. Inflammatory markers following resuscitation from out-of-hospital cardiac arrest-A prospective multicenter observational study. Resuscitation. 2016;103:117–24.
70. Matsui T, Tasaki M, Yoshioka T, Motoki Y, Tsuneoka H, Nojima J. Temperature and time-dependent changes in TLR2-activated microglial NF-kappaB activity and concentrations of inflammatory and anti-inflammatory factors. Intensive Care Med. 2012;38(8):1392–9.
71. Doll DN, Rellick SL, Barr TL, Ren X, Simpkins JW. Rapid mitochondrial dysfunction mediates TNF-alpha-induced neurotoxicity. J Neurochem. 2015;132(4):443–51.
72. Shichita T, Ito M, Yoshimura A. Post-ischemic inflammation regulates neural damage and protection. Front Cell Neurosci. 2014;14(8):319.
73. Kong Y, Le Y. Toll-like receptors in inflammation of the central nervous system. Int Immunopharmacol. 2011;11(10):1407–14.
74. Kahles T, Brandes RP. NADPH oxidases as therapeutic targets in ischemic stroke. Cell Mol Life Sci. 2012;69:2345–63.
75. Bolli R, Jeroudi MO, Patel BS, Aruoma OI, Halliwell B, Lai EK, et al. Marked reduction of free radical generation and contractile dysfunction by antioxidant therapy begun at the time of reperfusion. Evidence that myocardial stunning is a manifestation of reperfusion injury. Circ Res. 1989;65(3):607–22.
76. Khalid MA, Ashraf M. Direct detection of endogenous hydroxyl radical production in cultured adult cardiomyocytes during anoxia and reoxygenation. Is the hydroxyl radical really the most damaging radical species? Circ Res. 1993;72(4):725–36.
77. Chen H, Yoshioka H, Kim GS, Jung JE, Okami N, Sakata H, Maier CM, Narasimhan P, Goeders CE, Chan PH. Oxidative stress in ischemic brain damage: mechanisms of cell death and potential molecular targets for neuroprotection. Antioxid Redox Signal. 2011;14:1505–17.
78. Nagakannan P, Shivasharan BD, Thippeswamy BS, Veerapur VP. Effect of tramadol on behavioral alterations and lipid peroxidation after transient forebrain ischemia in rats. Toxicol Mech Methods. 2012;22:674–8.
79. Tuttolomondo A, Di Sciacca R, Di Raimondo D, Arnao V, Renda C, Pinto A, et al. Neuron protection as a therapeutic target in acute ischemic stroke. Curr Top Med Chem. 2009;9:1317–34.
80. Wong CH, Crack PJ. Modulation of neuro-inflammation and vascular response by oxidative stress following cerebral ischemia-reperfusion injury. Curr Med Chem. 2008;15:1–14.
81. Halliwell B. Free radicals, antioxidants, and human disease: curiosity, cause, or consequence. Lancet. 1994;344:721–4.
82. Sugawara T, Chan PH. Reactive oxygen radicals and pathogenesis of neuronal death after cerebral ischemia. Antioxid Redox Signal. 2003;5:597–607.
83. Huang Y, Rabb H, Womer KL. Ischemia-reperfusion and immediate T cell responses. Cell Immunol. 2007;248:4–11.

84. Jung JE, Kim GS, Chen H, Maier CM, Narasimhan P, Song YS, et al. Reperfusion and neurovascular dysfunction in stroke: from basic mechanisms to potential strategies for neuroprotection. Mol Neurobiol. 2010;41:172–9.
85. Lv M, Liu Y, Zhang J, Sun L, Liu Z, Zhang S, et al. Roles of inflammation response in microglia cell through toll-like receptors 2/interleukin-23/interleukin-17 pathway in cerebral ischemia/reperfusion injury. Neuroscience. 2011;176:162–72.
86. Yokobori S, Nakae R, Yokota H, Spurlock MS, Mondello S, Gajavelli S, Bullock RM. Subdural hematoma decompression model: a model of traumatic brain injury with ischemic-reperfusional pathophysiology: a review of the literature. Behav Brain Res. 2018;340:23–8.
87. Fan J, Li Y, Levy RM, Fan JJ, Hackam DJ, Vodovotz Y, Yang H, Tracey KJ, Billiar TR, Wilson MA. Hemorrhagic shock induces NAD(P)H oxidase activation in neutrophils: role of HMGB1-TLR4 signaling. J Immunol. 2007;178:6573–80.
88. Fujita T, Hirooka K, Nakamura T, Itano T, Nishiyama A, Nagai Y, Shiraga F. Neuroprotective effects of angiotensin II type 1 receptor (AT1-R) blocker via modulating AT1-R signaling and decreased extracellular glutamate levels. Invest Ophthalmol Vis Sci. 2012;53:4099–110.
89. Pamenter ME, Ali SS, Tang Q, Finley JC, Gu XQ, Dugan LL, Haddad GG. An in vitro ischemic penumbral mimic perfusate increases NADPH oxidase-mediated superoxide production in cultured hippocampal neurons. Brain Res. 2012;1452:165–72.
90. Dawson TM, Dawson VL, Snyder SH. A novel neuronal messenger in brain: the free radical, nitric oxide. Ann Neurol. 1992;32:297–311.
91. Dawson TM, Dawson VL. Nitric oxide: actions and pathological roles. Neuroscientist. 1995;1:7–18.
92. Samdani AF, Dawson TM, Dawson VL. Nitric oxide synthase in models of focal ischemia. Stroke. 1997;28:1283–8.
93. Dalkara T, Moskowitz MA. The role of nitric oxide in cerebral ischemia. In: Welch KMA, Caplan LR, Reis DJ, et al., editors. Primer on cerebrovascular disease. Philadelphia: Academic Press; 1997. p. 207–8.
94. Goto S, Xue R, Sugo N, et al. Poly(ADP-ribose) polymerase impairs early and long-term experimental stroke recovery. Stroke. 2002;33:1101–6.
95. Li Y, Chopp M, Jiang N, Yao F, Zaloga C. Temporal profile of in situ DNA fragmentation after transient middle cerebral artery occlusion in the rat. J Cereb Blood Flow Metab. 1995;15:389–97.
96. Mattson MP, Duan W, Pedersen WA, Culmsee C. Neurodegenerative disorders and ischemic brain diseases. Apoptosis. 2001;6:69–81.
97. Graham SH, Chen J. Programmed cell death in cerebral ischemia. J Cereb Blood Flow Metab. 2001;21:99–109.
98. Sugawara T, Fujimura M, Noshita N, et al. Neuronal death/survival signaling pathways in cerebral ischemia. NeuroRx. 2004;1:17–25.
99. Leist M, Nicotera P. Cell death: apoptosis versus necrosis. In: KMA W, Caplan LR, Reis DJ, et al., editors. Primer on cerebrovascular disease. Philadelphia: Academic Press; 1997. p. 101–4.
100. Li WL, Yu SP, Chen D, Yu SS, Jiang YJ, Genetta T, Wei L. Theregulatory role of NF-kappaB in autophagy-like cell death after focal cerebral ischemia in mice. Neuroscience. 2013b;244:16–30.
101. Li P, Nijha Wan D, Budihardjo I, Srinivasula SM, Ahmad M, Alnemri ES, Wang X. Cytochrome c and dATP-dependent formation of Apaf-1/caspase-9complex initiates an apoptotic protease cascade. Cell. 1997;91:479–89.
102. Shu Y, Yang Y, Zhang P. Neuroprotective effects of penehyclidine hydrochloride against cerebral ischemia/reperfusion injury in mice. Brain Res Bull. 2016;121:115–23.
103. Gozdecka M, Breitwieser W. The roles of ATF2 (activating transcription factor 2) in tumorigenesis. Biochem Soc Trans. 2012;40:230–4.

104. Alboni S, Tascedda F, Corsini D, Benatti C, Caggia F, Capone G, Barden N, Blom JM, Brunello N. Stress induces altered CRE/CREB pathway activity and BDNF expression in the hippocampus of glucocorticoid receptor-impaired mice. Neuropharmacology. 2011;60:1337–46.
105. Lu B, Nagappan G, Guan X, Nathan PJ, Wren P. BDNF-based synaptic repair as a disease-modifying strategy for neurodegenerative diseases. Nat Rev Neurosci. 2013;14:401–16.
106. Singh M, Su C. Progesterone, brain-derived neurotrophic factor and neuroprotection. Neuroscience. 2013;239:84–91.
107. Pardon MC, Roberts RE, Marsden CA, Bianchi M, Latif ML, Duxon MS, Kendall DA. Social threat and novel cage stress-induced sustained extracellular-regulated kinase1/2 (ERK1/2) phosphorylation but differential modulation of brain-derived neurotrophic factor (BDNF) expression in the hippocampus of NMRI mice. Neuroscience. 2005;132:561–74.
108. Hernandez-Jimenez M, Hurtado O, Cuartero MI, Ballesteros I, Moraga A, Pradillo JM, McBurney MW, Lizasoain I, Moro MA. Silent information regulator 1 protects the brain against cerebral ischemic damage. Stroke. 2013;44:2333–7.
109. Miao Y, Zhao S, Gao Y, Wang R, Wu Q, Wu H, Luo T. Curcumin pretreatment attenuates inflammation and mitochondrial dysfunction in experimental stroke: the possible role of Sirt1 signaling. Brain Res Bull. 2016;121:9–15.
110. Wan D, Zhou Y, Wang K, Hou Y, Hou R, Ye X. Resveratrol provides neuroprotection by inhibiting phosphodiesterases and regulating the cAMP/AMPK/SIRT1 pathway after stroke in rats. Brain Res Bull. 2016;121:255–62.
111. Alcendor RR, Kirshenbaum LA, Imai S, Vatner SF, Sadoshima J. Silentin formation regulator 2alpha a longevity factor and class III histone deacetylase, is an essential endogenous apoptosis inhibitor in cardiac myocytes. Circ Res. 2004;95:971–80.
112. Kaur H, Kumar A, Jaggi AS, Singh N. Pharmacologic investigations on the role of Sirt-1 in neuroprotective mechanism of postconditioning in mice. J Surg Res. 2015;197:191–200.
113. Mirzaei H, Momeni F, Saadatpour L, Sahebkar A, Goodarzi M, Masoudifar A, Kouhpayeh S, Salehi H, Mirzaei HR, Jaafari MR. MicroRNA: relevance to stroke diagnosis, prognosis and therapy. J Cell Physiol. 2017;233(2):856–65.
114. Yang F, Li T, Dong Z, Mi R. MicroRNA-410 is involved in mitophagy after cardiac ischemia/reperfusion injury by targeting high-mobility group box 1 protein. J Cell Biochem. 2018;119:2427–39.
115. Queliconi BB, Kowaltowski AJ, Gottlieb RA. Bicarbonate increases ischemia reperfusion damage by inhibiting mitophagy. PLoS One. 2016;11:e0167678.
116. Zhu T, Zhan L, Liang D, Hu J, Lu Z, Zhu X, Sun W, Liu L, Xu E. Hypoxia-inducible factor 1 alpha mediates neuroprotection of hypoxic postconditioning against global cerebral ischemia. J Neuropathol Exp Neurol. 2014;73:975–86.
117. Wang GL, Jiang BH, Rue EA, Semenza GL. Hypoxia-inducible factor 1 Isa basic-helix-loop-helix-PAS heterodimer regulated by cellular O2 tension. Proc Natl Acad Sci U S A. 1995;92:5510–4.
118. Liu BN, Han BX, Liu F. Neuroprotective effect of pAkt and HIF-1 alpha on ischemia rats. Asian Pac J Trop Med. 2014a;7:221–5.
119. Xiong ZG, Zhu XM, Chu XP, Minami M, Hey J, Wei WL, MacDonald JF, Wemmie JA, Price MP, Welsh MJ, Simon RP. Neuroprotection in ischemia: blocking calcium-permeable acid-sensing ion channels. Cell. 2004;118:687–98.
120. Pignataro G, Simon RP, Xiong ZG. Prolonged activation of ASIC1a and the time window for neuroprotection in cerebral ischaemia. Brain. 2007;130:151–8.

# Neuro-Prognostication After Cardiopulmonary Resuscitation

5

Jingyu He and Jing Wang

**Abstract**

Accurate conscious assessment for patients after cardiopulmonary resuscitation (CPR) is of great importance for avoiding futile treatment or avoiding premature withdrawal of life-sustaining treatment (WLST), especially in early ICU phase; however, common confounders (such as sedatives, muscle relaxants, and hypothermia) bring big challenges and interferences for clinical judgment and decision by clinicians and relatives of the patients. And how and when to evaluate is also a persistent problem.

Clinical neuro-prognostications start with physical examination and integrate with multimodal approaches subsequently, including electrophysiology, blood biomarkers, and neuroimaging, which are recommended to minimize the false-positive rate (FPR) in prediction. And also, treatment strategies with or without targeted temperature management (TTM) should be taken into deliberation during operational process.

**Keywords**

Cardiopulmonary resuscitation · Neuro-prognostication · Electroencephalography (EEG) · Somatosensory evoked potentials (SSEP) · Multimodal · Neuron-specific enolase (NSE) · Global cerebral ischemia reperfusion injury

## 5.1 Introduction

Delayed awakening (defined as coma for 72 h from targeted temperature management (TTM) and sedation withdrawal) is frequent among cardiac arrest patients [1]. Paul (2016) in a large single-center Parisian study found 30% of patients have

J. He · J. Wang (✉)
Emergency Department, Xuanwu Hospital, Capital Medical University, Beijing, China
e-mail: hejingyu@xwhosp.org; wj139113@xwhosp.org



H. Zhu (ed.), *Sudden Death*, https://doi.org/10.1007/978-981-15-7002-5_5

delayed awakening [2] and Mulder (2014) found up to 23% are persistently comatose at 1 week [3].

Prognosis evaluation to distinguish prolonged coma and irreversible cerebral damage for coma patients after cardiac arrest (CA), especially in early intensive care unit (ICU) stage, are essential for neurologists to inform family members about the chances of recovery. It is of great reference value to avoid futile treatment for the irreversible brain damage which prolonged suffering for patients and relatives and also to avoid premature withdrawal of life-sustaining treatment (WLST) following prognostication of a poor neurological outcome. However, when and how to accurately assess is the challenge for neurologists, because recovery process after resuscitation is dynamic and may continue for months following the arrest [4].

Neurologic assessment after cardiopulmonary resuscitation CPR should begin with a daily clinical neurological examination [5], which is the foundation for prognostication. A multimodal approach that combines clinical examination with electrophysiology (such as electroencephalography (EEG) and somatosensory evoked potentials (SSEP)), blood biomarkers (such as neuron-specific enolase (NSE), SB-100), and neuroimaging (magnetic resonance imaging (MRI) or computerized tomography (CT)) is recommended subsequently.

Optimal times for the assessment of neurological outcome after cardiac arrest are yet to be established. The general principle is that neuro-prognostication should be performed after the phase of TTM, and the patient is in normothermic state without interference of residual sedation, muscle relaxant, and other confounders. Current guidelines recommend performing prognostication no earlier than 72 h after the return of spontaneous circulation (ROSC) in all comatose patients with an absent or extensor motor response to pain, after having excluded confounders such as residual sedation that may interfere with clinical examination [6].

False-positive rate (FPR) is usually used to describe the reliability of test tools. (For example, FPR = 0.1, that means, in 10% of the patients with a good outcome, the test results predicted a poor outcome.) FPR is also defined as 1 minus specificity [7]. In an ideal state, FPR should be zero, or their specificity should be 100% [8, 9] while in real life, minimizing the risk of a falsely pessimistic prediction should be sustained attention; FPR has to be as low as possible, with a small 95% confidence interval (CI).

The aims of this part are to summarize practical recommendations on how to perform an accurate neuro-prognostication in patients suffering from CPR.

## 5.2 Cerebral Performance Categories Scale

The commonly used measure for reporting neurological outcome after CPR is represented by cerebral performance categories (CPCs) with 5 grading. CPC 1 corresponds to the best possible outcome with no or minor disabilities, CPC 2 represents moderate neurological disability, CPC 3 is defined as severe impairment, CPC 4 means vegetative status or comatose, and CPC 5 means dead [1, 6–9]. Investigators usually dichotomize neurological outcome as good or poor. However, there is no definite consensus in prognostication studies on what represents a poor neurological outcome. The latest version of the utstein guidelines on outcome reporting after OHCA defined that poor outcomes were as CPC 3-5; Scilicet poor neurological outcomes were as death, persistent vegetative state and severe neurological disability [6].

*Limitations*: CPC was debated to pay more attention to mental function and less information about body funcitons, activity and participation. This may explain the poor match between CPC and subjective quality of life [6, 7]. For clinical practice, pre-arrest health-related quality of life (HRQOL) is the ultimate goal of resuscitation. Inclusion of HRQOL among measured outcomes in future neuro-prognostication studies is desirable [6, 10].

### 5.2.1 Physical Clinical Examination

Physical clinical examination is the cornerstone of prognostic evaluation, which directly evaluates brain function, including brainstem reflexes (especially corneal and pupillary reflexes) and Glasgow Coma Scale motor response (GCS-M).

The reliability of clinical examination is low in the first days after resuscitation (false prediction for poor outcome is about 30%) [11], while the ability increases and reaches a maximum at 3 days from ROSC advent of TTM [12, 13]. However, it is postponed at about 72 h after ROSC or later in TH-treated or sedation-usage patients [14]; therefore, repeated assessments are often necessary.

#### 5.2.1.1 Pupillary Light Reflex (PLR)

Pupillary light reflex (PLR), defined as constriction of pupils to light, is a key component for clinical prognostication. It is not influenced by muscle relaxants, since is achieved via the parasympathetic action to the sphincter pupillae [15].

A bilaterally absent PLR is considered as a robust predictor for poor neurological outcome on day 3 after CA [12, 14, 16], in both TH-treated and non-TH-treated patients. (FPR 0.5%, 95%CI (0–2) vs. 0.5% (0–8)) [17–22]. However, the presence of pupillary reflexes at 72 h is not a strong indicator of good prognosis (predictive value was 61%, 95%CI (50–71)) [19]. A 2013 meta-analysis found that the true-positive rate of PLR with a favorable prognosis was as low as 20% [16].

Standard pupillary response is relatively inaccurate because of non-blinded measurements [23]. It was influenced by proficiency of the manipulator and was susceptible to self-fulfilling prophecy from clinicians, patient care, and WLST decision [24].

Quantitative PLR (expressed as the percentage of pupillary response to a calibrated light stimulus) by automated infrared pupillometry [25–27] provide an excellent accuracy than standard clinical evaluation [28–30] for coma prognostication in early phase. A European prospective international multicenter study (10 centers, 477 patients) testing the predictive value of automated infrared pupillometry (ClinicalTrials.gov Identifier NCT02607878) [31] found quantitative pupillometry [using the Neurological Pupil index (NPi)] had excellent ability to predict an unfavorable outcome from day 1 after CA, with no false positives and significantly higher specificity than standard manual pupillary examination. NPi $\leq 2$ ($n = 456$ patients) had a 51% (95%CI 49–53) negative-predictive value and a 100% positive-predictive value [PPV; 0% (0–2) false-positive rate], with a 100% (98–100) specificity and 32% (27–38) sensitivity for the prediction of unfavorable outcome). The addition of NPi to SSEP increased sensitivity of outcome prediction, while maintaining 100% specificity.

#### 5.2.1.2 Ocular Reflexes

Ocular reflexes as another prognosticators in coma after cardiac arrest is low, in fact only 20–30% of patients destined to a poor outcome show these signs. An absent corneal reflex is also usually associated with a poor outcome, but is slightly less specific than the pupillary reflex (FPR up to 5%) [26–28]. Similarly to pupillary reflexes, the main limitation of all neurological reflexes is their limited sensitivity in predicting a good recovery, true-positive rate of the present corneal reflexes which eventually showed a favorable prognosis was just 40% [32].

#### 5.2.1.3 Glasgow Coma Scale Motor Response (GCS-M)

The motor component of the Glasgow Coma Scale (GCS) score is useful and accurate for predicting the outcomes of comatose patients after CPR. A 2006 meta-analysis (10 studies, 1303 patients) showed that there were no false predictions of poor outcome for a GCS motor score $\leq 2$ (i.e., extensor or absent motor responses) 72 h after CPR (FPR = 0, 95%CI (0.00–0.06) [18].

In a 2013, systematic review and meta-analysis of several prognostication studies performed in individual centers across Europe and the United States showed that GCS-M less than 2 at 72 h after CA had a reduced accuracy in predicting poor prognosis [defined as severe disability, vegetative state and death; average FPR about 20%] [32].

GCS-M $\leq 2$ at $\geq 72$ h is sensitive but non-specific sign of poor outcome (FPR 10–40%) [17, 19, 20]. Like the corneal reflex, the motor response can be suppressed by the effects of sedatives opiates or neuromuscular blocking drugs [33]. It can also be postponed by reduced metabolic clearance (e.g., hypothermia or renal or liver dysfunction), or both [34].

#### 5.2.1.4 Myoclonus

Myoclonus is a CNS damage phenomenon consisting of sudden, brief, involuntary jerks caused by muscular contractions or inhibitions, which is related or not with epileptiform electrical activity [6]. Occasional myoclonus has limited value of poor prognosis and 9% patients finally showed a good prognosis during follow-up. Myoclonic status epilepticus defined as a continuous, repetitive, unrelenting, and generalized status, which involves face, limbs, and axial musculature; the presence of myoclonic status epilepticus often persistent for $\geq 30$ min. Early-onset ($\leq 48$ h after CA) of myoclonus is almost invariably associated and highly correlated with poor outcome. Myoclonus has less predictor than PLR or cornel reflex, and its use is recommended only in combination with other indices [9].

*Limitations*: First, as clinical examination is susceptible to interference from temperature and from residual effects of sedatives and/or neuromuscular blocking drugs, these confounders should be carefully ruled out before starting the prognostication process. Second, clinical examination lacks quantitative assessment, and timing and proficiency of the examination can greatly affect the elicited response.

**Recommended Chinese Expert Consensus in 2016**

Myoclonic status epilepticus 24 h after CPR (evidence from a 2013 meta-analysis, 6 studies, 764 patients, FPR = 0, 95%CI 0.00 ~ 0.03) [12, 14], absent pupillary light reflexes 72 h after CPR (evidence from a 2013 meta-analysis, 13 studies, 1188 patients, FPR = 0, 95%CI 0.00–0.08) [12, 14], and a GCS motor ≤2 score 72 h after CPR (evidence from a 2006-meta analysis, 10 studies, 1303 patients, FPR = 0, 95%CI 0.00–0.006) [18] were the appropriate predictors of poor prognosis. Absent oculovestibular reflexes 24 h after CPR (evidence from a 2013 meta-analysis, 13 studies, 1188 patients, FPR = 0, 95%CI 0.00–0.35) and absent corneal reflexes 48 h after CPR (evidence from a 2013 meta-analysis, 13 studies, 1188 patients, FPR = 0, 95%CI 0.00–0.22) can also be used to predict [12, 14]. Repeat assessments for clinical examinations must be performed whenever there is any doubt [35, 36].

### 5.2.2 Electroencephalogram (EEG)

Electroencephalographical signal is generated by cortical post-synaptic potentials [37]. Routine EEG is a common assessment for electrophysiological activity and neuronal function in coma patients after CA, and also a real-time tool for severity evaluation with easily acquired and repeated measurements, even bedsides [38, 39].

#### 5.2.2.1 Background Activity

Background activity that is a representative of global cerebral functioning is the first assessed EEG variable in clinical practice. EEG undergoing ischemia-reperfusion progress after CA showed decreased amplitude and slowing of background activity. Any of the following background activity may indicate a poor prognosis: such as low-voltage (<20 μV) or isoelectric (suppressed) background at 24 h after CA (FPR 0%, 95%CI 0–17) [40, 41], burst suppression at any time (FPR 0%, 95%CI 0–11) [40], burst suppression with identical bursts (FPR 0%, 95%CI 0–17) [42], and spontaneously discontinuous background during TTM (FPR 7%, 95%CI 0–24) [43]. These "Malignant" EEG patterns are appropriate for both TH-treated [44, 45] and non-TH-treated patients [40, 46]. Conversely, an early recovery of continuous background activity is an excellent early predictor of good neurological outcome [47], especially if combined with preserved EEG reactivity [37, 48]. For example, continuous background activity as soon as 12 h after CA [44] and a normal voltage background at 24 h are similarly associated with good outcomes [40]. The positive-predictive values (PPV) are 92% (80–98) and 72% (53–86), respectively. However, α -coma, which refers to an anterior prominent rhythm without reactivity was an exception and is associated with poor prognosis in up to 100% of patients [49].

The body temperature ranging from 32 to 36 °C has limited influence on EEG patterns, but the influence of sedation cannot be neglected and must to be taken into account [1].

#### 5.2.2.2 Background Reactivity

EEG reactivity is another assessment variable, which is defined as any reproducible change in amplitude or frequency by auditory or noxious stimuli; the character of EEG reactivity is either a transient attenuation or increase in electrical activity [37]. Absent reactivity showed correlation with poor prognostication, and the predictive value evolves dynamically over time. FPR was 7% (95%CI 1–15) after TTM [50, 51] and was 2% (95%CI 0–9) during TTM [45, 52]. Reproducible reactivity is associated with subsequent awakening when recorded during TTM (PPV 86% (77–92)) [52] and thereafter (78% (64–88)) [50]. Fifteen percent of patients after stimulation showed rhythmic, periodic, or ictal discharges and had poor prognosis (FPR 2%, 95%CI 0–11), particular during TTM or sedation [53]. EEG reactivity was found to have a better predictive value for neurological outcome than EEG patterns or evoked potentials [54].

*Limitations*: EEG reactivity with heavily subjective as stimuli administration and recording assessment; Standardized stimulation protocol might improve the predictive utility [37].

#### 5.2.2.3 Epileptiform Features

Epileptiform features such as sharp waves, spikes, poly-spikes, and waves after TTM are associated with poor outcome (FPR 9%, 95%CI 2–21) [50]. Thirty percent of patients undergoing electrographic seizures [55] after CA often but not always with poor prognosis [56] especially appearing after TTM and sedation weaning, with preserved brainstem reflexes, background reactivity, and somatosensory evoked potentials, might have reasonable functional recovery [57].

Continuous monitoring (cEEG) up to 48 h has been recommended by guidelines for accurate judgment, while intermittent EEG recordings is most commonly used in practice [1, 6]. Alvarez (2013) reported that two standard EEG recordings of 20–30 min duration within 48 h after CA are as informative as continuous EEG [58].

#### Recommended Chinese Expert Consensus in 2016

Generalized suppression or burst suppression on EEG, within 72 h after CPR, was an index of poor outcomes in comatose patients (evidence from a meta-analysis, 12 studies, 778 patients) (FPR = 0, 95%CI 0.00–0.24) [5]. The presence of an alpha coma pattern 24 h after CPR (PPV was 100% (95%CI 37–100) [5], EEG status epilepticus 72 h after CPR, the absence of EEG reactivity within 1–7 days after CPR, and an increased BSR within 1–7 days after CPR can also predict poor prognosis. The presence of generalized epileptiform activity or generalized periodic epileptiform complexes 24–48 h after CPR may be predictors of poor outcomes in comatose patients. EEG can be affected easily by drugs, greater attention should be focused to exclude false-positive reports by drugs [12, 14, 35].

### 5.2.3 Somatosensory Evoked Potentials (SSEPs)

The somatosensory evoked potentials (SSEP) is a small electrical signal which recorded noninvasively from skull after a series of electrical stimuli to peripheral nerves (median nerve is the most common used). It is the most commonly used and a nearly perfect predictors for poor neuro-prognostication after CPR. It had been used as a criterion to influence physicians' and families' decision for withdrawal of life-sustaining treatment (WLST). No matter in non-MTT-treated or MTT-treated or rewarming-treated patients, a bilateral absence of the N20 SSEP wave consistently predicts poor outcome [37]. A 2010 meta-analysis (25 studies, 2395 patients) showed the area under the receiver operating characteristic curve of SLSEP-N20 for poor outcomes was 0.891 within the first 24 h after CPR, and it was 0.912 at 48–72 h after CPR [59]. While, in a 2013 meta-analysis (12 studies, 1058 patients), during or after rewarming from hypothermia, the FPR of SLSEP-N20 was respectively 0 (95%CI 0.00–0.02) and 0 (95%CI 0.00–0.04) for poor outcomes [14]. However, a 2018 meta-analysis (35 studies, 2333 patients) [60] displayed that the survival in subjects with absent SSEP, though low, may be substantially higher than generally believed of 594 patients with absent SSEP, 14 had good functional outcomes. The rate of WLST for subjects with absent SSEP could be estimated in 14 of the 35 studies (mean 80%, median 100%); FPR in predicting poor neuro-prognosis is 7.7% (95%Cl 4–13%), rather than 0.7% [18]. The predictive sensitivity of absence SSEP is among 25–50% in heterogeneous studies. That means, many patients destined to a poor neurological outcome with bilaterally present N20 wave [6, 7, 15, 37]. In other words, presence of SSEP does not equate to a good prognosis, while absence of SSEP equates with a few chances for recovery.

SSEPs are less affected by hypothermia and sedation, but they may be impacted by electrical equipment and noise in ICU environment. Stimulus intensity and waveform are not uniform in different studies which might induce bias in clinical usage. Current guidelines recommend recording SSEP only after rewarming for TTM patients.

#### 5.2.3.1 Recommended Chinese Expert Consensus in 2016

Within 24 ~ 72 h after CPR, the bilateral absence of SLSEP-N20 can be used as an indicator of poor prognosis in patients, while presence of bilateral N20 is not equivalent to with a good prognosis (evidences from a 2010 meta-analysis, 25 studies, 2395 patients) [59, 61, 62] 7 days after CPR, bilateral N60 (or N70) exists or MMN can be used as indicators of regain consciousness.

### 5.2.4 Blood Biomarkers

The biomarkers used for neuro-prognostication after CA are from a presume that higher levels of biomarkers are associated with higher extents of CNS damage and with consequently lower chances of recovery [6].

Neuron-specific enolase (NSE) and SB100 are the most widely available and best documented biomarker of cerebral injury after CA, which were released by neurons and glial cells, respectively, and represent the corresponding damage of CNS. These markers showed advantages as: unlikely impacted by sedatives, easy to assess blindly, and suitable for patients with TTM treatment; continuous measurement or single point measurement showed good predictive value. In a large study on comatose survivors of CA (686 TTM-treated patients, 1823 samples assessed blind) [63]. NSE values corresponding to FPR <5% with the upper boundary of the 95%CI within 5% were 61, 46, and 35 ng/mL at 24, 48, and 72 h from ROSC, respectively. Their corresponding sensitivities were 24, 59, and 63%, and AUC were 0.75, 0.85, and 0.86, respectively. A single NSE measurement at 48 h (685 TTM-treated patients) also showed an accuracy of prediction (AUC 0.83, $P < 0.001$) [64].

*Limitations*: There was no uniform cut-off value for the prediction of poor outcome with 0% FPR in resuscitated comatose patients, because these continuous variables showed largely varying thresholds which can change with timing of measurement and heterogeneous detection techniques. For example, NSE threshold was 25–112.4 μg/L at 48 hours and 57.2–78.9 μg/L at 72 hours after ROSC in TTM treatment patients; while threshold ranged from 15 to 90 μg/L at 72 hours after ROSC in non-TTM patients [15]. SB-100 threshold was from 25 to 112.4ug/L in TTM patients [15]; In addition, NSE and S-100 have extracerebral sources (such as: erythrolysis, neuroendocrine tumors, and small cell carcinoma can release NSE [6, 37]; and muscle and adipose tissue can release S-100B after chest compressions [65]). These pitfalls might affect clinical judgment.

For ideally identifying a prognostic threshold for poor outcomes of CA, several considerations should be taken: First, sampling at multiple time points (especially at the first 72 h after ROSC) and combined with other indicators appears at present as the most prudent strategy to reduce the risk of a false-positive result and to assess reproducibility; Second, every clinical laboratory should validate its own biomarker thresholds for prediction; Third, serum biomarkers estimate cell injury irrespective of cell function which will be more relevant to prognostication [8, 15].

#### 5.2.4.1 Recommended Chinese Expert Consensus in 2016

Increased serum levels of NSE and S-100B protein predicts poor outcomes in comatose patients after CPR [35]. Without TTM treatment, 24 h NSE >33 μg/L (FPR = 0, 95%CI 0.00–0.08), 48 h NSE >65 μg/L (FPR = 0, 95%CI 0.00–0.03), and 72 h NSE >80 μg/L (FPR = 0, 95%CI 0.00–0.03), and 72 h S-100B protein >0.7 μg/L (FPR = 0, 95%CI 0.00–0.08) predict poor outcomes (evidence from a 2013 meta-analysis (10 studies, 935 patients)) [12]. While after TTM treatment, 48 h NSE ≥81.8 μg/L (FPR = 0, 95%CI 0.00–0.02), 72 h NSE ≥78.9 μg/L (FPR = 0, 95%CI 0.00–0.06), or 48 h S-100B ≥0.3 μg/L (FPR = 0, 95%CI 0.00–0.07) have shown good prediction (evidence from a meta-analysis, 12 studies, 976 patients) [14].

### 5.2.5 Neuroimaging

Neuroimaging studies after CPR is performed initially to rule out cerebral causes of coma (such as subarachnoid hemorrhage and massive cerebral stroke) and exclude contraindications of thrombolysis or/and anticoagulation. Recently, neuroimaging displays its prognostic value in brain ischemia-reperfusion injury.

#### 5.2.5.1 Computed Tomography (CT)

After CPR, diffuse cerebral edema appears through computed tomography (CT) as an attenuation of the gray matter (GM)/white matter (WM) interface, which has been measured as GWR (a density ratio between gray matter and white matter). By sampling GWR from basal ganglia, centrum semiovale, and high convexity, we can presume the brain injury [6, 7, 15, 37]. A GWR ranging between 1.16 and 1.22 predicted a poor neurological outcome (CPC 3–5) with 0% FPR and sensitivities ranging from 28 to 76% [66–73]. However, in a single-center study including 240 patients with brain CT performed within 24 h from ROSC [73], a GWR <1.22 predicted hospital mortality with 98% specificity but was unable to further distinguish survivors between poor vs. good outcomes. A cohort study (2017) [74] based on the TTM trial showed that GWR measurement predicted poor neurological outcome (CPC 3–5) with 97.6% specificity and 14.4% sensitivity within 24 h from ROSC. During 24 h to 7 days after ROSC, similar findings with the specificity and sensitivity increased to 100 (87.9–100.0)% and 56.5 (47.3–65.3)%, respectively.

Various studies performed heterogeneity of GWI in prediction with heterogeneous thresholds in different specificity and lower sensitivities. Combination of CT and other index improved sensitivity and specificity.

#### 5.2.5.2 Magnatic Resonance Imaging (MRI)

Diffusion-weighted imaging (DWI), one type of nuclear magnetic resonance sequence, optimally detected neuronal cytotoxic edema as hyperintense resulting from a reduction of energy-dependent water–protons transportation after CPR. These changes can be further quantified by apparent diffusion coefficient (ADC). Normal ADC values range between 700 and 800 × $10^{-6}$ $mm^2/s$ [75]. Mean ADC value of whole brain [66, 76], proportion of brain volume with decreased ADC [77, 78], and the lowest ADC value in specific brain areas (such as: occipital cortex, deep gray nuclei, hippocampus, and cerebellum) can be used to predict poor neurological outcomes [79]; however, there is no uniform threshold that predicts 0% FPR poor prognosis in prognostication studies.

Neuro-imaging studies are not affected by sedation and provide a topographic description for ischemia reperfusion injury. However, caution should be taken in using them for prognostication: First, results on imaging prediction introduced a selection bias because unstable patients were not enrolled in for their long inspection time and not a bedside tool; Second, report interpretation may be significantly affected by interobserver variability; Third, until today, evidences of neuroimaging for neuro-prognostication are lack of standardization and without consistency of quantitative control, imaging studies for prognostication should be in combination with other predictors and in centers where specific experience is available [75–79].

*Recommended Chinese Expert Consensus in 2016* [35]: GWI sampled from basal ganglia on brain CT <1.22 (FPR = 0.05, 95%CI 0.00–0.25) (evidence from a meta-analysis, 3 studies, 113 patients) [12, 14] and ADC <650 × $10^{-6}$ $mm^2/s$ in more than 10% of the brain volume on brain DWI 2–5 days after CPR could quantify diffuse brain swelling and predict poor outcomes (evidence from a cohort study: FPR was 0.00, 95%CI 0.00–0.78) [12, 14, 77].

*For TTM Patients, Recommended Chinese Expert Consensus in 2016* [35]: During hypothermia (32–34 °C) treatment, bilateral absence SLSEP-N20, BIS = 0, and higher biomarker threshold (NSE: 24 h ≥ 52.4 μg/L or S-100B:24 h ≥ 0.18–0.21 μg/L) predict poor outcome.

After rewarming from hypothermia, clinical examination (absence of pupillary light reflexes, absence of corneal reflexes, or presence of myoclonic status epilepticus, a GCS motor score ≤2), EEG (generalized suppression, burst suppression, status epilepticus), or the absence of EEG reactivity, and neurological biomarkers (48 h NSE ≥81.8 μg/L, 72 h NSE ≥78.9 μg/L, or 48 h S-100B ≥0.3 μg/L) predicts poor outcomes.

## 5.3 Conclusion

Early prognostication of neurological outcomes was an essential element in post-cardiac arrest evaluations and medical decision-making. Integrating clinical examination with electrophysiology, blood biomarkers, and neuroimaging, that means using multimodal prognostication, is the mainstream way to increase the accuracy of prediction. However, depending on the availability of expertise electrophysiological techniques and laboratory facilities, the multimodal approach used will vary among centers [7]. Making uniform evaluation algorithms and exploring quantitative methods are helpful to improve the accuracy and specificity of prediction.

## References

1. Oddoa M, Friberg H. Neuro- prognostication after cardiac arrest in the light of targeted temperature management. Curr Opin Crit Care. 2017;23:244–50.
2. Paul M, Bougouin W, Geri G, et al. Delayed awakening after cardiac arrest: prevalence and risk factors in the Parisian registry. Intensive Care Med. 2016;42:1128–36.
3. Mulder M, Gibbs HG, Smith SW, et al. Awakening and withdrawal of life sustaining treatment in cardiac arrest survivors treated with therapeutic hypothermia. Crit Care Med. 2014;42:2493–9.
4. Agarwal S, Presciutti A, Roth W, Matthews E, Rodriguez A, Roh DJ, Park S, Claassen J, Lazar RM. Determinants of long-term neurological recovery patterns relative to hospital discharge among cardiac arrest survivors. Crit Care Med. 2018;46(2):e141–50.

5. Sharshar T, Citerio G, Andrews PJ, Chieregato A, Latronico N, Menon DK, Puybasset L, Sandroni C, Stevens RD. Neurological examination of critically ill patients: a pragmatic approach. Report of an ESICM expert panel. Intensive Care Med. 2014;40:484–95.
6. Sandroni C, D'Arrigo S, Nolan JP. Prognostication after cardiac arrest. Crit Care. 2018;22(1):150.
7. Horn J, Cronberg T, Taccone FS. Prognostication after cardiac arrest. Curr Opin Crit Care. 2014;20(3):280–6.
8. Sandroni C, Cariou A, Cavallaro F, Cronberg T, Friberg H, Hoedemaekers C, Horn J, Nolan JP, Rossetti AO, Soar J. Prognostication in comatose survivors of cardiac arrest: an advisory statement from the European resuscitation council and the European Society of Intensive Care Medicine. Resuscitation. 2014;85:1779–89.
9. Nolan JP, Soar J, Cariou A, Cronberg T, Moulaert VR, Deakin CD, Bottiger BW, Friberg H, Sunde K, Sandroni C. European resuscitation council and European Society of Intensive Care Medicine Guidelines for post resuscitation care 2015: section 5 of the European resuscitation council guidelines for resuscitation 2015. Resuscitation. 2015;95:202–22.
10. Haywood K, Whitehead L, Nadkarni V, Beesems S, Bottinger BW, Brooks A, Castrén M, Ong MEH, Hazinski M, Koster RW, et al. Core outcome set for cardiac arrest (COSCA) in adults: an advisory statement from the international liaison committee on resuscitation. Circulation. 2018;137(22):e783–801.
11. Okada KOS, Otani N, Sera T, Mochizuki T, Aoki M, Ishimatsu S. Prediction protocol for neurological outcome for survivors of out-of-hospital cardiac arrest treated with targeted temperature management. Resuscitation. 2012;83:734–9.
12. Sandroni C, Cavallaro F, Callaway CW, et al. Predictors of poor neurological outcome in adult comatose survivors of cardiac arrest: a systematic review and meta-analysis. Part 1: patients not treated with therapeutic hypothermia. Resuscitation. 2013;84:1310–23. [PubMed: 23811182].
13. Zandbergen EG, Hijdra A, Koelman JH, et al. Prediction of poor outcome within the first 3 days of postanoxic coma. Neurology. 2006;66:62–8.
14. Sandroni C, Cavallaro F, Callaway CW, et al. Predictors of poor neurological outcome in adult comatose survivors of cardiac arrest: a systematic review and meta-analysis. Part 2: patients treated with therapeutic hypothermia. Resuscitation. 2013;84:1324–38.
15. Sandroni C, Geocadinb RG. Neurological prognostication after cardiac arrest. Curr Opin Crit Care. 2015;21(3):209–14.
16. Kamps MJ, Horn J, Oddo M, Fugate JE, Storm C, Cronberg T, Wijman CA, Wu O, Binnekade JM, Hoedemaekers CW. Prognostication of neurologic outcome in cardiac arrest patients after mild therapeutic hypothermia: a meta-analysis of the current literature. Intensive Care Med. 2013;39:1671–82.
17. Bouwes A, Binnekade JM, Kuiper MA, et al. Prognosis of coma after therapeutic hypothermia: a prospective cohort study. Ann Neurol. 2012;71:206–12.
18. Wijdicks EF, Hijdra A, Young GB, Bassetti CL, Wiebe S. Practice parameter: prediction of outcome in comatose survivors after cardiopulmonary resuscitation (an evidence-based review): report of the quality standards Subcommittee of the American Academy of neurology. Neurology. 2006;67:203–10.
19. Fugate JE, Wijdicks EF, Mandrekar J, et al. Predictors of neurologic outcome in hypothermia after cardiac arrest. Ann Neurol. 2010;68:907–14.
20. Golan E, Barrett K, Alali AS, et al. Predicting neurologic outcome after targeted temperature management for cardiac arrest: systematic review and meta-analysis. Crit Care Med. 2014;42:1919–30.
21. Sandroni C, Cariou A, Cavallaro F, et al. Prognostication in comatose survivors of cardiac arrest: an advisory statement from the European resuscitation council and the European Society of Intensive Care Medicine. Intensive Care Med. 2014;40:1816–31.
22. Greer DM, Yang J, Scripko PD, et al. Clinical examination for prognostication in comatose cardiac arrest patients. Resuscitation. 2013;84:1546–51.

23. Larson MD, Muhiudeen I. Pupillometric analysis of the 'absent light reflex'. Arch Neurol. 1995;52:369–72.
24. Sandroni C, Geocadin RG. Neurological prognostication after cardiac arrest. Curr Opin Crit Care. 2015;21:209–14.
25. Larson MD, Behrends M. Portable infrared pupillometry: a review. Anesth Analg. 2015;120:1242–53.
26. Couret D, Boumaza D, Grisotto C, et al. Reliability of standard pupillometry practice in neurocritical care: an observational, double-blinded study. Crit Care. 2016;20:99.
27. Olson DM, Stutzman S, Saju C, et al. Interrater reliability of pupillary assessments. Neurocrit Care. 2016;24:251–7.
28. Behrends M, Niemann CU, Larson MD. Infrared pupillometry to detect the light reflex during cardiopulmonary resuscitation: a case series. Resuscitation. 2012;83:1223–8.
29. Heimburger D, Durand M, Gaide-Chevronnay L, et al. Quantitative pupillometry and transcranial Doppler measurements in patients treated with hypothermia after cardiac arrest. Resuscitation. 2016;103:88–93.
30. Suys T, Bouzat P, Marques-Vidal P, et al. Automated quantitative pupillometry for the prognostication of coma after cardiac arrest. Neurocrit Care. 2014;21:300–8.
31. Oddo M, Sandroni C, Citerio G, et al. Quantitative versus standard pupillary light reflex for early prognostication in comatose cardiac arrest patients: an international prospective multicenter double-blinded study. Intensive Care Med. 2018;44:2102–11.
32. Kamps MJ, Horn J, Oddo M, et al. Prognostication of neurologic outcome in cardiac arrest patients after mild therapeutic hypothermia: a meta-analysis of the current literature. Intensive Care Med. 2013;39:1671–82.
33. Samaniego EA, Mlynash M, Caulfield AF, et al. Sedation confounds outcome prediction in cardiac arrest survivors treated with hypothermia. Neurocrit Care. 2011;15:113–9. [PubMed: 20680517].
34. Samaniego EA, Mlynash M, Caulfield AF, Eyngorn I, Wijman CA. Sedation confounds outcome prediction in cardiac arrest survivors treated with hypothermia. Neurocrit Care. 2011;15:113–9.
35. Neurocritical Care Committee of the Chinese Society of Neurology (NCC/CSN). The Chinese Expert Consensus on evaluation of coma after cardiopulmonary resuscitation. Chin Med J (Engl). 2016;129(17):2123–7.
36. Peberdy MA, Callaway CW, Neumar RW, Geocadin RG, Zimmerman JL, Donnino M, et al. Part 9: Post-cardiac arrest care: 2010. American Heart Association Guidelines for Cardiopulmonary Resuscitation and Emergency Cardiovascular Care. Circulation. 2010;122(18 Suppl 3):S768–86. https://doi.org/10.1161/CIRCULATIONAHA.110.971002.
37. Rossetti AO, Rabinstein AA, Oddo M. Neurological prognostication of outcome in patients in coma after cardiac arrest. Lancet Neurol. 2016;15:597–609.
38. Friberg H, Cronberg T, Dunser MW, et al. Survey on current practices for neurological prognostication after cardiac arrest. Resuscitation. 2015;90:158–62.
39. André-Obadiaa N, Zyss J, Gavaret M, et al. Recommendations for the use of Electroencephalography and evoked potentials in comatose patients. Neurophysiol Clin. 2018;48:143–69.
40. Sivaraju A, Gilmore EJ, Wira CR, et al. Prognostication of post-cardiac arrest coma: early clinical and electroencephalographic predictors of outcome. Intensive Care Med. 2015;41:1264–72.
41. Cloostermans MC, van Meulen FB, Eertman CJ, Hom HW, van Putten MJ. Continuous electroencephalography monitoring for early prediction of neurological outcome in postanoxic patients after cardiac arrest: a prospective cohort study. Crit Care Med. 2012;40:2867–75.
42. Kim F, Nichol G, Maynard C, et al. Effect of prehospital induction of mild hypothermia on survival and neurological status among adults with cardiac arrest: a randomized clinical trial. JAMA. 2014;311:45–52.
43. Rossetti AO, Carrera E, Oddo M. Early EEG correlates of neuronal injury after brain anoxia. Neurology. 2012;78:796–802.

44. Hofmeijer J, Beernink TM, Bosch FH, Beishuizen A, Tjepkema-Cloostermans MC, van Putten MJ. Early EEG contributes to multimodal outcome prediction of post anoxic coma. Neurology. 2015;85:137–43.
45. Oddo M, Rossetti AO. Early multimodal outcome prediction after cardiac arrest in patients treated with hypothermia. Crit Care Med. 2014;42:1340–7.
46. Smith K, Andrew E, Lijovic M, Nehme Z, Bernard S. Quality of life and functional outcomes 12 months after out-of-hospital cardiac arrest. Circulation. 2015;131:174–81.
47. Rundgren M, Westhall E, Cronberg T, et al. Continuous amplitude-integrated electroencephalogram predicts outcome in hypothermia-treated cardiac arrest patients. Crit Care Med. 2010;38:1838–44.
48. Ben-Hamouda N, Taccone FS, Rossetti AO, Oddo M. Contemporary approach to neurologic prognostication of coma after cardiac arrest. Chest. 2014;146:1375–86.
49. Berkhoff M, Donati F, Bassetti C. Postanoxic alpha (theta) coma: a reappraisal of its prognostic significance. Clin Neurophysiol. 2000;111:297–304.
50. Rossetti AO, Oddo M, Logroscino G, Kaplan PW. Prognostication after cardiac arrest and hypothermia: a prospective study. Ann Neurol. 2010;67:301–7.
51. Thenayan EA, Savard M, Sharpe MD, Norton L, Young B. Electroencephalogram for prognosis after cardiac arrest. J Crit Care. 2010;25:300–4.
52. Tsetsou S, Oddo M, Rossetti AO. Clinical outcome after a reactive hypothermic EEG following cardiac arrest. Neurocrit Care. 2013;19:283–6.
53. Alvarez V, Oddo M, Rossetti AO. Stimulus-induced rhythmic, periodic or ictal discharges (SIRPIDs) in comatose survivors of cardiac arrest: characteristics and prognostic value. Clin Neurophysiol. 2013;124:204–8.
54. Thenayan EA, Savard M, Sharpe MD, et al. Electroencephalogram for prognosis after cardiac arrest. J Crit Care. 2010;25:300–4.
55. Seder DB, Sunde K, Rubertsson S, et al. Neurologic outcomes and postresuscitation care of patients with myoclonus following cardiac arrest. Crit Care Med. 2015;43:965–72.
56. Backman S, Westhall E, Dragancea I, et al. Electroencephalographic characteristics of status epilepticus after cardiac arrest. Clin Neurophysiol. 2017;128:681–8.
57. Rossetti AO, Oddo M, Liaudet L, Kaplan PW. Predictors of awakening from postanoxic status epilepticus after therapeutic hypothermia. Neurology. 2009;72:744–9.
58. Alvarez V, Sierra-Marcos A, Oddo M, Rossetti AO. Yield of intermittent versus continuous EEG in comatose survivors of cardiac arrest treated with hypothermia. Crit Care. 2013;17:R190.
59. Lee YC, Phan TG, Jolley DJ, Castley HC, Ingram DA, Reutens DC. Accuracy of clinical signs, SEP, and EEG in predicting outcome of hypoxic coma: a meta-analysis. Neurology. 2010;74:572–80. https://doi.org/10.1212/WNL.0b013e3181cff761.
60. Amorim E, Ghassemi MM, Lee JW, Greer DM, Kaplan PW, Cole AJ, Cash SS, Bianchi MT, Westover MB. Estimating the false positive rate of absent somatosensory evoked potentials in cardiac arrest prognostication. Crit Care Med. 2018;46(12):e1213–21. https://doi.org/10.1097/CCM.0000000000003436.
61. Rothstein TL. The role of evoked potentials in anoxic-ischemic coma and severe brain trauma. J Clin Neurophysiol. 2000;17:486–97. https://doi.org/10.1097/00004691-200009000-00007.
62. Logi F, Fischer C, Murri L, Mauguière F. The prognostic value of evoked responses from primary somatosensory and auditory cortex in comatose patients. Clin Neurophysiol. 2003;114:1615–27. https://doi.org/10.1016/S1388-2457(03)00086-5.
63. Stammet P, Collignon O, Hassager C, Wise MP, Hovdenes J, Aneman A, et al. Neuron-specific Enolase as a predictor of death or poor neurological outcome after out-of-hospital cardiac arrest and targeted temperature management at 33 degrees C and 36 degrees C. J Am Coll Cardiol. 2015;65(19):2104–14.
64. Wiberg S, Hassager C, Stammet P, Winther-Jensen M, Thomsen JH, Erlinge D, Wanscher M, Nielsen N, Pellis T, Aneman A, et al. Single versus serial measurements of neuron-specific Enolase and prediction of poor neurological outcome in persistently unconscious patients after out-of-hospital cardiac arrest—a TTM-trial substudy. PLoS One. 2017;12:e0168894.

65. Anderson RE, Hansson LO, Nilsson O, et al. High serum S100B levels for trauma patients without head injuries. Neurosurgery. 2001;48:1255–8. discussion 1258-60. [PubMed: 11383727].
66. Jeon CH, Park JS, Lee JH, Kim H, Kim SC, Park KH, Yi KS, Kim SM, Youn CS, Kim YM, et al. Comparison of brain computed tomography and diffusionweighted magnetic resonance imaging to predict early neurologic outcome before target temperature management comatose cardiac arrest survivors. Resuscitation. 2017;118:21–6.
67. Choi SP, Park HK, Park KN, Kim YM, Ahn KJ, Choi KH, Lee WJ, Jeong SK. The density ratio of grey to white matter on computed tomography as an early predictor of vegetative state or death after cardiac arrest. Emerg Med J. 2008;25:666–9.
68. Torbey MT, Selim M, Knorr J, Bigelow C, Recht L. Quantitative analysis of the loss of distinction between gray and white matter in comatose patients after cardiac arrest. Stroke. 2000;31:2163–7.
69. Lee BK, Kim WY, Shin J, Oh JS, Wee JH, Cha KC, Park Y, Choi JH, Jeung KW. Prognostic value of gray matter to white matter ratio in hypoxic and non-hypoxic cardiac arrest with non-cardiac etiology. Am J Emerg Med. 2016;34:1583–8.
70. Scheel M, Storm C, Gentsch A, Nee J, Luckenbach F, Ploner CJ, Leithner C. The prognostic value of gray-white-matter ratio in cardiac arrest patients treated with hypothermia. Scand J Trauma Resusc Emerg Med. 2013;21:23.
71. Choi SP, Youn CS, Park KN, et al. Therapeutic hypothermia in adult cardiac arrest because of drowning. Acta Anaesthesiol Scand. 2012;56:116–23. [PubMed: 22091986].
72. Kim SH, Choi SP, Park KN, et al. Early brain computed tomography findings are associated with outcome in patients treated with therapeutic hypothermia after out-of-hospital cardiac arrest. Scand J Trauma Resusc Emerg Med. 2013;21:57. [PubMed: 23870424].
73. Metter RB, Rittenberger JC, Guyette FX, Callaway CW. Association between a quantitative CT scan measure of brain edema and outcome after cardiac arrest. Resuscitation. 2011;82:1180–5. [PubMed: 21592642].
74. Moseby-Knappe M, Pellis T, Dragancea I, Friberg H, Nielsen N, Horn J, Kuiper M, Roncarati A, Siemund R, Unden J, et al. Head computed tomography for prognostication of poor outcome in comatose patients after cardiac arrest and targeted temperature management. Resuscitation. 2017;119:89–94.
75. Wijdicks EF, Campeau NG, Miller GM. MR imaging in comatose survivors of cardiac resuscitation. AJNR Am J Neuroradiol. 2001;22:1561–5.
76. Wu O, Sorensen AG, Benner T, Singhal AB, Furie KL, Greer DM. Comatose patients with cardiac arrest: predicting clinical outcome with diffusion weighted MR imaging. Radiology. 2009;252:173–81.
77. Wijman CA, Mlynash M, Caulfield AF, Hsia AW, Eyngorn I, Bammer R, Fischbein N, Albers GW, Moseley M. Prognostic value of brain diffusion weighted imaging after cardiac arrest. Ann Neurol. 2009;65:394–402.
78. Hirsch KG, Mlynash M, Eyngorn I, Pirsaheli R, Okada A, Komshian S, Chen C, Mayer SA, Meschia JF, Bernstein RA, et al. Multi-center study of diffusion weighted imaging in coma after cardiac arrest. Neurocrit Care. 2016;24:82–9.
79. Choi SP, Park KN, Park HK, Kim JY, Youn CS, Ahn KJ, Yim HW. Diffusion-weighted magnetic resonance imaging for predicting the clinical outcome of comatose survivors after cardiac arrest: a cohort study. Crit Care. 2010;14:R17.

# Progress in Cardiorespiratory Ischemia-Reperfusion Injury

# 6

Chang Pan, Qiuhuan Yuan, and Feng Xu

**Abstract**

Sudden cardiac arrest (SCA) is a common cause of death in emergency departments, although SCA treatment has been improved with the improvement of medical and health care, the improvement of cardiopulmonary resuscitation technology, and the use of drugs and other therapeutic measures. However, the survival and discharge rate is still not optimistic. Post-cardiac arrest syndrome (PCAS) is a complex combination of pathophysiological processes, consisting of post-cardiac arrest brain injury, post-cardiac arrest myocardial dysfunction, systemic ischemia-reperfusion response, and persistent precipitating pathology. This part will focus on the latest progress of post-resuscitation myocardial dysfunction, mainly focusing on the mechanism of ischemia-reperfusion injury, to provide basis for clinical treatment.

C. Pan · Q. Yuan · F. Xu (✉)
Department of Emergency Medicine and Chest Pain Center, Qilu Hospital of Shandong University, Jinan, China

Shandong Provincial Clinical Research Center for Emergency and Critical Care Medicine, Institute of Emergency and Critical Care Medicine of Shandong University, Qilu Hospital of Shandong University, Jinan, China

Key Laboratory of Emergency and Critical Care Medicine of Shandong Province, Key Laboratory of Cardiopulmonary-Cerebral Resuscitation Research of Shandong Province, Shandong Provincial Engineering Laboratory for Emergency and Critical Care Medicine, Qilu Hospital of Shandong University, Jinan, China

The Key Laboratory of Cardiovascular Remodeling and Function Research, Chinese Ministry of Education, Chinese Ministry of Health and Chinese Academy of Medical Sciences; The State and Shandong Province Joint Key Laboratory of Translational Cardiovascular Medicine, Qilu Hospital of Shandong University, Jinan, China



H. Zhu (ed.), *Sudden Death*, https://doi.org/10.1007/978-981-15-7002-5_6

**Keywords**

Post-resuscitation myocardial dysfunction (PRMD) · Post-cardiac arrest syndrome (PCAS) · Sudden cardiac arrest (SCA) · Ischemia-reperfusion injury

## 6.1 Introduction

Successful cardiopulmonary resuscitation (CPR) attempts and subsequent return of spontaneous circulation (ROSC) are the first important steps to achieve the goal of complete recovery from SCA. The term post-cardiac arrest syndrome (PCAS) is caused by the pathophysiologic process after the whole-body intense ischemia during prolonged SCA and the subsequent reperfusion injuries after successful resuscitation. Despite continuous efforts are made to minimize the damages caused by CPR, the prognosis of patients with SCA is still frustrating, and the pathophysiological mechanisms of CPR are not fully understood. Myocardial dysfunction, with myocardial stunning and cardiogenic hemodynamic instability being major causes of mortality after resuscitation, occurs usually within the first few hours after ROSC. Till now, ischemia-reperfusion injury is the main mechanism of myocardial dysfunction post-cardiopulmonary resuscitation. This section will review the research progress of pathophysiological mechanisms of myocardial ischemia-reperfusion injury after CPR in recent years.

## 6.2 Intracellular Ion Homeostasis Abnormalities

### 6.2.1 Intracellular $Ca^{2+}$ Overload

$Ca^{2+}$ overload is an important mechanism of ischemia-reperfusion injury post-cardiorespiratory resuscitation. The high oxygen demand of the fibrillating heart, combined with the interrupted coronary artery flow, produces an extremely severe imbalance of oxygen in the myocardium. The decrease in oxygen supply results in a rise of intracellular $Ca^{2+}$ followed by left ventricular diastolic and systolic dysfunction. Increased $Ca^{2+}$ sparks during ischemia serve as the subcellular events underlying $Ca^{2+}$ overload and are converted to $Ca^{2+}$ waves to mediate elevated $Ca^{2+}$ during early diastole of reperfusion [1]. The dysfunction of $Ca^{2+}$ relevant proteins, such as $Na^+$/$Ca^{2+}$ exchange protein, $Na^+$/$H^+$ exchange protein, L-type voltage-dependent $Ca^{2+}$ channel (L-VDCC), and sarco−/endoplasmic reticulum ATPase 2a (SERCA2a)/phospholamban (PLB) contributes to intracellular $Ca^{2+}$ overload [2]. During myocardial ischemia reperfusion, calcium/calmodulin-dependent II (CaMK II), an intracellular $Ca^{2+}$ sensor, is activated. Especially, CaMKII activation promotes L-VDCC opening by phosphorylation of its α-subunit, which in turn controls cardiac myocyte apoptosis [3]. The consequences of $Ca^{2+}$ overload include mitochondrial dysfunction, phospholipase activation, transient inward ion current through $Na^+$/$Ca^{2+}$ exchange protein, free radical production, myofibril contracture and rupture, mechanical damage of biofilm, destruction of cytoskeleton, and so on [4].

$Na^+/Ca^{2+}$ exchange protein is the main channel of $Ca^{2+}$ entering cardiomyocytes, which is responsible for $Ca^{2+}$ overload during ischemia-reperfusion injury [5]. The activity of $Na^+/Ca^{2+}$ exchange protein is mainly regulated by the concentration of transmembrane $Na^+$, and it is also affected by the concentration of $Ca^{2+}$, ATP, $Mg^{2+}$, and $H^+$ [6]. When cardiac arrest occurs, cessation of blood flow rapidly causes intense myocardial ischemia, activation of the sarcolemmal $Na^+/H^+$ exchanger isoform-1 (NHE1) [7], and decrease of intracellular ATP content, which can drive $Na^+$ into the cells in exchange for $H^+$ with the exchange rate intensified during reperfusion. The accumulation of $Na^+$ in the cytosol drives $Ca^{2+}$ entry through the $Na^+/Ca^{2+}$ exchange protein, leading to cytosolic and mitochondrial $Ca^{2+}$ overload and myocardial injury by compromising mitochondrial bioenergetic functions [8].

### 6.2.2 Drop in pH with Rapid Normalization Upon Reperfusion

During ischemia or hypoxia, due to the enhancement of anaerobic metabolism, $H^+$ production increases acutely, and pH value in both of tissue fluid and intracellular fluid decreases significantly. However, after reperfusion, the concentration of $H^+$ in tissue fluid decreases rapidly, but intracellular $H^+$ concentration is still high, which forms a gradient of transmembrane $H^+$ concentration. The difference of $H^+$ concentration on both sides of cell membrane can activate myocardial $Na^+/H^+$ exchange protein, promoting intracellular $H^+$ excretion and extracellular $Na^+$ influx [9]. Moreover, regional acidosis can locally inhibit but remotely stimulate $Ca^{2+}$ waves in ventricular myocytes [10].

In addition to energy deficiency, ischemia can also bring out the accumulation of $CO_2$ and $H^+$, resulting in serious acidosis in the myocardium. However, acidosis is considered to exert a protective effect. Recent studies have shown that in an animal model of reperfusion after cardiac arrest in pigs, hypocalcemia and mild acidosis can alleviate myocardial edema at the beginning of reperfusion [9]. Intracellular acidosis at the time of reperfusion appears to prevent mitochondrial permeability transition pores(mPTP) opening.

## 6.3 Mitochondrial Injuries

Mitochondria play a crucial role in regulating normal metabolism of cells and in the susceptibility to ischemia-reperfusion injury. The inner membrane of mitochondria is highly impermeable to water and folds inward into the mitochondrial matrix forming multiple cristae on which proteins that are responsible for oxidative phosphorylation reside. The outer membrane of mitochondria is rich in channel forming proteins, such as voltage-dependent anion channels (VDAC), so it is more permeable. Destruction of the inner membrane permeability leads to the collapse of the $H^+$ gradient, damaging the proton forces required for ATP synthesis, and causes a large amount of mitochondrial swelling, but this swelling may be reduced to some extent after post-resuscitation reperfusion. These changes lead to ultrastructural abnormalities in mitochondria, with the accumulation of intramyocellular droplets and glycogen deposits which may be a sign that mitochondria are unable to utilize energy substrates [11, 12]. There are higher serum levels of mitochondrial injury markers, such as cytochrome c and mitochondrial DNA, in patients with cardiac arrest versus healthy controls and higher levels in non-survivors versus survivors after cardiac arrest [13].

### 6.3.1 The Opening of mPTP

Under physiological conditions, the inner mitochondrial membrane is impermeable to most ions and metabolites, and the mPTP are closed. Following the ischemia-reperfusion, the restoration of blood flow after a period of ischemia promotes $Ca^{2+}$ overload, excessive production of reactive oxygen species (ROS), depletion of adenine nucleotide, and correction of intracellular pH, all of which increase the susceptibility of mPTP opening [14–16]. The opening of mPTP leads to rapid dissipation of mitochondrial membrane potential, uncoupling of the respiratory chain with possible fatal decline in ATP levels, and the release of mitochondrial ROS and pro-apoptotic factors, leading to cardiomyocyte death [14, 16, 17]. Water also enters via the opening pores, leading to mitochondrial swelling and lysis and even cell death. In addition, mPTP activation can also lead to $Ca^{2+}$ pump dysfunction caused by ATP hydrolysis, resulting in $Ca^{2+}$ overload in the cytoplasm, and $Ca^{2+}$ can pass through mitochondrial calcium uniporter (MCU) and mitochondrial inorganic polyphosphate mediated mPTP opening.

## 6.4 Free Radical Formation and ROS

Reperfusion after resuscitation from cardiac arrest can increase the production of ROS and lead to oxidative stress. The alterations that occurred during cardiac arrest brought about a great deal of free radical during the first minutes of post-arrest phase. There are high plasma biomarkers of oxidative damage, such as isoprostanes (IsoP), a marker of lipid peroxidation, and 8-hydroxyguanosine (8-OHG), a marker of DNA oxidative damage. The mechanisms include increased production of xanthine oxidase (XO), respiratory burst of neutrophils, impaired mitochondrial function, "ROS induced by ROS," and so on [18, 19].

### 6.4.1 XO

When myocardial tissue is hypoxic, due to the decrease in ATP production and the dysfunction of membrane pumps, $Ca^{2+}$ enters the cells and activates $Ca^{2+}$-dependent proteases, thus triggering the conversion of xanthine dehydrogenase (XD) into XO. At the same time, ATP is in turn decomposed into ADP, AMP, adenosine, inosine, and hypoxanthine. As a result, hypoxanthine can't be metabolized into xanthine under hypoxic condition, leading to excessive hypoxanthine accumulation. During reperfusion, the ischemic tissue regains oxygen, and the hypoxanthine accumulated during ischemia is converted into xanthine under the action of XO, which is then catalyzed into uric acid [20]. These reactions lead to a large amount of $O_2^-$ and $H_2O_2$ production.

### 6.4.2 Neutrophils

Under normal physiological conditions, neutrophils are not in contact with vascular endothelial cells. Myocardial reperfusion can produce a series of pro-inflammatory factors, such as tumor necrosis factor-α (TNF-α), interleukin (IL)-1β, IL-6, and IL-21, and a large number of chemokines, such as IL-8 and macrophage inflammatory proteins (MIPs), which can induce neutrophils adhering to vascular endothelial cells and thus causing respiratory bursts [21–24]. In addition, tissue ischemia can activate complement system or produce a variety of molecules with chemotactic activity through cell membrane decomposition, such as C3 fragments, leukotrienes, to attract and activate neutrophils. Activated neutrophils consume more oxygen during reperfusion, producing plenty of oxygen free radicals, which is called respiratory bursts or oxygen bursts [25]. The activated neutrophils can release a large number of enzymes through degranulation reaction explosively, leading to impaired endothelial cell structure and function.

### 6.4.3 Mitochondria

Mitochondria are the most important source of free radicals, and tricarboxylic acid cycle enzymes and oxidative phosphorylation are sensitive to ROS damage. mPTP opening can induce the production of ROS, and excessive ROS can in turn cause the opening of more mPTPs. This leads to a positive feedback loop of mitochondrial extra free radical release, "ROS-induced ROS release," which aggravates myocardial damage [26, 27]. A great deal of mitochondrial ROS directly lead to myocardial apoptosis and necrosis, while moderate mitochondrial ROS levels cause a slight opening of mPTP and give rise to ischemic preconditioning and other effects [28].

### 6.4.4 $Ca^{2+}$

Besides, during ischemia and hypoxia, $Ca^{2+}$ entry into mitochondria reduces manganese superoxide dismutase, thus reducing its ability to scavenge free radicals and further increasing the production of oxygen free radicals [29].

## 6.5 Cell Death

Recently, research has shed new light on the mechanisms of cell injury and death during cardiorespiratory ischemia-reperfusion injury. The largest fraction of cardiomyocyte death associated with reperfusion occurs during the initial minutes of reflow, with the mechanisms originating in cardiomyocytes rather than vascular or blood-derived cells, and can be prevented by interventions applied at the time of reperfusion [30]. Ischemia-reperfusion leads to the activation of cell death program, mainly including necrosis, apoptosis, and autophagy-related cell death [31].

Necrosis is characterized by swelling of cells and organelles, followed by rupture of membranes, leading to leakage of proteins and lysosomes [32]. Necrotic mediators, such as ROS, $Ca^{2+}$, poly-ADP-ribose polymerase (PARP), $Ca^{2+}$-activated non-lysosomal proteases (calpains), and cathepsins, mediate necrosis [33]. Necrotic cells can further cause the infiltration of inflammatory cells and production of cytokines [32].

Apoptosis is regulated by multiple signaling pathways, such as Fas/FasL signaling pathway [34]. Oxygen-free radicals, $Ca^{2+}$ overload, and mPTP opening can lead to mitochondrial swelling and rupture, releasing apoptotic-related proteins such as apoptotic inducible factors and cytochrome c and further initiating the caspase cascade to induce apoptosis [31]. In addition, studies have shown that ATP released from apoptotic cells through the pannexin channel is a "self-discovery" signal that attracts phagocytes [35].

Autophagy is a physiological response of the body during ischemia-reperfusion injury. Ischemia can induce autophagy through AMPK-mTOR and PI3K-Akt signaling pathways, and inhibiting apoptosis may play a protective role against ischemia [36]. Excessive autophagy in the reperfusion phase is not conducive to cell survival and can aggravate cell damage and even lead to cell death [37]. The mechanism is mainly related to the interaction between Beclin1 and Beclin2 [38].

In addition, several other types of cell death have recently been found to be associated with ischemia-reperfusion injury, such as oncosis, pyroptosis, ferroptosis, and parthanatos [39]. The process of oncosis ultimately causes depletion of cellular energy stores and failure of the ionic pumps in the plasma membrane. Changed intracellular $Ca^{2+}$ levels may regulate oncotic cell death. Increased cytoplasmic $Ca^{2+}$ concentrations can activate cysteine proteases of the calpain family that mediate plasma membrane breakdown through the proteolysis of cytoskeletal and plasma membrane proteins. Intracellular ATP levels can also affect the way of cell death. If the energy supply is insufficient, the program of apoptosis is unable to be accomplished, and the cells can turn to oncosis. The more serious the I/R injury was, the greater the mPTP opening was, and the lower the intracellular ATP content was, the more likely the cells were to oncosis [40]. Pyroptosis and ferroptosis may also be important during ischemia and reperfusion; however, it is not clear whether these entities act as an independent death procedure or as an amplification mechanism for necrotic cell death. Pyroptosis is pro-inflammatory programmed cell death that is caspase-1-dependent [41]. Ferroptosis is a cell death that depends on iron and ROS, and its cytological changes include decreased or vanished mitochondria cristae, ruptured outer mitochondrial membrane, and condensed mitochondrial membrane. These abnormalities are due to the loss of selective permeability of plasma membranes caused by strong membrane lipid peroxidation and oxidative stress [42]. Parthanatos (PARP-1-dependent cell death) is a new form of programmed cell death and ROS can induce parthanatos. ROS overproduction will lead to endoplasmic reticulum (ER) calcium release, causing mitochondria depolarization with the loss of mitochondrial membrane potential. Mitochondria depolarization lead mitochondria to release more ROS, which, in turn, contributes to parthanatos [43].

## 6.6 Endothelial Dysfunction

Endothelial dysfunction occurred in the early stages of post-resuscitation, with multiple mechanisms including cytotoxicity caused by pH change [44], production of ROS, inhibition of eNOS-NO, etc [45]. Recent studies have provided new insights into the molecular mechanisms of endothelial dysfunction caused by reperfusion, such as the regulation of ion channels and gap junction proteins [46].

During ischemia-reperfusion, cardiomyocytes, endothelial cells, and inflammatory cells can produce a large amount of ROS. Activation of endothelial cells by oxidative stress can promote micro-thrombosis, blood flow reduction, and inflammatory cell activation. The expression of E-selectin, P-selectin, and intercellular adhesion molecules (ICAMs) on the surface of activated endothelial cells can promote the recruitment of neutrophils, which are the main effector cells of inflammation during ischemia-reperfusion [47]. In addition, there is an increase in endothelial microparticles (EMPs) in endothelial dysfunction. Nuclear factor kappa-B (NF-κB) plays a key role in the activation of endothelial cells induced by ischemia-reperfusion injury. Tyrosine phosphorylation of IκB induced by oxidative stress leads to the dissociation of the inhibitor from NF-κB, thus resulting in NF-κB nuclear translocation and transcription of pro-inflammatory and procoagulant factors and initiating ischemia-reperfusion injury. Oxidative stress can also activate MAPKs to phosphorylate the subunit of NF-κB and regulate the transactivation activity of NF-κB [48]. In addition to being the target of ROS, endothelial cells are also an important source of ROS. ROS produced by endothelial cells via XO, NADH/NADPH oxidase, and uncoupled endothelial nitric oxide synthase (eNOS) can significantly contribute to vascular dysfunction after ischemia-reperfusion [49, 50].

Besides, endothelial permeability obviously increases after myocardial ischemia-reperfusion. The loss of endothelial cell barrier function can be attributed to ROS released by activated leukocytes, which can cause the changes in endothelial cell skeleton structure and promote the formation of intercellular space. Endothelial barrier dysfunction promotes the migration of neutrophils and other inflammatory cells to damage myocardium and further aggravates ischemia-reperfusion injury [51].

## 6.7 Dysregulated NO Metabolism

Nitric oxide (NO), an important vasodilator, is mainly catalyzed by NO synthase (NOS). NO synthase includes endothelial cell type, neuron type, and inducible type (eNOS, nNOS, and iNOS). NO itself is a highly reactive free radical, which can be oxidized into nitrate or nitrite and can further combine with peroxide groups to form nitrite oxide, which has a strong cytotoxic effect. Therefore, the role of NO during ischemia-reperfusion remains controversial [52].

In response to myocardial ischemia, the level of cardiac nNOS is upregulated, which in turn inhibits xanthine oxidoreductase, leading to the suppression of superoxide generation. Additionally, L-VDCC is downregulated by nNOS overexpression, attenuating $Ca^{2+}$ overload due to ischemia, thus protecting the heart against ischemia-reperfusion injury.

The induction of iNOS produces excessive NO, accompanied by increased production of ROS, including superoxide and peroxynitrite ($OONO^-$), which are harmful to the heart [53]. The expression of iNOS is also correlated positively with the expression of pro-inflammatory cytokines and severity of cardiac dysfunction. In response to myocardial ischemia, the upregulated iNOS-derived NO enhances the levels of intracellular cGMP, leading to the decrease of $Ca^{2+}$ influx, thus depressing the sensitivity of myofilament to $Ca^{2+}$ and subsequently attenuating cardiac contractile function [54]. During the late stage of ischemia-reperfusion injury, high-output inducible iNOS/NO pathway is activated and further aggravates left ventricular dysfunction and increases myocardial infarct size [55]. Moreover, enhanced amount of NO induced by upregulated iNOS contributes to the formation of $OONO^-$ in the circulation system and the heart, subsequently leading to severe myocardial apoptosis [56].

Low levels of eNOS-derived NO physiologically regulate normal vascular tone within the sinusoids, prevent the adhesion of leukocyte, and reduce the production of ROS, thus playing a beneficial role in ischemia-reperfusion injury. The level of eNOS is upregulated within minutes during ischemia, which is reduced with the prolonged cardiac ischemia [57].

## 6.8 Platelet Aggregation and Microembolism

$Ca^{2+}$ overload can promote platelet adhesion and aggregation, thus promoting the formation of thrombus. Superoxide and hydrogen peroxide produced by XO can activate phospholipase to induce the production of platelet-activating factor (PAF), which can rapidly trigger or exacerbate inflammation in venules [58].

Tissue ischemia-reperfusion can activate complement system and produce multiple chemotactic substances, such as C3 fragment and leukotriene. This attracts and activates neutrophils to aggregate in the blood vessels of ischemic area and enter the tissues, triggering inflammation and causing slow blood flow or no reflux [59]. Activated neutrophils release TNF-$\alpha$, IL-1, and IL-6 and cause the exposure of adhesion molecules on vascular endothelial cells and leukocytes. With the prolongation of reperfusion time, the release of inflammatory factors and leukocyte activating factors, such as IL-8, thromboxane A2, and PAF, increases, further promoting the adhesion and activation of neutrophils. The adherent neutrophils and vascular endothelial cells further activate, synthesize, and release more chemotactic inflammatory mediators, forming a vicious cycle, leading to microvascular mechanical blockage. The components of microembolism include aggregated platelets, fibrin, lipid fragments (including cholesterol crystals), matrix components, etc [60].

Tissue ischemia-reperfusion can also lead to microcirculation disorders, which are mainly related to leukocyte infiltration, migration, vasodilation dysfunction, increased vascular permeability, thrombosis, and neovascularization [61]. The microcirculation disturbance will lead to no reflow in ischemic area after reperfusion. No-reflow phenomenon refers to the phenomenon that blood perfusion does not occur in some or all ischemic tissues during ischemia-reperfusion. Myocardial no-reflow phenomenon may be related to the following factors. Firstly, cardiomyocyte swelling. Because ischemia causes the dysfunction of $Na^+$-$K^+$ pump in cell membrane, $Na^+$ and water are retained in cells, and myocardial cells in ischemic area swell and compress microvessels during reperfusion. Secondly, vascular endothelial cell swelling. Endothelial cell swelling also occurs during ischemia-reperfusion. Endothelial cells protrude into the lumen, resulting in lumen stenosis and obstruction of blood perfusion. The swelling of endothelial cells is caused by the increase of oxygen free radicals [62]. Oxygen free radicals can damage the endothelial cell membrane. $Na^+$ enters the endothelial cells and causes cell edema. Thirdly, cardiomyocyte contraction oppresses microvessels, preventing some parts of ischemic area from being reperfused with blood. Swelling and contraction of cardiomyocytes can coexist. Finally, platelets, thrombus, and neutrophils clog microvessels. Capillary embolism caused by neutrophils may be the main cause of no reflow [63].

Intravascular hemolysis releases acellular hemoglobin (Hb) into plasma. Oxygenated Hb (Oxy-Hb) consumes vascular NO via dioxidation to form methemoglobin and nitrate, an inert NO metabolite. Plasma Oxy-Hb depletion of vascular NO promotes vasoconstriction, thrombosis, and inflammation, thus damaging tissue perfusion [64].

## 6.9 Immune Response and Inflammatory Cytokines

### 6.9.1 Immune Responses

Cardiorespiratory ischemia-reperfusion usually occurs in a sterile environment, which activates immune system rapidly and thus triggers myocardial inflammation and injury [23]. This sterile immune response involves signaling pathways through pattern recognition molecules, which include Toll-like receptors (TLRs), and recruitment and activation of immune cells of the innate and adaptive immune system [59].

TLRs play an important role in innate immune system and have been demonstrated to be involved in the pathogenesis of cardiorespiratory ischemia-reperfusion injury. Once ligands bind to TLRs, they can activate downstream signaling pathways, such as NF-κB, MAPK, and type I interferon pathways, thereby inducing the production of pro-inflammatory cytokines and chemokines [65]. TLR2 is a membrane surface receptor activated by bacterial peptidoglycan, which is expressed in inflammatory cells, such as monocytes/macrophages, dendritic cells, B lymphocytes, and T lymphocytes. Generally, TLR2 signaling pathway leads to the production of TNF-α and NF-κB. It was shown that a humanized anti-TLR2 antibody could decrease myocardial ischemia-reperfusion injury in pigs, and deficiency of TLR2 could improve survival and neurological function in mice after circulatory arrest [66, 67]. TLR3 also plays an important role in cardiorespiratory injury induced by ischemia-reperfusion, involving the activation of apoptotic signaling and increased NF-κB activity [68]. TLR3 deficiency could attenuate lung ischemia-reperfusion injury and improve pulmonary function, and deletion of TLR3 could reduce cytokine expression both in serum and lung tissues and inhibit pulmonary apoptosis following ischemia-reperfusion [69]. TLR4, one of the most widely studied pattern recognition receptors, mediates inflammatory response of Gram-negative bacteria through lipopolysaccharide activation. Oxidative stress can enhance the activation of TLR4 and redistribute TLR4 to lipid rafts in plasma membrane. In the TLR4 signaling pathway, loss of myeloid differentiation protein 1 (MD1) enhances the activation of TLR-4/NF-κB pathway, thus increasing inflammatory response and apoptosis and aggravating reperfusion injury [70].

Neutrophils are recruited by chemotactic mediators which are released from ischemic myocardium to reperfusion myocardium. The chemotactic mediators, such as TNF-α, IL-18, IL-6, PAF, complement, and leukotriene, can activate the adhesion of neutrophils and endothelium. In the early stage of reperfusion, the aggregation of neutrophils is closely related to the development of reperfusion injury. The mechanisms of rapid recruitment of neutrophils include the production of oxygen free radicals and the release of degranulation products, arachidonic acid metabolites, and PAFs. Neutrophils can produce large quantities of superoxide anions, hydrogen peroxide, and hydroxyl radicals. These oxygen free radicals promote endothelial cells to release inflammatory mediators, express adhesion molecules, and increase endothelial permeability [71].

At the later stage of reperfusion, monocytes and macrophages exudate to the myocardial tissue, aggravating the injury and affecting the tissue repair process.

In addition, ischemia-reperfusion can cause a strong adaptive immune response [59]. Several studies show that T cells and regulatory T cells (Tregs) are also involved in immune disorders after ROSC. Human leukocyte antigen-DR (HLA-DR) is a valuable marker of cardiac arrest. Recent studies have shown that after ROSC, the expression of HLA-DR on monocytes and B and T lymphocytes are decreased [72]. Studies of mouse lines deficient in specific populations of lymphocytes showed that both $CD4^+$ and $CD8^+$ T cells have an adverse effect in myocardial ischemia-reperfusion. During the early period of successful cardiopulmonary resuscitation, Th1/Th2/Th17 subsets and Th1/Th2 cell ratio are imbalance.

### 6.9.2 Inflammatory Cytokines

Some cytokines are elevated post-resuscitation, inhibiting adrenal cortisol synthesis and increasing the risk of early refractory shock [73, 74]. It is worth to point out that the levels of TNF-α and IL-8 are upregulated obviously. TNF-α disruptes $Ca^{2+}$ homeostasis and induced b-adrenergic signaling defects, resulting in catecholamine refractoriness, whereas IL-8 aggravates myocardial injury through inducing neutrophil infiltration. Besides, IL-6 can trigger endothelial activation and damage and glycocalyx damage, which leads to capillary leakage and increased vascular permeability, contributing to hemodynamic instability [75–77]. In addition, matrix metalloproteinases (MMPs) also play an important role in the ischemia-reperfusion injury. MMP-2 and MMP-9 can disrupt type IV collagen, gelatin, and elastin, allow inflammatory cells to infiltrate tissues, and contribute to the loss of vasculature integrity [78].

## References


1. Mattiazzi A, Argenziano M, Aguilar-Sanchez Y, Mazzocchi G, Escobar AL. Ca2+ Sparks and Ca2+ waves are the subcellular events underlying Ca2+ overload during ischemia and reperfusion in perfused intact hearts. J Mol Cell Cardiol. 2015;79:69–78.
2. Nascimento AM, Lima EM, Brasil GA, et al. Serca2a and Na(+)/Ca(2+) exchanger are involved in left ventricular function following cardiac remodelling of female rats treated with anabolic androgenic steroid. Toxicol Appl Pharmacol. 2016;301:22–30.
3. Rusciano MR, Sommariva E, Douin-Echinard V, Ciccarelli M, Poggio P, Maione AS. CaMKII activity in the inflammatory response of cardiac diseases. Int J Mol Sci. 2019;20(18):4374.
4. Tribulova N, Seki S, Radosinska J, et al. Myocardial Ca2+ handling and cell-to-cell coupling, key factors in prevention of sudden cardiac death. Can J Physiol Pharmacol. 2009;87(12):1120–9.
5. Liu T, Takimoto E, Dimaano VL, et al. Inhibiting mitochondrial Na+/Ca2+ exchange prevents sudden death in a Guinea pig model of heart failure. Circ Res. 2014;115(1):44–54.
6. Bondarenko A, Svichar N, Chesler M. Role of Na+-H+ and Na+-Ca2+ exchange in hypoxia-related acute astrocyte death. Glia. 2005;49(1):143–52.
7. Ayoub IM, Kolarova J, Yi Z, et al. Sodium-hydrogen exchange inhibition during ventricular fibrillation: beneficial effects on ischemic contracture, action potential duration, reperfusion arrhythmias, myocardial function, and resuscitability. Circulation. 2003;107(13):1804–9.
8. Gazmuri RJ, Radhakrishnan J, Ayoub IM. Sodium-Hydrogen Exchanger Isoform-1 inhibition: a promising pharmacological intervention for resuscitation from cardiac arrest. Molecules. 2019;24(9):1765.
9. White C, Ambrose E, Muller A, et al. Impact of reperfusion calcium and pH on the resuscitation of hearts donated after circulatory death. Ann Thorac Surg. 2017;103(1):122–30.
10. Ford KL, Moorhouse EL, Bortolozzi M, Richards MA, Swietach P, Vaughan-Jones RD. Regional acidosis locally inhibits but remotely stimulates Ca2+ waves in ventricular myocytes. Cardiovasc Res. 2017;113(8):984–95.
11. Fang X, Huang Z, Zhu J, et al. Ultrastructural evidence of mitochondrial abnormalities in postresuscitation myocardial dysfunction. Resuscitation. 2012;83(3):386–94.
12. Xu W, Fu Y, Jiang L, et al. Cardiopulmonary resuscitation ameliorates myocardial mitochondrial dysfunction in a cardiac arrest rat model. Am J Emerg Med. 2020;38:65–72.

13. Donnino MW, Liu X, Andersen LW, et al. Characterization of mitochondrial injury after cardiac arrest (COMICA). Resuscitation. 2017;113:56–62.
14. Bernardi P, Di Lisa F, Fogolari F, Lippe G. From ATP to PTP and Back: a dual function for the mitochondrial ATP synthase. Circ Res. 2015;116(11):1850–62.
15. van Vuuren D, Lochner A. Ischaemic postconditioning: from bench to bedside. Cardiovasc J Afr. 2008;19(6):311–20.
16. Alam MR, Baetz D, Ovize M. Cyclophilin D and myocardial ischemia-reperfusion injury: a fresh perspective. J Mol Cell Cardiol. 2015;78:80–9.
17. Cour M, Gomez L, Mewton N, Ovize M, Argaud L. Postconditioning: from the bench to bedside. J Cardiovasc Pharmacol Ther. 2011;16(2):117–30.
18. Poprac P, Jomova K, Simunkova M, Kollar V, Rhodes CJ, Valko M. Targeting free radicals in oxidative stress-related human diseases. Trends Pharmacol Sci. 2017;38(7):592–607.
19. Zorov DB, Filburn CR, Klotz LO, Zweier JL, Sollott SJ. Reactive oxygen species (ROS)-induced ROS release: a new phenomenon accompanying induction of the mitochondrial permeability transition in cardiac myocytes. J Exp Med. 2000;192(7):1001–14.
20. Patil KD, Halperin HR, Becker LB. Cardiac arrest. Circ Res. 2015;116(12):2041–9.
21. Wang K, Wen S, Jiao J, et al. IL-21 promotes myocardial ischaemia/reperfusion injury through the modulation of neutrophil infiltration. Br J Pharmacol. 2018;175(8):1329–43.
22. Eltzschig HK, Carmeliet P. Hypoxia and inflammation. N Engl J Med. 2011;364(7):656–65.
23. Laubach VE, Sharma AK. Mechanisms of lung ischemia-reperfusion injury. Curr Opin Organ Transplant. 2016;21(3):246–52.
24. Li RJ, Ji WQ, Pang JJ, Wang JL, Chen YG, Zhang Y. Alpha-lipoic acid ameliorates oxidative stress by increasing aldehyde dehydrogenase-2 activity in patients with acute coronary syndrome. Tohoku J Exp Med. 2013;229(1):45–51.
25. Eisenhardt SU, Weiss JB, Smolka C, et al. MicroRNA-155 aggravates ischemia-reperfusion injury by modulation of inflammatory cell recruitment and the respiratory oxidative burst. Basic Res Cardiol. 2015;110(3):32.
26. Zorov DB, Juhaszova M, Sollott SJ. Mitochondrial ROS-induced ROS release: an update and review. Biochim Biophys Acta. 2006;1757(5–6):509–17.
27. Nickel A, Kohlhaas M, Maack C. Mitochondrial reactive oxygen species production and elimination. J Mol Cell Cardiol. 2014;73:26–33.
28. Bagheri F, Khori V, Alizadeh AM, Khalighfard S, Khodayari S, Khodayari H. Reactive oxygen species-mediated cardiac-reperfusion injury: mechanisms and therapies. Life Sci. 2016;165:43–55.
29. Macmillan-Crow LA, Cruthirds DL. Invited review: manganese superoxide dismutase in disease. Free Radic Res. 2001;34(4):325–36.
30. García-Dorado D. Myocardial reperfusion injury: a new view. Cardiovasc Res. 2004;61(3):363–4.
31. Hotchkiss RS, Strasser A, McDunn JE, Swanson PE. Cell death. N Engl J Med. 2009;361(16):1570–83.
32. Turer AT, Hill JA. Pathogenesis of myocardial ischemia-reperfusion injury and rationale for therapy. Am J Cardiol. 2010;106(3):360–8.
33. Conus S, Simon HU. Cathepsins: key modulators of cell death and inflammatory responses. Biochem Pharmacol. 2008;76(11):1374–82.
34. Liu XM, Yang ZM, Liu XK. Fas/FasL induces myocardial cell apoptosis in myocardial ischemia-reperfusion rat model. Eur Rev Med Pharmacol Sci. 2017;21(12):2913–8.
35. Chekeni FB, Elliott MR, Sandilos JK, et al. Pannexin 1 channels mediate 'find-me' signal release and membrane permeability during apoptosis. Nature. 2010;467(7317):863–7.
36. Lu J, Shen Y, Liu LJ, Qian HY, Zhu CL. Combining epinephrine and Esmolol attenuates excessive autophagy and Mitophagy in rat Cardiomyocytes after cardiac arrest. J Cardiovasc Pharmacol. 2015;66(5):449–56.
37. Wei H, Yin M, Lu Y, et al. Mild hypothermia improves neurological outcome in mice after cardiopulmonary resuscitation through Silent Information Regulator 1-actviated autophagy. Cell Death Discov. 2019;5:129.

38. Xue D, Wang Q, Chen Z, et al. 3-Anhydro-6-hydroxy-ophiobolin A, a fungal sesterterpene from Bipolaris oryzae induced autophagy and promoted the degradation of α-synuclein in PC12 cells. Bioorg Med Chem Lett. 2015;25(7):1464–70.
39. Del Re DP, Amgalan D, Linkermann A, Liu Q, Kitsis RN. Fundamental mechanisms of regulated cell death and implications for heart disease. Physiol Rev. 2019;99(4):1765–817.
40. Liu LF, Qian ZH, Qin Q, et al. Effect of melatonin on oncosis of myocardial cells in the myocardial ischemia/reperfusion injury rat and the role of the mitochondrial permeability transition pore. Genet Mol Res. 2015;14(3):7481–9.
41. Fink SL, Cookson BT. Apoptosis, pyroptosis, and necrosis: mechanistic description of dead and dying eukaryotic cells. Infect Immun. 2005;73(4):1907–16.
42. Mou Y, Wang J, Wu J, et al. Ferroptosis, a new form of cell death: opportunities and challenges in cancer. J Hematol Oncol. 2019;12(1):34.
43. Zhong H, Song R, Pang Q, et al. Propofol inhibits parthanatos via ROS-ER-calcium-mitochondria signal pathway in vivo and vitro. Cell Death Dis. 2018;9(10):932.
44. Meyer AS, Ostrowski SR, Kjaergaard J, Johansson PI, Hassager C. Endothelial Dysfunction in Resuscitated Cardiac Arrest (ENDO-RCA): safety and efficacy of low-dose prostacyclin administration and blood pressure target in addition to standard therapy, as compared to standard therapy alone, in post-cardiac arrest syndrome patients: study protocol for a randomized controlled trial. Trials. 2016;17:378.
45. Asai M, Takeuchi K, Saotome M, et al. Extracellular acidosis suppresses endothelial function by inhibiting store-operated Ca2+ entry via non-selective cation channels. Cardiovasc Res. 2009;83(1):97–105.
46. Yang Q, He GW, Underwood MJ, Yu CM. Cellular and molecular mechanisms of endothelial ischemia/reperfusion injury: perspectives and implications for postischemic myocardial protection. Am J Transl Res. 2016;8(2):765–77.
47. Bro-Jeppesen J, Johansson PI, Kjaergaard J, et al. Level of systemic inflammation and endothelial injury is associated with cardiovascular dysfunction and vasopressor support in post-cardiac arrest patients. Resuscitation. 2017;121:179–86.
48. Jones WK, Brown M, Ren X, He S, McGuinness M. NF-kappaB as an integrator of diverse signaling pathways: the heart of myocardial signaling? Cardiovasc Toxicol. 2003;3(3):229–54.
49. Reyes LA, Boslett J, Varadharaj S, et al. Depletion of NADP(H) due to CD38 activation triggers endothelial dysfunction in the postischemic heart. Proc Natl Acad Sci U S A. 2015;112(37):11648–53.
50. Troelsen TT, Granfeldt A, Secher N, Tonnesen EK, Simonsen U. Impaired NO-mediated vasodilatation in rat coronary arteries after asphyxial cardiac arrest. Acta Anaesthesiol Scand. 2015;59(5):654–67.
51. Fink K, Schwarz M, Feldbrugge L, et al. Severe endothelial injury and subsequent repair in patients after successful cardiopulmonary resuscitation. Crit Care. 2010;14(3):R104.
52. Morgan RW, Sutton RM, Karlsson M, et al. Pulmonary vasodilator therapy in shock-associated cardiac arrest. Am J Respir Crit Care Med. 2018;197(7):905–12.
53. Yu X, Ge L, Niu L, Lian X, Ma H, Pang L. The dual role of inducible nitric oxide synthase in myocardial ischemia/reperfusion injury: friend or foe? Oxid Med Cell Longev. 2018;2018:8364848.
54. Mendez-Carmona N, Wyss RK, Arnold M, et al. Differential effects of ischemia/reperfusion on endothelial function and contractility in donation after circulatory death. J Heart Lung Transplant. 2019;38(7):767–77.
55. Zhang H, Wu Q, Wan Z, Cao Y, Zeng Z. Preconditioning but not postconditioning treatment with resveratrol substantially ameliorates postresuscitation myocardial dysfunction through the PI3K/Akt signaling pathway. Mol Med Rep. 2019;20(2):1250–8.
56. Wang G, Zhang Q, Yuan W, Wu J, Li C. Sildenafil protects against myocardial ischemia-reperfusion injury following cardiac arrest in a porcine model: possible role of the renin-angiotensin system. Int J Mol Sci. 2015;16(11):27015–31.
57. Xue L, Yang F, Han Z, et al. ALDH2 mediates the dose-response protection of chronic ethanol against endothelial senescence through SIRT1/p53 pathway. Biochem Biophys Res Commun. 2018;504(4):777–83.

58. Schanze N, Bode C, Duerschmied D. Platelet contributions to myocardial ischemia/reperfusion injury. Front Immunol. 2019;10:1260.
59. Eltzschig HK, Eckle T. Ischemia and reperfusion—from mechanism to translation. Nat Med. 2011;17(11):1391–401.
60. Mezger M, Nording H, Sauter R, et al. Platelets and immune responses during thromboinflammation. Front Immunol. 2019;10:1731.
61. Hidalgo A, Chang J, Jang JE, Peired AJ, Chiang EY, Frenette PS. Heterotypic interactions enabled by polarized neutrophil microdomains mediate thromboinflammatory injury. Nat Med. 2009;15(4):384–91.
62. Carden DL, Granger DN. Pathophysiology of ischaemia-reperfusion injury. J Pathol. 2000;190(3):255–66.
63. Yellon DM, Hausenloy DJ. Myocardial reperfusion injury. N Engl J Med. 2007;357(11):1121–35.
64. Hayashida K, Miyazaki Y, Yu B, et al. Depletion of vascular nitric oxide contributes to poor outcomes after cardiac arrest. Am J Respir Crit Care Med. 2019;199(10):1288–90.
65. Asmussen A, Fink K, Busch HJ, et al. Inflammasome and toll-like receptor signaling in human monocytes after successful cardiopulmonary resuscitation. Crit Care. 2016;20(1):170.
66. Arslan F, Houtgraaf JH, Keogh B, et al. Treatment with OPN-305, a humanized anti-Toll-Like receptor-2 antibody, reduces myocardial ischemia/reperfusion injury in pigs. Circ Cardiovasc Interv. 2012;5(2):279–87.
67. Bergt S, Guter A, Grub A, et al. Impact of toll-like receptor 2 deficiency on survival and neurological function after cardiac arrest: a murine model of cardiopulmonary resuscitation. PLoS One. 2013;8(9):e74944.
68. Chen C, Feng Y, Zou L, et al. Role of extracellular RNA and TLR3-Trif signaling in myocardial ischemia-reperfusion injury. J Am Heart Assoc. 2014;3(1):e000683.
69. Zhang XY, Chen C, Zhang YB, et al. Role of toll-like receptor 3 in lung ischemia-reperfusion injury. Shock. 2016;46(4):405–11.
70. Jiang X, Kong B, Shuai W, et al. Loss of MD1 exacerbates myocardial ischemia/reperfusion injury and susceptibility to ventricular arrhythmia. Eur J Pharmacol. 2019;844:79–86.
71. Podolec J, Trabka-Zawicki A, Badacz R, et al. Chemokine RANTES and IL-1beta in mild therapeutic hypothermia-treated patients after out-of-hospital sudden cardiac arrest. Postepy Kardiol Interwencyjnej. 2019;15(1):98–106.
72. Qi Z, An L, Liu B, et al. Patients with out-of-hospital cardiac arrest show decreased human leucocyte antigen-DR expression on monocytes and B and T lymphocytes after return of spontaneous circulation. Scand J Immunol. 2018;88(4):e12707.
73. El-Menyar AA. The resuscitation outcome: revisit the story of the stony heart. Chest. 2005;128(4):2835–46.
74. Tulaimat A, Patel A, Wisniewski M, Gueret R. The validity and reliability of the clinical assessment of increased work of breathing in acutely ill patients. J Crit Care. 2016;34:111–5.
75. Bro-Jeppesen J, Johansson PI, Hassager C, et al. Endothelial activation/injury and associations with severity of post-cardiac arrest syndrome and mortality after out-of-hospital cardiac arrest. Resuscitation. 2016;107:71–9.
76. Chelazzi C, Villa G, Mancinelli P, De Gaudio AR, Adembri C. Glycocalyx and sepsis-induced alterations in vascular permeability. Crit Care. 2015;19:26.
77. Li XX, Zhao L, Chang Y, et al. Ezetimibe prevents myocardial remodeling in an obese rat model by inhibiting inflammation. Acta Biochim Pol. 2018;65(3):465–70.
78. Jou C, Shah R, Figueroa A, Patel JK. The role of inflammatory cytokines in cardiac arrest. J Intensive Care Med. 2020;35(3):219–24.

# Progress in Reperfusion Injury of Other Important Organs in Cardiovascular Events

7

Li Zhao and Qian Wang

**Abstract**

Ischemia-reperfusion injury is one of the most common and complicated phenomena in clinical process, which causes different kinds of injury in different organs, especially in cardiovascular events. We analyze and summarize new progress and researches in this chapter.

**Keywords**

Ischemia-reperfusion injury · Mechanisms · Brain · Myocardium · Kidney

## 7.1 Introduction

Ischemia-reperfusion (I/R) can cause irreversible injury to different tissues and organ, which is characterized by insufficient oxygen supply and subsequent restoration of blood flow. The word ischemia comes from the Greek "iskhein," which means the absence of blood supplies in different organs, because of blood vessel obstruction or organ transplantation. Some clinical conditions, acute coronary syndrome, organ transplantation, limb damage, and so on, may cause tissue hypoperfusion. Reperfusion of the tissue or organs is the return of the blood flow and the reoxygenation of the tissue or organs. However, clinical prognosis after restoration of blood supply to ischemic tissue or organs is not optimal. Some studies have revealed that reperfusion has the potential impairments to induce subsequent injury in ischemic tissue or organs, and this is named ischemia/reperfusion (I/R) injury.

Different factors could damage the organs in I/R processes, for instance, reduced ATP levels, loss of nutrients, inflammation, and oxidative stress. The I/R injury is a major reason for the prognosis. For example, the reperfusion of the kidneys increases

L. Zhao (✉) · Q. Wang
Emergency Dpartment of Fu Xing Hospital, Capital Medical University, Beijing, China



H. Zhu (ed.), *Sudden Death*, https://doi.org/10.1007/978-981-15-7002-5_7

the recruitment of neutrophils into the kidney, which will exacerbate the inflammatory reaction [1].

Mechanisms underlying I/R injury are complex and multifactorial. Some clinical conditions can induce ischemia and cause hypoxia and hypoperfusion, just like atherosclerosis and acute myocardial infarction.

Ischemic injury may cause hypoxia and hyponutrition. Once cell is damaged owing to prolonged I/R injury, apoptosis, autophagy, and necroptosis will appear as bad outcomes. In addition, moderate I/R injury may lead to cell dysfunction by autophagy, as well as activate recovery systems for survival.

A research reveals necrosis occurs when cells are subjected to excessive external stress [2]. In fact, necrosis is a form of cell death with early plasma membrane permeation and organelle swelling. Necrosis is a common and usual pathological condition in human, such as ischemic cerebrovascular disease, but the mechanism of necrosis regulation in I/R injury is not clear. According to necroptosis in mouse models of inflammation and I/R injury, the role of necrosis has been confirmed. Obstruction of blood flow can induce local ischemia into associated tissue, with less supply of oxygen and nutrients, which may disturb energy metabolism and cause cell death. The reperfusion rises the supply of oxygen and the production of reactive oxygen species (ROS), which induces cell death.

## 7.2 Mechanisms of Ischemia/Reperfusion Injury

Many animal experiments have been established to evaluate the pathogenesis and mechanisms of intestinal I/R injury. Increases in cellular calcium and ROS are proved to be the significant mediators of reperfusion injury. What is more, mitochondrial dysfunction also plays an important role in its process. Addition, polyubiquitination of the proteins require some specific proteins, E1 (ubiquitin-activating), E2 (ubiquitin-conjugating), and E3 (ubiquitin-ligating) enzymes [3, 4] and so on, in the conjugation ubiquitin to the targeted protein. Except that, the level of 26S proteasome is lower during the ischemia period, which actually plays antioxidative effect. Endoplasmic reticulum and peroxisomes associates with production of ROS, which can be harmful to cell metabolism once cellular levels are higher.

In reperfusion period, the production of ROS and the formation of oxidized proteins rise because of the oxygen supply, which uncovers that proteasome activation could decrease the toxic concentration of oxidized proteins during the reperfusion period. When the ROS level slightly increases in the cells, the activity of the 26S proteasome increases to remove oxidized proteins, by a ubiquitin-dependent degradation pathway [5].

The higher ROS can cause liver cell death by enhancing the inflammatory response with activating IL-4. It was surprising that the expression of superoxide dismutase (SOD) and glutathione peroxidase continued to decrease after the reoxygenation of the heart, when it was expected that the oxygen should reverse the ischemia effect on their expression [6]. Inflammatory cascades and oxidative stress may subsequently lead to a cytokine storm, which damages cellular structures and promotes cell death eventually. The reperfusion period is changed and may last for several days.

## 7.3 Character of Different Organs

Many studies have investigated I/R injury in cardiac, cerebral, and kidney diseases, as well as intestinal injury and transplantation.

### 7.3.1 Brain

In all of the body organs, the brain shows the highest sensitivity to ischemia, because it has the highest metabolic activity per unit weight of any organ. What is more, the brain needs consistent supply of glucose as a sufficient resource to meet its metabolic demands. Neuronal glutamate and dopamine are excessive release in the cerebral I/R injury, which cause neuronal calcium overload and subsequent cytotoxicity because of ischemia-induced injury of downstream signaling. As a consequence of I/R injury in the brain, microvascular permeability could change, which can cause edema formation and increased interstitial fluid pressure. Not only edema formation enlarges the diffusion distance for oxygen and nutrients, but also the up in tissue pressure contributes to no reflow by physically compressing microvessels.

### 7.3.2 Myocardium

Like the brain, the myocardium is also exquisitely sensitive to ischemia. In all of the cardiovascular events, myocardial I/R injury is a critical issue also for forensic pathologists since sudden death may occur despite timely reperfusion following acute myocardial infarction, which is one of the most frequently litigated areas of cardiology practice [7].

But, the time window before the beginning of irreversible injury is slightly longer and starts to show the damage after about 20 min of ischemia in both humans and animal models. As in the brain or any other organ, the sooner the impaired coronary arteries are reopened, the better for survival of viable cardiomyocytes. In fact, reperfusion itself may promote additional myocardial injury, except generated by ischemia alone. In the heart, fibrosis occurs after I/R injury by processes invoked by fibroblasts and mast cells and modulated by T cell subsets. Depending on their polarization into Th1 versus Th2 cells, CD4+ T lymphocytes modulate the activity of fibroblasts to influence fibrosis and scar formation [8]. In contrast, fibrosis is absence in postischemic brain. In fact, apoptosis of myocardial cells is an important mechanism of I/R injury.

## 7.3.3 Kidney

The kidneys are the third most susceptible organ system to ischemia, with lasting damage if the duration of ischemia is more than 30 min in humans. Renal cortical cells are susceptible to ischemia, because renal oxygen levels are highest in this region. Just like the brain, microvascular permeability changes could appear as a result of I/R injury in the kidneys. The available data does not confirm the efficacy of remote ischemic preconditioning in reducing renal I/R injury in patients undergoing major cardiac and vascular surgery [9].

### 7.3.3.1 Introduction About I/R Injury in Kidneys

Kidney I/R injury emerges in various clinical settings as a great problem complicating the course and outcome.

I/R injury is a leading cause of acute kidney injury (AKI), which is not only associated with high morbidity and mortality but also increased costs of treatment. The incidence of AKI in hospitalized patients has been reported to be between 2 and 7% and even greater than 10% in intensive care unit (ICU) patients contributing to increased mortality rate [10]. Comprehensive influence about pathophysiological processes with inflammation, abnormal repair, and fibrosis makes AKI an essential risk factor for development of chronic kidney disease.

I/R injury is an important risk factor for developing chronic kidney disease (CKD), which is defined as abnormalities of kidney structure or function, at least 3 months, and interruption of the renal blood flow followed by the subsequent restoration of perfusion, just like sudden heart arrest with resuscitation, vascular and cardiac operation, and so on.

### 7.3.3.2 Mechanisms and Potential Therapy

Initial hypoxic injury with subsequent production of ROS, due to reoxygenation, initiates events in I/R injury, leading to apoptosis, necrosis, and a profound inflammatory response [11]. Besides ROS, reactive nitrogen species (RNS), such as nitric oxide, are produced in kidney I/R injury via the activity of inducible NO synthase (iNOS), which is considered as one of the inflammatory mediators [12]. iNOS and a lot of proinflammatory cytokines are mainly induced by the action of NF-κB.

The detrimental role of Th17 cells in pathogenesis of kidney IR injury has recently been confirmed [13, 14], because noncanonical NF-κB activation directs the development of Th17 cell immune response, so it may be inhibited by the IKK2-mediated canonical NF-κB pathway.

It has been shown that NF-κB activation in renal tubular epithelial cells aggravated tubular injury and exacerbated inflammation in a mouse model of kidney I/R injury [15]. This promotes researchers to explore NF-κB-based treatments of I/R injury.

In the future, mitochondria-targeted antioxidants may be one therapeutic method for treatment of kidney I/R injury, which represents a new way and strategy, especially in clinical practice in whose kidney I/R injury could be prevented or improved.

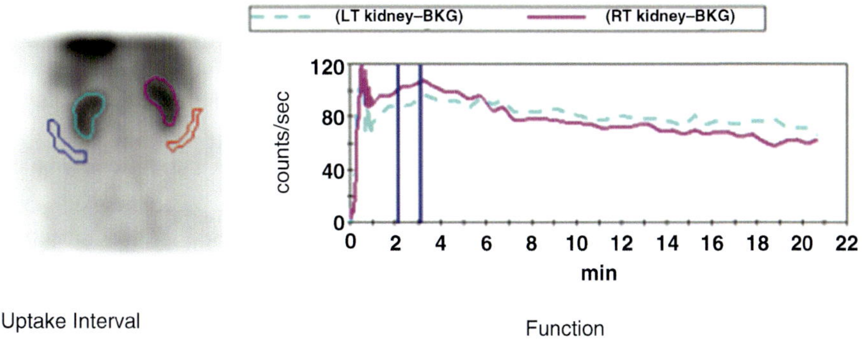


**Fig. 7.1** The function of kidney under ECT

Kidney resident cells and recruited inflammatory cells can produce proinflammatory and anti-inflammatory mediators, which determine renal injury, tissue repair, and progression to CKD. In animal experiments, it has been shown that mice subjected to kidney I/R injury and treated with TJ-M2010–2, which restrained MyD88 homodimerization, had higher survival rate than non-treated animals. Additionally, treatment with TJ-M2010–2 markedly attenuated inflammatory response and ameliorated tubular interstitial fibrosis in mice subjected to kidney I/R injury [16].

In clinical practice, we also can use ECT (emission computed tomography) to evaluate the function of kidney (Fig. 7.1).

Some details are still unknown, for instance, what on earth are the different inflammatory cell roles in I/R injury and how they work in progression of AKI to CKD and why researches in animals targeting some inflammatory pathways have proved helpful, but clinical studies intervening the same pathways have not succeeded. Except, berberine showed better renoprotective function in renal I/R injury. Berberine nanoparticles (BBR-NP) can be used in therapy to reduce oxidative stress and subsequent apoptosis in renal I/R injury. Administration of BBR-NP resulted in protection both morphologically and functionally and is superior to BBR alone [17].

#### 7.3.3.3 Biomarkers of AKI

AKI diagnostic criteria are a sudden decrease in renal function (<48 h), with an increase in absolute serum creatinine ≥0.3 mg/dL (26.4 μmol/L), an increase of >50% (1.5 times the baseline value), and urine volume < 0.5 mL/kg/h > for more than 6 h. AKI is classified into one, two, and three phases.

Serum creatinine and urine volume are still the broadest markers of AKI. Creatinine (Cr) is a protein metabolite that is almost completely cleared by the kidneys. However, its sensitivity and specificity are low.

With the discovery and research of new biomarkers, the diagnosis of AKI is no longer limited to changes in SCr and urine volume. It brings new hopes for the early diagnosis and treatment of AKI. These new biomarkers include low molecular weight proteins, for instance, retinol binding protein (RBP), β2-microglobulin (β2-MG), N-acetyl-β-D-glucosaminidase (NAG), and cysteine protease inhibitor cystatin C (CysC). In recent years, studies have shown that serum RBP is a sensitive indicator reflecting the development and outcome of liver and kidney diseases, and its degree of change can reflect the degree of liver function and damage of proximal tubular function. Increased RBP in urine has an early diagnostic value for renal diseases, especially tubular damage. The increase in urinary β2-MG concentration is mostly due to renal tubular reabsorption due to proximal convoluted tubule injury. Roos et al. [18] showed that changes in β2-MG were associated with endogenous creatinine clearance (Ccr) and were a mature indicator for evaluating glomerular filtration (GFR).

And other cytokines are suitable as an early indicator of the diagnosis of AKI, such as interleukin-18 (IL-18), keratinocyte-derived chemokine (KC), and keratinocyte-derived chemokine isoform (Gro-α). In recent years, studies have found that IL-18 is an important indicator for predicting the occurrence and development of AKI. Washburn et al. [19] found that urine IL-18 concentration testing not only facilitates the early effective diagnosis of AKI patients in the ICU but also predicts the mortality rate. Molls et al. [20] determined the concentration of 18 cell cytokines in I/R injury mice at 3, 24, and 72 h after ischemia and found that KC was the earliest and elevated cytokine.

In addition, neutrophil gelatinase-associated lipocalin (NGAL), kidney injury molecule-1 (KIM-1), sodium-hydrogen exchanger 3 (NHE-3), homocysteine (Cyr61), and atrial natriuretic peptide (ANP) are also used for the diagnosis of AKI. Devarajan [21] found that NGAL was detected in urine samples 3 h after renal injury by studying the model of kidney damage caused by nephrotoxicity, which was significantly earlier than that of SCr. Studies have found that in the injury of renal tubules, the elevated level of NHE-3 is consistent with SCr. ATN patients are significantly higher than patients with pre-renal azotemia, while patients with renal solid ARF are not significantly elevated. And in recent years, studies have found that the expression of Cyr61 is significantly upregulated in kidney ischemia animal model. Cyr61 can be detected in urine samples after 3–6 h of renal ischemia, until the expression reaches its peak after 6–9 h of ischemia, and it can still be detected continuously within 24 h [22].

### 7.3.4 Intestinal

Intestinal I/R injury destroys tight junctions between epithelial cells of the mucosal layer and impaired intestinal mucosal barrier, which may cause transport of bacteria or enterotoxins from the lumen to the interstitial space of the affected bowel. If ischemia is severe or the volume of ischemic mesenteric tissue is large, sepsis and multiple organ failure will occur.

Acute mesenteric ischemia (AMI) is a typical intestinal I/R injury-related disease that is caused by rapid interruption of blood flow in the mesenteric vessel. Nonocclusive mesenteric ischemia (NOMI) is a common type. Usually, patients with NOMI are critically ill with severe heart failure, hemodialysis, aortic insufficiency, septic shock, or myocardial infarction, and the mortality rate exceeds 50% [23]. Guidelines of the *European Journal of Trauma and Emergency Surgery* recommend that broad-spectrum antibiotics should be administered because bacterial translocation is an early event in the progress of AMI [24]. Mucosal barrier function is destroyed and vascular permeability is increased during the formation of the I/R injury.

The increased vascular permeability allows the activation and adhesion of inflammatory cells. These inflammatory cells release ROS, proinflammatory chemokines, and protein kinases. A large number of bacteria exist in the human gastrointestinal tract, especially in the colon. Many diseases, like diabetes, IBD, and nonsteroidal anti-inflammatory drug (NSAID)-induced small intestinal damage, were associated with abnormalities of the gut microbiome, called dysbiosis.

A representative TLR4 ligand [25] decreased intestinal I/R injury by preventing an increase in intestinal permeability through TNF-α signaling. Moreover, the TLR4 signaling pathway is the aggravating factor against intestinal I/R injury.

### 7.3.5 Skin and Skeletal

The skin and skeletal muscle can bear much longer ischemic time than other organs. Compared with the heart, brain, and kidneys, skeletal muscles contain satellite cells, which can regenerate muscle tissue even after widespread injury.

Except that we mentioned before, injury of other organs often occurs on reperfusion process after localized tissue ischemia, which is called remote organ injury (ROI). The ROI can progress to acute respiratory distress syndrome (ARDS) and systemic inflammatory response syndrome (SIRS), which are critical stages to multiple organ dysfunction syndrome (MODS), especially when the volume of tissue impaired is severe. For instance, cardiac I/R injury may lead to MODS, if pump function is reduced to a so low degree that cannot supply sufficient perfusion to other organs. In the future, lncRNAs in I/R injury may provide new therapy for patients.

## 7.4 Conclusion

For young people, sudden unexpected death is most often suspected to sudden cardiac death (SCD). SCD can be described as a natural death induced by sudden malignant arrhythmia often happening without previous warning or symptoms.

In many of these cases, structural abnormalities of the heart, cardiomyopathies, such as hypertrophic cardiomyopathy, are revealed owing to autopsy. What is more, in which no structural cardiovascular or other anatomical abnormalities are also observed or are equivocal at autopsy, a fatal arrhythmogenic disorder should be suspected according to clinical, historical, family, or other detailed information. Heritable genetic variants have been suggested as the cause of up to a third of SCD cases [26].

I/R affects many regulatory systems at the cellular level. Underlying factors of I/R involve dysfunction of energy metabolism, cellular changes of the mitochondria and cellular membranes, initiation of different forms of cell death-like apoptosis, and so on. Chemokines and cytokines together with other factors promote the inflammatory response leading to activation of the innate immune system as well as the adaptive immune system. And it is a relevant factor in determining high morbidity and mortality in several diseases among which are myocardial infarction, ischemic stroke, AKI, and trauma [27].

## References


1. Yago T, Petrich BH, Zhang N, et al. Blocking neutrophil integrin activation prevents ischemia-reperfusion injury. J Exp Med. 2015;212:1267–81. https://doi.org/10.1084/jem.20142358.
2. Saeed WK, Jun DW, Jang K, et al. Does necroptosis have a crucial role in hepatic ischemia-reperfusion injury? PLoS One. 2017;12:e0184752.
3. Bedford L, Lowe J, Dick LR, et al. Ubiquitin-like protein conjugation and the ubiquitin-proteasome system as drug targets. Nat Rev Drug Discov. 2011;10:29–46. https://doi.org/10.1038/nrd3321.
4. Buetow L, Huang DT. Structural insights into the catalysis and regulation of E3 ubiquitin ligases. Nat Rev Mol Cell Biol. 2016;17:626–42. https://doi.org/10.1038/nrm.2016.91.
5. Pajares M, Jimenez-Moreno N, Dias IH, et al. Redox control of protein degradation. Redox Biol. 2015;6:409–20. https://doi.org/10.1016/j.redox.2015.07.003.
6. Yuan X, Niu HT, Wang PL, et al. Cardioprotective effect of licochalcone D against myocardial ischemia/reperfusion injury in langendorff-perfused rat hearts. PLoS One. 2015;10:e0128375. https://doi.org/10.1371/journal.pone.0128375.
7. Neri M, Riezzo I, Pascale N, et al. Ischemia/reperfusion injury following acute myocardial infarction: a critical issue for clinicians and forensic pathologists. Mediators Inflamm. 2017;2017:7018393. [PMID: 28286377].
8. Ramos G, Hofmann U, Frantz S. Myocardial fibrosis through the lenses of T-cell biology. J Mol Cell Cardiol. 2016;92:41–5. [PubMed: 26804387].
9. Menting TP, Wever KE, Ozdemir-van Brunschot DMD, et al. Ischaemic preconditioning for the reduction of renal ischaemia reperfusion injury. Cochrane Database Syst Rev. 2017;3:CD010777. [PMID:28258686].
10. Chertow GM, Burdick E, Honour M, et al. Acute kidney injury, mortality, length of stay, and costs in hospitalized patients. J Am Soc Nephrol. 2005;16(11):3365–70. https://doi.org/10.1681/ASN.2004090740.
11. Devarajan P. Update of mechanisms of ischemic acute kidney injury. J Am Soc Nephrol. 2006;17(6):1503–20.
12. Walker M, York JL, Imam SZ, et al. Oxidative stress and reactive nitrogen species generation during renal ischemia. Toxicol Sci. 2001;63(1):143–8. https://doi.org/10.1093/toxsci/63.1.143.
13. Guo L, Lee HH, Noriega ML, et al. Lymphocyte-specific deletion of IKK2 or NEMO mediates an increase in intrarenal Th17 cells and accelerates renal damage in an ischemia-reperfusion injury mouse model. Am J Physiol Renal Physiol. 2016;311(5):F1005–14. https://doi.org/10.1152/ajprenal.00242.2016.
14. Patil CN, Wallace K, LaMarca BD, et al. Low-dose testosterone protects against renal ischemia-reperfusion injury by increasing renal IL-10-to-TNF-α ratio and attenuating T-cell infiltration. Am J Physiol Renal Physiol. 2016;311(2):F395–403. https://doi.org/10.1152/ajprenal.00454.2015.
15. Markó L, Vigolo E, Hinze C, et al. Tubular epithelial NF-κB activity regulates ischemic AKI. J Am Soc Nephrol. 2016;27(9):2658–69. https://doi.org/10.1681/ASN.2015070748.

16. Zhang LM, Liu JH, Xue CB, et al. Pharmacological inhibition of MyD88 homodimerization counteracts renal ischemia reperfusion-induced progressive renal injury in vivo and in vitro. Sci Rep. 2016;6:26954.
17. Xie D, Xu Y, Jing W, et al. Berberine nanoparticles protects tubular epithelial cells from renal ischemia-reperfusion injury. Oncotarget. 2017;8(15):24154–62. https://doi.org/10.18632/oncotarget.16530.
18. Roos JF, Doust J, Tett SE, et al. Diagnostic accuracy of cystatin C compared to serum creatinine for the estimation of renal dysfunction in adults and children: a meta-analysis. Clin Biochem. 2007;40(5/6):383–91.
19. Washburn KK, Zappitelli M, Arikan AA, et al. Urinary interleukin-18 is an acute kidney injury biomarker in critically ill children. Nephrol Dial Transplant. 2008;23(2):566–72.
20. Molls RR, Savransky V, Liu M, et al. Keratinocyte-derived chemokine is an early biomarker of ischemic acute kidney injury. Am J Physiol Renal Physiol. 2006;290(5):1187–93.
21. Devarajan P. Neutrophil gelatinase-associated lipocalin (NAGL): a new marker of kidney disease. Scand J Clin Lab Invest Suppl. 2008;241(4):89–94.
22. Muramatsu Y, Tsujie M, Kohda Y, et al. Early detection of cysteine rich protein 61 (CYR61, CCN1) in urine following renal ischemic reperfusion injury. Kidney Int. 2002;62(5):1601–10.
23. Muschitz GK, Fochtmann A, Keck M, et al. Non-occlusive mesenteric ischaemia: the prevalent cause of gastrointestinal infarction in patients with severe burn injuries. Injury. 2015;46:124–30.
24. Tilsed JV, Casamassima A, Kurihara H, et al. ESTES guidelines: acute mesenteric ischaemia. Eur J Trauma Emerg Surg. 2016;42:253–70.
25. Nadatani Y, Huo X, Zhang X, et al. NOD-like receptor protein 3 inflammasome priming and activation in Barrett's epithelial cells. Cell Mol Gastroenterol Hepatol. 2016;2:439–53.
26. Nicole D, Methner R, Scherer SE, Welch K, et al. Postmortem genetic screening for the identification, verification, and reporting of genetic variants contributing to the sudden death of the young. Genome Res. 2016;26(9):1170–7. https://doi.org/10.1101/gr.195800.115. Epub 2016 Jul 19.
27. Salvadori M, Rosso G, Bertoni E. Update on ischemia-reperfusion injury in kidney transplantation: pathogenesis and treatment. World J Transplant. 2015;5(2):52–67. Published online 2015 Jun 24. https://doi.org/10.5500/wjt.v5.i2.52.

# Part II

# Diagnosis of Sudden Cardiac Death

# Improvement in Diagnosis of Sudden Cardiac Death

8

Zhenzhen Gao, Fang Zhang, Changxiao Yu, and Ziren Tang

**Abstract**

Sudden death (SD) is often the first clinical manifestation of an underlying disease in previously asymptomatic, apparently "healthy" subjects. Various criteria have been used to define sudden cardiac arrest and sudden cardiac death in the medical literature. The 2006 American College of Cardiology/American Heart Association/Heart Rhythm Society (ACC/AHA/HRS Writing Committee to establish data standards for electrophysiology) included definitions to guide documentation in research and clinical practice. "[Sudden] cardiac arrest is the sudden cessation of cardiac activity so that the victim becomes unresponsive, with no normal breathing and no signs of circulation. If corrective measures are not taken rapidly, this condition progresses to sudden death. Cardiac arrest should be used to signify an event as described above, that is reversed, usually by CPR and/or defibrillation or cardioversion, or cardiac pacing. Sudden cardiac death should not be used to describe events that are not fatal." Correct identification of future SCD victims is especially important as there is an effective treatment, namely, defibrillation via an external or internal (implanted) defibrillator. Currently, the commonly used SCD risk score based on left ventricular ejection fraction can only predict some cardiac arrest events. There is an urgent need for more effective and reliable SCD risk early warning methods. The rapid development of ECG signals, genetic markers, and a combination of multiple index risk scoring models, including the foregoing two, have opened new paths for SCD early warning diagnosis.

**Keywords**

Sudden cardiac death (SCD) · Sudden cardiac arrest (SCA) · Definition · Genetic markers · Risk score

Z. Gao · F. Zhang · C. Yu · Z. Tang (✉)
Emergency Department, Beijing Chao-Yang Hospital, Beijing, China



H. Zhu (ed.), *Sudden Death*, https://doi.org/10.1007/978-981-15-7002-5_8

Sudden cardiac death (SCD) refers to sudden accidental death within 1 or 24 h after the onset of symptoms and to exclude death caused by arrhythmia or hemodynamic reasons [1]. Epidemiological investigations have shown that SCD is still a serious public health issue, although significant progress has been made in high-risk patients with implantable cardioverter-defibrillator (ICD) implantation and coronary heart disease prevention. Cardiac arrest and its main outcome, SCD, account for 50% of cardiovascular deaths, causing serious health threats and huge social burdens worldwide [2]. Survival analysis shows that the survival rate of patients with cardiac arrest outside the hospital is less than 10%, and even if the cardiac arrest occurs in the hospital, the incidence of survival to hospital rescue is less than 25% [3]. Therefore, the early diagnosis of SCD is particularly important, and a reliable and effective early diagnosis method of SCD is urgently needed to improve the severe social health status of SCD diagnosis and treatment.

Left ventricular ejection fraction (LVEF) is an important indicator for clinical evaluation of left ventricular systolic function and has been widely used as an indication criterion for ICD treatment. The latest US SCD prevention management guidelines released in September 2018 have once again emphasized the importance of LVEF as an early warning indicator of SCD and an indicator of whether or not to implant CD [1]. However, there is evidence that more than 50% of patients with high-risk SCD after myocardial infarction often do not show a decrease in LVEF or show only a slight decrease in LVEF [4]. In addition, even in high-risk SCD populations with significantly reduced LVEF, only 10–30% of patients can benefit from ICD treatment [5]. Therefore, the results of more and more large clinical studies show that the effectiveness of LVEF as an indicator of SCD risk stratification faces major challenges. The direct cause of SCD is mainly malignant arrhythmia events, which are mostly manifested as ventricular tachycardia, ventricular fibrillation, cardiac arrest, etc., and the cardiac function index LVEF is not sufficient to sensitively reflect changes in the patient's ECG activity. Because SCD mainly comes from malignant arrhythmias, the SCD warning value of ECG signals has great potential.

At present, the field of ECG detection technology continues to develop, and a variety of ECG characteristics have played an important role in predicting sudden cardiac death in the clinic.

## 8.1 Heart Rate

1. Resting heart rate is a simple indicator commonly used in clinical practice. High-level resting heart rate has been reported by many studies to be related to the risk of sudden cardiac death. A prospective study in Paris showed that those with a high level of resting heart rate (75 beats/min) had a risk of sudden cardiac death approximately four times as high as those with low resting heart rate (<65 beats/min) [6].
2. Heart rate turbulence: Heart rate turbulence describes a short-term change in heart rate caused by ventricular premature beats (VVTs). It usually manifests as a significant acceleration of the heart rate (T0) followed by a gradual heart rate

deceleration (TS). Abnormal heart rate turbulence has been reported to be significantly associated with all-cause death and sudden cardiac death, especially in patients with heart failure after myocardial infarction [7]. Similarly, some studies have shown that heart rate turbulence is significantly related to cardiovascular death and can effectively predict the occurrence of sudden cardiac death in patients after acute myocardial infarction, and its prediction efficiency has significantly improved after combining with other ECG characteristics [8].

3. Heart rate variability: Heart rate variability refers to the frequency variation between heart beats, which reflects the state of cardiac autonomic nerve function, and can predict the occurrence of sudden cardiac death in patients with chronic heart failure [9].

## 8.2 12-Lead ECG

### 8.2.1 Deep Negative of P Wave in Lead V1

Deep terminal negativity of P wave in V1 (DTNPVl) is a marker of atrial abnormality, defined as biphasic P wave detected by resting 12-lead ECG, and negative P wave amplitude>1 mm. DTNPV1 is closely related to all-cause death, cardiovascular disease death, and ischemic heart disease death in the adult population. It is a simple but effective prognostic indicator [10, 11].

### 8.2.2 QT Interval

Corrected QT interval (QTc) is a classic indicator for the diagnosis of cardiac ion channel diseases (such as long QT syndrome and short QT syndrome, etc.), but its clinical value is not limited to the diagnosis of cardiac ion channel disease. It can be extended to the risk diagnosis of heart failure, diabetes, and other diseases [12]. The prolongation of the QT interval reflects the prolongation of the action potential of cells, which in turn leads to the activation of L-type calcium ion channels, which eventually leads to cardiovascular events [13].

### 8.2.3 QRS Wave

1. In a follow-up study in Finland, the risk of sudden cardiac death in patients with QRS duration (QRSd) ≥110 ms was 2.5 times higher than in patients with QRSd <96 ms [14]. QRSd is an independent risk factor for cardiovascular death, and an increase in QRSd every 10 ms results in an 18% increase in the risk of cardiovascular death [15].
2. QRS dispersion (QRS dispersion) refers to the maximum QRSd and minimum QRSd in a 12-lead ECG. Difference. QRSd has been reported as an independent predictor of sudden cardiac death in arrhythmic right ventricular cardiomyopa-

thy populations [16]. In patients with heart failure, QRSd is significantly associated with left ventricular systolic dysfunction and can effectively predict sudden cardiac death [17].

3. Fragmented QRS (fQRS) refers to a multiphase QRS wave that appears in two or more adjacent leads of a 12-lead ECG and complete or incomplete bundle branch block and complete right bundle branch block. Studies have reported that fQRS can be used as a predictor of myocardial scars and also predict arrhythmic events in non-ischemic cardiomyopathy [18].
4. QRS. The QRS-T angle refers to the angle between the QRS wave and the T-wave electrical axis and can be divided into a space angle and a frontal angle. A case-control study showed that the positive QRS-T angle was significantly associated with sudden cardiac death and that its predictive value was independent of the left ventricular ejection fraction [19–21].
5. QRS points are scores composed of the Q, R, and S wave amplitude, time history, and notch of each lead. In ischemic cardiomyopathy, QRS scores are still highly reliable in the evaluation of myocardial scars compared to the myocardial nuclear magnetic resonance that is currently prevalent [22]. Increased QRS scores have been shown to be closely related to ventricular arrhythmias, the occurrence of ICD discharges, and decreased left ventricular inverse remodeling [23].

### 8.2.4 T Wave

T wave alternans (TWA) refers to the phenomenon in which the shape, amplitude, and polarity of T waves alternately change step by step in an electrocardiogram. TWA is mainly produced by the alternating repolarization of a single myocardial cell. Other possible mechanisms include calcium imbalance, myocardial memory, and mechanical-electrical feedback [24]. TWA can be observed in various disease states, such as myocardial infarction, heart failure, long QT syndrome, and Brugada syndrome. TWA is highly consistent with intracardiac electrophysiology in predicting sudden cardiac death and can be used as a predictor of sudden cardiac death [25].

### 8.2.5 Others

(1) Index of cardiac electrophysiological balance (iCEB) is calculated from the ratio of QT interval to QRSd (iCEB = QT/QRSd), which can effectively predict arrhythmia events caused by multiple drugs [26]. (2) Ventricular ectopic QRS interval (VEQSI) refers to the maximum interval between ventricular ectopic fluctuations. A health-based study in Italy found that VEQSI is significantly associated with structural heart disease and can help predict all-cause mortality [27]. (3) Waveform heterogeneity is the rapid development of computer image recognition technology, which makes the digitization of ECG and more complicated calculation indicators possible. Some studies have used the residual algorithm to evaluate the

heterogeneity of R waves and T waves on each lead and provided a better predictive model for the risk of arrhythmia than conventional ECG [28]. There are also studies that used the second-order central moment analysis method to process the electronic 12-lead ECG of 5618 adults, and the results show that the increase in R wave, J wave, and T wave heterogeneity is significantly related to the occurrence of sudden cardiac death, and even after adjusting for conventional risk factors, the heterogeneity of J wave and T wave is still significantly associated with sudden cardiac death, suggesting that waveform heterogeneity can provide more ECG information and help assess the risk of sudden cardiac death [29].

In recent decades, with the rapid development of high-throughput sequencing technology, more and more whole-genome association studies (GWAS) have been implemented, and the genetic markers of SCD have gained more recognition. For example, in hypertrophic cardiomyopathy, mutations in the myocardial sarcomere gene can explain about 60% of the etiology of hypertrophic cardiomyopathy, with MYBPC3 and MYH7 being the most common. Studies have confirmed that patients with hypertrophic cardiomyopathy who carry multiple mutations in disease-causing genes will face a higher risk of SCD and a worse disease prognosis [30]. Long QT syndrome often shows autosomal dominant inheritance, and the exact pathogenic genes can be detected in more than 85% of patients. More than 15 gene mutations are closely related to the disease. In familial long QT syndrome, even carriers of genetic mutations who are asymptomatic and have normal ECG examinations have a risk of developing cardiac events about ten times higher than those of non-mutated carriers [31]. Therefore, this increasing evidence suggests that genetic testing can play an extremely important role in SCD risk warning [32].

In addition to the above cardiac function indicators, ECG signals, and genetic markers, there are still many other factors that may be related to SCD risk, such as age, gender, ethnicity, and disease history. Combining multiple predictive factors into a scoring system can more improve the prediction of SCD risk. For example, the CHA2DS2-VASc score that has been used clinically to assess the risk of stroke in patients with atrial fibrillation (AF) has been reported to be significantly associated with SCD events in patients with AF [33]. Based on the well-known ARIC cohort study, some researchers have proposed a SCD risk scoring system that includes a variety of traditional risk factors. The scoring system includes age, gender, total cholesterol, lipid-lowering drugs, hypertension drugs, systolic blood pressure, and diastolic blood pressure. Ten risk factors including smoking status, smoking status, diabetes, and body mass index build an index function prediction model, which predicts the risk of SCD in the community population and the actual observed risk is very close: And this study also used the Framingham cohort to verify the scoring system, suggesting the scoring system can effectively predict community SCD high-risk populations [34].

Obviously, in the routine diagnosis and treatment work, high-risk patients need to get an arrhythmia risk assessment quickly. At the same time, in view of the current SCD risk assessment's complete reliance on LVEF and the high medical costs of ICD treatment, other clinical-based, predictive indicators that are independent of LVEF are urgently needed. Electrocardiogram as a routine examination has the advantages of being simple, fast, effective, and inexpensive, and it is also very suitable for capturing the electrophysiological abnormalities of patients with high-risk SCD. We have reason to believe that with the rapid development of computer science, next-generation sequencing technology, and big data science, various new types of ECG characteristics, genetic markers, and a scoring system composed of multiple risk factors are likely to provide SCD warnings. More valuable information. In addition, the rapid popularization of wireless signal transmission technology and wearable devices has made it possible to extract and analyze remote ECG features, which will greatly expand the individualization, real time, and effectiveness of SCD risk prevention and control based on ECG monitoring. It is expected that SCD early warning for the general population will be truly realized in the near future.

## 8.3 The Evolution of Diagnostic Criteria of Sudden Cardiac Death

Sudden death (SD) is usually the first clinical manifestation of an underlying disease in previously asymptomatic, apparently "healthy" subjects [35]. Sudden death is a major problem that has significant impact on public health. Many conditions can predispose to sudden cardiac death (SCD) and sudden cardiac arrest (SCA) [36, 37]. Various criteria have been used to define sudden cardiac arrest and sudden cardiac death in the medical literature [38]. Difficulties in deriving a specific definition include the following:

- Events are witnessed in only two-thirds of cases, which makes the diagnosis difficult to establish in many instances.
- It is too hard to restrict the definition of SCA to documented cases of VF since the cardiac rhythm at clinical presentation is unknown in so many cases.
- The duration of symptoms prior to SCA generally defines the suddenness of death. However, the duration of symptoms is unknown in approximately one-third of cases.

Therefore operational criteria for SCA and SCD have been proposed that do not rely on the cardiac rhythm at the right time of the event. The criteria focus on the out-of-hospital occurrence of a presumed sudden pulseless condition and the absence of evidence of a noncardiac condition (e.g., central airway obstruction, intracranial hemorrhage, pulmonary embolism) as the cause of cardiac arrest.

An international multidisciplinary conference held at the Utstein Abbey near Stavanger in June 1990. The purpose of this meeting was to develop uniform terms and definitions for out-of-hospital resuscitation. The term "Utstein style" is synonymous with consensus reporting guidelines for resuscitation from then on [38, 39]. The original Utstein recommendations focused on patients with non-emergency medical services—witnessed cardiac arrest of presumed cardiac cause, with ventricular fibrillation at the point of first rhythm analysis. At that time, cardiac arrest was defined as the cessation of cardiac mechanical activity, which confirmed by pulseless, by unresponsiveness, and by apnea (or agonal, gasping respirations). For the purposes of the Utstein style, no comment on time or "suddenness" was recommended [40].

The Utstein definitions were revised in 2004 with the purposes of reducing complexity and updating data elements based on advances in resuscitation science [41]. The Utstein 2004 revision broadened this focus on including all EMS-treated cardiac arrests no matter what the first monitored rhythm is and whether or not the arrests were witnessed. Other changes in 2004 related to the definition of cardiac arrest (transition from carotid pulse to signs of circulation), including defibrillation attempts by bystanders, and extension of the template to include reporting of in-hospital cardiac arrest (IHCA) in adults and children in the same template [41, 42]. The 2004 Utstein resuscitation registry template for out-of-hospital cardiac arrest was updated in 2015, which balances the necessity of uniform collection of evidence-based factors associated with outcome and the challenges of real-life data collection and validation. Because substantial between in-hospital and out-of-hospital epidemiology, process of care, and treatments are different, a decision was made again to use separate reporting templates [43]. And a 2019 update was focused on in-hospital cardiac arrest [44].

The Utstein elements of the latest out-of-hospital cardiac arrest were grouped into five domains. Each domain contained both core and supplemental elements. Some important subgroups are identified which allow an estimate of the specific contribution of rhythm and bystander actions that are the key determinants of outcome [43].

The 2006 American College of Cardiology/American Heart Association/Heart Rhythm Society (ACC/AHA/HRS Writing Committee to establish data standards for electrophysiology) included definitions to guide documentation in research and clinical practice [45].

The following definitions of SCA and SCD were presented:

> "[Sudden] cardiac arrest is the sudden cessation of cardiac activity so that the victim becomes unresponsive, with no normal breathing and no signs of circulation. If corrective measures are not taken rapidly, this condition progresses to sudden death. Cardiac arrest should be used to signify an event as described above, that is reversed, usually by CPR and/or defibrillation or cardioversion, or cardiac pacing. Sudden cardiac death should not be used to describe events that are not fatal."

Sudden cardiac death is unexpected death within 1 h of symptoms [46]. It is a devastating and tragic outcome of numbers of underlying cardiovascular diseases. While coronary artery disease and acute myocardial infarction are the most probable causes of SCD in older populations, genetic cardiac disorders comprise a substantial proportion of SCD cases aged ≤40. It includes primary arrhythmogenic disorders such as long QT syndromes and inherited cardiomyopathies. In 30% of young SCD, no cause of death is identified at postmortem, which is called autopsy-negative or sudden arrhythmic death syndrome (SADS). Since these disorders rarely cause structural change to the heart, postmortem is often "negative." That means no cause of death is identified at postmortem, including normal histopathology and normal toxicology analysis [47].

Worldwide, less than 1% of those who experience sudden cardiac arrest can finally survive [48]. Widespread accessibility of automated external defibrillators and effective utilization of public defibrillation programs can improve management of out-of-hospital cardiac arrest [49]. The investigation of sudden death involves five steps:

1. Clinical features, including the history and circumstances of death.
2. Autopsy examination and histology.
3. Further laboratory tests including toxicology.
4. Formulation of a diagnosis.
5. Recommendation for family screening by specialized cardiologists [46].

SCD pressingly requires primary prevention since the first clinical event is always fatal, especially in patients with ventricular tachyarrhythmias. Patients with acute bradyarrhythmias usually retain a basal circulation. Accordingly, the appropriate treatment (such as pacemaker) can be deployed in time to prevent irreversible MODS when a sudden bradyarrhythmia occurs. However, VF often results in a rapid and complete loss of blood circulation. This condition will result in irreversible organ (especially the brain) damage after a few minutes if untreated timely. Only a very small proportion of patients suffering from VF can leave the hospital alive even in the regions with highly developed emergency medical care systems. Despite recent efforts to improve the treatment in the community setting by using semiautomatic external defibrillators, primary prevention of SCD is such a diagnostic challenge that it requires identification of future sudden death victims prior to the first arrhythmia episode. Correct identification of future SCD victims is important, cause there is an effective treatment, which is called defibrillation via an external or internal (implanted) defibrillator [50].

## References


1. Al Khatib SM, Stevenson WG, Ackerman MJ, et al. 2017 AHA/ACC/HRS guideline for management of patients with ventricular arrhythmias and the prevention of sudden cardiac death. Circulation. 2018;138(13):272–391.
2. Thomas H, Diamond J, Vieco A, et al. Global atlas of cardiovascular disease 2000–2016: the path to prevention and control. Glob Heart. 2018;13(3):143–63.
3. Benjamin EJ, Blaha MJ, Chiuve SE, et al. Heart disease and stroke Statistics-2017 update: a report from the American Heart Association. Circulation. 2017;135(10):e146–603.
4. Chow T, Kereiakes DJ, Onufer J, et al. Does microvolt T-wave Alternans testing predict ventricular Tachyarrhythmias in patients with ischemic cardiomyopathy and prophylactic defibrillators?: the MASTER (microvolt T wave Alternans testing for risk stratification of post-myocardial infarction patients) trial. J Am Coll Cardiol. 2008;52(20):1607–15.
5. Jouven X, Zureik M, Desnos M, et al. Resting heart rate as a predictive risk factor for sudden death in middle-aged men. Cardiovasc Res. 2001;50(2):373–8.

6. Gorgels A. Out-of-hospital cardiac arrest-the relevance of heart failure. The Maastricht circulatory Arrest registry. Eur Heart J. 2003;24(13):1204–9.
7. Cygankiewicz I. Heart rate turbulence. Prog Cardiovasc Dis. 2013;56(2):160–71.
8. Disertori M, Mase M, Rigoni M, et al. Heart rate turbulence is a powerful predictor of cardiac death and ventricular arrhythmias in postmyocardial infarction and heart failure patients: a systematic review and meta-analysis. Circ Arrhythm Electrophysiol. 2016;9(12):e004610.
9. Al-Zaiti SS, Pietrasik G, Carey MG, et al. The role of heart rate variability, heart rate turbulence, and deceleration capacity in predicting cause-specific mortality in chronic heart failure. J Electrocardiol. 2019;52(1):70–4.
10. Tereshchenko LG, Shah AJ, Li Y, et al. Electrocardiographic deep terminal negativity of the P wave in V1 and risk of mortality: the National Health and nutrition examination survey III. J Cardiovasc Electrophysiol. 2014;25(11):1242–8.
11. Tereshchenko LG, Henrikson CA, Sotoodehnia N, et al. Electrocardiographic deep terminal negativity of the P wave in V(1) and risk of sudden cardiac death: the atherosclerosis risk in communities (ARIC) study. J Am Heart Assoc. 2014;3(6):e001387.
12. Stettler C, Bearth A, Allemann S, et al. QTc interval and resting heart rate as long-term predictors of mortality in type 1 and type 2 diabetes mellitus: a 23-year follow-up. Diabetologia. 2007;50(1):186–94.
13. January CT, Riddle JM. Early after depolarizations: mechanism of induction and block. A role for L-type Ca2+ current. Circ Res. 1989;64(5):977–90.
14. Kurl S, Makikallio TH, Rautaharju P, et al. Duration of QRS complex in resting electrocardiogram is a predictor of sudden cardiac death in men. Circulation. 2012;125(21):2588–94.
15. Desai AD, Yaw TS, Yamazaki T, et al. Prognostic significance of quantitative QRS duration. Am J Med. 2006;119(7):600–6.
16. Turrini P, Corrado D, Basso C, et al. Dispersion of ventricular depolarization-repolarization: a noninvasive marker for risk stratification in arrhythmogenic right ventricular cardiomyopathy. Circulation. 2001;103(25):3075–2080.
17. Kountouris E, Korantzopoulos P, Karanikis P, et al. QRS dispersion: an electrocardiographic index of systolic left ventricular dysfunction in patients with left bundle branch block. Int J Cardiol. 2004;97(2):321–2.
18. Das MK, Zipes DP. Fragmented QRS: a predictor of mortality and sudden cardiac death. Heart Rhythm. 2009;6(3):S8–14.
19. Chua KC, Teodorescu C, Reinier K, et al. Wide QRS-T angle on the 12-Lead ECG as a prediction of sudden death beyond the LV ejection fraction. J Cardiovasc Electrophysiol. 2016;27(7):833–9.
20. Lingman M, Hartford M, Karlsson T, et al. Value of the QRS-T area angle in improving the prediction of sudden cardiac death after acute coronary syndromes. Int J Cardiol. 2016;218(1):1–11.
21. Laukkanen JA, Di Angelantonio E, Khan H, et al. T-wave inversion, QRS duration, and QRS/T angle as electrocardiographic predictors of the risk for sudden cardiac death. Am J Cardiol. 2014;113(7):1178–83.
22. Mewton N, Strauss DG, Rizzi P, et al. Screening for cardiac magnetic resonance scar features by 12-Lead ECG, in patients with preserved ejection fraction. Ann Noninvasive Electrocardiol. 2016;21(1):49–59.
23. Sweeney MO, van Bommel RJ, Schalij MJ, et al. Analysis of ventricular activation using surface electrocardiography to predict left ventricular reverse volumetric remodeling during cardiac resynchronization therapy. Circulation. 2010;121(5):626–34.
24. Takasugi N, Goto H, Kuwahara T, et al. Sudden paradoxical QT-interval prolongation exacerbating T-wave alternans in a patient with type 3 long QT syndrome. Ann Noninvasive Electrocardiol. 2015;20(3):290–1.
25. Narayan SM. T-wave alternans and the susceptibility to ventricular arrhythmias. J Am Coll Cardiol. 2006;47(2):269–81.

26. Lu HR, Yan GX, Gallacher DJ. A new biomarker—index of cardiac electrophysiological balance (iCEB) – plays an important role in drug-induced cardiac arrhythmias: beyond QT-prolongation and Torsades de pointes (TdPs). J Pharmacol Toxicol Methods. 2013;68(2):250–9.
27. Gallagher MM, Padula M, Sgueglia M, et al. Electrocardiographic markers of structural heart disease and predictors of death in 2332 unselected patients undergoing outpatient Holter recording. Europace. 2007;9(12):1203–8.
28. Bastiaenen R, Pantazis A, Gonna H, et al. The ventricular ectopic QRS interval (VEQSI): diagnosis of arrhythmogenic right ventricular cardiomyopathy in patients with incomplete disease expression. Heart Rhythm. 2016;13(7):1504–12.
29. Kentta TV, Nearing BD, Porthan K, et al. Prediction of sudden cardiac death with automated high-throughput analysis of heterogeneity in standard resting 12-lead electrocardiograms. Heart Rhythm. 2016;13(3):713–20.
30. Driest SLV, Vasile VC, Ommen SR, et al. Myosin binding protein C mutations and compound heterozygosity in hypertrophic cardiomyopathy. J Am Coll Cardiol. 2004;44(9):1903–10.
31. Goldenberg I, Horr S, Moss AJ, Lopes CM, et al. Risk for life-threatening cardiac events in patients with genotype-confirmed long-QT syndrome and normal-range corrected QT intervals. J Am Coll Cardiol. 2011;57(1):51–9.
32. Bezzina CR, Lahrouchi N, Priori SG. Genetics of sudden cardiac death. Circ Res. 2015;116(12):1919.
33. Kuo L, Chao TF, Liu CJ. Usefulness of the CHA2DS2-VASc score to predict the risk of sudden cardiac death and ventricular arrhythmias in patients with atrial fibrillation. Am J Cardiol. 2018;122(12):2049–54.
34. Bogle BM, Ning H, Goldberger JJ, et al. A simple community-based risk prediction score for sudden cardiac death. Am J Med. 2018;131(5):532–9.
35. Basso C, et al. Guidelines for autopsy investigation of sudden cardiac death: 2017 update from the Association for European Cardiovascular Pathology. Virchows Arch. 2017;471(6):691–705.
36. Estes NA III, De Nofrio D. The challenge of prediction and prevention of sudden cardiac death in congestive heart failure. J Interv Card Electrophysiol. 2001;5(1):5–8.
37. Morin DP, Homoud MK, Estes NAM 3rd. Prediction and prevention of sudden cardiac death. Card Electrophysiol Clin. 2017;9(4):631–8.
38. Schmidt G. Sudden cardiac death: diagnostic help from chaos research? Prof. Dr. med. Georg Schmidt, Munich, on preventive diagnostic criteria. Interview by Beatrice Wagner. Fortschr Med. 1996;114(1–2):14, 16–7.
39. Nolan J, Soar J. Images in resuscitation: the ECG in hypothermia. Resuscitation. 2005;64(2):133–4.
40. Cummins RO, et al. Recommended guidelines for uniform reporting of data from out-of-hospital cardiac arrest: the Utstein style. A statement for health professionals from a task force of the American Heart Association, the European resuscitation council, the Heart and Stroke Foundation of Canada, and the Australian resuscitation council. Circulation. 1991;84(2):960–75.
41. Jacobs I, et al. Cardiac arrest and cardiopulmonary resuscitation outcome reports: update and simplification of the Utstein templates for resuscitation registries. A statement for healthcare professionals from a task force of the international liaison committee on resuscitation (American Heart Association, European Resuscitation Council, Australian Resuscitation Council, New Zealand Resuscitation Council, Heart and Stroke Foundation of Canada, InterAmerican Heart Foundation, Resuscitation Council of Southern Africa). Resuscitation. 2004;63(3):233–49.
42. Nishiyama C, et al. Apples to apples or apples to oranges? International variation in reporting of process and outcome of care for out-of-hospital cardiac arrest. Resuscitation. 2014;85(11):1599–609.
43. Perkins GD, et al. Cardiac arrest and cardiopulmonary resuscitation outcome reports: update of the Utstein Resuscitation Registry Templates for Out-of-Hospital Cardiac Arrest: a statement for healthcare professionals from a task force of the International Liaison Committee on

Resuscitation (American Heart Association, European Resuscitation Council, Australian and New Zealand Council on Resuscitation, Heart and Stroke Foundation of Canada, InterAmerican Heart Foundation, Resuscitation Council of Southern Africa, Resuscitation Council of Asia); and the American Heart Association Emergency Cardiovascular Care Committee and the Council on Cardiopulmonary, Critical Care, Perioperative and Resuscitation. Resuscitation. 2015;96:328–40.
44. Nolan JP, et al. Cardiac arrest and cardiopulmonary resuscitation outcome reports: update of the Utstein Resuscitation Registry Template for In-Hospital Cardiac Arrest: a consensus report from a Task Force of the International Liaison Committee on Resuscitation (American Heart Association, European Resuscitation Council, Australian and New Zealand Council on Resuscitation, Heart and Stroke Foundation of Canada, InterAmerican Heart Foundation, Resuscitation Council of Southern Africa, Resuscitation Council of Asia). Circulation. 2019;140(18):e746–57.
45. Kirchhof P, Breithardt G, Eckardt L. Primary prevention of sudden cardiac death. Heart. 2006;92(12):1873–8.
46. Sheppard MN. The pathological investigation of sudden cardiac death. Br J Hosp Med (Lond). 2010;71(11):604–5.
47. Semsarian C, Ingles J, Wilde AA. Sudden cardiac death in the young: the molecular autopsy and a practical approach to surviving relatives. Eur Heart J. 2015;36(21):1290–6.
48. Pochmalicki G, et al. Management of sudden death in a semi-rural district, seine-et-Marne: the DEFI 77 study. Arch Mal Coeur Vaiss. 2007;100(10):838–44.
49. Sukhija R, et al. Implantable cardioverter defibrillators for prevention of sudden cardiac death. Clin Cardiol. 2007;30(1):3–8.
50. Priori SG, et al. Update of the guidelines on sudden cardiac death of the European Society of Cardiology. Eur Heart J. 2003;24(1):13–5.

# Chronic Fatigue Stress and Sudden Death

9

Haiyan Zhu and Guoxin Han

**Abstract**

With the development of today's society, the pace of people's work and life is accelerating. This common negative stress that people currently suffer is caused by long-term physical fatigue and excessive mental load, as well as the depression and irritability. The sudden death led by chronic fatigue has not only brought huge disasters to their families but also had serious negative effects on social production. This chapter mainly describes chronic fatigue stress and sudden death.

**Keywords**

Sudden death · Chronic fatigue · Stress

## 9.1 Definition of Stress

The word stress is heard every day and is a polysemous word used to express multiple meanings. Since the middle of the twentieth century, stress scientist H. Selye has expounded on the diversity and non-specificity of the definition and explanation of stress. Stress is caused by the stabs, certain events, and certain conditions caused by the increase of physical and mental load. The external stimuli that cause stress

H. Zhu (✉)
Emergency Department, The First Medical Center of Chinese PLA General Hospital, Beijing, China

Emergency Department, Hainan Hospital of Chinese PLA General Hospital, Haitangwan Bay, Sanya City, Hainan Province, China

G. Han
Emergency Department of Strategic Support Force Special Medical Center, Chaoyang, Beijing, China



H. Zhu (ed.), *Sudden Death*, https://doi.org/10.1007/978-981-15-7002-5_9

are called stress. Stress is categorized into too much stress and too little stress and qualitatively divided into beneficial stress and harmful stress. There are many kinds of stress such as physical, chemical, physical, psychological, and social environmental. Regardless of the type of stress, stress is a non-specific response of the body and is a systemic adaptation syndrome mediated by the hypothalamus-pituitary-adrenal cortex system. Later, in the body response caused by stress, it is related to endocrine, autonomic nervous system, and neuro-immunity [1].

Modern medicine believes that stress is an emotional state caused by dangerous or unexpected changes in external conditions and is a psychological factor that may arise in decision-making psychological activities [2]. Stress-causing stimuli can be physical, psychological, and sociocultural. However, these stimuli usually do not directly cause stress, and there are many intermediary factors between stimulus and stress, such as human health, personality characteristics, life experience, coping ability, cognitive evaluation, beliefs, and the quality of social support received, which can play an important regulatory role. During stress, a series of changes occur in the internal organs. After the central brain receives external stimuli, the information is transmitted to the hypothalamus, secretes corticotropin-releasing factor (CRF), and then stimulates the pituitary gland to secrete corticotropin, so that the body is fully mobilized. Significant changes in muscle tension, metabolic levels, etc. increase the strength of the body's activity to cope with emergencies.

### 9.1.1 Stress Structure

A stressor is a stimulus that causes stress or tension; stress itself is a special state of physical and mental tension; stress response is a physical and psychological response to a stressor, also known as physiological and psychological stress [3].

### 9.1.2 Performance of Stressors

There are mainly two performances of stress. One is activity suppression or complete disorder, or even errors in sensory memory, showing an unadaptive response, such as stunned, confused, and distressed; the other is the mobilization of various forces to deal with emergencies, such as to act quickly and get out of trouble. Under stress, the biochemical system undergoes drastic changes, the secretion of adrenaline and glands increases, and the body's vitality increases, so that the entire body is fully mobilized to cope with unexpected changes. Being in a state of stress for a long time is harmful to human health and may even be dangerous.

In 1974, a study by Canadian physiologist G. Selye showed that the continuous state of stress can defeat a person's biochemical protection mechanism, reduce the person's resistance, and easily cause psychosomatic diseases. He referred to the stress response as systemic adaptation syndrome and divided it into three phases: (1) The alarm phase is manifested by increased adrenaline secretion; increased heart rate; decreased body temperature and muscle elasticity, anemia, and blood glucose levels; and a temporary increase in gastric acidity which may lead to shock. (2) The impedance phase shows the disappearance of symptoms in the panic phase. The body mobilizes many protective systems to resist the causes of the crisis. At this time, the level of systemic metabolism increases and the liver releases a large amount of blood sugar. If the time is too long, a large amount of sugar can be consumed in the body, and excessive activities of the hypothalamus, pituitary, and adrenal system will cause physical damage to the internal organs and symptoms such as gastric ulcer and thymus degeneration. (3) The exhaustion stage is manifested by the almost exhaustion of various storages in the body, and the body is in a crisis state, which can lead to serious illness or death. Therefore, it is necessary to minimize and avoid unnecessary stress states and learn to treat stress states scientifically.

## 9.2 Chronic Fatigue Stress

Fatigue is a very common phenomenon and is associated with a considerable degree of physical and mental illness. Fatigue is a common complaint in primary and specialty medicine. Fatigue is the main symptom of chronic fatigue syndrome (CFS), which is related to many acute and chronic diseases such as rheumatoid arthritis, cancer, and multiple sclerosis [4]. It is also commonly found in certain medical treatments, such as radiotherapy or chemotherapy. In many of these cases, fatigue is often one of the most important causes of disability, and patients with severe health conditions often treat it as one of the most serious symptoms. Fatigue can be a normal response to activity or stress, but it can also be a sign of certain illnesses. In this sense, fatigue can be considered physiological or pathological. For healthy individuals, fatigue is a physiological response to strenuous and prolonged activity; it is predictable and short-lived and can be relieved after a break without affecting daily activities. Jason defined pathological fatigue as a fatigue that lasts more than 3 months and is more intense than the fatigue experienced previously, affecting daily activities and quality of life. Due to the lack of accurate definitions of fatigue and differences in measurement techniques, there are significant differences in reported prevalence. The prevalence of fatigue in primary care is between 7% and 45%. An epidemiological study in the United States found that 24% of people suffer from fatigue. Addington's analysis of epidemiological follow-up samples found that the unexplained lifetime prevalence of fatigue is 20% and the duration is 2 weeks or more. Some community epidemiological studies have reported high fatigue rates in the general population. For example, Norwegian prevalence is 22%, Dutch prevalence is 25%, UK prevalence is 18%, and US prevalence is 20%, and data on fatigue rates in China are currently lacking [5–7].

Chronic fatigue stress refers to the stress state of the human body under long-term exposure to fatigue, which is a kind of physiological fatigue. Also known as fatigue subhealth, chronic fatigue stress is common in countries and regions with developed economies and fierce social competition. The number of people has been increasing year by year, and it has become one of the hot topics in the international medical community. The proposition of the concept of chronic fatigue stress is not accidental. It is the embodiment of the new health concept that modern people pay attention to preventing the disease from happening or developing. Although sub-health manifests problems in the medical field in terms of symptoms, as a whole, it is inseparable from the social environment; economic, cultural, and psychological factors; and physical quality. Chronic fatigue stress can also be called the third state of the human body, including no clinical symptoms or mild feelings, but there is already underlying pathological information [6]. It has a wide range of connotations. It is people's emotional experience about health or subhealth. The chronic fatigue stress state is constantly changing and developing, and it can be transformed into a healthy state or a disease state, which depends on the self-care measures and the immunity to the disease. And the transition to a healthy state requires measures such as precautions, self-care awareness, and properly adjusting the dietary structure. Chronic fatigue stress has a large space-time span. Research on it is still in its infancy, and several issues remain to be explored. Due to differences in people's age, adaptability, immunity, sociocultural level, etc., the symptoms of chronic fatigue stress are intricate and complex. The more common are reduced vitality response ability, adaptive ability and immunity, physical fatigue, cold, tiredness after a short movement, sweating, loss of appetite, headache, insomnia, anxiety, uncoordinated interpersonal relationships, family harmony, sexual dysfunction, etc. The symptoms of chronic fatigue stress include chronic fatigue syndrome, excess information syndrome, neurasthenia, and obesity.

### 9.2.1 Epidemiology of Chronic Fatigue Stress

The population in a state of subhealth disease is increasing in many countries and regions. According to statistics, six million people in the United States are suspected of being sub-healthy every year, and they are between 20 and 45 years old [8]. China has more than 700 million people in a sub-health state, accounting for 60% to 70% of the country's total population. Middle-aged people in China are a sub-healthy population. As early as the 1970s and 1980s, fatigue became a serious health problem in developed countries [9]. A survey in the United States found that 14% of adult men and 20% of women show significant fatigue, and one in eight develops chronic fatigue syndrome [10]. Surveys in the United Kingdom show that approximately 20% of men and 25% of women always experience fatigue, of which approximately a quarter may be chronic fatigue syndrome. At present, the number of people with chronic fatigue syndrome is increasing year by year. The number of people in the United States is mostly among young whites with a higher socioeconomic status. Medical staff, especially nurses, have a higher incidence than the general population. Japanese medical experts listed 27 kinds of symptoms and factors of excessive fatigue [11]. Among them, more than seven of them are those who are at risk for excessive fatigue, and those with more than ten items may suffer from overwork at any time. The word "overwork" first appeared in Japan during the economic boom of the 1970s and 1980s. It is not a clinical medical name but belongs to the category of social medicine [12]. In Japan, it is defined as exacerbating underlying diseases such as hypertension due to excessive workload and then causing acute circulatory organ disorders such as cerebrovascular or cardiovascular diseases, which puts patients into a state of death. The cause of death from overwork is the accelerated work rhythm, increased mental stress, and long-term overload work, which exceeds the limits of human physical and mental capacity and leads to overwork [13]. Surveys in China show that the incidence of chronic fatigue syndrome in urban emerging industry populations ranges from 10% to 20% and up to 50% in certain industries, such as technology, news, public servants, entertainers, and taxi drivers. Japan's special survey on fatigue shows that as high as 60% of people are feeling "very tired." Among them, 44% were due to heavy workload, heavy housework, and mental stress, and many people could not explain why. Another survey of 130,000 employees confirmed that the fatigue of "workers" seems to be stronger. Seventy-two percent of people claim to feel very tired at work, and 75% often feel listless or have headaches and dizziness [14]. The reasons are often "interpersonal tension," "promotion too slow," or "too much to learn." Between 1987 and 1989, there were only 180 cases of overwork deaths reported in Japan. Within 1 year in 1995, the general managers of 12 major companies including Kawasaki Steel Co., Ltd., a well-known Japanese company, Seiko, and Japan Airlines all died suddenly, mostly between the ages of 40 and 50. Medical scientists consider their premature death to be caused by overwork. Sociologists believe that a nation's excessive fatigue can affect its national strength, and they emphasize that Japan's suicide rate, divorce rate, and violent crime rate remain high. It is related to the general and persistent fatigue of the people.

### 9.2.2 Diagnosis of Chronic Fatigue Stress

#### 9.2.2.1 Standard Diagnosis of Symptoms

The United States and Japan, which paid close attention to chronic fatigue stress and sub-health problems, have developed diagnostic standards for the most common chronic fatigue syndrome in sub-health states. The US standards consider it necessary to introduce some criteria. People who meet two major fatigue criteria and six or more symptom criteria plus two or more physical symptoms criteria, or a simple symptom criteria of more than 8 criteria, can be diagnosed as chronic fatigue syndrome. On the basis of revising and supplementing the US diagnostic criteria, Japan has determined the criteria for the diagnosis of chronic fatigue syndrome. It should be pointed out that the diagnosis of chronic fatigue syndrome is an exclusion diagnosis. It should be performed on the basis of the belief that other diseases are excluded, and the specific diagnosis cannot be based on medical history or laboratory examination.

#### 9.2.2.2 Quantitative Diagnostics

Chronic fatigue is mostly based on personal feelings. Physical examinations have no positive signs, and various laboratory tests are negative, which makes diagnosis difficult. Therefore, comprehensive quantitative analysis is needed. Inspections are divided into primary inspections and secondary inspections. The first-level examination is a general physical examination. If the symptoms are obvious and the primary examination cannot detect the cause, perform secondary examinations, such as exercise experiments, electroencephalograms, 24 h ambulatory blood pressure monitoring, and psychological status tests on standard scales. Microscopic methods can also be used for individualized physical examination. For example, the body's immune cell function test, blood ultrahigh magnification morphological examination, and disease-related DNA and gene PCR examinations can all find small physiological changes in the human body.

#### 9.2.2.3 MDI Health Assessment

Many scholars use the world's popular MDI health assessment method to carry out quantitative research on chronic fatigue status. It was originally used by WHO to measure the indicators suggested by the diseases that are most harmful to human death and evaluated according to the actual detection status of the subject's scoring (take a 100-point scale, with a perfect score of 100 points), corresponding to WHO's definition of health. The criteria are 85 or higher for health, 70 or lower for disease, and 70–85 for sub-health (third status). MDI-based assessment includes cardiovascular and cerebrovascular disease monitoring and stroke prediction, malignant tumor signs, organ lesions, blood and allergic diseases, blood pollution, endocrine system examination, limb damage detection, and medication effect. Physical indicators, such as detection, and psychological and social disorders increased in recent years. Cai Ronglin's team has two criteria for determining fatigue sub-health. Its contents are the same as what was included in "Clinical Guidelines for Sub-Health Chinese Medicine," including persistent discomfort, or a marked decline in adaptability, which lasts more than 3 months, but can maintain normal work, no major organic diseases and mental and psychiatric diseases, and failure to meet the clinical diagnosis although laboratory test results deviate. The different contents are as follows: using the fatigue scale (FS-14) to evaluate, the total fatigue score is $\geq$3 points; using the fatigue self-assessment scale (FSAS) to evaluate, the score is $\geq$3 points.

## 9.3 Chronic Fatigue Stress and Sudden Death

With the continuous development of today's society, the pace of people's work and life is accelerating, and the physical and mental pressure on young people who are the main productive groups of society is increasing. Long-term physical fatigue and excessive mental load, as well as the consequent depression, irritability, and other bad psychological emotions, together constitute the current state of adverse stress that young people generally suffer. Sudden deaths of young people caused by chronic fatigue stress are common, especially in first-tier cities such as Beijing, Shanghai, Guangzhou, and Shenzhen. The premature death of these lives has not only brought huge disasters to their families but also caused serious negative effects on social production and has created a huge medical and social burden. This article summarizes the content of chronic fatigue stress and sudden cardiac death in young people.

### 9.3.1 Epidemiology of Sudden Cardiac Death in Young People

Surveys show that about 80% of white-collar workers in China are in an overworked state. Among people aged 30 to 50 who died prematurely, 95.7% died of fatal diseases caused by excessive fatigue, of which 80% were sudden cardiac death. Sudden cardiac death (SCD) refers to sudden death due to cardiovascular causes, with or without structural heart disease. SCD is generally considered to be death within 1 h of sudden onset or within 24 h from the last known stable state. The most common causes are acute coronary syndrome, dilated cardiomyopathy, genetic-related rhythm disorders (such as long QT syndrome, Brugada syndrome, and catecholamine-related polymorphic ventricular tachycardia), various types of cardiomyopathy (such as stress cardiomyopathy), and so on [15]. According to statistics, the total number of sudden cardiac deaths in the United States is 300,000 per year, with an annual incidence rate of 0.1%–0.2%. The incidence in Europe is similar to that in the United States. The epidemiological survey of sudden death in the Chinese population shows that the incidence of sudden death in China is 41.84 cases per 100,000 people per year, and the incidence rate is about 0.04% of the general population, which is lower than that of European and American countries. However, based on the country's 1.3 billion people, it is estimated that nearly 544,000 people die suddenly each year in China, with an average of about 1500 people per day. Subject to China's prehospital rescue level and emergency transfer system, the out-of-hospital rescue rate for sudden death in China is less than 1%. Therefore, in-depth study of the relationship between the adverse stress caused by long-term fatigue and sudden death of young people helps to clarify the mechanism of sudden death of young people, and taking effective preventive measures is of great significance to the individual, family, and society [16].

### 9.3.2 Bridge Role of Stress in Sudden Cardiac Death

Stress refers to the physical and psychological tension and response caused by the imbalance between actual or cognitive requirements and the ability to adapt and cope with the body's adaptation to various adverse factors in the living environment [17]. With the advancement of modern medicine, humans have become increasingly aware that the health depends on the biological effects of the interaction between the environment and the body [18]. Environmental factors are one of the important factors in the occurrence of diseases. According to statistics, about 70%–90% of the risk can be attributed to the effects of environmental exposure, while stress is an important interface for the interaction between the environment and the body. Sudden death, as the most serious result of stress diseases, especially the sudden death of young people caused by stress, has been a hot spot in the research of stress diseases at home and abroad in recent years. Similar problems exist in animals. Animals often die quickly when they cannot escape, when they are placed in a place where it is expected that there will be too many strong stimuli, and when the spouse dies. It has been reported that when a camel was shot dead, his spouse died within minutes. The prelude to sudden cardiac death is often arrhythmia, leading to cardiac arrest. Lown puts forward four related hypotheses about the mechanism of stress-induced sudden cardiac death: the direct cause of sudden death is ventricular fibrillation; electrical instability exists long before sudden death; the index reflecting electrical instability is some kind of premature ventricular contractions; and stress can cause electrical instability and increase susceptibility to ventricular fibrillation [19–21]. In addition, long-term intense stimulation of chronic fatigue stress on sympathetic nerves can reduce the pre-contraction stimulation threshold of experimental animals and the threshold of electrical stimulation that causes ventricular fibrillation. Therefore, the sympathetic nerves also play an important role in sudden cardiac death.

### 9.3.3 Chronic Fatigue Stress and Coronary Heart Disease in Young People

Coronary heart disease accounts for 65–80% of sudden cardiac death [22]. As the most important cause of sudden cardiac death, chronic fatigue stress often causes sudden cardiac death in young patients with coronary heart disease. Chronic fatigue stress is not only the cause of early coronary heart disease in young people but also the cause of sudden cardiac death in young patients with coronary heart disease. According to a large number of studies, the occurrence and development of coronary heart disease are related to many biological, psychological, and social factors, including genetics, hypertension, hyperlipidemia, smoking, alcoholism, obesity, type A behavioral patterns, social relationship inconsistency, depression, etc. [23] Disorders of lipid metabolism, hemodynamic changes, and changes in the arterial wall itself are the direct factors of coronary heart disease. Psychological and social factors can affect the above three processes through neuroendocrine mediating mechanisms, thereby affecting the occurrence and development of coronary heart disease. Studies have shown that under chronic fatigue stress conditions such as long working hours, heavy burdens, and performing more than two different jobs, it may increase the incidence and mortality of coronary heart disease. Young patients with coronary heart disease have been chronically fatigued for a long time, causing the accumulation of inflammatory factors and leukocytes to destroy the vascular endothelial structure of the coronary arteries and prompting inflammatory cells in the body to release interleukin and tumor necrosis factor and degrade the extracellular matrix of coronary atheroma. The stability of the plaque is reduced, which leads to acute myocardial infarction due to coronary reocclusion; in addition, the large coronary artery is rich in the distribution of α-adrenergic receptors, and chronic fatigue stress states continue to activate the brain region of the plaque nucleus, which is rich in noradrenergic neurons. Sympathetic nerve tension continues to increase, catecholamine secretion increases, and coronary alpha receptors are excited, causing coronary spasm and prompting recurrence of myocardial infarction in young patients with coronary heart disease, increasing the risk of sudden cardiac death.

### 9.3.4 Chronic Fatigue Stress and Stress Cardiomyopathy in Young People

Stress-induced cardiomyopathy (SCM), also known as Takotsubo cardiomyopathy, is a type of mental or physical stress that is related to temporary abnormalities in the movement of the left ventricle (and possibly the right ventricle). ECG and clinical manifestations of heart disease are very similar to those of acute coronary syndrome. A meta-study found that about 1%–2% of patients admitted to the hospital for diagnosis of acute coronary syndrome, heart failure, and arrhythmia are stress cardiomyopathy, which is currently misdiagnosed due to insufficient clinician knowledge and missed diagnosis [24]. Stress cardiomyopathy is also one of the main causes of sudden cardiac death. Physical stress and mental stress are considered to be the main causes of stress cardiomyopathy. With the increasing pressure of work and life in modern society, young people, as the main force of social productivity, have been in chronic fatigue stress for a long time, leading to the increasing incidence of stress cardiomyopathy. Stress cardiomyopathy, as one of the causes of sudden cardiac death, has gradually attracted the attention of experts and scholars. In a systematic review of young stress cardiomyopathy, Wang Yueyue et al. [25] found that physical stress is the main predisposing factor for young patients with stress cardiomyopathy; the incidence of young women is higher than that of young men, which may be related to the heart of women. It is more sensitive to sympathetic nerves and more prone to systolic dysfunction, and women have more fragile and sensitive traits than men. The mechanism of chronic fatigue stress in the pathophysiological process of stress cardiomyopathy in young people is not clear. The possible pathogenesis is that chronic fatigue stress may cause changes in the brain structure. The human body affects the hypothalamus-pituitary-adrenal cortex. The response sensitivity of the axis is reduced, and the secretion of adrenocorticotropic hormone and glucocorticoid is increased to improve the body's metabolic function activities to cope with the external damaging stress. At the same time, the adrenocorticotropic hormone enhances the release of adrenal medulla adrenaline and norepinephrine leading to the body. Catecholamines remain at high levels for a long time, and the toxic effects of superphysiological amounts of catecholamines on the heart promote the occurrence of stress cardiomyopathy in young people [26–28].

### 9.3.5 Pathogenesis of Arrhythmia Caused by Chronic Fatigue Stress

When the human body is in a state of fatigue stress for a long time, mitochondria produce excessively active molecules such as reactive oxygen species (ROS), and the degree of oxidation exceeds the ability of scavenging oxides, leading to a series of changes in myocardial ion channels leading to ventricularity [29]. Arrhythmia occurs. ROS has been shown to affect Na ion channel function through multiple pathways. At the transcription level, ROS reduces the expression of Nav1.5 sodium channel genes by reducing mRNA expression. At the protein level, ROS directly makes methionine in Nav1.5 sodium channel proteins. Oxidative inactivation leads to a decrease in the peak value of Na ion channel current. ROS can also increase the probability of Na ion channel opening, leading to changes in cardiac rhythm caused by increased sodium current in the later period, including action potential, prolonged depolarization in the early stage, and calcium ion overload [29]. ROS can also affect sodium channel phosphorylation by indirectly changing the membrane lipid environment or by activating signaling molecules such as protein kinase C and calmodulin-dependent protein kinase II to reduce sodium current peaks, leading to arrhythmia. Activation of calmodulin-dependent protein kinase II can also phosphorylate subunits of the Cav1.2 calcium channel, opening up L-type calcium ion channels, increasing calcium influx, and increasing myocardial cell reactivity to isoproterenol, leading to delayed depolarization and systolic dysfunction [30–32]. In addition, excessive ROS in the cell can reduce the current repolarization of potassium ions and prolong the duration of the action potential and the early period of post-depolarization, increasing the electrical heterogeneity of myocardial cells and the susceptibility to arrhythmia. Finally, ROS-induced mitochondrial dysfunction can also cause mitochondrial membrane potential depolarization, leading to the opening of the sarcKATP channel, which in turn forms a sink current that propagates depolarized waves, increasing the possibility of conduction block and arrhythmia [33, 34]. In summary, chronic fatigue stress may cause ventricular arrhythmias by increasing the production of ROS, leading to changes in myocardial ion channels, which may cause sudden cardiac death.

### 9.3.6 Mitochondrial Gene Mutation and Sudden Death in Young People

Mitochondrion is the cell's energy factory. It consumes 98% of oxygen in the body to provide energy for human life activities [35]. It is the core organelle of the cell's redox. Its main function is realized by the electron transfer system of the respiratory chain. The electron transfer chain is composed of four kinds of complexes, including complexes I, II, III, and IV (i.e., NADH dehydrogenase, succinate dehydrogenase, cytochrome C reductase, and cytochrome C oxidase) [36]. During human development, mitochondrial gene mutations are random in human tissues, but as defective mitochondria are destroyed by free radicals for a long time, the average value of mitochondrial mutation ratios in organs or tissues gradually increases. Mutations in the mitochondrial genome follow this pattern. Heterogeneity is a feature, most of which are family clusters, and its related diseases usually occur in tissues and organs that consume large amounts of oxygen, such as the heart, skeletal muscle, pancreas, and nerve tissue. To date, more than 100 diseases such as cardiovascular disease, deafness, and mitochondrial myopathy are related to mitochondrial gene mutations [36–38]. The relationship between mt-DNA point mutation and cardiovascular disease has become a hot spot in the field of genetics. Meta-research has found that nearly 20 kinds of mitochondrial gene single nucleotide mutations are related to the occurrence and development of coronary heart disease.

Through a comparative analysis of mitochondrial gene scanning in young patients with coronary heart disease, Han et al. found that mitochondrial mutations C8414T, A8508G, and A8701G are related to the development of coronary heart disease in young people. Both C8414T and A8508G are located in the ATP8 gene [39–41]. The ATP8 gene corresponds to the 8386–8572 base pair of the mitochondrial genome and encodes the A6L subunit located in the neck of the complex V. Meta-research found that mutations in the ATP8 gene mainly cause dysfunction of the complex V and cause mitochondrial dysfunction, mainly affecting the heart, kidney, nervous system, and other organs or tissues with high energy metabolism [42]. Jonckheere reported that a mitochondrial mutation in a patient with G8529A caused hypertrophic cardiomyopathy, speech, dyskinesia, and reduced tendon reflexes. Ware et al. reported that four unrelated T8258C mutations were associated with hypertrophic cardiomyopathy and congestive heart failure [43]. Under normal human conditions, complex V produces ATP by phosphorylating ADP in the mitochondrial matrix, and most of the ATP powers the body through the mitochondrial inner membrane through ANP [44]. Similarly, ANT transports ADP back to the mitochondrial matrix for phosphorylation. Mitochondrial C8414T and G8584A mutations may lead to deficiency of complex V energy supply, insufficient phosphorylation level of complex V, and ATP production obstacles. At the same time, the increase of mitochondrial membrane potential is accompanied by an increase in active oxygen content produced by the mitochondrial respiratory chain, insufficient energy supply, and oxidative stress [38, 45]. The surge has contributed to the development of coronary heart disease. Yu et al. established a mouse model of the mouse ATP8 gene G7778A gene mutation and performed functional studies to indicate changes in mitochondrial structure, increased $H_2O_2$ synthesis, enhanced CD4 + T cell activity, and increased adaptability of CD4 + T cells to mitochondrial oxidative phosphorylation damage [46]. Experiments have confirmed that CD4 + T cells play an important role in the formation and expansion of atherosclerotic plaques. CD4 + T cells express CD40 ligand (CD40L). CD40L induces endothelial cells, vascular smooth muscle cells, and macrophages to express procoagulant factors [47, 48]. The CD40L system plays a decisive role in cardiovascular inflammation. It is speculated that mitochondrial C8414T and A8508G mutations may also promote the occurrence of coronary atherosclerosis by increasing the activity of CD4 + T cells [43].

In the mitochondrial gene A8701G mutation, the 59th amino acid at ATPase6 (F0 subunit of complex V) was replaced by threonine and alanine. Studies have confirmed that changes in the base AG are often associated with increased reactive oxygen species [44]. Kazuno et al. found the A8701G mutation changes the pH of the mitochondrial matrix, causing calcium overload and increased reactive oxygen species production, and calcium plays an important role in the development of coronary heart disease [49]. Active oxygen can open mPTP channels to induce cardiomyocyte apoptosis. A large number of reactive oxygen species open mPTP channels to induce myocardial cell apoptosis. Opening mPTP channels induces myocardial cell apoptosis; activated calcium-dependent potassium channels act on vascular endothelial cells to participate in the process of atherosclerosis by coupling PKG-1α signaling in smooth muscle cells [43]. Using voltage-dependent potassium channels and thiol redox signaling inhibits the formation of coronary collateral circulation. Increased calcium ions promote ROS generation [50]. Excessive ROS can further increase calcium and ROS levels by triggering mitochondrial calcium ion signals and regulating calcium regulatory proteins. Finally, positive feedback of calcium ions and ROS is formed. Calcium ions are triggered by activating the mPTP pathway. In addition to mitochondrial dysfunction, Ca/calmodulin-dependent protein kinase II (CaMII) can be activated and elevated through the $Ca^{2+}$/CaM-dependent activation pathway [51]. CaMII can prolong the duration of action potentials by inducing action and cause early rhythm after depolarization. The abnormality causes cardiomyocytes to apoptosis, which in turn causes continuous damage to the cardiomyocytes and electrophysiological disorders (see Fig. 9.1).

Chronic fatigue has become a "modern disease" common in high-speed modern society, and it is an important cause of sudden cardiac death in young people under high stress. It is urgent to do the in-depth research on the relationship between

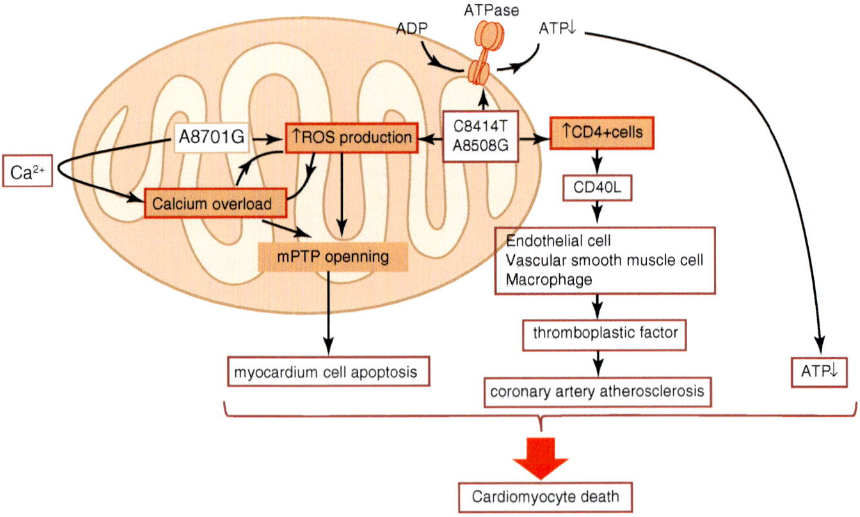


**Fig. 9.1** Mitochondrial gene mutation and sudden death in young people

chronic fatigue stress and sudden cardiac death in young people and study early warning mechanism of sudden fatigue caused by chronic fatigue stress, so as to screen high-risk groups of young people under chronic fatigue stress and take early prevention measures to provide insurance for young people who are the backbone of society and make some contributions to protecting their health.

## 9.4 Sudden Female Death

### 9.4.1 Difference between Sudden Female Death and Male Death

Sudden death of women is 30% of that of men, and sudden death of women is 10–20 years later than men [52]. Coronary heart disease is considered to be the main cause of sudden death, but the proportion of women with sudden death, coronary heart disease, structural heart disease, and left heart failure is lower than that of men. Only 37% of women with sudden death have a history of coronary heart disease. The proportion of coronary heart disease in men with sudden death is 56% [53]. At the same time, women with coronary heart disease have a lower risk of sudden death than men. The Framingham study showed that half of men with coronary heart disease died of sudden death, compared with only one quarter of women. With the improvement of primary and secondary prevention measures of coronary heart disease in recent years, the mortality of coronary heart disease has gradually decreased, and the incidence of sudden death of men has also decreased by 2.8%. However, the incidence of sudden death among young women of the same age increased by 21%.

### 9.4.2 Risk Factors Related to Sudden Death in Women

Smoking is an important cause of death from cardiovascular disease. Nurses' Health Study follow-up data for 101,018 women through 2011 show that amount and length of smoking are linearly related to sudden death. The risk of sudden death in women without coronary heart disease is 1.84 times that of nonsmokers. The risk of sudden death in heavy smokers is 3.3 times that of nonsmokers. This is equivalent to the risk of sudden death in patients with myocardial infarction. The risk of sudden death increases by 8% for each additional 5 years, and the risk of sudden death decreases significantly after stopping smoking. Women with coronary heart disease are at higher risk of sudden death from smoking, and even after quitting, they have a higher risk of sudden death. Smoking is an independent risk factor for women with sudden death. The effects of smoking on sudden death include, in addition to coronary atherosclerosis, the direct arrhythmic effects of nicotine. Nicotine can increase the release of catecholamines, change the potassium ion channel, and enhance transient platelet adhesion, thereby reducing the ventricular fibrillation threshold. Therefore, actively quitting smoking is important for preventing sudden death in women.

### 9.4.3 Sports

It is well known that exercise has many benefits, but there are also many records of sudden death caused by exercise. The Nurses' Health Study followed 69,693 women without cardiovascular disease for 18 years, and the results showed that the risk of sudden death from moderate- to high-intensity exercise was very low, about 1 in every 36.5 million hours of exercise [54, 55]. Compared with non-exercise and light exercise, moderate- to high-intensity exercise will cause a transient increase in the risk of sudden death, but long-term adherence to medium- to high-intensity exercise will reduce this transient risk [56]. When you exercise for 2 h or more per week, this risk will disappear. Medium- to high-intensity exercise will reduce the risk of sudden death in the long run, and the reduction in risk of sudden death is more significant in women who exercised regularly for more than 4 h per week. The Physicians' Health Study study showed that the relative risk of sudden death from strenuous exercise in men was 19 times that of women in the study. This is in line with the conclusions of a smaller retrospective study in the United States and Finland, which showed that men are nine to 14 times more likely to suffer sudden death from strenuous exercise than women. Therefore, it is suggested that women insist on long-term regular exercise instead of short-term vigorous exercise to reduce the occurrence of sudden death.

### 9.4.4 Drinking

Moderate drinking can reduce the incidence of hypertension, coronary heart disease, stroke, and death in women. In the Nurses' Health Study, 85, 067 women were followed for 26 years. The results showed that there was a U-shaped relationship between ethanol intake and sudden death. The incidence of sudden death was lower in mild to moderate drinkers. The risk of sudden death was lowest when drinking 5.0 to 14.9 g daily, and the risk of sudden death was similar for both non-drinkers and heavy drinkers [57]. There was no significant relationship between the type of simultaneous drinking and sudden death.

### 9.4.5 Depression and Anxiety

Depression and anxiety are the most common mental illnesses that affect cardiovascular disease. Studies have found that the incidence of sudden death also increases sharply when major events such as earthquakes and wars occur [58]. Depression is a risk factor for poor prognosis and decreased survival in patients with myocardial infarction, which is mainly related to the arrhythmia caused by depression. A prospective study by William et al. showed that as the depression scale score decreases (heavier depression), the risk of sudden death gradually increases. The relative hazard ratio of sudden death for severely depressed patients compared with those without depression is 2.33:1, and depression is an independent risk factor for sudden death. A study of patients with ICD showed that depressive symptoms were closely related to the number of ventricular arrhythmias recorded and the occurrence of sudden death [59]. This may be related to sympathetic hyperexcitation, increased resting heart rate, increased QT interval dispersion, and decreased heart rate variability in depressed patients. At the same time, antidepressants taken by depressed patients may also cause sudden death increase. For example, fluoxetine may prolong QT interval and induce apical torsional ventricular tachycardia. Tricyclic antidepressants may also prolong QT interval to induce ventricular arrhythmias.

### 9.4.6 Saturation and Types of Fatty Acids

The relationship between fatty acids and arrhythmias varies depending on the length of the fatty chain and its saturation. Saturated fatty acids have arrhythmogenic effects, while N-3 and N-6 polyunsaturated fatty acids have antiarrhythmic effects. In the Nurses' Health Study, 91,981 women were included. After 30 years of follow-up, it was found that the relative risk ratio of sudden death was 1.44 compared with women with more saturated fatty acids and less intake. The relative hazard ratio of sudden death in the group was 0.57, and N-3 and N-6 polyunsaturated fatty acids were closely related to the reduction in sudden death. Trans-fatty acids have arrhythmogenic effects. The Nurses' Health Study found that trans-18:2, but not trans-18:1, fatty acids were positively correlated with sudden death in women during a 26-year follow-up of 86,762 women. Coronary heart disease subgroup analysis showed that women with coronary heart disease consumed the most total trans-fatty acids. The relative hazard ratio of sudden death in the group and the least group was 3.24, which suggests that trans-fatty acids significantly increase the risk of sudden death in women with coronary heart disease. Studies have suggested that polyunsaturated fatty acids can affect atherosclerosis by affecting blood lipids, blood pressure, endothelial cell function, inflammatory response, thrombosis, and myocardial cells' use of oxygen and thus indirectly affect the occurrence of sudden death. At the same time, polyunsaturated fatty acids in the cell membrane can directly affect the occurrence of sudden death by affecting the stability of myocardial cells' electrical activity and changing their susceptibility to ventricular arrhythmias [60]. This suggests that improving the quality of fatty acids in the diet, such as replacing saturated fatty acids with N-3 and N-6 polyunsaturated fatty acids, and reducing the content of trans-fatty acids may be beneficial in reducing sudden death.

### 9.4.7 Diet and Serum Magnesium Content

Magnesium has an antiarrhythmic effect, and chronic magnesium deficiency can cause arrhythmias. Epidemiological and etiology studies of drinking water hardness and sudden death have shown that there is a negative correlation between magnesium ion concentration and the occurrence of fatal ventricular arrhythmias, and autopsy studies have also shown that magnesium ion concentrations in cardiac muscle cells of patients with sudden death have decreased. The 26-year follow-up of 88,375 women in the Nurses' Health Study showed that women with high levels of magnesium and low levels of diet and serum had a significantly lower risk of sudden death compared with women and that serum magnesium concentrations were inversely proportional to sudden death. For every 0.10 mmol/L increase in serum magnesium ion, the risk of sudden death is reduced by 41%. Magnesium ion is an ATPase activator of cardiomyocyte sodium ion channel and plays a very important role in maintaining electrophysiological activities such as resting membrane potential, cell membrane stability, and excitability of cardiomyocytes [61]. Magnesium ion can inhibit the depolarization of myocardial cells and reduce the repolarization dispersion. It plays an important role in the treatment of polymorphic ventricular tachycardia and apical torsional ventricular tachycardia. At the same time, magnesium ions can also indirectly affect the occurrence of sudden death by improving vascular tension, fat metabolism, endothelial cell function, and inflammatory response and inhibiting platelet function [62].

Our current traditional methods for predicting sudden death may not be suitable for women, and it is necessary to find risk stratification methods that can more accurately predict sudden death for these people. At present, there are few researches in this area in China. More epidemiological investigations and clinical studies are needed to explore the risk stratification methods of female sudden death, so as to better prevent the sudden death of female high-risk groups.

## References


1. Perez-Polo JR. Epigenetics: stress and disease. Int J Dev Neurosci. 2017;62:54–5.
2. Cohen S, Gianaros PJ, Manuck SB. A stage model of stress and disease. Perspect Psychol Sci. 2016;11:456–63.
3. Maiuri MC, Kroemer G. Autophagy in stress and disease. Cell Death Differ. 2015;22:365–6.
4. Zou J, Shi HF, Cai YM. Epidemiologic study on basic TCM syndrome in the subhealth population in the Zhengzhou area. Zhongguo Zhong Xi Yi Jie He Za Zhi. 2008;28:610–3.
5. Bunkenborg M. Subhealth: questioning the quality of bodies in contemporary China. Med Anthropol. 2014;33:128–43.
6. Li G, Xie F, Yan S, Hu X, Jin B, Wang J, Wu J, Yin D, Xie Q. Subhealth: definition, criteria for diagnosis and potential prevalence in the central region of China. BMC Public Health. 2013;13:446.
7. Li ZP, Su Y, Shen HY, Zhang XT, Fan L. An analysis of subhealth status based on partial least squares. Zhong Xi Yi Jie He Xue Bao. 2011;9:148–52.
8. Tsai SY, Chen HJ, Chen C, Lio CF, Kuo CF, Leong KH, Wang YT, Yang TY, You CH, Wang WS. Increased risk of chronic fatigue syndrome following psoriasis: a nationwide population-based cohort study. J Transl Med. 2019;17:154.
9. Shi J, Shen J, Xie J, Zhi J, Xu Y. Chronic fatigue syndrome in Chinese middle-school students. Medicine (Baltimore). 2018;97:e9716.
10. Estevez-Lopez F, Castro-Marrero J, Wang X, Bakken IJ, Ivanovs A, Nacul L, Sepulveda N, Strand EB, Pheby D, Alegre J, Scheibenbogen C, Shikova E, Lorusso L, Capelli E, Sekulic S, Lacerda E, Murovska M. Prevalence and incidence of myalgic encephalomyelitis/chronic fatigue syndrome in Europe-the euro-epiME study from the European network EUROMENE: a protocol for a systematic review. BMJ Open. 2018;8:e20817.

11. Loades ME, Rimes KA, Ali S, Lievesley K, Chalder T. The presence of co-morbid mental health problems in a cohort of adolescents with chronic fatigue syndrome. Clin Child Psychol Psychiatry. 2018;23:398–408.
12. Borren NZ, van der Woude CJ, Ananthakrishnan AN. Fatigue in IBD: epidemiology, pathophysiology and management. Nat Rev Gastroenterol Hepatol. 2019;16:247–59.
13. Olimulder MA, Galjee MA, Wagenaar LJ, van Es J, van der Palen J, Visser FC, Vermeulen RC, von Birgelen C. Chronic fatigue syndrome in women assessed with combined cardiac magnetic resonance imaging. Neth Heart J. 2016;24:709–16.
14. Loades ME, Sheils EA, Crawley E. Treatment for paediatric chronic fatigue syndrome or myalgic encephalomyelitis (CFS/ME) and comorbid depression: a systematic review. BMJ Open. 2016;6:e12271.
15. Meng XX, Wang RL, Gao S, Xie H, Tan JT, Qian YB. Effect of ulinastatin on paraquat-induced-oxidative stress in human type II alveolar epithelial cells. World J Emerg Med. 2013;4:133–7.
16. Olson KA, Patel RB, Ahmad FS, Ning H, Bogle BM, Goldberger JJ, Lloyd-Jones DM. Sudden cardiac death risk distribution in the United States population (from NHANES, 2005 to 2012). Am J Cardiol. 2019;123:1249–54.
17. Willett WC. Balancing life-style and genomics research for disease prevention. Science. 2002;296:695–8.
18. Zhang S. Sudden cardiac death in China: current status and future perspectives. Europace. 2015;17(Suppl 2):i14–8.
19. Mellor G, Raju H, de Noronha SV, Papadakis M, Sharma S, Behr ER, Sheppard MN. Clinical characteristics and circumstances of death in the sudden arrhythmic death syndrome. Circ Arrhythm Electrophysiol. 2014;7:1078–83.
20. Palmiere C, Lesta MM, Vanhaebost J, Mangin P, Augsburger M, Vogt P. Early repolarization, acute emotional stress and sudden death. J Forensic Sci. 2014;59:836–40.
21. Heidbuchel H, Prior DL, La Gerche A. Ventricular arrhythmias associated with long-term endurance sports: what is the evidence? Br J Sports Med. 2012;46(Suppl 1):i44–50.
22. Hoshuyama T. Overwork and its health effects—current status and future approach regarding Karoshi. Sangyo Eiseigaku Zasshi. 2003;45:187–93.
23. Sweeting J, Semsarian C. Sudden cardiac death in athletes. Heart Lung Circ. 2018;27:1072–7.
24. Yao HM, Sun TW, Wan YD, Zhang XJ, Fu X, Shen DL, Zhang JY, Li L. Domestic versus imported drug-eluting stents for the treatment of patients with acute coronary syndrome. World J Emerg Med. 2014;5:175–81.
25. Wang Y, Xia L, Shen X, Han G, Feng D, Xiao H, Zhai Y, Chen X, Miao Y, Zhao C, Wang Y, Guo M, Li T, Zhu HY. A new insight into sudden cardiac death in young people: a systematic review of cases of Takotsubo cardiomyopathy. Medicine (Baltimore). 2015;94:e1174.
26. Lyon AR, Rees PS, Prasad S, Poole-Wilson PA, Harding SE. Stress (Takotsubo) cardiomyopathy—a novel pathophysiological hypothesis to explain catecholamine-induced acute myocardial stunning. Nat Clin Pract Cardiovasc Med. 2008;5:22–9.
27. Garrett JE, Wellman CL. Chronic stress effects on dendritic morphology in medial prefrontal cortex: sex differences and estrogen dependence. Neuroscience. 2009;162:195–207.
28. Redfors B, Shao Y, Omerovic E. Stress-induced cardiomyopathy (Takotsubo)—broken heart and mind? Vasc Health Risk Manag. 2013;9:149–54.
29. Bybee KA, Kara T, Prasad A, Lerman A, Barsness GW, Wright RS, Rihal CS. Systematic review: transient left ventricular apical ballooning: a syndrome that mimics ST-segment elevation myocardial infarction. Ann Intern Med. 2004;141:858–65.
30. Shang LL, Sanyal S, Pfahnl AE, Jiao Z, Allen J, Liu H, Dudley SJ. NF-kappaB-dependent transcriptional regulation of the cardiac scn5a sodium channel by angiotensin II. Am J Physiol Cell Physiol. 2008;294:C372–9.
31. Gao G, Xie A, Zhang J, Herman AM, Jeong EM, Gu L, Liu M, Yang KC, Kamp TJ, Dudley SC. Unfolded protein response regulates cardiac sodium current in systolic human heart failure. Circ Arrhythm Electrophysiol. 2013;6:1018–24.

32. Kassmann M, Hansel A, Leipold E, Birkenbeil J, Lu SQ, Hoshi T, Heinemann SH. Oxidation of multiple methionine residues impairs rapid sodium channel inactivation. Pflugers Arch. 2008;456:1085–95.
33. Ma JH, Luo AT, Zhang PH. Effect of hydrogen peroxide on persistent sodium current in Guinea pig ventricular myocytes. Acta Pharmacol Sin. 2005;26:828–34.
34. Song Y, Shryock JC, Wagner S, Maier LS, Belardinelli L. Blocking late sodium current reduces hydrogen peroxide-induced arrhythmogenic activity and contractile dysfunction. J Pharmacol Exp Ther. 2006;318:214–22.
35. Duchen MR. Mitochondria in health and disease: perspectives on a new mitochondrial biology. Mol Aspects Med. 2004;25:365–451.
36. El-Hattab AW, Scaglia F. Mitochondrial cardiomyopathies. Front Cardiovasc Med. 2016;3:25.
37. Monsalve M, Borniquel S, Valle I, Lamas S. Mitochondrial dysfunction in human pathologies. Front Biosci. 2007;12:1131–53.
38. Akar FG, O'Rourke B. Mitochondria are sources of metabolic sink and arrhythmias. Pharmacol Ther. 2011;131:287–94.
39. Han GX, Xia L, Li SS, Jin QH, Song Y, Shen H, Wang LL, Kong LJ, Li TS, Zhu HY. The association between the C5263T mutation in the mitochondrial ND2 gene and Coronary heart disease among young Chinese Han people. Biomed Environ Sci. 2017;30:280–7.
40. Han GXSYCL. The role of mitochondrial DNA mutations in a Han Chinese population on sepsis pathogenesis. Eur Rev Med Pharm. 2017;21:3247–52.
41. Shen XHGLS. Association between the T6459C point mutation of the mitochondrial MT-CO1 gene and susceptibility to sepsis among Chinese Han people. J Cell Mol Med. 2018;22:5257–64.
42. Gallego-Delgado M, Cobo-Marcos M, Bornstein B, Hernandez-Lain A, Alonso-Pulpon L, Garcia-Pavia P. Mitochondrial cardiomyopathies associated with the m.3243A>G mutation in the MT-TL1 gene: two sides of the same coin. Rev Esp Cardiol (Engl Ed). 2015;68:153–5.
43. Liu Y, Zhao H, Li H, Kalyanaraman B, Nicolosi AC, Gutterman DD. Mitochondrial sources of H2O2 generation play a key role in flow-mediated dilation in human coronary resistance arteries. Circ Res. 2003;93:573–80.
44. Pung YF, Sam WJ, Stevanov K, Enrick M, Chen CL, Kolz C, Thakker P, Hardwick JP, Chen YR, Dyck JR, Yin L, Chilian WM. Mitochondrial oxidative stress corrupts coronary collateral growth by activating adenosine monophosphate activated kinase-alpha signaling. Arterioscler Thromb Vasc Biol. 2013;33:1911–9.
45. Song J, Liu X, Zhai P, Huang J, Lu L. A putative mitochondrial calcium uniporter in A. fumigatus contributes to mitochondrial Ca(2+) homeostasis and stress responses. Fungal Genet Biol. 2016;94:15–22.
46. Yu X, Wester-Rosenlof L, Gimsa U, Holzhueter SA, Marques A, Jonas L, Hagenow K, Kunz M, Nizze H, Tiedge M, Holmdahl R, Ibrahim SM. The mtDNA nt7778 G/T polymorphism affects autoimmune diseases and reproductive performance in the mouse. Hum Mol Genet. 2009;18:4689–98.
47. Wu T, Guo R, Zhang B. Developments in the study of CD40/CD40L gene and its polymorphism in atherosclerosis. Zhong Nan Da Xue Xue Bao Yi Xue Ban. 2012;37:413–8.
48. Haig D. Intracellular evolution of mitochondrial DNA (mtDNA) and the tragedy of the cytoplasmic commons. Bioessays. 2016;38:549–55.
49. Kazuno AA, Munakata K, Nagai T, Shimozono S, Tanaka M, Yoneda M, Kato N, Miyawaki A, Kato T. Identification of mitochondrial DNA polymorphisms that alter mitochondrial matrix pH and intracellular calcium dynamics. PLoS Genet. 2006;2:e128.
50. Sobenin IA, Sazonova MA, Ivanova MM, Zhelankin AV, Myasoedova VA, Postnov AY, Nurbaev SD, Bobryshev YV, Orekhov AN. Mutation C3256T of mitochondrial genome in white blood cells: novel genetic marker of atherosclerosis and coronary heart disease. PLoS One. 2012;7:e46573.
51. Sazonova MA, Sinyov VV, Barinova VA, Ryzhkova AI, Zhelankin AV, Postnov AY, Sobenin IA, Bobryshev YV, Orekhov AN. Mosaicism of mitochondrial genetic variation in atherosclerotic lesions of the human aorta. Biomed Res Int. 2015;2015:825468.

52. Chugh SS, Reinier K, Teodorescu C, Evanado A, Kehr E, Al SM, Mariani R, Gunson K, Jui J. Epidemiology of sudden cardiac death: clinical and research implications. Prog Cardiovasc Dis. 2008;51:213–28.
53. Haukilahti M, Holmstrom L, Vahatalo J, Kentta T, Tikkanen J, Pakanen L, Kortelainen ML, Perkiomaki J, Huikuri H, Myerburg RJ, Junttila MJ. Sudden cardiac death in women. Circulation. 2019;139:1012–21.
54. Bertoia ML, Triche EW, Michaud DS, Baylin A, Hogan JW, Neuhouser ML, Freiberg MS, Allison MA, Safford MM, Li W, Mossavar-Rahmani Y, Rosal MC, Eaton CB. Long-term alcohol and caffeine intake and risk of sudden cardiac death in women. Am J Clin Nutr. 2013;97:1356–63.
55. Whang W, Manson JE, Hu FB, Chae CU, Rexrode KM, Willett WC, Stampfer MJ, Albert CM. Physical exertion, exercise, and sudden cardiac death in women. JAMA. 2006;295:1399–403.
56. Albert CM, Mittleman MA, Chae CU, Lee IM, Hennekens CH, Manson JE. Triggering of sudden death from cardiac causes by vigorous exertion. N Engl J Med. 2000;343:1355–61.
57. Chiuve SE, Rimm EB, Mukamal KJ, Rexrode KM, Stampfer MJ, Manson JE, Albert CM. Light-to-moderate alcohol consumption and risk of sudden cardiac death in women. Heart Rhythm. 2010;7:1374–80.
58. Whang W, Kubzansky LD, Kawachi I, Rexrode KM, Kroenke CH, Glynn RJ, Garan H, Albert CM. Depression and risk of sudden cardiac death and coronary heart disease in women: results from the Nurses' health study. J Am Coll Cardiol. 2009;53:950–8.
59. Albert CM, Chae CU, Rexrode KM, Manson JE, Kawachi I. Phobic anxiety and risk of coronary heart disease and sudden cardiac death among women. Circulation. 2005;111:480–7.
60. Chiuve SE, Rimm EB, Sandhu RK, Bernstein AM, Rexrode KM, Manson JE, Willett WC, Albert CM. Dietary fat quality and risk of sudden cardiac death in women. Am J Clin Nutr. 2012;96:498–507.
61. Shechter M. Magnesium and cardiovascular system. Magnes Res. 2010;23:60–72.
62. Chiuve SE, Korngold EC, Januzzi JJ, Gantzer ML, Albert CM. Plasma and dietary magnesium and risk of sudden cardiac death in women. Am J Clin Nutr. 2011;93:253–60.

# The Children and Infant Sudden Death 10

Zhichun Feng, Qiuping Li, Xiangyong Kong,
and Xiaoyang Hong

**Abstract**

The sudden unexpected infant death (SUID) usually occurs in a healthy infant and children, and the cause of death remains unclear. Sudden infant and children death syndrome (SICDS) cannot be completely prevented, but it is thought that risk can be decreased by sleeping safely. SICDS is associated with a variety of risk factors, including maternal, infant, and environmental factors. The sudden infant death rates were significantly declined from the late 1980s to early 1990s, after prevention campaigns were introduced across many countries. These campaigns appear to affect some part of our population and resulted in behavioral change; this is not totally successful. The principles and evidence for public health approaches to prevention are based on different strategies. The interventions must focus on a limited number of simple feasible interventions and deliver through programs. The programs should be resourced appropriately, based on the long term and taken on long-term leadership which could make the target communities engagement and authorization. These programs must have been performed in robust monitoring and evaluation.

**Keywords**

Sudden unexpected infant death (SUID) · Sudden infant and children death syndrome (SICDS) · Preventive strategy

Z. Feng (✉) · Q. Li · X. Kong · X. Hong
Bayi Children's Hospital, The Seventh Medical Center, PLA General Hospital, Beijing, China



H. Zhu (ed.), *Sudden Death*, https://doi.org/10.1007/978-981-15-7002-5_10

## 10.1 Epidemiology of Sudden Death in Infant and Children

The sudden unexpected infant death (SUID) usually occurs in a formerly healthy infant and children, and the cause of death remains hard to fully explain despite a thorough case analysis, including autopsy, death investigation, and evaluation of the clinical history.

In the USA, about 4000 infants die per year due to sleep-related deaths, indicated as sudden unexpected infant deaths (SUIDs) [1]. These deaths take place suddenly and may be explained or unexplained among infants less than 1 year of age, and they are usually reported as sudden infant and children death syndrome (SICDS), death from unexplained cause, and death from accidental apnea and asphyxia in bed. SICDS includes about 50% of all SUIDs and is characterized by the sudden death during the sleep of the infants and children. Most SICDS deaths take place during the first 6 months of age, especially between ages 2 and 4 months. Since the sponsor of the Back to Sleep campaign in 1994 by the American Academy of Pediatrics (AAP), the total SICDS rate has declined by more than 50% in the USA. The number of death has declined from 130 per 100,000 live births in 1990 to 40 per 100,000 live births in 2015 [1]. Nonetheless, SICDS still is the second leading cause of early infant death and the fourth leading cause of infant and children mortality in the USA [2]. In recent years, the mortality rate of SICDS has become invariant unless major public health efforts were made to improve infant's sleep environment and aimed at focusing on high-risk groups. SICDS affects families of all social, economic, culture, and ethnic spheres. However, it is more likely to occur in infants born to mothers with few or inadequate antenatal care, mothers smoking during pregnancy, male infants, prone and side-lying position during sleep, and premature and low birth weight infants [3]. SICDS is not completely prevented, but it is considered that the risks could be avoided by following the basic "ABC" of safe sleep pattern. It means having the infant sleep "alone" and not with the parents or other people and not sleep with too soft pillows or unfixed blankets, having the infant on his or her "back" and not in prone or side-lying position during sleep, and having the infant sleep in his or her own "crib" and not on an adult bed, sofa, or other very soft surface.

## 10.2 Etiology and Risk Factors of Sudden Death in Children and Infant

A lot of risk factors are known to cause SICDS. They can be summarized as maternal, infant, and environmental factors (see Table 10.1). Statistically, the proportion of SICDS cases related to at least one risk factor exceeds 95%. And in a number of cases, factors leading to SICDS are modificable. Among these factors, sleep posture, sleep environment, and parental smoking are more often to be altered [4]. We will discuss these risk factors and related protection factors in detail in this chapter.

**Table 10.1** Risk factors of SICDS

| Maternal factors | Infant and environmental factors |
|---|---|
| Young age<br>Cigarette smoke<br>Alcohol or drug abuse<br>Pregnancy complications | Premature delivery and/or low birth weight<br>Prone sleep posture<br>Twins<br>Genetic polymorphisms<br>Sleeping environment<br>Sibling of SICDS victim<br>History of apnea<br>Overheating |

### 10.2.1 Maternal Risk Factors

#### 10.2.1.1 Young Maternal Age

Many studies have found that young maternal age is related to the risk of SICDS [5, 6]. A research conducted by the USA points out that after the neonatal period, SICDS occurred in 5.2 out of every 1000 infants born to teenage mothers, while the incidence in infants born by the older mothers was 1.0 per 1000 [6]. Another case-control study conducted by the Netherlands shows that the younger age of mother is an important risk factor for SICDS [7]. Compared with older mothers, very young mothers may differ in the way they take care of their children, and perhaps they have more things to worry about.

#### 10.2.1.2 Maternal Smoking

Maternal smoking can significantly increase the risk of SICDS and is positively correlated with the amount of smoking [8]. Cigarette smoking during pregnancy would bring the most distinct impact on babies, and second-hand smoke exposure is another independent risk factor for SICDS [9]. A great deal of studies have suggested that the babies were more susceptible to SICDS if their mothers smoke during the gestation period, and smoking prevention/intervention program could greatly reduce the risk of SICDS [8, 10]. According to a case-control study of KC Schoendorf et al., infants who were surviving had less exposure to maternal smoking, compared with those who died of SICDS. They also concluded that the odds ratio (OR) for passive exposure among normal birth weight infants of black race and white race was 2.4 and 2.2, respectively, but that of combined exposure was 2.9 and 4.1. By adjusting the demographic risk factors, the ratio for SICDS in these two races went consistent. The ratio for passive exposure was approximately 2, and the value for passive exposure became 3 [11]. Another prospective follow-up study found that there were 0.8 cases of SICDS per 1000 live births ($n = 20$). Maternal cigarette smoke significantly increased the children's risk of SICDS by more than three times (OR = 3.5; 95% CI 1.4–8.7), and the higher the number of cigarettes smoked every day, the higher the risk of SICDS ($p < 0.05$) [12]. Whether in the fetal period or after birth, tobacco can hinder the normal development of physiological functions and anatomical structures, thereby greatly increasing the risk of SICDS.

#### 10.2.1.3 Maternal Alcohol Use or Drug Abuse

Alcohol abuse by mothers can significantly increase SICDS risk [13]. A population-based case-control study of Northern Plains American Indians showed the significant associations between SICDS and pre-pregnancy maternal drinking (adjusted OR = 6.2; 95% CI 1.6–23.3), and between SICDS and early pregnancy bibulosity (adjusted OR = 8.2; 95% CI 1.9–35.3) [14]. Drug abuse by mothers can also increase the risk of SICDS [15]. Infants of mothers abusing methadone, heroin, cocaine, and other drugs during pregnancy can reach an incidence of SICDS of 5.89%, which is 4.19 times higher than infants born to mothers without drug abuse. Different drugs have different risks of increasing SICDS. Among them, SICDS risk for babies of cocaine-abusing mothers has increased threefold, heroin has increased fivefold, and methadone has increased sevenfold.

#### 10.2.1.4 Pregnancy Complications

A variety of complications may occur during pregnancy, including placenta previa, placental abruption, premature rupture of membranes, and elevated maternal alpha-fetoprotein. The ones listed above are currently regarded as maternal-related risk factors of SICDS [15–18]. Premature delivery is another common complication of pregnancy, but does not appear to increase the risk of SICDS.

### 10.2.2 Infant Risk Factors

#### 10.2.2.1 Prematurity

Compared with full-term delivery, premature delivery puts the babies at higher risk of SICDS [19, 20]. One study indicated that SICDS occurred three to four times more frequently in infants who are born with a low weight or a very low weight than that of full-term infants [21]. Donna R. Halloran et al. reported that length of gestation was closely related to the incidence of SICDS. Among all groups, infants between 28 and 32 weeks of gestation had the highest risk of SICDS (adjusted OR, 2.9; 95% CI, 2.6–3.2). The adjusted average age of postnatal SICDS death for infants born at 22 to 27 weeks was 20.9 (SD = 0.8) weeks, 28 to 32 weeks was 15.3 (SD = 0.5) weeks ($p \leq 0.002$), and 40 to 41 weeks was 14.5 (SD = 0.4) weeks [22]. From the above data, it can be seen that the mean death age of babies born at older gestational age decreased instead. Compared with term ones, very preterm infants died at an age 6 weeks later.

#### 10.2.2.2 Low Birth Weight

SICDS risk is raised in small for gestational age infants [23, 24]. Gestational age, maternal cigarette smoke, and hypertension are all related to low birth weight. And regardless of whether these factors are adjusted or not, borning at a low weight is still weakly but significantly associated with the risk of SICDS.

#### 10.2.2.3 Twins

Cohort studies indicated that the sudden death risk in twins was about twice as high as that in singletons [25–27]. The risk elevates partly because the proportion of premature births and low birth weight of twins is higher than that of singletons. However, other studies found that the SICDS risk for twins with gestational age of 37w and birth weight of 3000 g or more was still higher [28].

#### 10.2.2.4 Genetic Polymorphisms

Sudden infant death syndrome has a certain correlation with genes. The existence of some unknown gene polymorphisms and gene mutations may lead to a series of different responses of individuals to the external environment and the internal body, thus increasing the rate of sudden death. Neubauer et al. recently sequenced 161 SICDS infants in 2017 and found potential pathogenic gene variations in 20% of SICDS cases. These diseases are related to ion channel diseases (9%), myocardial diseases (7%), and metabolic diseases (1%) [29].

#### 10.2.2.5 Sleep Position

The majority of sudden deaths in infants are sleep-related, but it doesn't matter when they sleep. Sudden infant death syndrome deaths do not occur at a specific time within a day [30]. Prone sleep posture, which can cause extra physiological pressure on the cardiopulmonary system, leads to SICDS and plays a more important role than any other environmental or "external" factors. In fact, an infant's risk of SICDS in this sleeping position may be 14 times that of other sleeping positions [31]. The death mechanism attributed to prone sleep is usually asphyxia, but asphyxia cannot explain all deaths. Other mechanisms involve the changes of the blood flow, body temperature, etc. Firstly, the composition of air inhaled by the infants in the prone position changes. The oxygen they inhale decreases and the carbon dioxide increases, resulting in hypoxemia and hypercapnia. Secondly, prone position is prone to airway obstruction. Thirdly, infants may have less sleep arousal response and require more stimulation to wake them up, especially external stimuli. Fourthly, their cardiovascular capacity will change and blood flow to the brain will decrease. Finally, elevated infant body temperature can cause death, and splinting of the diaphragm is another related mechanism [32]. In contrast, supine position can reduce the risk of SICDS in premature infants. In the past, some people worried that supine position of premature infants might reduce oxygen cooperation, but two small research projects didn't support this theory, at least in babies over 32 weeks after menstruation [33, 34]. Even some studies have shown that compared with prone sleep posture, brain oxygenation is improved when lying on your back [35]. Based on the above evidence, the American Academy of Pediatrics (AAP) suggests a supine position for the premature babies. They had better start supine position from 32 weeks or earlier after menstruation [36]. In addition, side sleep may also lead to increased risk of SICDS, as side sleep can easily be converted to prone position sleep.

#### 10.2.2.6 Sibling of SICDS Victim

Siblings of SICDS victims increased the risk of SICDS by five- to sixfold [31, 37]. However, there is no need to worry too much, because the incidence rate of SICDS is extremely low (0.06%), and the SICDS incidence rate in subsequent siblings for most families after the risk increases is less than 1%.

#### 10.2.2.7 History of Apnea

Apnea or other respiratory dysfunction may be the final common pathway of many possible mechanisms of SICDS. Although apnea history, obvious life-threatening events (ALTE), or other respiratory pattern abnormalities cannot effectively predict the risk of SICDS, even the timely detection of apnea by a standard cardiopulmonary monitor cannot achieve a decreased SICDS risk. According to a case-control study, the history of apnea or cyanosis did not particularly increase among SICDS victims [38]. Another prospective study found no respiratory problems that could explain the elevated risk of SICDS [39].

#### 10.2.2.8 Sleep Environment

The environment around a sleeping baby may also be related to SICDS. Pay attention to the softness of the bed surface when the baby sleeps, the pajamas, the items on the bed, the ambient temperature, and whether the baby shares a bed or a room with his or her parents. Several studies have shown that the use of soft sleep surfaces can significantly increase the risk of SICDS [40, 41]. SICDS risk can also elevate by up to five times when infants use loose bedding, especially for older infants. This association is unrelated to sleep posture and appears to be caused by soft objects covering the head or blocking airflow. In addition, studies have shown that crib bumper pads are also associated with infant deaths due to "asphyxia" [42, 43]. Therefore, the AAP and Canadian Academy of Pediatrics both advise infants not to use crib bumper pads [36, 44]. Several studies have reported that the risk of SICDS was related to bed sharing, especially for babies in the first 3 months of life [41, 45–47]. A meta-analysis used 11 case-control studies on SICDS and bed sharing and calculated an odds ratio value of 2.89, with 95% confidence interval, 1.99–4.18 [47]. Combined with other factors leading to SICDS, such as bottle feeding, parental tobacco smoke, and alcohol use, the SICDS risk of bed-sharing infants will be 15-fold higher [48]. AAP suggests infants sleeping in the same room as their parents, but not in the same bed [36]. It is a good choice to put a crib or cradle beside the parents' bed.

#### 10.2.2.9 Overheating

Too high room temperature, or too much wrapped clothing, can cause the baby to overheat, thus increasing the SICDS risk. A study by North American Plains Indians found a significant correlation between the incidence of SICDS and wearing at least two layers of clothing (adjusted odds ratio 6.2, 95% confidence interval 1.4–26.5) [14].

## 10.3 Prevention of Sudden Death in Infant and Children

The sudden infant death rates significantly declined from the late 1980s to early 1990s, after prevention campaigns were introduced across many countries, which has been marked as one of the great public health success stories in the twentieth century [49, 50]. SICDS rates in many countries during the time of introduction of the prevention programs could be seen with falls of between 42% and 92%. These campaigns appear to have effectively changed some segments of our population in behavior, this is not universal. We will summarize the principles of public health approaches to prevention and the evidence base for different strategies in this chapter. We will consider the evidence for current approaches for reducing the risk of SICDS.

### 10.3.1 Principle of Preventive Strategies

SICDS is a complicated phenomenon caused by multiple, interacting risk factors. As such, any single preventive approach will hardly achieve universal success. Rather, more complex and multifaceted community-based approaches may lead to further reductions in SICDS mortality. From public health approaches to injury prevention, much can be learned [50–52]. Injury prevention approaches include three domains: education, environmental modification, and enforcement of legislation or regulations [51]. Now, there can be a fourth aspect, named empowerment.

The SICDS prevention approaches can be educational most commonly. If the public are clear what are the health-promoting behaviors, they are willing to follow them. When there has some effect, they tend to be limited in their impact. It is inconsistent between changes in knowledge and actual behavior [51]. This can be demonstrated in the persistence of unsafe sleeping and parental smoking (both risk factors of SICDS), especially in some of the most vulnerable groups [53].

In SICDS prevention, approaches must be based on environmental or product modification and on enforcing legislation, which have typically been shown to have a greater improvement on outcomes [51]. Many examples exist within the published literature of successful interventions which have resulted in reductions in mortality and morbidity. As has been seen in the impact of seat belt and motorcycle helmet legislation in many countries, environmental measures are most successful when combined with legislation.

Compared with educational approaches, environmental modification or legislation are more passive approaches: once implemented, individuals do not need to repeat their behavioral changes [51]. In contrast, educational approaches depend on individuals learning the lessons, and they will consistently be implemented when they are on every occasion of potential risk.

## 10.3.2 Educational Approaches

### 10.3.2.1 Public Health Campaigns

In the late 1980s and early 1990s, the first mass public health campaigns for promoting supine sleeping were conducted after two decades of high sudden infant death rates in some countries, a period that has been described as "SICDS pandemic" [54]. At that time to avoid aspiration of vomit, prone position sleep was recommended for infants. However, observational studies found a growing evidence that SICDS was linked to prone sleeping at mid-1980s. By 1991 in the UK, Australia, and New Zealand, campaigns were conducted to encourage parents to sleep infants supine, following earlier examples in the Netherlands and Norway [49].

### 10.3.2.2 Sleep Supine

The prevention campaign became known as "Back to Sleep" and was conducted by the Department of Health in conjunction with the Foundation for the Study of Infant Deaths in the UK (FSID, now known as The Lullaby Trust). In this campaign, professionals can receive mass mail-outs of information and public service announcements on the radio and television [55]. This campaign successfully brought a rapid and marked decline in rate of SICDS. The successful reasons are as follows. Primarily, the intervention of sleeping infant's supine is powerful. The SICDS rates declined dramatically with more and more parents sleeping their infant prone, which suggested the intervention was effective and responsible for the drop of SICDS deaths [56]. Second, the key message of campaigns was easy to understand and implement: avoid sleeping your infant prone. Third, the media and influential spokespeople participated in these campaigns, and public awareness and emotive case studies were heightened, which effectively conveyed that no infants are "immune" and all are at risk of SICDS [57].

SICDS is now most likely to occur in low-income families, with infants often sleeping supine and in bed-sharing situations with hazardous circumstances [54]. Recently in one study, 10–21% of infants were found to sleep on a non-recommended surface, 14–33% slept non-supine, and 87–93% were placed on loose or soft bed or other items nearby [58]. Safer sleep education and guidance are a continuous work. Noting the incidence of "sleep-related deaths" and moving away from focusing only on SICDS to a safe sleep environment, the risk of all sleep-related infant deaths can be reduced, including SICDS [59].

## 10.3.3 Safer Sleep Week

In 2015 a campaign named "Back to Sleep" was renewed campaigning efforts to Safer Sleep Week, which was a weeklong campaign held every March. The aim was to promote safer sleep advice for parents, professionals, and any babysitter. Activities were held during the Safer Sleep Week, which include press releases nationally and locally. Displaying the toolkits for disseminations at health and children's centers and educational talks were also included in the activities. Safer Sleep Week successfully raised awareness of ways to reduce the risk of SICDS.

#### 10.3.3.1 Support for High-Risk Families

There is a debate of universal provision versus targeted services in SICDS prevention. Maternal and child health service provision is significantly different among high-income countries, with models ranging from universal services free at the point of access to insurance-based provision requiring a financial contribution. The identification of populations who need to be labeled "at risk" or "in need" of service interventions is controversial. At best, targeted service provision focuses resources and supports on the more vulnerable populations to a great extent; at worst these populations are labeled and look down upon.

Young and disadvantaged mothers are usually considered a potential high-risk group, as they require targeted intervention and monitoring for lacking in parenting skills. Mothers in these groups are often supposed to be resistant to changing their behavior or infant care practices. Hence professionals have difficulty in understanding and identifying what motivates individuals in different groups, what affects behavioral change in different populations, and what kind of interventions are relevant and acceptable to different population groups. As the next section shows, several interventions successfully improved outcomes for groups with increasing risk for sudden unexpected death in infancy in varying degrees.

#### 10.3.3.2 Parenting Support Interventions

Educational interventions that have been regarded as successful in modifying parental behavior include the Family-Nurse Partnership (FNP) model that originates from the USA [60]. This program is targeted for vulnerable, young, first-time parents and can provide intensive home visiting from early pregnancy to 1 year after childbirth. In an area of Sydney, Australia, a study that evaluated a parent support program through home visits and supported with young disadvantaged parents described the experiences of staff and identified important components that contributed to program success [61]. This intervention acknowledges that parenting happens within the context of other priorities for parents with low income and poor resources. Dealing with these issues promotes resilience and supports parents to raise their children in a safe and nurturing environment.

#### 10.3.3.3 Support for Families with a Previous Unexpected Infant Death

Siblings born subsequently to an infant who died of SICDS in the family carry an increased risk of sudden infant death, both from explained and unexplained causes [62]. Families who have an infant who died of SICDS are more likely to have significant risk factors, including smoking, being a younger mother of higher parity, and low income, which likely exist persistently for subsequent children [63]. These factors, combined with strong feelings of anxiety at the prospect of a new infant [64], mean that families were a vulnerable group of SICDS and needed support and could be benefit from targeted preventative interventions.

A study in 2011 confirmed an overrepresentation of risk factors: the smoke rate was twice in the parents and the unemployed rate was five times than the national averages and those families had a higher chance to give births [65]. Family support, such as intensive home visiting by professionals, has been proved to reduce prevalence of sudden infant death in high-risk families [66].

#### 10.3.3.4 Peer Support Programs

At the beginning of the chapter, interventions that are modified for a specific populations are more likely to be effective and sustainable, if the populations engaged in design and implementation. However, very little research focuses on community involvement using peer educators in SICDS risk-reduction strategies. One community of particular interest is young parents whose ages are under 20. Particularly young mothers have been usually associated with an increased risk of SICDS in their children [67]. Peer support programs would reduce prevalence of sudden death in high-risk infants.

### 10.3.4 Approaches Based on Engineering, Environmental Modification, and Enforcement

All kinds of approaches including engineering and environmental modification have been developed to ensure safe sleep environments for infants. Equipment such as sleeping bags and safe cribs/bassinettes are provided for infants and tools to support parents for early recognition of illness.

#### 10.3.4.1 Safe Sleep Environments

##### Sleeping Bags

However, there is not any prospective studies until now that have evaluated the value of providing or using sleeping bags as a SICDS prevention measure for infant. Just like the risks related to prone sleeping and thick or loose bedding, intuitively at least, infant sleeping bags are a great potential approach for prevention. Thick bedding and bedding that can cover an infant's head have been shown to be risk factors for SICDS [68]. In a study, the risk of SICDS of infants using a duvet doubled compared to that sleeping with a sleeping bag or light cotton blanket [69]. However, evidence for using sleeping bags as a preventive measure for SICDS is limited until now. As a study from the Netherlands showed, cotton sleeping sacks have a protective effect [70]. Another UK study showed that sleeping bags were used more commonly in control group than that in SICDS group, but this was not significant on multivariate analysis [71].

#### 10.3.4.2 Baby Boxes

Effective interventions can combine culture and tradition which will encourage parental behavioral change, such as the distribution of "baby boxes," an old tradition in Finland since 1938 [72]. A cardboard box, modified and repurposed as a bed, contains a mattress and fitted sheet is used for neonates by every woman during her first pregnancy. Although these boxes were used before the SICDS "pandemic" of the 1970s and 1980s and were not associated with SICDS prevention, the low infant mortality rate in Finland [73] has been seen and noted by other countries. In recent years programs called copy-cat cardboard baby box schemes have been set up in other countries, including the USA, Scotland, and England. Some interventions are covered by the healthcare system, as in Finland, such as pilot schemes in two regions of Scotland [74], in London [75], and in Alaska [76].

#### 10.3.4.3 Tools for Recognition of Illness

Many infants who die of SICDS, for either explained or unexplained reasons, show signs and symptoms of SICDS in the immediate 24 h before death [77]. They are most likely to present during doctors' surgeries or in the weeks after admission to hospital [78]. Both parents and professionals can ignore the signs of serious illness sometimes, even the symptoms such as fever that can invoke in parents with high anxiety [79]. A system for assessing seriousness of illness accurately can support parents and help professionals to treat appropriately, which may help to prevent sudden infant death.

#### 10.3.4.4 Combined Strategies for Behavioral Change: Smoking Cessation in Pregnancy

Following prone sleeping, maternal smoking is wildly acknowledged as the next most important modifiable risk factor for SICDS [80]. While smoking rates in the common populations of developed countries have decreased steadily over the last 40 years, Lumley et al. identified what kinds of populations were more likely to continue to smoke and the characteristics of these groups which include lower socioeconomic status, lower educational achievement, poverty, younger women, and psychologically resilient or more marginalized and unsupported [81]. In Fleming and Blair's study, the prevalence of smoking during pregnancy was found to decrease in the common population between1984 and 2003 from 30% to 20%, but the proportion of smoking during pregnancy in SICDS mothers increased from 50% to 80% [82]. Thus, reducing maternal smoking among these most vulnerable populations should be a priority for SICDS prevention.

#### 10.3.4.5 Telephone and Internet Support

It is unclear whether or not telephone and Internet-based support is successful for antenatal smoking cessation. A systematic review found there was no evidence that telephone support was more likely to have reduced, or stopped smoking at the end of pregnancy, or during the postnatal period. Even telephone support could not reduce the probability of smoking relapse [83]. Another systematic review evaluated the supportive effect of telephone helplines for smoking cessation, which found that telephone helplines can promote people to stop. However, these helplines only increase the likelihood of some persons who are ready and intend to stop smoking or want to resist relapse. So, they had more willingness than those who didn't contact the helplines [84]. This review also revealed a "dose-response" effect in a number of helpline contacts. Compared to a minimal intervention such as providing brief advice, standard self-help materials, or NRT, three or more calls increased the likelihood of stopping. Telephone counseling and helplines make support accessible for those who want to seek help, and therefore such interventions may be useful and measurable benefit compared to brief advice and self-help interventions.

#### 10.3.4.6 Real-Time Feedback

Ultrasound monitoring provides visual evidence and measurement of fetal development in antenatal care, which presents an opportunity to discuss maternal behavior related to the health and development of the fetus. A study with 129 participants found that women who received detailed feedback about the growth and development of the fetus during their scan appointment were more likely to stop smoking and avoid alcohol during pregnancy [85]. However, a systematic review revealed that there was insufficient evidence to suggest that both low and high detailed feedback could result in behavioral change during the scan appointment [86].

#### 10.3.4.7 Nicotine Replacement Therapy (NRT)

NRT may be a reasonable option to support smoking cessation during pregnancy [87]. Nicotine has significant deleterious effects on the developing fetus; it will metabolize much more quickly during pregnancy, which may protect the fetus through decreased toxic levels of circulating nicotine. Therefore, nicotine replacement products seem to be safer than smoking during pregnancy due to the reduction of exposure to the toxic levels of circulating nicotine [88]. The efficacy and safety of NRT for smoking cessation was confirmed by a systematic review of five randomized controlled trials (RCTs); there was no sufficient evidence of both efficacy and safety of its use in pregnancy with or without behavioral support [89]. However, the compliance of treatment was low across all studies, and most participants did not complete the recommended course of NRT. A subsequent meta-analysis by Myung et al. found that late pregnant smokers using NRT presented an abstinence rate 1.8 times higher than the control group; however, compared to the non-pregnant smoking population, pregnant smokers who used NRT had lower cessation rates [90]. The conclusion revealed that there was no significant impact on the birth outcomes of infants between the subject and control groups. There may be clinical supportive evidence for using NRT, and NRT was usually safe for use with pregnant women in Myung's conclusion.

#### 10.3.4.8 Electronic Cigarettes

Since 2007, electronic cigarettes (EC) have been available and used by smokers as a cessation treatment. EC was also a more socially acceptable habit and substitute for cigarettes than cigarette smoking for non-smokers in public places [91]. Early studies have found some physiological benefits of using ECs over cigarette smoking, as they contain fewer of the toxic substance and less carbon monoxide than normal cigarettes [92]. Pregnant women may be advised by healthcare practitioners to move to ECs as a safer and more socially acceptable substitute that can encourage them for smoking cessation [93].

## 10.4 Conclusion

In this part, we have reviewed the epidemiology, etiology, and risk factors and the strategies of prevention of SICDS. In the 1990s, the great successes of the initial public health strategies demonstrate what can be achieved through concerted national efforts. However, after the initial rapid declines, the SICDS mortality has plateaued now. It seems clear that the approaches will now only have little effects, especially for the families with highest risk of SICDS. If we focus on those most at risk, we should understand behavioral change deeply and ensure that our interventions are more feasible toward empowerment of individuals. High levels of professional support may be required over prolonged time frames.

As we reduce the risks of SICDS further in our efforts, sound public health principles are more important than ever for risk reduction. The successful strategies should promote more creative thinking about how we can engage with, and empower, those at highest risk. We need a limited number of simple achievable interventions. These interventions are composed of combined programs that are appropriately resourced and long term in nature. Strong leadership is recruited and engaged and empowered the target communities in these programs. Finally, we must confirm that these programs are performed under robust monitoring and evaluation.

## References

1. Centers for Disease Control and Prevention. About sudden unexpected infant death and sudden infant death syndrome. https://www.cdc.gov/SICDS/aboutsuidandSICDS.htm. Accessed 23 Nov 2019.
2. Shapiro-Mendoza CK, Camperlengo L, Ludvigsen R, et al. Classification system for the sudden unexpected infant death case registry and its application. Pediatrics. 2014;134(1):e210–9.
3. Heron M. Deaths: leading causes for 2014. Natl Vital Stat Rep. 2016;65(5):1–86.
4. Ostfeld BM, Esposito L, Perl H, Hegyi T. Concurrent risks in sudden infant death syndrome. Pediatrics. 2010;125(3):447–53.
5. Daltveit AK, Oyen N, Skjaerven R, Irgens LM. The epidemic of SICDS in Norway 1967-93: changing effects of risk factors. Arch Dis Child. 1997;77(1):23–7.
6. Babson SG, Clarke NG. Relationship between infant death and maternal age. Comparison of sudden infant death incidence with other causes of infant mortality. J Pediatr. 1983;103(3):391–3.
7. l'Hoir MP, Engelberts AC, van Well GT, et al. Case-control study of current validity of previously described risk factors for SICDS in the Netherlands. Arch Dis Child. 1998;79(5):386–93.
8. MacDorman MF, Cnattingius S, Hoffman HJ, Kramer MS, Haglund B. Sudden infant death syndrome and smoking in the United States and Sweden. Am J Epidemiol. 1997;146(3):249–57.
9. Golding J. Sudden infant death syndrome and parental smoking—a literature review. Paediatr Perinat Epidemiol. 1997;11(1):67–77.
10. Taylor JA, Sanderson M. A reexamination of the risk factors for the sudden infant death syndrome. J Pediatr. 1995;126(6):887–91.
11. Schoendorf KC, Kiely JL. Relationship of sudden infant death syndrome to maternal smoking during and after pregnancy. Pediatrics. 1992;90(6):905–8.
12. Wisborg K, Kesmodel U, Henriksen TB, Olsen SF, Secher NJ. A prospective study of smoking during pregnancy and SICDS. Arch Dis Child. 2000;83(3):203–6.
13. O'Leary CM, Jacoby PJ, Bartu A, D'Antoine H, Bower C. Maternal alcohol use and sudden infant death syndrome and infant mortality excluding SICDS. Pediatrics. 2013;131(3):e770–8.

14. Iyasu S, Randall LL, Welty TK, et al. Risk factors for sudden infant death syndrome among northern plains Indians. JAMA. 2002;288(21):2717–23.
15. Rosen TS, Johnson HL. Drug-addicted mothers, their infants, and SICDS. Ann N Y Acad Sci. 1988;533:89–95.
16. Klonoff-Cohen HS, Srinivasan IP, Edelstein SL. Prenatal and intrapartum events and sudden infant death syndrome. Paediatr Perinat Epidemiol. 2002;16(1):82–9.
17. Li DK, Wi S. Maternal pre-eclampsia/eclampsia and the risk of sudden infant death syndrome in offspring. Paediatr Perinat Epidemiol. 2000;14(2):141–4.
18. Smith GC, Wood AM, Pell JP, White IR, Crossley JA, Dobbie R. Second-trimester maternal serum levels of alpha-fetoprotein and the subsequent risk of sudden infant death syndrome. N Engl J Med. 2004;351(10):978–86.
19. Malloy MH, Hoffman HJ. Prematurity, sudden infant death syndrome, and age of death. Pediatrics. 1995;96(3 Pt 1):464–71.
20. Thompson JM, Mitchell EA. Are the risk factors for SICDS different for preterm and term infants. Arch Dis Child. 2006;91(2):107–11.
21. Bigger HR, Silvestri JM, Shott S, Weese-Mayer DE. Influence of increased survival in very low birth weight, low birth weight, and normal birth weight infants on the incidence of sudden infant death syndrome in the United States: 1985-1991. J Pediatr. 1998;133(1):73–8.
22. Halloran DR, Alexander GR. Preterm delivery and age of SICDS death. Ann Epidemiol. 2006;16(8):600–6.
23. Blair PS, Platt MW, Smith IJ, Fleming PJ. Sudden infant death syndrome and sleeping position in pre-term and low birth weight infants: an opportunity for targeted intervention. Arch Dis Child. 2006;91(2):101–6.
24. Malloy MH. Size for gestational age at birth: impact on risk for sudden infant death and other causes of death, USA 2002. Arch Dis Child Fetal Neonatal Ed. 2007;92(6):F473–8.
25. Pharoah PO, Platt MJ. Sudden infant death syndrome in twins and singletons. Twin Res Hum Genet. 2007;10(4):644–8.
26. Malloy MH, Freeman DH. Sudden infant death syndrome among twins. Arch Pediatr Adolesc Med. 1999;153(7):736–40.
27. Beal S. Sudden infant death syndrome in twins. Pediatrics. 1989;84(6):1038–44.
28. Platt MJ, Pharoah PO. The epidemiology of sudden infant death syndrome. Arch Dis Child. 2003;88(1):27–9.
29. Neubauer J, Lecca MR, Russo G, et al. Post-mortem whole-exome analysis in a large sudden infant death syndrome cohort with a focus on cardiovascular and metabolic genetic diseases. Eur J Hum Genet. 2017;25(4):404–9.
30. Beal SM, Blundell HK. Recurrence incidence of sudden infant death syndrome. Arch Dis Child. 1988;63(8):924–30.
31. Oyen N, Skjaerven R, Irgens LM. Population-based recurrence risk of sudden infant death syndrome compared with other infant and fetal deaths. Am J Epidemiol. 1996;144(3):300–5.
32. Carpenter RG, Waite A, Coombs RC, et al. Repeat sudden unexpected and unexplained infant deaths: natural or unnatural. Lancet. 2005;365(9453):29–35.
33. Kassim Z, Donaldson N, Khetriwal B, et al. Sleeping position, oxygen saturation and lung volume in convalescent, prematurely born infants. Arch Dis Child Fetal Neonatal Ed. 2007;92(5):F347–50.
34. Elder DE, Campbell AJ, Galletly D. Effect of position on oxygen saturation and requirement in convalescent preterm infants. Acta Paediatr. 2011;100(5):661–5.
35. Fyfe KL, Yiallourou SR, Wong FY, Odoi A, Walker AM, Horne RS. Cerebral oxygenation in preterm infants. Pediatrics. 2014;134(3):435–45.
36. Moon RY. SICDS and other sleep-related infant deaths: evidence base for 2016 updated recommendations for a safe infant sleeping environment. Pediatrics. 2016;138(5):e20162938.
37. Guntheroth WG, Lohmann R, Spiers PS. Risk of sudden infant death syndrome in subsequent siblings. J Pediatr. 1990;116(4):520–4.
38. Hoffman HJ, Damus K, Hillman L, Krongrad E. Risk factors for SICDS. Results of the National Institute of Child Health and Human Development SICDS cooperative epidemiological study. Ann N Y Acad Sci. 1988;533:13–30.

39. Hoppenbrouwers T, Hodgman JE, Ramanathan A, Dorey F. Extreme and conventional cardiorespiratory events and epidemiologic risk factors for SICDS. J Pediatr. 2008;152(5):636–41.
40. Mitchell EA, Scragg L, Clements M. Soft cot mattresses and the sudden infant death syndrome. N Z Med J. 1996;109(1023):206–7.
41. Erck LAB, Parks SE, Cottengim C, Faulkner M, Hauck FR, Shapiro-Mendoza CK. Sleep-related infant suffocation deaths attributable to soft bedding, overlay, and wedging. Pediatrics. 2019;143(5):e20183408.
42. Thach BT, Rutherford GW, Harris K. Deaths and injuries attributed to infant crib bumper pads. J Pediatr. 2007;151(3):271–4, 274.e1–3.
43. Scheers NJ, Woodard DW, Thach BT. Crib bumpers continue to cause infant deaths: a need for a new preventive approach. J Pediatr. 2016;169:93–7.e1.
44. Moon RY. SICDS and other sleep-related infant deaths: updated 2016 recommendations for a safe infant sleeping environment. Pediatrics. 2016;138(5):e20162940.
45. Trachtenberg FL, Haas EA, Kinney HC, Stanley C, Krous HF. Risk factor changes for sudden infant death syndrome after initiation of Back-to-sleep campaign. Pediatrics. 2012;129(4):630–8.
46. Blair PS, Fleming PJ, Smith IJ, et al. Babies sleeping with parents: case-control study of factors influencing the risk of the sudden infant death syndrome. CESDI SUDI Research Group. BMJ. 1999;319(7223):1457–61.
47. Vennemann MM, Hense HW, Bajanowski T, et al. Bed sharing and the risk of sudden infant death syndrome: can we resolve the debate. J Pediatr. 2012;160(1):44–8.e2.
48. Carpenter R, McGarvey C, Mitchell EA, et al. Bed sharing when parents do not smoke: is there a risk of SICDS? An individual level analysis of five major case-control studies. BMJ Open. 2013;3(5):e002299.
49. Ponsonby AL, Dwyer T, Cochrane J. Population trends in sudden infant death syndrome. Semin Perinatol. 2002;26(4):296–305. https://doi.org/10.1053/sper.2002.34774.
50. Rivara FP, Johnston B. Effective primary prevention programs in public health and their applicability to the prevention of child maltreatment. Child Welfare. 2013;92(2):119–39.
51. Deal LW, Gomby DS, Zippiroli L, Behrman RE. Unintentional injuries in childhood: analysis and recommendations. Future Child. 2000;10(1):4–22. https://doi.org/10.2307/1602823.
52. Towner E, Dowswell T. Community-based childhood injury prevention interventions: What works? Health Promot Int. 2002;17(3):273–84. https://doi.org/10.1093/heapro/17.3.273.
53. Blair PS, Sidebotham P, Berry PJ, Evans M, Fleming PJ. Major epidemiological changes in sudden infant death syndrome: a 20-year population-based study in the UK. Lancet. 2006;367(9507):314–9. https://doi.org/10.1016/S0140-6736(06)67968-3.
54. Van Wouwe JP, Hirasing RA. Prevention of sudden unexpected infant death. Lancet. 2006;367(9507):277–8. https://doi.org/10.1016/S0140-6736(06)67969-5.
55. NIH. Safe to Sleep public education campaign. https://www.nichd.nih.gov/sts/Pages/default.aspx. Accessed 5 May 2017.
56. Blair P. Sudden infant death syndrome. In: Sidebotham P, Fleming P, editors. Unexpected death in childhood: a handbook for practitioners. Chichester: Wiley; 2007. p. 41–60. https://doi.org/10.1002/9780470988176.ch4.
57. Moon RY, Hauck FR, Colson ER. Safe infant sleep interventions: what is the evidence for successful behavior change? Curr Pediatr Rev. 2016;12(1):67–75. https://doi.org/10.2174/1573396311666151026110148.
58. Batra EK, Teti DM, Schaefer EW, Neumann BA, Meek EA, Paul IM. Nocturnal video assessment of infant sleep environments. Pediatrics. 2016;138(3):e20161533. https://doi.org/10.1542/peds.2016-1533.
59. Task Force On Sudden Infant Death Syndrome. SICDS and other sleep-related infant deaths: updated 2016 recommendations for a safe infant sleeping environment. Pediatrics. 2016;138(5).
60. Olds DL, Henderson CR Jr, Tatelbaum R, Chamberlin R. Improving the delivery of prenatal care and outcomes of pregnancy: a randomized trial of nurse home visitation. Pediatrics. 1986;77(1):16–28.

61. Mills A, Schmied V, Taylor C, Dahlen H, Schuiringa W, Hudson ME. Connecting, learning, leaving: supporting young parents in the community. Health Soc Care Community. 2012;20(6):663–72. https://doi.org/10.1111/j.1365-2524.2012.01084.x.
62. Hunt CE. Sudden infant death syndrome and other causes of infant mortality: diagnosis, mechanisms, and risk for recurrence in siblings. Am J Respir Crit Care Med. 2001;164(3):346–57. https://doi.org/10.1164/ajrccm.164.3.9910045.
63. Campbell MJ, Hall D, Stephenson T, Bacon C, Madan J. Recurrence rates for sudden infant death syndrome (SICDS): the importance of risk stratification. Arch Dis Child. 2008;93(11):936–9. https://doi.org/10.1136/adc.2007.121350.
64. Brooten D, Youngblut JM, Hannan J, Caicedo C, Roche R, Malkawi F. Infant and child deaths: parent concerns about subsequent pregnancies. J Am Assoc Nurse Pract. 2015;27(12):690–7. https://doi.org/10.1002/2327-6924.12243.
65. Waite A, McKenzie A, Daman-Willems C. CONI: confirmation of continuing relevance after 20 years. Community Pract. 2011;84(1):25–9.
66. Taylor EM, Spencer NJ, Carpenter RG. Evaluation of attempted prevention of unexpected infant death in very high-risk infants by planned health care. Acta Paediatr. 1993;82(1):83–6. https://doi.org/10.1111/j.1651-2227.1993.tb12522.x.
67. Caraballo M, Shimasaki S, Johnston K, Tung G, Albright K, Halbower AC. Knowledge, attitudes, and risk for sudden unexpected infant death in children of adolescent mothers: a qualitative study. J Pediatr. 2016;174:78–83.e2.
68. Carpenter RG, Irgens LM, Blair PS, England PD, Fleming P, Huber J, et al. Sudden unexplained infant death in 20 regions in Europe: case control study. Lancet. 2004;363(9404):185–91. https://doi.org/10.1016/S0140-6736(03)15323-8.
69. Vennemann MM, Bajanowski T, Brinkmann B, Jorch G, Sauerland C, Mitchell EA, et al. Sleep environment risk factors for sudden infant death syndrome: the German sudden infant death syndrome study. Pediatrics. 2009;123(4):1162–70. https://doi.org/10.1542/peds.2008-0505.
70. L'Hoir MP, Engelberts AC, van Well GT, McClelland S, Westers P, Dandachli T, et al. Risk and preventive factors for cot death in the Netherlands, a low-incidence country. Eur J Pediatr. 1998;157(8):681–8. https://doi.org/10.1007/s004310050911.
71. Blair PS, Sidebotham P, Evason-Coombe C, Edmonds M, Heckstall-Smith EM, Fleming P. Hazardous cosleeping environments and risk factors amenable to change: case-control study of SICDS in south West England. BMJ. 2009;339:b3666. https://doi.org/10.1136/bmj.b3666.
72. Moon RY, Task Force On Sudden Infant Deaths. SICDS and other sleep-related infant deaths: evidence base for 2016 updated recommendations for a safe infant sleeping environment. Pediatrics. 2016;138(5):e20162940. https://doi.org/10.1542/peds.2016-2940.
73. Statistics Finland. Causes of death: Appendix table 3. Mortality during infant and perinatal period 1987–2015. http://www.stat.fi/til/ksyyt/2015/ksyyt_2015_2016-12-30_tau_005_en.html. Accessed 11 Oct 2017.
74. Ross L. Baby boxes: improving wellbeing outcomes in Scotland. J Health Visiting. 2017;5(4):172–5. https://doi.org/10.12968/johv.2017.5.4.172.
75. Murphy M. UK's first Baby Box programme launched at London NHS Trust. Br J Midwifery. 2016;24(7):521–2. https://doi.org/10.12968/bjom.2016.24.7.521.
76. Demer L. Rash of sleep-related infant deaths troubles health officials. Alaska Dispatch News [internet]. 2015. https://www.adn.com/health/article/rash-infant-deaths-related-sleeping-alarms-health-officials/2015/02/15/. Accessed 1 Jun 2017.
77. Ward Platt M, Blair PS, Fleming PJ, Smith IJ, Cole TJ, Leach CE, et al. A clinical comparison of SICDS and explained sudden infant deaths: How healthy and how normal? CESDI SUDI Research Group. Confidential Inquiry into Stillbirths and Deaths in Infancy study. Arch Dis Child. 2000;82(2):98–106. https://doi.org/10.1136/adc.82.2.98.
78. Ford RP, Mitchell EA, Stewart AW, Scragg R, Taylor BJ. SICDS, illness, and acute medical care. New Zealand cot death study group. Arch Dis Child. 1997;77(1):54–5. https://doi.org/10.1136/adc.77.1.54.
79. Wilkinson A. Pre-hospital assessment of a child under one year old with fever. Emerg Nurse. 2017;24(10):28–33. https://doi.org/10.7748/en.2017.e1663.

80. Mitchell EA, Milerad J. Smoking and the sudden infant death syndrome. Rev Environ Health. 2006;21(2):81–103. https://doi.org/10.1515/REVEH.2006.21.2.81.
81. Lumley J, Chamberlain C, Dowswell T, Oliver S, Oakley L, Watson L. Interventions for promoting smoking cessation during pregnancy. Cochrane Database Syst Rev. 2009;8(3):CD001055. https://doi.org/10.1002/14651858.CD001055.pub3.
82. Fleming P, Blair PS. Sudden infant death syndrome and parental smoking. Early Hum Dev. 2007;83(11):721–5. https://doi.org/10.1016/j.earlhumdev.2007.07.011.
83. Lavender T, Richens Y, Milan SJ, Smyth RM, Dowswell T. Telephone support for women during pregnancy and the first six weeks postpartum. Cochrane Database Syst Rev. 2013;7:CD009338. https://doi.org/10.1002/14651858.CD009338.pub2.
84. Stead LF, Hartmann-Boyce J, Perera R, Lancaster T. Telephone counselling for smoking cessation. Cochrane Database Syst Rev. 2013;8:CD002850. https://doi.org/10.1002/14651858.CD002850.pub3.
85. Reading AE, Campbell S, Cox DN, Sledmere CM. Health beliefs and health care behavior in pregnancy. Psychol Med. 1982;12(2):379–83. https://doi.org/10.1017/S0033291700046717.
86. Nabhan AF, Faris MA. High feedback versus low feedback of prenatal ultrasound for reducing maternal anxiety and improving maternal health behavior in pregnancy. Cochrane Database Syst Rev. 2010;4:CD007208.
87. Dempsey D, Jacob P 3rd, Benowitz NL. Accelerated metabolism of nicotine and cotinine in pregnant smokers. J Pharmacol Exp Ther. 2002;301(2):594–8. https://doi.org/10.1124/jpet.301.2.594.
88. Benowitz N, Dempsey D. Pharmacotherapy for smoking cessation during pregnancy. Nicotine Tob Res. 2004;6(Suppl 2):S189–202. https://doi.org/10.1080/14622200410001669169.
89. Coleman T, Chamberlain C, Cooper S, Leonardi-Bee J. Efficacy and safety of nicotine replacement therapy for smoking cessation in pregnancy: systematic review and meta-analysis. Addiction. 2011;106(1):52–61. https://doi.org/10.1111/j.1360-0443.2010.03179.x.).
90. Myung SK, Ju W, Jung HS, Park CH, Oh SW, Seo H, et al. Efficacy and safety of pharmacotherapy for smoking cessation among pregnant smokers: a meta-analysis. BJOG. 2012;119(9):1029–39. https://doi.org/10.1111/j.1471-0528.2012.03408.x.
91. Etter JF. Electronic cigarettes: a survey of users. BMC Public Health. 2010;10:231. https://doi.org/10.1186/1471-2458-10-231.
92. Breland A, Soule E, Lopez A, Ramoa C, El-Hellani A, Eissenberg T. Electronic cigarettes: what are they and what do they do? Ann N Y Acad Sci. 2017;1394(1):5–30. https://doi.org/10.1111/nyas.12977.
93. England LJ, Anderson BL, Tong VT, Mahoney J, Coleman-Cowger VH, Melstrom P, et al. Screening practices and attitudes of obstetricians-gynecologists toward new and emerging tobacco products. Am J Obstet Gynecol. 2014;211(6):695 e1–7.

# Part III

# Treatment and Progress of Sudden Cardiac Death

# Prevention of Sudden Cardiac Death

# 11

Yanfen Chai, Songtao Shou, and Yonggang Gui

**Abstract**

Sudden death refers to death that occurs unexpectedly within 6 h of the onset of symptoms and in a normal state of health before. Mortality from sudden cardiac death (SCD) exceed the combined mortality of all major cancers. SCD mostly occurs outside the hospital, and most of them are asymptomatic before the onset of event. SCD has the characteristics of burstiness and unpredictability. The out-of-hospital cardiac arrest survival chain emphasizes timely identification and call for help, mainly chest compressions, defibrillation as soon as possible, and waiting for the professional team to transfer to the hospital as soon as possible after arriving. The hospital cardiac arrest survival chain emphasizes strengthening monitoring, establishing a rapid response system, and multidisciplinary and multi-team collaboration. SCD prevention should focus on high-risk populations. Efforts are made to help patients remove the etiology, take effective measures to control risk factors, detect changes in the condition of high-risk patients, and reduce the incidence of SCD.

**Keywords**

Sudden cardiac death · Treatment · Prevention

## 11.1 Definition

Sudden death (SD) refers to a sudden and unexpected death. At present, the defined duration from the onset of symptoms to death is still un-uniform. This definition is advocated by the World Health Organization (WHO): [1–3]. In 2015, the European Society of Cardiology (ESC) defined SD as death occurs unexpectedly within 1 h of

Y. Chai (✉) · S. Shou · Y. Gui
Emergency Department, General Hospital, Tianjin Medical University, Tianjin, China



H. Zhu (ed.), *Sudden Death*, https://doi.org/10.1007/978-981-15-7002-5_11

the onset of symptoms caused by non-traumatic, accidental fatal events [4, 5]. Generally, SD is clinically divided into sudden cardiac death (SCD) and non-SD cardiac death (NSCD). SCD accounts for nearly 80% of SD and NSCD accounts for approximately 20% of SD [6]. The definition of SCD is also constantly being updated. In 2008, ESC, the American Heart Association (AHA), and the American College of Cardiology (ACC) jointly revised the definition of SCD as an unexpected death due to cardiac causes that occurs within 1 h of the onset of symptoms, heralded by abrupt loss of consciousness [7]. In 2015, the ESC updated the definition of SCD as: a congenital or acquired, potentially fatal cardiac condition known to be present during life, or autopsy has identified a cardiac or vascular abnormality as the probable cause of the event or no obvious extra-cardiac causes have been identified by post-mortem, and therefore an arrhythmia event is a likely cause of death [4].

## 11.2 Epidemiology

SCD is the number one killer in United States. The incidence of SCD in the adult population is 0.1%–0.2% per year and is estimated to cause 17,0000 to 45,0000 deaths annually. Mortality from SCD exceed the combined mortality of all major cancers (lung, breast, colorectal, and prostate). It is estimated that there are 544,000 cases of SCD annually in China. The study predicts that the number of cardiovascular deaths will increase to 7.7 million in China by 2030, and SCD will account for more than half of all cardiovascular deaths [5, 8].

Etiologic factors causing SCD vary depending on an individual's age. There is a general increase in SCD risk beginning around age 35 years, which correlates with the increased prevalence of CHD over time. The annual incidence rate is 0.01% for persons <35 years of age, 1% for the age of 35–40 years, 2% for the age of 60 years, and 25% for the elderly. Most of the SCD occurred among people older than 65-year-old in China [9]. In Italy, investigators in the Veneto region conducted a prospective cohort study showing the annual incidence of SD in young athletes is higher than that in similar-aged non-athletes (0.23% years vs. 0.09% years), and the intensity of the activity is core risk factor [10]. In the Framingham SCD study, lifetime risk of SCD was higher in men than in women. Before 65 years of age, the incidence of SCD in men is almost four to seven times that of women. After that, the male to female ratio for SCD remained around 2:1, and this difference gradually diminished over time [1, 11].

## 11.3 Etiology and Pathogenesis of SCD

SCD is the result of an unresuscitated cardiac arrest, and its occurrence is closely related to cardiovascular disease. Preexisting heart disease is present in nearly 80% of patients with SCD. The causes of SCD could be broadly categorized as structural heart diseases (aortic disease, coronary artery disease, nonischemic cardiomyopathy, valvular heart disease, congenital heart disease, and conduction system disease), functional (hemodynamic instability, ischemia and reperfusion, electrolyte abnormalities, autonomic fluctuations, pharmacologic and toxic cardiac effects), electrogenic (ion channel disease), and other causes. According to European SCD guidelines, anatomical studies have found that coronary atherosclerotic disease is the main cause of SCD in the elderly, and about half of sudden death in the young is caused by cardiomyopathy. The pathogenesis of SCD is more complicated. It is mainly related to the internal environment, cardiac mechanism, ventricular depolarization, and abnormal repolarization [12, 13].

From the perspective of pathophysiology, SCD is divided into arrhythmic SCD and circulatory failure SCD. Underlying arrhythmias are thought to be the mechanism of death in SCD. Most cardiac arrests are due to life-threatening arrhythmia, such as ventricular tachycardia, fibrillation, or extremely slow arrhythmia. In patients undergoing ambulatory electrocardiographic monitoring at the time of SCD, ventricular tachycardia (VT) and ventricular fibrillation (VF) made up approximately 85% of SCD events, whereas bradyarrhythmias accounted for the remaining 15%. Sudden arrhythmic death is further divided into three categories according to the cause: (1) arrhythmias caused by organic heart disease, (2) malignant arrhythmias caused by secondary cardiac electrical activity disorder, and (3) arrhythmias due to ion channel defects [1, 14].

### 11.3.1 Coronary Artery Disease

The single most important cause of SCD among adults is coronary artery disease, with or without previous myocardial infarction, accounting for more than 75% of cases of SCD. In the coronary heart disease population, 50% of SCD events represent the first clinical manifestation of cardiovascular disease. Coronary artery disease includes coronary atherosclerosis, coronary arteritis, and congenital coronary artery abnormalities. Coronary atherosclerotic heart disease is the most common cause of sudden cardiac death, mostly manifested as acute coronary syndromes [15]. Coronary heart disease causes SCD involving two different pathophysiology mechanisms: acute ischemia and chronic ischemia. Acute myocardial infarction has a close relationship with the onset of SCD. Ischemic heart disease causes the change of ion channels between ischemic and normal myocardium, forming unstable currents and causing local electrophysiological disorders and excitement of ectopic rhythms, leading to fatal arrhythmias, especially ventricular fibrillation [16]. In chronic ishemic heart disease, the interaction of ischemia with the arrhythmias in the presence of autonomic nervous system abnormalities, LV dysfunction, and metabolic abnormal, genetic, and environmental influences are relevant factors in the occurrence of fatal arrhythmia [7].

### 11.3.2 Cardiomyopathies

Cardiomyopathy includes dilated cardiomyopathy, hypertrophic cardiomyopathy, arrhythmogenic right ventricular cardiomyopathy, etc., which are also common causes of SCD [17]. Dilated cardiomyopathy is a unilateral or bilateral ventricular enlargement, decreased myocardial contractility, and unexplained diseases with or without congestive heart failure, and about 70% of patients with dilated cardiomyopathy die from SCD. The degree of ventricular dilatation is positively correlated with the risk of developing SCD. Dilated cardiomyopathy, ventricular muscle scars, fibrosis, and focal necrosis promote ventricular arrhythmia via heterogeneous conduction and electrical reentry. Myocardial cells of patients with dilated cardiomyopathy have changes in the electrophysiological properties of ion channels and abnormal calcium concentrations inside and outside the cardiomyocytes, which increase the occurrence of fatal arrhythmias and then SCD. Hypertrophic cardiomyopathy is classified into obstructive hypertrophy and nonobstructive hypertrophic cardiomyopathy according to the pressure of left ventricular outflow tract. It is characterized by asymmetric LV hypertrophy, restricted left ventricular filling, and diastolic compliance decline. Disorders of myocardial cells in patients with hypertrophic cardiomyopathy and unstable electrical activity between hypertrophic myocardium cause recurrent arrhythmias. These factors can lead to SCD caused by ventricular fibrillation [18]. Arrhythmogenic right ventricular cardiomyopathy is an autosomal dominant hereditary disease characterized by progressive fibrofatty replacement of right ventricular myocardium. In the progressive fibrofatty replacement, patchy myocardial atrophy and repair by fibrofatty replacement may become the basis for reentrant ventricular arrhythmia [19].

### 11.3.3 Valvular Heart Disease

Valvular heart diseases may result from degenerative changes, inflammation, trauma, congenital malformations, and ischemic necrosis of the valve, which has structural and functional abnormalities of single or multiple valves, leading to stenosis and/or regurgitation. In China, the most common cause of valvular heart disease is rheumatic carditis. The mitral valve is most commonly affected, followed by the aortic valve. In pure mitral stenosis (MS), left atrial (LA) pressure increases to maintain cardiac output. The LA gradually enlarges and hypertrophies as a consequence of LA hypertension. When mitral stenosis is severe, transvalvular pressure and left atrial pressure increase significantly. Pulmonary venous pressure rises with LA pressure increase, which result in pulmonary edema; SCD also occurs [20–22].

### 11.3.4 Primary Electrical Abnormalities

Underlying arrhythmias are thought to be the mechanism of death in SCD. In patients undergoing ambulatory electrocardiographic monitoring at the time of SCD, ventricular tachycardia (VT) and ventricular fibrillation (VF) made up approximately 85% of SCD events, whereas bradyarrhythmias accounted for the remaining 15%.

In patients without structural heart disease, severe functional abnormalities can also lead to fatal arrhythmia, such as sinus node disease and abnormalities in the conduction system (Lenegre disease, WPW syndrome, Brugada syndrome, long Q-T interval syndrome, etc.) which can induce SCD. When the heart's conduction system is abnormal, it may induce myocardial impulse and conduction disorders, eventually leading to complete atrioventricular block and even SCD resulting from ventricular fibrillation. Such problems are generally classified as ion channel diseases, which include potassium and/or sodium ion channel problem, which often interferes with the electrical activity of the heart and produces fatal ventricular arrhythmias. It is more common in young people, and its clinical manifestations are hidden and varied, which is related to genetic mutations [23].

### 11.3.5 Other Causes

Other causes include heart rupture, massive acute pulmonary embolism, acute pericardial tamponade, intracardiac thrombus or tumor occlusion, aortic dissection, cardiac pacemaker failure, etc. These diseases cause cardiovascular collapse due to acute hemodynamic disorders, which cause SCD.

## 11.4 Clinical Manifestation

The cardiac arrest itself is characterized by abrupt loss of consciousness owing to inadequate cerebral blood flow, due to VF/VT, bradyarrhythmia/asystole, or EMD. The cause of SCD is more subtle. Because the human body has a strong ability to compensate, patients are often asymptomatic or have only mild symptoms before onset and can engage in normal daily activities. Most deaths occur at home, at rest, or during sleep. Prodromal symptoms such as sudden chest pain, chest tightness, dyspnea, weakness or fatigue, palpitations, dizziness, syncope, and a number of unspecific complaints may presage coronary events, particularly myocardial infarction and SCD. Thirty-one to forty-six percent of SCD victims consulted the medical system weeks to months before SCD, and from one-third to one-fourth of them had consulted a physician because of symptoms which appeared to be related to the heart.

A history of previous infarction and congestive heart failure complicating the infarction is useful to identify patients at increased mortality risk [24, 25].

## 11.5 Risk Factors

SCDs occur in patients with underlying heart disease, and the risk factors for SCD can induce or promote the sudden deterioration of underlying diseases in patients.

1. **Family history and genetic factors**: SCD and fatal ventricular arrhythmias are family susceptible. Some cardiomyopathy is an autosomal dominant genetic disease.

2. **Dietary structure**: Dietary structure is related to the incidence of SCD. Moderate intake of deep-sea fish can increase the content of omega-3 fatty acids in the body, which adjusts blood lipids to reduce the incidence of myocardial infarction. Deficiency of magnesium ion can cause coronary artery spasm and arrhythmia. Magnesium ions reduce the risk of SCD through antiarrhythmic effects. Increased dietary magnesium intake is associated with a reduced risk of SCD.
3. **Atrial fibrillation, kidney disease, and obstructive sleep apnea syndrome**: The use of oral anticoagulants has significantly reduced the death caused by embolism in patients with atrial fibrillation, but cannot prevent the SCD. Patients with chronic kidney disease have a high incidence of SCD. Triggers such as electrolyte disorders, left ventricular hypertrophy, hypertension, high blood volume, anemia, abnormal blood glucose, vitamin deficiency, low albumin, and increased sympathetic nerve function may precipitate an event. Obstructive sleep apnea syndrome is a recurrent, intermittent, severe, sleep-related respiratory disease that is characterized by apnea and hypoxemia caused by upper airway collapse and is an independent risk factor of SCD.
4. **Obesity**: The obesity is prone to cause hypertension, hyperlipidemia, and hyperglycemia, which are independent risk factors for coronary heart disease and can predispose to SCD.
5. **Mental factors**: There are many reports linking depression, anxiety, and excessive psychological stress to SCD.
6. **Overworked**: Overworked and vigorous exercise can lead to sympathetic and parasympathetic dysfunction, which can cause electrolyte imbalance and hypoglycemia and precipitate SCD.
7. **Bad living habits**: Staying up late for a long time leads to sympathetic and parasympathetic nerve dysfunction and induces premature heartbeat and other arrhythmias, causing SCD. Smoking and drinking are risk factors for coronary heart disease and trigger the onset of coronary heart disease. High stress in life can cause hypertension, coronary heart disease, and many other diseases, which can increase the risk of SCD due to arrhythmia and coronary artery spasm. Long-term exposure to severely polluted air is also the risk factor of SCD [9, 26, 27].

## 11.6 Differential Diagnosis

SCD often needs to be distinguished from sudden deaths caused by other diseases, mainly including respiratory diseases, central nervous system diseases, digestive system diseases, and tumor diseases.

1. **Respiratory diseases**: Respiratory diseases can also cause sudden death, foreign body obstruction, laryngospasm, acute exacerbation of chronic obstructive pulmonary disease, tension pneumothorax, massive acute pulmonary embolism, and persistent asthma which can cause asphyxia, hypoxia, and abnormal V/Q, which cause SCD.
2. **Central nervous system diseases**: Central nervous system diseases can induce sudden death; cerebral hemorrhage is most common, followed by cerebral

infarction and subarachnoid hemorrhage. Intracerebral hemorrhage can cause intracranial hyperpressure, compression of brain tissue, and shift of the midline structure, resulting in cerebral hernia. Epilepsy, epidemic cerebrospinal meningitis, and epidemic encephalitis B can also contribute to SCD.

3. **Digestive system diseases**: Massive upper gastrointestinal bleeding result in hypovolemia shock or asphyxiation caused by vomiting which are the main causes of sudden death. Severe acute pancreatitis develops rapidly and the mortality rate is high. Patients can progress to multiple organ dysfunction syndrome and die in a short period of time. Hepatic coma, toxic acute bacterial dysentery, and other digestive diseases can also induce sudden death.
4. **Tumors**: Malignant arrhythmias and massive pulmonary embolism are common causes of sudden death in patients with malignant tumors. Cancer cell invasion and dissemination by blood and multiple organ damage caused by lymphatic metastases can also cause sudden death, and tumor rupture and bleeding can also induce sudden death, most commonly lung cancer, followed by gastric cancer, esophageal cancer, liver cancer, and colon cancer.
5. **Obstetrics and gynecology diseases**: Hemorrhagic shock and amniotic fluid embolism caused by ectopic pregnancy rupture and hemorrhage can be the cause of SCD.

## 11.7 SCD Treatment

SCD mostly occurs outside the hospital, and most of them are asymptomatic before the onset of event. Timely and effective rescue can protect brain cells to a certain extent, even prevent the development of brain death. Timely and effective first aid is the final step to prevent SCD. The "2015 International Cardiopulmonary Resuscitation Guide Update" detailed the cardiac arrest survival chain and divided it into two parts: in-hospital cardiac arrest survival chain and out-of-hospital cardiac arrest survival chain. The purpose is to distinguish between patients with cardiac arrest in and out of the hospital and give different treatments according to different circumstances to ensure that patients can get the most effective management [28]. The out-of-hospital cardiac arrest survival chain emphasizes timely identification and call for help, mainly chest compressions, defibrillation as soon as possible, and waiting for the professional team to transfer to the hospital as soon as possible after arriving. The hospital cardiac arrest survival chain emphasizes strengthening monitoring, establishing a rapid response system, and multidisciplinary and multi-team collaboration [29].

### 11.7.1 Out-of-Hospital Cardiac Arrest

Witnesses at the scene to give CPR to patients with cardiac arrest in a timely manner are of vital importance. Government departments should improve the emergency medical service system, popularize CPR knowledge, train CPR skills to the entire public, and raise the awareness of participating in first aid. Call for help and cardiopulmonary resuscitation as soon as the cardiac arrest is diagnosed. In the order of C-A-B, C is Circulation, artificial circulation; A is Airway, keeping the airway unobstructed; and B is Breathing, artificial respiration. Chest compression refers to pressing the left palm with the middle and lower 1/3 of the patient's chest and sternum. The two palms overlap, the fingers are raised, the upper body is leaning forward, the shoulders are directly above the patient's sternum, and the arms are straight. The hip joint is used as a fulcrum, and the upper body is used to press down vertically with the force of gravity. The compression frequency is 100 to 120 times per minute. The compression depth for adults is 5 to 6 cm, and the compression depth for infants is 4 cm. After compression, ensure that the thorax fully rebounds. When opening the airway, in order to ensure effective artificial respiration, the patient's head should be tilted to one side, oral secretions and dentures should be removed, and the airway should be opened by raising the jaw. Keep the patient's airway unobstructed, pinch the patient's nose with thumb and forefinger, tightly wrap the mouth around the patient's mouth, slowly blow for 1 s, and observe the patient's thorax lift (the artificial breathing frequency is eight to ten times/min) The compression breathing ratio is 30:2. After five cycles of high-efficiency CPR, it is necessary to determine whether the resuscitation is effective, observe whether the patient has thoracic undulations, and touch the carotid artery for pulsation. The emergency rescue chain for out-of-hospital cardiac arrest includes five aspects: (1) effective identification and rapid activation of the emergency response system, (2) high-quality cardiopulmonary resuscitation, (3) rapid electrical defibrillation, (4) basic and advanced emergency medical services, and (5) advanced life support, post-arrest treatment [30–33].

### 11.7.2 In-Hospital Cardiac Arrest First Aid

The survival chain of in-hospital cardiac arrest also includes five aspects: (1) monitoring and prevention, (2) identifying and activating an emergency response system, (3) instant high-quality cardiopulmonary resuscitation, (4) rapid defibrillation, and (5) advanced life support treatment after sudden arrest. After the patient has a cardiac arrest in the hospital, the monitoring system can identify it immediately, and the medical staff quickly activates the in-hospital emergency response system to notify the trained professional resuscitation team to perform cardiopulmonary resuscitation. The "2015 International Cardiopulmonary Resuscitation Guide Update" states that in-hospital emergency-related personnel and organizations should pay attention to the formation of resuscitation teams and organize related training in the form of teams to ensure that first-aid patients with cardiac arrest can be implemented in a timely and efficient manner. Advanced life support mainly includes (1) establishment of artificial airways, (2) mechanical ventilation, (3) establishment of effective circulation, (4) rational and effective application of drugs, (5) electrical defibrillation, (6) evaluation of disease and efficacy, and (7) maintenance of various organ functions after resuscitation. For patients with cardiac arrest and pulseless electrical activity, epinephrine 1 mg/time is recommended for intravenous injection every 3 to 5 min. For both ventricular fibrillation and pulseless ventricular tachycardia, single-phase wave 360 J or bi-phase wave 200 J is recommended for one electric defibrillation, chest compressions immediately after defibrillation, and five cycles of cardiopulmonary resuscitation (approximately 2 min) to check for appearance. Autonomous cycle recovery. When preparing the defibrillator, chest compressions should be performed immediately to minimize interruption of chest compressions, and the defibrillator should be defibrillated as soon as possible after the defibrillator is ready. For patients with defibrillation-unresponsive ventricular fibrillation or pulseless ventricular tachycardia, cardiac amiodarone or lidocaine is recommended. Routine use of magnesium is not recommended. For torsional ventricular tachycardia, magnesium can be considered [30, 34, 35].

### 11.7.3 Treatment after Cardiac Arrest

After cardiac arrest, the blood supply to various organs in the body is interrupted, and organ function is severely damaged. Therefore, treatment after cardiac arrest and resuscitation is critical to patient survival and prognosis. Post-cardiac arrest treatment is a comprehensive treatment that includes multiple disciplines. These include the following:

1. Target temperature management. Mild hypothermia has a protective effect on the recovery of nerve function in patients with spontaneous circulation after cardiac arrest. For patients with in-hospital cardiac arrest and out-of-hospital cardiac arrest caused by cardioplegia or pulseless electrical activity, patients with unconscious recovery from cardiopulmonary resuscitation after cardiopulmonary resuscitation can still control their body temperature at 32–36 °C for at least 24 h.
2. Hemodynamics and ventilation optimization. Through rehydration, vasoactive drugs, and positive inotropic drugs, the mean arterial pressure is ≥65 mmHg, and proper cardiac output and systemic perfusion are maintained. By adjusting the ventilation rate and oxygen concentration to maintain arterial oxygen saturation ≥94%, end-expiratory carbon dioxide reached 35–40 mmHg, and arterial blood carbon dioxide reached 40–45 mmHg.
3. Immediate coronary reperfusion through percutaneous coronary intervention. All ST-segment elevation or non-ST-segment elevation with hemodynamic or ECG instability should be transferred to a medical center with percutaneous coronary intervention for emergency surgery.
4. Blood sugar control. The patient's blood glucose can be controlled at 8–10 mmol/L. The ultimate goals of cardiac arrest system treatment include (1) maximizing the recovery of patient's neurological function, controlling the patient's body temperature, and improving the survival rate; (2) identifying and treating ACS; (3) choosing the appropriate mechanical ventilation method to reduce lung injury; (4) prevention of multiple organ failure syndrome; (5) assessment of prognosis for resuscitation; and (6) provision of systematic rehabilitation for surviving SCD patients [30, 36].

## 11.8 SCD Prevention

SCD has the characteristics of burstiness and unpredictability. SCD prevention should focus on high-risk populations suffering from coronary artery disease, cardiomyopathy, valvular heart disease, and cardiac electrophysiological abnormality. Efforts are made to help patients remove the etiology, take effective measures to control risk factors, detect changes in the condition of high-risk patients, and reduce the incidence of SCD.

### 11.8.1 Prediction of SCD

#### 11.8.1.1 The Early Identification of High-Risk Patients with SCD

(1) People with the family history of SCD; (2) chest distress, palpitations, and dizziness during rest or activity; (3) people with the family history of hypertension, hyperlipidemia, diabetes, obesity, and premature cardiovascular disease; and (4) people with heart disease [37].

#### 11.8.1.2 The Early Warning Indicators of SCD

1. ECG, Holter, and ECG exercise test: ECG and Holter can determine the likelihood of SCD by detecting the slow or rapid arrhythmias and myocardial ischemia. For the patients with angina pectoris during activity and normal ECG in resting state, the ECG exercise test can confirm whether angina pectoris is caused by myocardial ischemia during activity.
2. Ultrasonic testing bedside ultrasound plays an important role in the rapid assessment and treatment of patients with acute critical illness. It has the advantages of simplicity, rapidity, effectiveness, noninvasiveness, and repeatability and has been described as the visible stethoscope of clinicians [38]. Echocardiography can accurately measure the size of cardiac structure and quantitatively evaluate cardiac function in real time and judge the severity of cardiac function and structural abnormality. Echocardiography can confirm the diagnosis of underlying structural heart disease (cardiomyopathy, cardiac valvular disease, congenital heart disease) and identify the cause of SCD. Simpson method, m-type method, and two-dimensional echocardiography were used to measure left ventricular ejection fraction (LVEF), which reflects the left ventricular pumping function and is the most commonly used indicator of left ventricular systolic function. SCD accounts for about 30–50% of deaths in patients with heart failure. SCD occurs in about 25% of patients within 2.5 years of diagnosis of symptomatic heart failure. LVEF is less than 30% in the approximately 45% of cardiac arrest patients. In the patients with ischemic or nonischemic cardiomyopathy, LVEF less than or equal to 35% has an increased risk of SCD and needs further evaluation for ICD therapy. These patients are at increased risk for SCD and need to be further evaluated for ICD therapy. Patients with LVEF ranging from 36% to 40%, previous myocardial infarction, and non-persistent VT should also be fur-

ther evaluated for ICD therapy [2]. LVEF is the only effective predictor of SCD and the main criterion for applying appropriate measures to prevent SCD [39].

Bedside ultrasound can quickly assist the diagnosis of severe hypovolemic, tension pneumothorax, pericardial tamponade, pulmonary embolism, and myocardial infarction. Subxiphoid or parasternal long axis sections of the right and left ventricles showing flat collapse heights indicate insufficient blood volume [40]. Pneumothorax can be excluded when the ultrasonic probe is placed in the forechest for quick scanning and the lung sliding sign appears. If the unilateral sliding sign of the lung disappears with the disappearance of line B, the height indicates the possibility of pneumothorax. The echogenic zone between the epicardium and parietal pericardium and diastolic right ventricular or right atrial collapse seen by the sonography under the xiphoid process can diagnose pericardial tamponade. Ultrasound can accurately and quickly locate the pericardial puncture point and improve the success rate of puncture [41]. Pulmonary embolism can be diagnosed by detecting a large embolus in the pulmonary trunk and left and right branches. Sonographic signs of pulmonary embolism include relative enlargement of the right ventricle, flat collapse of the left ventricle, d-shaped heart, right ventricle/left ventricular >1, inferior vena cava dilation with loss of respiratory variability, and subpleural nodules. Pulmonary embolism cannot be diagnosed by right ventricular enlargement alone and should be comprehensively determined by combining medical history, physical signs, and other laboratory tests [42]. The ultrasonic signs of myocardial infarction include dyssynchrony of ventricular wall motion, decrease of motion amplitude, paradoxical motion, and enhancement of normal segment ventricular wall motion.

3. Brain natriuretic peptide: The increase of brain natriuretic peptide is associated with SCD, which is a predictor of CD risk. Brain natriuretic peptides have predictive value for SCD not only in patients with coronary heart disease and heart failure but also in healthy people at potential risk [43].
4. Stiffness of the aorta and limb blood pressure examination: It can check the elasticity of the aorta, limb synchronous blood pressure, and limb synchronous blood flow state and is an effective method for early screening of atherosclerosis.
5. Coronary CT and coronary angiography: It can be used to clearly diagnose ischemic heart disease and guide whether to conduct myocardial revascularization. Ischemic heart disease is a serious threat to human health. The myocardial scar and cardiac dysfunction caused by ischemic heart disease can give rise to electrophysiological disorder and induce malignant arrhythmia, which is the main cause of SCD. Active detection of ischemic heart disease is the key to preventing SCD [44].
6. Ventricular late potential (VLP): It is located at the end of QRS wave at high frequency and low-amplitude fragmentation potential, which is the expression of electrical activity of non-synchronous depolarization and delayed conduction in ventricular myocardium. VLP has high sensitivity and specificity in predicting myocardial infarction with malignant arrhythmia. LVEF combined with VLP increases the predictive value of arrhythmia events and is an independent predictor of ventricular arrhythmia in patients with heart disease.

## 11.8.2 Preventive Measures of SCD

### 11.8.2.1 Surgery Prevention

Implantable cardioverter-defibrillator (ICD) is considered to be the best and most effective way to treat and prevent SCD. It can quickly identify patients with ventricular arrhythmias in a few seconds and can automatically defibrillate to save patient's lives. Compared with antiarrhythmic drugs, ICD can reduce the incidence of malignant ventricular arrhythmias and significantly reduce the incidence of SCD. For patients with persistent ventricular tachycardia, ICD can prevent the occurrence of SCD, significantly improve the prognosis, and improve the survival rate of patients [45]. Due to China's economic level and the reasons that medical insurance policies cannot fully cover the cost of patients, there is still a certain gap between the application of ICD and developed countries in Europe and the United States. The public's awareness of ICD and the necessity of ICD for SCD should be universally popularized to increase the possibility of patients using ICD. Patients with significant left heart failure should be implanted with ICD to prevent SCD. ICD is the treatment of choice for patients with dilated cardiomyopathy and hypertrophic cardiomyopathy of SCD who have previously experienced ventricular fibrillation and ventricular tachycardia, which can effectively prevent the occurrence of SCD [46]. In patients with previous cardiac arrest and syncope, the effect of drug treatment is not clear, and ICD is the first choice. Implantation of ICD with arrhythmogenic right ventricular cardiomyopathy with persistent ventricular tachycardia and syncope in the past can prevent the occurrence of SCD. Patients with grade IV cardiac function often die from malignant ventricular arrhythmias due to decompensated heart failure. ICD can also prevent SCD and reduce mortality.

Automatic external defibrillator China's public places have gradually been equipped with automatic external defibrillator (AED), but insufficient public education on the use of SCD and AED, resulting in the limited use of AED, not only caused a waste of resources but, more importantly, sudden death on those who did not receive timely and effective treatment. Patients with cardiac arrest due to ventricular fibrillation after 48 h of acute myocardial infarction are at high risk of reoccurrence of cardiac arrest after successful resuscitation. Vascular recanalization should be performed first. Coronary heart disease, especially patients with acute myocardial infarction, should undergo percutaneous coronary intervention as soon as possible to open the coronary vessels to restore myocardial blood supply and prevent SCD from recurring to improve the prognosis. However, the 2017 AHA/ACC/HRS Guidelines for the Management of Patients with Ventricular Arrhythmias and Prevention of Sudden Cardiac Death states that for patients with ischemic heart disease and persistent monomorphic ventricular tachycardia, coronary revascularizatio is not effective in preventing SCD. For patients with severe heart failure without malignant arrhythmias, cardiac resynchronization therapy may be preferred to improve cardiac function and reduce SCD. Catheter ablation is recommended to prevent SCD in patients with persistent ventricular tachycardia after myocardial infarction or patients with ventricular tachycardia or ventricular fibrillation storms who cannot tolerate amiodarone or other antiarrhythmic drugs [29].

#### 11.8.2.2 Drug

Although ICD is the preferred method for preventing and treating SCD, it is difficult to achieve the popularity of ICD in the short term according to China's national conditions. Drug prevention of SCD is still indispensable. Drug therapy plays an important role in stopping SCD caused by malignant arrhythmia.

1. Beta-blockers: It can reduce mortality and reduce the incidence of cardiovascular events in patients after myocardial infarction. For patients with coronary heart disease, β-receptor blockers can reduce myocardial oxygen consumption by slowing heart rate and controlling blood pressure and extend diastole, improve coronary perfusion, increase myocardial oxygen supply, and reduce fatal heart rhythm disorders to reduce the incidence of SCD. For patients with heart failure, β-receptor blockers can delay or reverse myocardial remodeling and reduce SCD by antagonizing the sympathetic nervous system, renin-angiotensin aldosterone system, and over-activated neurohumoral factors. Beta-blockers have become a safe first-line treatment for the prevention of malignant ventricular arrhythmia [47].
2. Amiodarone: It is a class III antiarrhythmic drug. Amiodarone plays an anticardiac rhythm aberrant effect by extending the effective refractory period of myocardial cells to eliminate reentry stimuli, inhibiting the influx of fast sodium ions in myocardial conductive fibers, slowing the conduction speed, and reducing the sinoatrial node autonomy. Amiodarone is the drug of choice for the treatment of malignant arrhythmias and the prevention of SCD. Amiodarone is the first choice for the treatment of malignant arrhythmia and the prevention of SCD. Amiodarone can also be used to prevent SCD in patients with coronary heart disease, atrial fibrillation with heart failure, and symptomatic, nonpersistent ventricular tachycardia [48, 49].
3. Angiotensin-converting enzyme inhibitors It can counteract left ventricular remodeling, increase vagal tone, and reduce the concentration of angiotensin II, which is involved in adrenergic transmission. Angiotensin-converting enzyme inhibitors can reduce the occurrence of SCD in diabetic patients with left ventricular dysfunction after myocardial infarction and improve the prognosis [50].
4. Aldosterone receptor antagonist: Aldosterone is involved in myocardial interstitial fibrosis and myocardial cell hypertrophy. Blocking aldosterone receptor can prevent myocardial remodeling and improve heart rate variability. Spironolactone significantly reduced SCD in patients with LVEF $<40\%$ [50].
5. Statins: Statins are effective in primary and secondary prevention of coronary heart disease and stroke [51]. Statins can reduce the risk of ventricular tachycardia and ventricular fibrillation in patients with coronary heart disease with ventricular arrhythmias, thereby reducing the incidence of SCD. Statins also can reduce the risk of arrhythmia and death in patients with nonischemic cardiomyopathy who require ICD [52].
6. The 2017 AHA/ACC/HRS Guidelines for the Management and Prevention of Sudden Cardiac Death in Patients with Ventricular Arrhythmias recommends that for patients with heart failure (LVEF«40%), β-receptor blockers, aldoste-

rone receptor antagonists, and angiotensin-converting enzyme inhibitors/angiotensin receptor antagonists/angiotensin receptor-enkephalinase inhibitors can reduce the incidence of SCD [29].

#### 11.8.2.3 Other Precautions

There are many risk factors for SCD, and effective control of risk factors has a certain effect on reducing the occurrence of SCD. Improving the diet structure, reducing the intake of sugars and fats, and increasing the intake of cellulose and deep-sea fish; maintaining blood pressure, blood sugar, and blood lipids at optimal level; actively controlling weight; avoiding depression, anxiety, excessive psychological stress, and excessive emotional fluctuations; avoiding overwork and strenuous exercise; and improving bad habits such as smoking, drinking, and staying up late can all reduce the incidence of SCD.

## References


1. Kuriachan VP, Sumner GL, Mitchell LB. Sudden cardiac death. Curr Probl Cardiol. 2015;40(4):133–200.
2. Tonnis T, Tack C, Kuck KH. Sudden cardiac death in athletes and its prevention. Herz. 2015;40(3):379–85.
3. Al Khatib SM, Sanders GD, Carlson M, et al. Preventing tomorrow's sudden cardiac death today:dissemination of effective therapies for sudden cardiac death prevention. Am Heart J. 2008;156(4):613–22.
4. Priori SG, Blomstrom-Lundqvist C, Mazzanti A, et al. 2015 ESC guidelines for the management of patients with ventricular arrhythmias and the prevention of sudden cardiac death. Eur Heart J. 2015;36(41):2793–867.
5. Krokhaleva Y, Vaseghi M. Update on prevention and treatment of sudden cardiac arrest. Trends Cardiovasc Med. 2019;29(7):394–400.
6. Al-Khatib SM, Yancy CW, Solis P, et al. 2016 AHA/ACC clinical performance and quality measures for prevention of sudden cardiac death. J Am Coll Cardiol. 2017;69(6):712–44.
7. Estes NAM. Predicting and preventing sudden cardiac death. Circulation. 2011;124(5):651–6.
8. Zhang S. Sudden cardiac death in China: current status and future perspectives. Europace. 2015;17(Suppl 2):ii14–8.
9. Jazayeri MA, Emert MP. Sudden cardiac death: who is at risk? Med Clin North Am. 2019;103(5):913–30.
10. Winkel BG, Jabbari R, Tfelt-Hansen J. How to prevent SCD in the young? Int J Cardiol. 2017;237:6–9.
11. Bergau L, Seegers J, Zabel M. Sex differences in ICD benefit. J Electrocardiol. 2014;47(6):869–73.
12. Wong CX, Brown A, Lau DH, et al. Epidemiology of sudden cardiac death: global and regional perspectives. Heart Lung Circ. 2019;28(1):6–14.
13. Goyal V, Jassal DS, Dhalla NS. Pathophysiology and prevention of sudden cardiac death. Can J Physiol Pharmacol. 2016;94(3):237–44.
14. Wasfy MM, Hutter AM, Weiner RB. Sudden cardiac death in athletes. Methodist Debakey Cardiovasc J. 2016;12(2):76–80.
15. Morin DP, Homoud MK, Estes NAM 3rd. Prediction and prevention of sudden cardiac death. Card Electrophysiol Clin. 2017;9(4):631–8.
16. Sara JD, Eleid MF, Gulati R, Holmes DR Jr. Sudden cardiac death from the perspective of coronary artery disease. Mayo Clin Proc. 2014;89(12):1685–98.

17. Magi S, Lariccia V, Maiolino M, Amoroso S, Gratteri S. Sudden cardiac death: focus on the genetics of channelopathies and cardiomyopathies. J Biomed Sci. 2017;24(1):56.
18. Kruska M, El-Battrawy I, Behnes M, Borggrefe M, Akin I. Biomarkers in cardiomyopathies and prediction of sudden cardiac death. Curr Pharm Biotechnol. 2017;18(6):472–81.
19. Calkins H, Corrado D, Marcus F. Risk stratification in arrhythmogenic right ventricular cardiomyopathy. Circulation. 2017;136(21):2068–82.
20. Haude M. Management von Herzklappenerkrankungen: ESC/EACTS-Leitlinie 2017 [Management of valvular heart disease: ESC/EACTS guidelines 2017]. Herz. 2017;42(8):715–20.
21. Mrsic Z, Hopkins SP, Antevil JL, Mullenix PS. Valvular heart disease. Prim Care. 2018;45(1):81–94.
22. Iung B, Vahanian A. Epidemiology of acquired valvular heart disease. Can J Cardiol. 2014;30(9):962–70.
23. Abriel H, Rougier JS, Jalife J. Ion channel macromolecular complexes in cardiomyocytes: roles in sudden cardiac death. Circ Res. 2015;116(12):1971–88.
24. Rabinstein AA. Sudden cardiac death. Handb Clin Neurol. 2014;119:19–24.
25. Schmied C, Borjesson M. Sudden cardiac death in athletes. J Intern Med. 2014;275(2):93–103.
26. Shenasa M, Shenasa H. Hypertension, left ventricular hypertrophy, and sudden cardiac death. Int J Cardiol. 2017;237:60–3.
27. Shah M. Hypertrophic cardiomyopathy. Cardiol Young. 2017;27(S1):S25–30.
28. Nolan JP. International CPR guidelines-perspective in CPR. Best Pract Res Clin Anaesthesiol. 2013;27(3):317–25.
29. Al-Khatib SM, Stevenson WG, Ackerman MJ, et al. 2017 AHA/ACC/HRS guideline for management of patients with ventricular arrhythmias and the prevention of sudden cardiac death: executive summary: a report of the American College of Cardiology/American Heart Association task force on clinical practice guidelines and the Heart Rhythm Society [published correction appears in heart rhythm. 2018 Sep 26]. Heart Rhythm. 2018;15(10):e190–252.
30. Neumar RW, Shuster M, Callaway CW, et al. Part 1: executive summary: 2015 American Heart Association guidelines update for cardiopulmonary resuscitation and emergency cardiovascular care. Circulation. 2015;132(18 Suppl 2):S315–67.
31. Idris AH, Guffey D, Pepe PE, et al. Chest compression rates and survival following out-of-hospital cardiac arrest. Crit Care Med. 2015;43(4):840–8.
32. Ringh M, Rosenqvist M, Hollenberg J, et al. Mobile-phone dispatch of laypersons for CPR in out-of-hospital cardiac arrest. N Engl J Med. 2015;372(24):2316–25.
33. Smith CM, Wilson MH, Ghorbangholi A, et al. The use of trained volunteers in the response to out-of-hospital cardiac arrest – the GoodSAM experience. Resuscitation. 2017;121:123–6.
34. Moler FW, Silverstein FS, Holubkov R, et al. Therapeutic hypothermia after in-hospital cardiac arrest in children. N Engl J Med. 2017;376(4):318–29.
35. Sandroni C, Nolan J, Cavallaro F, Antonelli M. In-hospital cardiac arrest: incidence, prognosis and possible measures to improve survival. Intensive Care Med. 2007;33(2):237–45.
36. Andersen LW, Holmberg MJ, Berg KM, Donnino MW, Granfeldt A. In-hospital cardiac arrest: a review. JAMA. 2019;321(12):1200–10.
37. Fishman GI, Chugh SS, Dimarco JP, et al. Sudden cardiac death prediction and prevention: report from a National Heart, lung, and blood institute and Heart Rhythm Society workshop. Circulation. 2010;122(22):2335–48.
38. Huis In't Veld MA, Allison MG, Bostick DS, et al. Ultrasound use during cardiopulmonary resuscitation is associated with delays in chest compressions. Resuscitation. 2017;119:95–8.
39. John RM, Tedrow UB, Koplan BA, et al. Ventricular arrhythmias and sudden cardiac death. Lancet. 2012;380(9852):1520–9.
40. Atkinson P, Bowra J, Milne J, et al. International Federation for Emergency Medicine Consensus Statement: sonography in hypotension and cardiac arrest (SHoC): an international consensus on the use of point of care ultrasound for undifferentiated hypotension and during cardiac arrest. CJEM. 2017;19(6):459–70.

41. Steiger HV, Rimbach K, Muller E, et al. Focused emergency echocardiography: lifesaving tool for a 14-year-old girl suffering out-of-hospital pulseless electrical activity arrest because of cardiac tamponade. Eur J Emerg Med. 2009;16(2):103–5.
42. Chowdhury MA, Moza A, Siddiqui NS, et al. Emergent echocardiography and extracorporeal membrane oxygenation: lifesaving in massive pulmonary embolism. Heart Lung. 2015;44(4):344–6.
43. Cao ZP, Xue JJ, Zhang Y, et al. Differential expression of B-type natriuretic peptide between left and right ventricles, with particular regard to sudden cardiac death. Mol Med Rep. 2017;16(4):4763–9.
44. Jappar IA, Chua T, Htoo MM, et al. Diagnosis of anomalous origin and course of coronary arteries using non-contrast cardiac CT scan and detection features. J Cardiovasc Comput Tomogr. 2012;5:335–45.
45. Deniz A, Demir M. Comments on 2015 ESC guidelines for the Management of Patients with ventricular arrhythmias and the prevention of sudden cardiac death. Turk Kardiyol Dern Ars. 2016;44(1):9–14.
46. Podriguez-Manero M, Barrio-Lopez MT. Primary prevention of sudden death in patients with valvular cardiomyopathy. Rev Esp Cardiol (Engl Ed). 2016;69(3):272–8.
47. Tsuji Y, Ishikawa T, Makiya N. Molecular mechanisms of heart failure progression associated with implantable cardioverter-defibrillator shocks for ventricular tachyarrhythmias. J Arrhythmia. 2014;30(4):235–41.
48. Wyllie J, Perlman JM, Kattwinkel J, et al. Part 7: Neonatal resuscitation: 2015 International consensus on cardiopulmonary resuscitation and emergency cardiovascular care science with treatment recommendations. Resuscitation. 2015;95:e169–201.
49. Finn JC, Bhanji F, Lockey A, et al. Part 8:Education, implementation, and teams: 2015 International consensus on cardiopulmonary resuscitation and emergency cardiovascular care science with treatment recommendations. Resuscitation. 2015;95:e203–24.
50. Peck KY, Lim YZ, Hopper I, et al. Medical therapy versus implantable cardioverter-defibrillator in preventing sudden cardiac death in patients with left ventricular systolic dysfunction and heart failure: a meta-analysis of >35000 patients. Int J Cardiol. 2014;173(2):197–203.
51. Chrispin J, Martin SS, Hasan RK, Joshi PH, Minder CM, McEvoy JW, Kohli P, Johnson AE, Wang L, Blaha MJ, Blumenthal RS. Landmark lipid-lowering trials in the primary prevention of cardiovascular disease. Clin Cardiol. 2013;36:516–23.
52. Goldberger JJ, Subacius H, Schaechter A, Howard A, Berger R, Shalaby A, Levine J, Kadish AH, DEFINITE Investigators. Effects of statin therapy on arrhythmic events and survival in patients with nonischemic dilated cardiomyopathy. J Am Coll Cardiol. 2006;48:1228–33.

# Cardiopulmonary Resuscitation 12

Xuelian Yin, Haiyan Zhu, Yang Yang, and Hong Shen

**Abstract**

High-quality cardiopulmonary resuscitation (CPR) improves the rate return of spontaneous circulation and survival in patients with cardiac arrest. Despite well-established recommendations of the guidelines, high-quality CPR remains a challenge in the clinical practice. As our understanding of cardiac arrest and resuscitation physiology has developed, more and more new techniques and devices have emerged, which involved in most parts of CPR: compression, defibrillation, and airway management. Development of the Internet and health service systems facilitates integration of basic life support measures with prehospital care. These advances may improve the prognosis of cardiac arrest and will be integrated into new cardiac arrest protocols in the future. Large-scale randomized controlled clinical trials are awaited to verify the effectiveness of these new resuscitation techniques and strategies. On the other hand, organ protection to reduce systemic ischemia-reperfusion injury induced by cardiac arrest and resuscitation is the focus of CA treatment.

X. Yin
Emergency Department, Tongren Hospital, Capital Medical University, Beijing, China

H. Zhu
Emergency Department, The First Medical Center of Chinese PLA General Hospital, Beijing, China

Emergency Department, Hainan Hospital of Chinese PLA General Hospital, Haitangwan Bay, Sanya City, Hainan Province, China

Y. Yang
Emergency Department, 900 Joint Logistics Support Force Hospital of PLA, Fuzhou, China

H. Shen (✉)
The General Hospital of People's Liberation Army, Beijing, China
e-mail: shenhong@em120.com



H. Zhu (ed.), *Sudden Death*, https://doi.org/10.1007/978-981-15-7002-5_12

**Keywords**

Cardiopulmonary resuscitation · Chest compressions · Mitochondria · Sarcoplasmic Anisodamine · Epinephrine

## 12.1 Introduction

Cardiac arrest (CA) is defined as the sudden unexpected termination of cardiac activity within 24 h. It is a life-threatening emergency and one of the largest causes of mortality in the world. In the USA, CA affects 350,000 to 450,000 individuals per year [1]. Approximately 395,000 cases occur out of hospital (OHCA) [2] and 200,000 cases occur in hospital (IHCA) [3] annually. Clinical studies indicate the survival rate for OHCA is 12% and for IHCA is 24.8% in the USA. A multicenter prospective observational study in China showed the survival of sudden CA in emergency department was still poor. The rate of return of spontaneous circulation (ROSC) in IHCA patients was higher than that in OHCA patients [37.3% (154/413) vs. 27.0% (54/200)]. But there was no statistic difference in 28-day survival rate between the two groups ([3.6% (15/413) vs. 2.5% (5/200)] [4].

Coronary artery disease is the most common underlying etiology for the sudden cardiac death, as seen in approximately 80% of OHCA in the USA. Non-cardiac origin CA may occur in suffocation, drowning, pulmonary disease, and stroke.

Cardiopulmonary resuscitation (CPR) is a skill that can rescue the life of human body when the process of death begins. The American Heart Association and the European Resuscitation Council formed the International Liaison Committee on Resuscitation (ILCOR) for the development of international guidelines in 1992. In 2019, the ILCOR has initiated the third annual summary of the International Liaison Committee on Resuscitation International Consensus on Cardiopulmonary Resuscitation and Emergency Cardiovascular Care Science with Treatment Recommendations (CoSTR) [5]. The consensus generally includes the following topics: Basic life support; Advanced life support (ALS); Pediatric life support; Neonatal life support (NLS); Education, Implementation, and Teams (EIT); and ALS. Early and high-quality CPR is closely associated with the survival rate of patients with CA 10 min after CA, and the survival rate falls down to 4.5% . If the CPR is initiated in 5 min, the survival rate is 37.5%. However, if the CPR is done 10 min after CA, the survival rate falls down to 4.5% Early electric defibrillation, manual chest compression, CA that occurred in hospital or in ambulance, and witness CPR can improve the ROSC rate of CA patients. Excessive use of adrenaline is not beneficial to patients with CA.

In this chapter, we review the history and progress on adult CPR, focusing on four skills; chest compressions, defibrillation, airway and ventilation management, and drug use.

## 12.2 High-Quality Chest Compressions

High-quality chest compressions are thought as a key element in the cardiac arrest chain of survival.

In 1960, Kouwenhoven et al. [6] at Johns Hopkins Hospital first showed that closed-chest cardiac massage of the lower portion of the sternum maintained an adequate circulation. They found this technique increases peak blood pressure to 80 mmHg and gives rise to survival rate to 70% on 20 patients. However, 50 years after publication of this landmark article, only a minority of cardiac arrest patients survive to hospital discharge.

The primary purpose of chest compression is to artificially establish circulation by increasing thoracic pressure and squeezing heart. By providing blood flow to the whole body, high-quality CPR might rescue varied energy-depleted organs. In a clinical study, 90 s of chest compression to persons with out-of-hospital ventricular fibrillation (VF) prior to defibrillation was associated with increased survival. This result suggests improved myocardial reperfusion is necessary to achieve successful resuscitation. Coronary perfusion pressure (CPP), which is the difference between aortic relaxation ("diastolic") pressure and right atrial relaxation ("diastolic") pressure, is a surrogate for myocardial perfusion. During CA, higher CPP consistently improved the outcome [7]. Paradis et al. [8] found that a CPP >15 mmHg was required for successful ROSC. In 2011, Zhou [9], from the research group led by professor Shen, firstly showed sustained abdominal aorta compression-cardiopulmonary resuscitation (SAAC-CPR) can rapidly and reversibly raise the CPP as much as epinephrine in swine models can. This maneuver is especially suitable for out-of-hospital CPR. To perform high-quality CPR with effective chest compressions, the latest adult CPR guidelines [5] recommend as follows: (a) push chest quickly (100–120/min), (b) compress appropriately (5–6 cm), (c) relax chest fully (complete chest recoil), (d) avoid interruption of compression, and (e) avoid hyperventilation (30:2 chest compression/ventilation ratio prior to advanced airway; 10 breaths/min with advanced airway). In 2011, Dai [10] measured the distance from inter-nipple line (INL) to anterior mitral valve (AMV) plane of 1002 adult patients and the width of hand heel (WHH) in 100 volunteers. The distance from INL to AMV plane was within WHH value in about 96% of patients. These data support that the center of the chest between the nipples is the appropriate compression position in adult CPR. Idris [11] found a curvilinear association between chest compression rate and return of spontaneous circulation (ROSC). ROSC peaked at a compression rate of 125/min and then declined. Edelson [12] and colleagues reported compression depth is linearly related to survival too. Hellevuo [13] indicated when chest compression depth is >6 cm, risk for CPR-related injury increases significantly.

High-quality manual chest compression is challenged by several factors such as fatigue and physical strength of the rescuer. Besides, in special situations such as ambulance transportation, primary percutaneous coronary intervention, extracorporeal CPR, high-quality manual chest compression cannot be safely delivered. To solve those defects, mechanical CPR devices are invented [14]. A number of devices are currently available in markets, such as Thumper, AutoPulse, and the LUCAS chest compressors. They can provide stable and long-lasting chest compression in an automated way. However, it is still uncertain whether the use of mechanical devices improves outcomes in CA patients. In a systematic review analysis, Zhu [15] indicated there is no significant difference in terms of the ROSC rate, the rate of survival to hospital discharge, and neurological function between mechanical and manual chest compression in OHCA patients. They suggested that manual chest compression be applied in the early stage of CPR for OHCA patients, while mechanical compression can be used as part of advanced life support in the late stage. Further trials are needed to evaluate the use of mechanical CPR devices in IHCA.

In 2019 CoSTR, ILCOR [5] addresses the effect of dispatchers providing CPR instruction to callers/bystanders (DA-CPR) on outcomes for patients in OHCA.

## 12.3 Defibrillation

The major cause of CA is cardiovascular origin. Over 20% of OHCA patients present with a shockable rhythm initially (ventricular fibrillation, VF, or pulseless ventricular tachycardia, VT), while the incidence of non-pulsed electrical activity (PEA) is 19–23%, and asystole is 50%, respectively. Outcome of OHCA patients who have non-shockable initial rhythm is worse than those with shockable rhythm. Defibrillation [16] refers to passing an electrical current across myocardium to depolarize the muscle, which terminates arrhythmia and results in a sinus rhythm. Defibrillation is the definitive treatment for shockable arrhythmia. In 1956, Zoll [17] terminates ventricular fibrillation in man through externally applied electric counter shock. Now this method has been applied universally for CA patients by trained medical staff.

Refractory VF [15] refers to persisting VF despite three shocks. It has been shown that significant coronary artery disease (>70% stenosis) was noted in greater than 80% of patients with refractory VF OHCA. In 2002, Weisfeldt [18] speculated if the circulation is stopped for more than 10 min, defibrillation may fail to terminate VF or VF may change to non-shockable rhythm because of global metabolic failure. High-quality chest compression improves the chances of successful defibrillation by providing blood flow to the myocardium.

Besides, defibrillation requires stopping CPR for rhythm analysis and shock delivery. Coult [19] suggested waveform measures during CPR combined with prior return of organized rhythm (ROR) exceeded the predictive capability of CPR-free waveform measures alone. Ideally, the shocks can be timed to maximize the likelihood of resuscitation and to limit the interruption of CPR.

Since the 1990s, automated external defibrillators (AEDs) have been increasingly applied for prehospital defibrillation of patients. A meta-analysis showed that CPR + AED improve outcome of prehospital CA patients compared with CPR-only group. A retrospective analysis indicated the use of on-site AEDs and non-emergency medical service (EMS) defibrillation increases survival rate of patients with a shockable initial rhythm. Shen and Nguyen [20] reported that machine learning technique improves certainly the detection performance of the proposed shock advice algorithm (SAA) applied in the AED.

## 12.4 Airway Management

In 1958, Safar [21] described effective pulmonary ventilation by mouth-to-mouth breathing without an artificial airway. After cardiac origin CA, chest compressions and defibrillation are thought to take priority over airway and ventilation interventions [22]. When asphyxial cardiac arrest occurs, appropriate, earlier airway and ventilation interventions to restore adequate oxygenation to the vital organs may be preferable.

Basic airway interventions refer to mouth-to-mouth ventilation, mouth-to-mask ventilation and bag-mask ventilation (with or without an oropharyngeal airway). Advanced airway interventions include supraglottic airways (SGAs) and tracheal intubation using direct or video laryngoscopy. Voss [23] reported that which airway intervention an OHCA patient may receive is according to the skills of the rescuer present and the time point during resuscitation. Nichol [24] reported bag-mask ventilation without pausing compressions did not increase survival rate in OHCA compared with pausing for ventilation after every 30 compressions.

Advanced airway management enables chest compressions to continue uninterrupted and protect the lungs from aspiration of gastric contents. SGA insertion is easier to learn than tracheal intubation and feasible with fewer and shorter interruptions in chest compression. A meta-analysis showed patients with OHCA who receive endotracheal intubation (ETI) by EMS are more likely to obtain ROSC, survive to hospital admission, and survive neurologically intact when compared to SGA. Compared to classic laryngeal airway mask (cLMA), the second-generation SGAs (e.g., i-gel and LMA Supreme (LMAS)) provide patients with more optimal pharyngeal seal pressure, esophageal drainage tubes, and integrated bite blocks. Large RCTs that compare second-generation SGAs with tracheal intubation during OHCA are awaited [25]. Besides, video laryngoscopy (VL) use has potential advantages over conventional laryngoscopy during CPR [26].

Detection of $CO_2$ in exhaled air following intubation is the most specific criterion for confirming endotracheal tube placement during CPR. End-tidal carbon dioxide ($ETCO_2$) concentration is also a reliable index of effective chest compression during CPR [27], which is associated with cardiac output. $ETCO_2$ levels $<10$ mmHg are consistently associated with a poor outcome.

## 12.5 Drug Therapy

### 12.5.1 Epinephrine

Epinephrine (adrenaline) increases aortic diastolic pressure through activating$\alpha$-adrenergic receptors during CPR; thereby it augments coronary blood flow [28]. However, $\beta$-adrenergic activation causes dysrhythmias and increased myocardial oxygen demand. Early administration of epinephrine in patients with a non-shockable rhythm is associated with better outcomes. In contrast, for CA patients with shockable rhythm, epinephrine leads to worse prognosis. Recently, Perkins [29] et al. found that although epinephrine resulted in a significantly higher rate of

30-day survival than the use of placebo, more survivors had severe neurologic impairment in the epinephrine group. They speculated the neurologic impairment is associated with cerebral microcirculation dysfunction induced by$\alpha$-adrenergic stimulation. Epinephrine has been shown to significantly decrease the sublingual, myocardial, and cerebral cortical microcirculation in pigs [30, 31]. These data support that although the use of epinephrine during CPR can increase CPP, the blood supply of tissues does not increase because of the reduction of microcirculation blood flow caused by epinephrine.

### 12.5.2 Antiarrhythmic Drugs

The North American Resuscitation Outcomes Consortium (ROC)-Amiodarone, Lidocaine, or Placebo Study (ALPS) (ROC-ALPS) [32] is the largest RCT to evaluate the effects of antiarrhythmic drugs on OHCA. For treatment of refractory VF/pVT, this study reported no difference in survival to hospital discharge or neurological outcome. In patients with witnessed arrest, survival was improved with amiodarone 300 mg and lidocaine 120 mg compared to placebo (amiodarone 27.7%, lidocaine 27.8%, and placebo 22.7%). Antiarrhythmic drugs also decreased the number of shocks required to terminate VF/pVT and increased the rate of ROSC by hospital arrival. For non-shockable-turned-shockable OHCA, ROC/ALPS study showed after adjusted absolute differences, survival with amiodarone vs. placebo was 2.3% (−0.3, 4.8), $p = 0.08$, and for lidocaine vs. placebo 1.2% (−1.1, 3.6), $p = 0.30$. These data support that there does not appear to be any clear survival benefit for amiodarone or lidocaine in OHCA. Recently, a retrospective study via Wang indicated for patients with IHCA and shock-refractory VF/pVT that the amiodarone-first strategy was associated with a higher probability of terminating VF/pVT within three shocks (OR, 11.61; 95% confidence interval 1.34e100.84; $p$ value = 0.03).

### 12.5.3 Anisodamine

Anisodamine [33–35] is an alkaloid extracted from the root of scopolamine tangkula. It is a non-subtype-selective muscarinic and also a nicotinic cholinoceptor antagonist. It can relieve the smooth muscle spasm by non-selectively blocking M cholinergic receptor. It can also relieve microvasospasm, increase coronary blood flow, and improve tissue microcirculation. The mechanisms seem to include inhibiting ACh-induced endothelial cell activation, $\alpha$1-adrenoceptor blockade, and antithrombotic and fibrinolytic effects. Anisodamine also has been shown to possess an antioxidant and anti-inflammatory action. Alpha-7 nicotinic ACh receptors ($\alpha$7nAChRs) may play an important role in the cholinergic anti-inflammatory responses. Recently, Xing [36] found anisodamine reduced cardiomyocyte apoptosis in a rat model of ischaemia-reperfusion. Since one decade ago, the research team led by professor Shen has conducted a series of studies and proved the protective effect of anisodamine on various cardiac arrest and cardiopulmonary resuscitation

(CA/CPR) animal models. Now, growing evidence supports that anisodamine has the beneficial effects on CA/CPR.

In 2008, Sun [37] (see Table 12.1) reported firstly that administration of epinephrine plus anisodamine at the beginning of treatment for cardiac arrest could improve ROSC rate and 3-h survival rate in rats after ventricular fibrillation (VF) or asystole was induced by transesophageal alternating current stimulation. In 2011, Yin [38] also showed 24-h survival rate was significantly different between epinephrine plus anisodamine group and epinephrine group (see Fig. 12.1).

In 2011, Zhou [39] found that in alternating current-induced VF swines, administration of anisodamine in combination with epinephrine at the beginning of CA could improve CPP (see Fig. 12.2) and success rate of ROSC. Zhou reported that the level of $PETCO_2$ in anisodamine + epinephrine group was significantly higher than anisodamine group ($n$ = 9, 18.14 ± 1.35 mmHg vs. 13.17 ± 1.35 mmHg) before

**Table 12.1** Comparison of the number of return of spontaneous circulation (ROSC) and 3-h survival rate in each group

| Group | $n$ | ROSC | 30-min survival | 3-h survival |
|---|---|---|---|---|
| Control | 15 | 1 (6.7) | 0 | 0 |
| Epinephrine | 15 | 7 (46.6) | 5 (33.3)* | 1* |
| Epinephrine+anisodamine | 15 | 14 (93.3) | 12 (80)*,# | 10 (67)*,# |

Note: *compared with the control group ($p < 0.05$), #compared with the epinephrine group

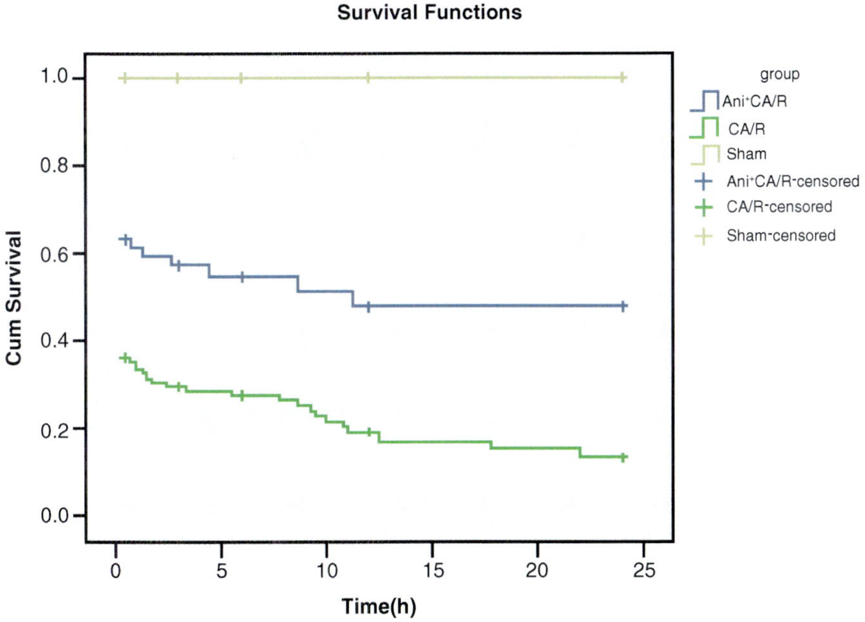


**Fig. 12.1** Survival curve of each group of rats after cardiac arrest

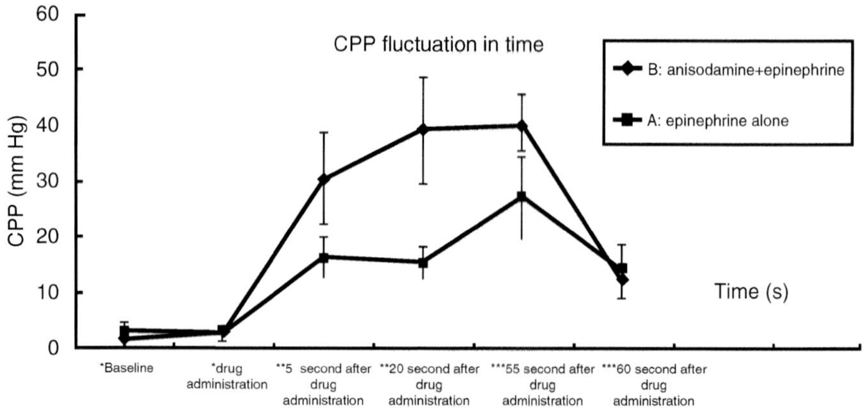


**Fig. 12.2** Mean coronary perfusion pressure (CPP) fluctuation for animals receiving 1 min of CPR after intravenous drug administration in time in two groups

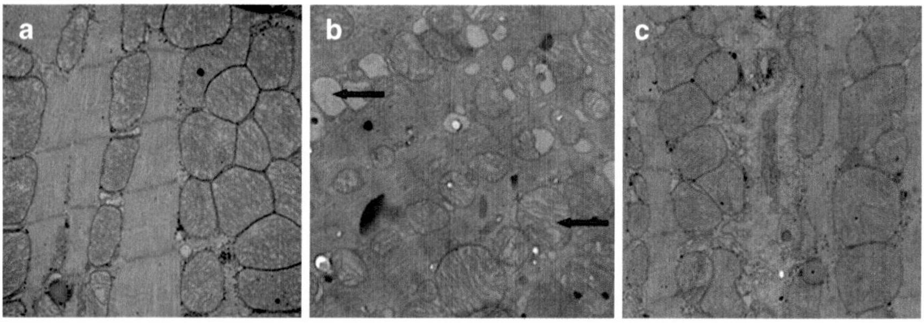


**Fig. 12.3** Mitochondria in rat cardiomyocytes 3 h after CPR (×20,000). (**a**) Sham operation group: complete mitochondria with rich and complete cristae. (**b**) Epinephrine group: mitochondria swelling with partial vacuolization and sparse cristae; (**c**) Epinephrine + anisodamine group: swollen and complete mitochondria with cristae fuzzy

first-shock defibrillation (after 9 min of untreated prolonged VF with 1 min of chest compression).

Further studies found that anisodamine reduced ischemic/reperfusion injury induced by CA/CPR in various tissues such as myocardium, lung, intestine, and brain [37–44]. Cells were well preserved, and less ultrastructural damage was observed in anisodamine plus epinephrine group compared with epinephrine-only group, as shown by Yang [40] (Fig. 12.3), Yin [41] (Fig. 12.4), and Dai [42] (Fig. 12.5).

This group of researchers also found that anisodamine may exert its protective effects on CA and CPR through multiple pathways.

Firstly, anisodamine can improve microcirculation and tissue metabolism. Jia [45] found that after ROSC, the proportion of mesenteric recanalization, microvascular diameter, blood flow velocity, and intestinal wall tissue perfusion volume in

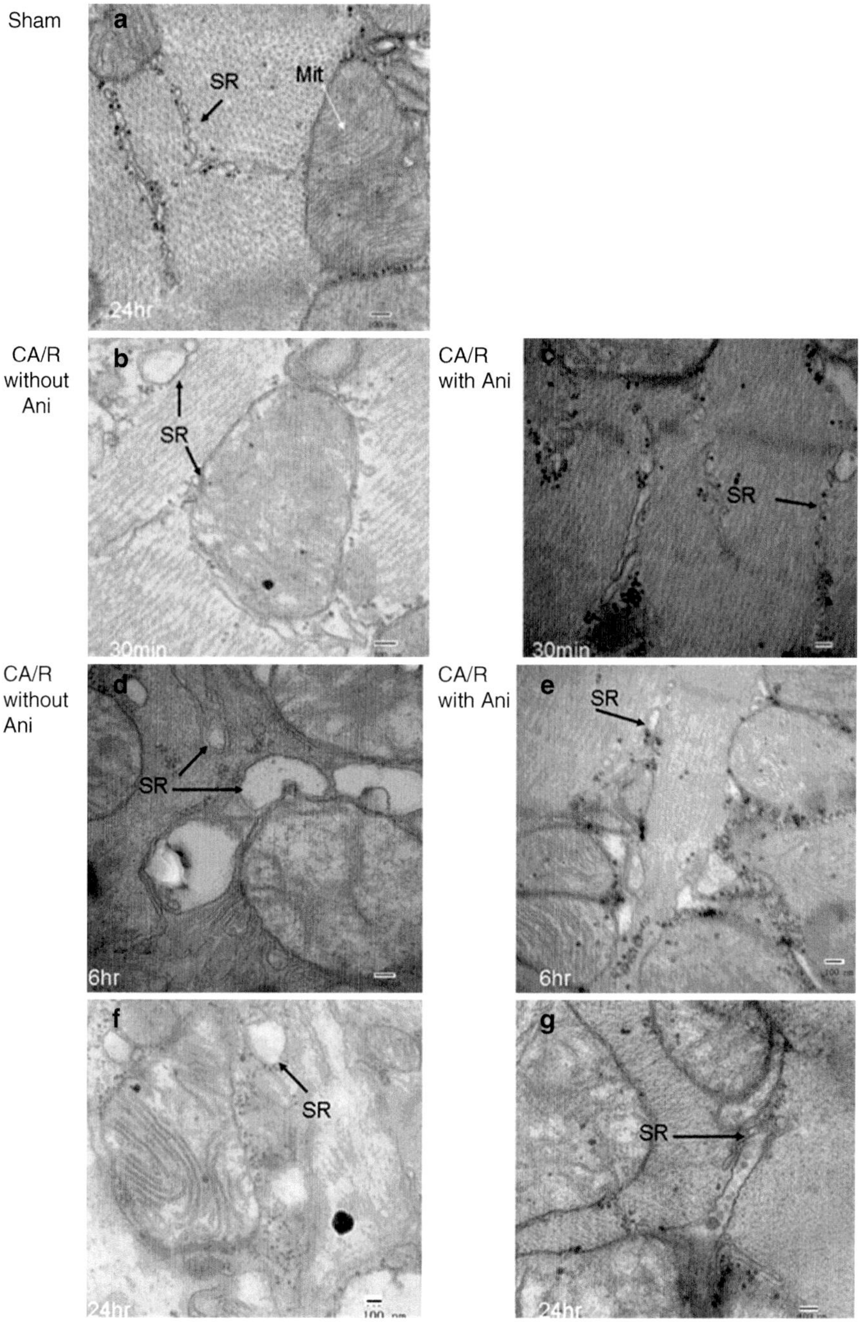


**Fig. 12.4** Sarcoplasmic (SR) in cardiomyocytes after cardiac arrest and ROSC (×60,000). (**a**) Sham operation group: normal structure of SR (↑). (**b**, **d**, **f**) Epinephrine group at 30 min, 6 h, and 24 h after ROSC: mitochondria and SR edema or disruption gets worse over time. (**c**, **e**, **g**) Epinephrine + anisodamine group: swollen and deformation of SR and mitochondria

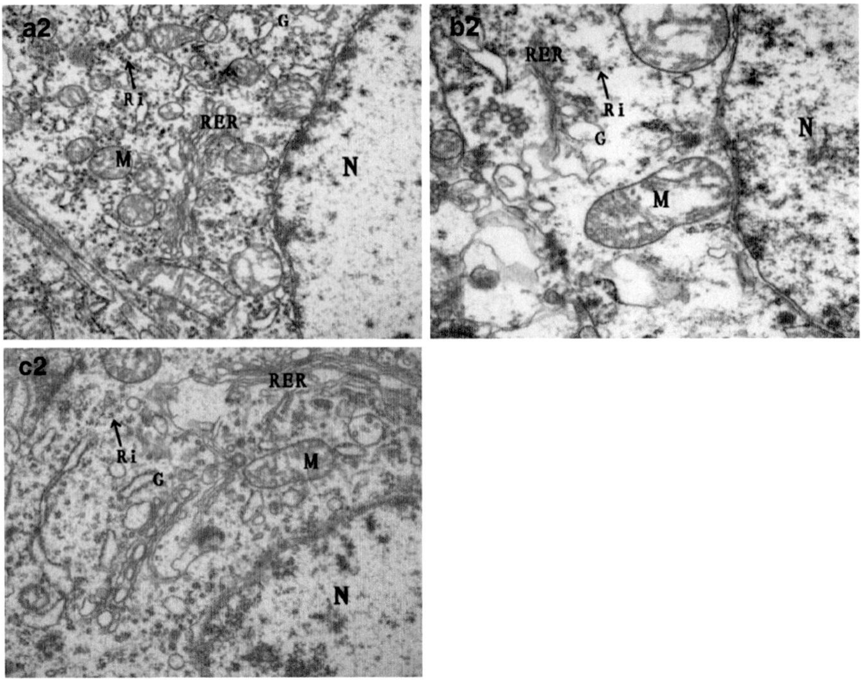


**Fig. 12.5** Ultrastructure of cortical neurons in each group under electron microscope (×24,000). A2 control group: Neuron nucleus (N) has low and uniform electron density, little heterochromatin, Golgi body (G), rough endoplasmic reticulum (RER), and mitochondria (M) have complete and clear morphology, nuclear chromatin particles are relatively uniform, ribosome (Ri). B2 adrenalin group: Nucleus chromatin concentration, edge set, nuclear membrane folding, Golgi body, and RER obvious expansion, vacuolization; mitochondria swollen ridge rupture, ribosome content decreased significantly. C2 Epinephrine + anisodamine group

anisodamine plus epinephrine group were significantly higher than those of epinephrine and control group (as seen in Fig. 12.6). In rabbits after VF, Zhou [39] reported that administration of epinephrine decreased the heart local tissue oxygen saturation ($rSO_2$) with relation to decrease of myocardial blood flow. Epinephrine combined with anisodamine can increase the heart $rSO_2$ with relation to increase of myocardial blood flow. Jia [46] also reported that epinephrine plus anisodamine increases the success rate of ROSC in rats after cardiac arrest by improving the energy metabolism of myocardium and brain tissue. Yang [40] found the ATP levels in rat myocardial mitochondria after CA/CPR were all significantly decreased within 24 h. However, the recovery of the ATP levels in group adrenaline + anisodamine was higher at 12 h (1.88 ± 0.26 vs. 1.23 ± 0.16 μmol/L, $p < 0.05$) and 24 h (2.09 ± 0.25 vs. 1.02 ± 0.12 μmol/L, $p < 0.05$) after CA/CPR than those of group adrenaline accordingly (see Fig. 12.7). Besides, anisodamine has been shown to protect myocardium conduction structure and function by upregulating the ratio of gap junction protein p-Cx43and Cx43 in myocardium [47].

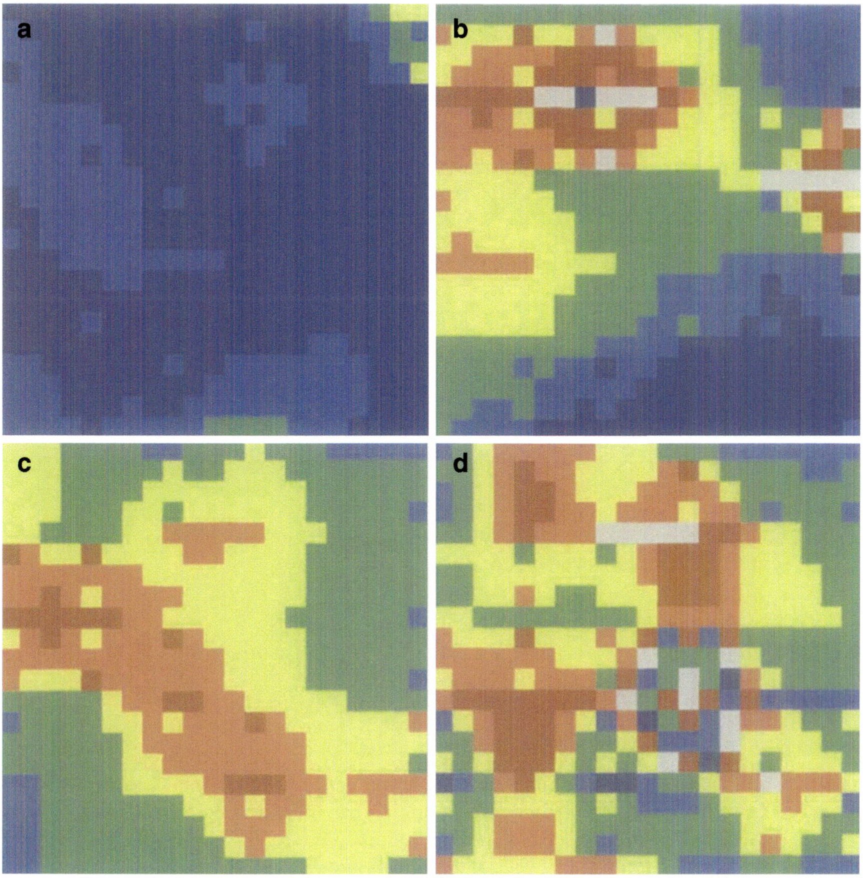


**Fig. 12.6** Blood perfusion volume of rat intestinal wall tissue after cardiac arrest was measured by laser Doppler blood flow imager. (**a**) at cardiac arrest; (**b**) epinephrine (200 μg/kg) group after ROSC; (**c**) epinephrine + low anisodamine (5 mg/kg) group after ROSC; (**d**) epinephrine + high anisodamine (10 mg/kg). The two-dimensional color-coded image shows tissue perfusion images. Red represented areas with high blood flow, green represented areas with decreased blood flow, blue represented areas with further decreased blood flow, and dark blue represented areas with near zero blood flow

Secondly, anisodamine has been shown to exert its positive effects through regulating inflammatory response and scavenge oxygen free radical. Liu [47] found the blood malondialdehyde (MDA) of both CPR groups was higher than that of control group ($p < 0.01$, but the MDA level of anisodamine + epinephrine group was lower than epinephrine group in ROSC 30 min and ROSC 24 h ($p < 0.05$) (seen in Table 12.2). On the other hand, the blood enzyme activity of superoxide dismutase (SOD) of both CPR groups was lower than that of control group ($p < 0.05$) after CA. But there are no differences between two CPR groups at the same point ($p > 0.05$) (as seen in Table 12.3). The myocardium SOD activity of Ani + CA/R group was higher than CA/R group ($p < 0.01$) (seen in Table 12.4). Yang found

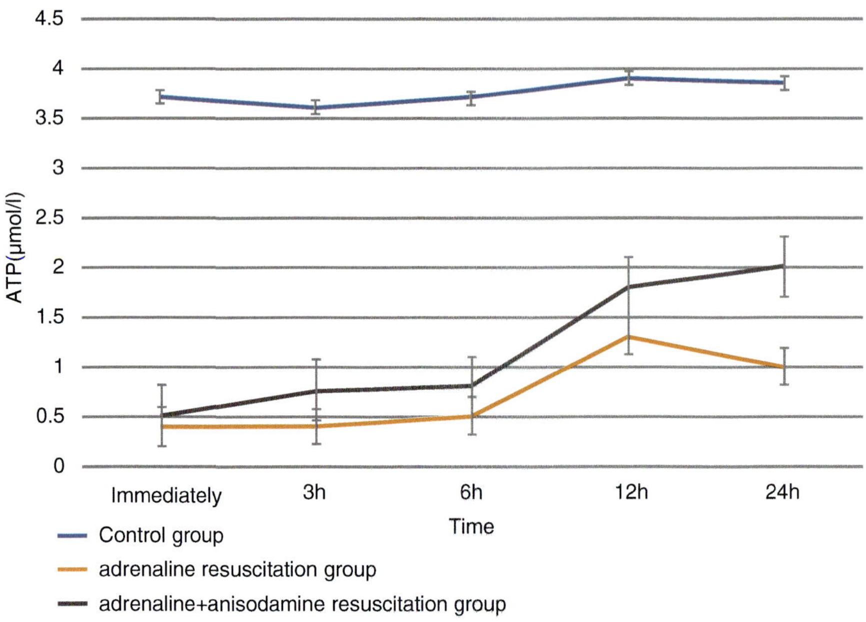


**Fig. 12.7** Changes in ATP levels in myocardial tissues at different time points

**Table 12.2** The plasma MDA content in swine ($x \pm s$, μM)

| Group | *n* | At base | CA 8 min | ROSC | ROSC 30 min | ROSC 24 h |
|---|---|---|---|---|---|---|
| Sham | 5 | 14.73 ± 2.59 | 12.66 ± 2.88 | 14.08 ± 3.93 | 15.94 ± 4.38 | 15.35 ± 3.28 |
| Epi | 5 | 13.38 ± 2.87 | 52.06 ± 6.43$^{**}$ | 56.78 ± 10.91$^{**}$ | 55.47 ± 10.97$^{**}$ | 55.47 ± 7.85$^{**}$ |
| Ani + epi | 7 | 13.21 ± 4.22 | 52.51 ± 6.05$^{**}$ | 56.05 ± 11.12$^{**}$ | 43.38 ± 8.12$^{**\#}$ | 43.38 ± 6.04$^{**\#}$ |

Compared with sham group $^{**}P < 0.01$; compared with epinephrine group $^{**}P < 0.01$, $^{\#}P < 0.05$

**Table 12.3** The plasma SOD activity in swine ($\overline{x} \pm s$, U)

| Group | *n* | At base | CA 8 min | ROSC | ROSC 30 min | ROSC 24 h |
|---|---|---|---|---|---|---|
| Sham | 5 | 7.40 ± 2.25 | 7.17 ± 1.96 | 7.31 ± 2.24 | 7.55 ± 2.44 | 7.22 ± 2.26 |
| Epi | 5 | 7.55 ± 1.93 | 5.07 ± 1.34$^{*}$ | 1.45 ± 0.43$^{**}$ | 1.29 ± 0.60$^{**}$ | 1.88 ± 0.88$^{**}$ |
| Ani + epi | 7 | 7.36 ± 1.89 | 4.64 ± 0.93$^{*}$ | 1.95 ± 0.84$^{**}$ | 2.18 ± 0.93$^{**}$ | 2.90 ± 1.36$^{**}$ |

Compared with sham group: $^{**}P < 0.01$, $^{*}P < 0.05$

**Table 12.4** The myocardial SOD activity in swine ($\overline{x} \pm s$, U/mg)

| Group | *n* | ROSC 24 h |
|---|---|---|
| Sham | 5 | 0.95 ± 0.34 |
| Epi | 5 | 0.54 ± 0.19 |
| Ani + epi | 7 | 1.35 ± 0.50$^{\#\#}$ |

Compared with Epi group: $^{\#\#}P < 0.01$

reactive oxygen species (ROS) levels in rat myocardium increased after CPR, but the level of ROS in adrenaline + anisodamine group was significantly lower than that of adrenaline group (seen in Table 12.5).

These data suggest anisodamine can ameliorate the metabolic disorder of oxygen radicals after CA and CPR. In swine VF model, Zhang [43] showed SOD content of lung tissue of epinephrine plus anisodamine group (C group) was statistically significantly higher than that of epinephrine group (B group), while MDA, MPO, TNF-α, water content, and W/D of C group were statistically significantly lower than those of B group ($p < 0.05$). Light microscope found alveolar wall capillaries expanded, alveolar exudate elevated, and infiltration of inflammatory cells of B group, while above features of C group were relatively relieved. Zhang suggested anisodamine can relieve lung injury after CPR in pigs with CA through inhibiting the excessive release of TNF-α and alleviating lipid peroxidation.

Thirdly, they found anisodamine reduced mitochondrial calcium overload induced by CA and CPR, thus inactivating the mitochondrial apoptotic pathway. Yang [40] found in myocardium in rats after resuscitation, the content of calcium ions in the mitochondria increased significantly and the level of mitochondrial membrane potential (MMP) decreased in the adrenaline resuscitation group compared with the control group. Administration of anisodamine can significantly reduce mitochondrial calcium overload (seen Fig. 12.8) and thus maintain mitochondrial membrane potential (see Table 12.6, Fig. 12.9) and decrease mitochondrial permeability (see Table 12.7, Fig. 12.10).

**Table 12.5** Results of ROS levels in purified myocardial mitochondria at different time points ($\bar{x} \pm s$, RFU, $n = 8$)

| Group | Immediately | 3 h | 6 h | 12 h | 24 h |
|---|---|---|---|---|---|
| Control group | 65.4 ± 4.9 | 68.3 ± 8.9 | 63.3 ± 6.1 | 63.5 ± 4.9 | 64.2 ± 6.1 |
| Adrenaline group | 87.2 ± 5.1$^{*}$ | 104.8 ± 8.1$^{*}$ | 103.4 ± 7.5$^{*}$ | 98.2 ± 6.7$^{*}$ | 92.2 ± 4.8$^{*}$ |
| Adrenaline + anisodamine group | 77.6 ± 6.8$^{*\#}$ | 88.9 ± 6.9$^{*\#}$ | 93.2 ± 9.2$^{*\#}$ | 81.9 ± 5.3$^{*\#}$ | 78.3 ± 7.9$^{*\#}$ |

Note: $^{*}P \leq 0.05$ compared with the control group; $^{\#}P \leq 0.05$ compared with the adrenaline resuscitation group

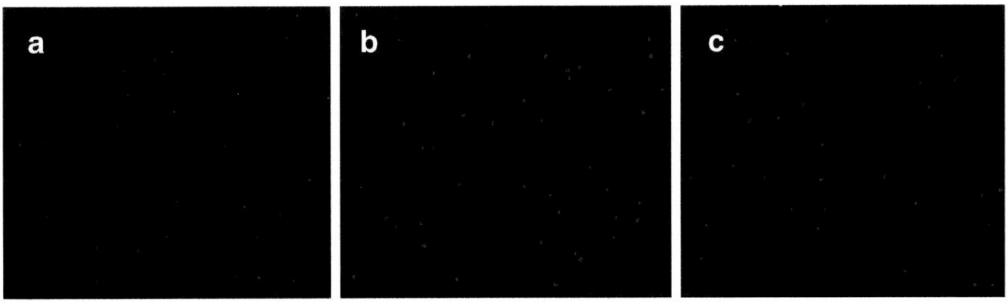


**Fig. 12.8** Calcium ions in mitochondria detected by laser copolymerization focus (**a**) control; (**b**), epinephrine group; (**c**), anisodamine plus epinephrine group

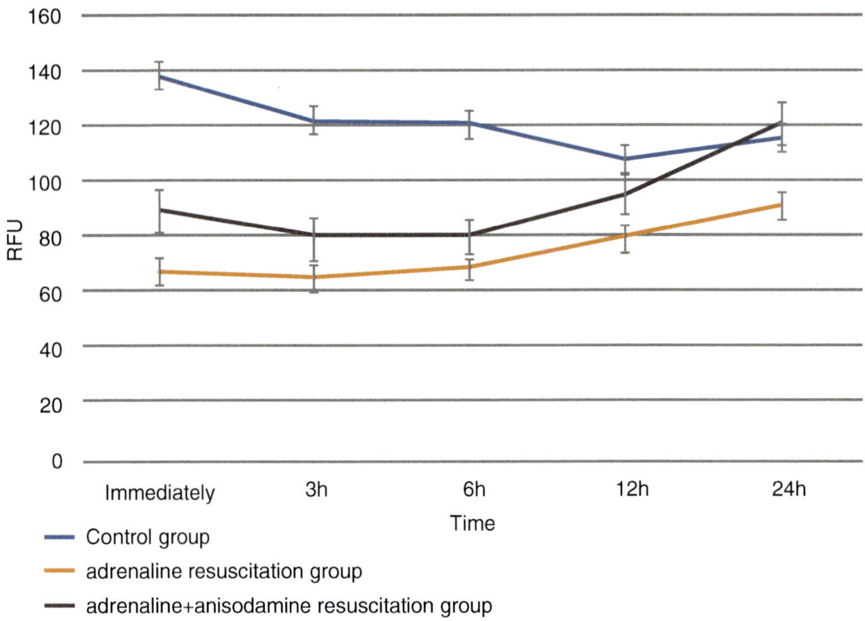


**Fig. 12.9** Changes in the membrane potential of purified myocardial mitochondria at different time points

**Table 12.6** Changes in the membrane potential of purified myocardial mitochondria at different time points ($\overline{x} \pm s$, RF, $n = 8$)

| Group | Immediately | 3 h | 6 h | 12 h | 24 h |
|---|---|---|---|---|---|
| Control group | 137.5 ± 26.2 | 123.2 ± 18.9 | 121.8 ± 16.3 | 106.1 ± 10.4 | 115.4 ± 20.4 |
| Adrenaline group | 67.1 ± 5.2* | 63.9 ± 9.5* | 67.8 ± 8.8* | 78.4 ± 4.7* | 91.2 ± 14.6* |
| Adrenaline + anisodamine group | 90.6 ± 8.0*# | 81.2 ± 6.0*# | 79.5 ± 5.1*# | 95.7 ± 15.0# | 123.1 ± 17.3# |

Note: *$P \leq 0.05$ compared with the control group; #$P \leq 0.05$ compared with the adrenaline resuscitation group

**Table 12.7** Membrane permeability levels of purified myocardial mitochondria at different time points ($\overline{x} \pm s$, RFU, $n = 8$)

| Group/time | Immediately | 3 h | 6 h | 12 h | 24 h |
|---|---|---|---|---|---|
| Control group | 287.8 ± 9. 8 | 291.0 ± 13.7 | 283.5 ± 17.0 | 291.5 ± 9.9 | 285.7 ± 17.2 |
| Adrenaline group | 168.6 ± 45.9* | 115.7 ± 39.1* | 125.5 ± 48.1* | 174.1 ± 31.6* | 190.6 ± 34.8* |
| Adrenaline + anisodamine group | 200.7 ± 28.9* | 174.3 ± 34.6*# | 194.1 ± 33.4*# | 239.8 ± 37.0*# | 258.5 ± 40.2# |

Note: *$P \leq 0.05$ compared with the control group; #$P \leq 0.05$ compared with the adrenaline resuscitation group

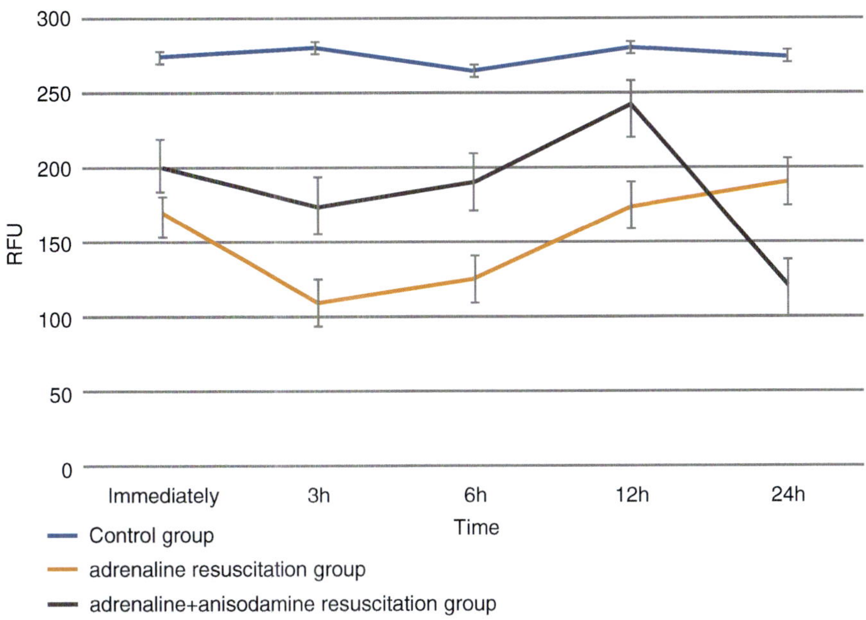


**Fig. 12.10** Membrane permeability levels of purified myocardial mitochondria at different time points

Liu [47] also found that anisodamine can protect the myocardial ultrastructure and restrain the mitochondria-induced cell apoptosis after resuscitation in swines by decreasing the protein content of cytochrome C (Cyt C) and reducing the extent of damage to myocardial mitochondria.

In a rat resuscitation model, anisodamine markedly decreased the number of apoptotic cardiomyoctes. Yin [41] found endoplasmic reticulum chaperones GRP78 and calreticulin were significantly elevated in the I/R group. In addition, ER stress-related apoptotic pathway was activated, which manifested as upregulated CHOP. Anisodamine treatment abrogated myocardial injury and the upregulation of GRP78, calreticulin, and CHOP. After that Liu [47] showed that anisodamine decreased the expression of endoplasmic reticulum stress-associated proteins including JNK, calpain, and caspase 12 (see Fig. 12.11) and thus reduced the ultra-structural damage and apoptosis (Fig. 12.12) in cardiomyocytes in swine CA model.

In conclusion, anisodamine is a multifunctional bio-alkaloid. In animal models, it seems to relieve the side effect of epinephrine on circulation and reduce ischemia/reperfusion (I/R) injury induced by cardiac arrest and resuscitation. The efficacy of anisodamine in the treatment of cardiac arrest in combination with epinephrine should be further evaluated, both in the experimental and the clinical settings.

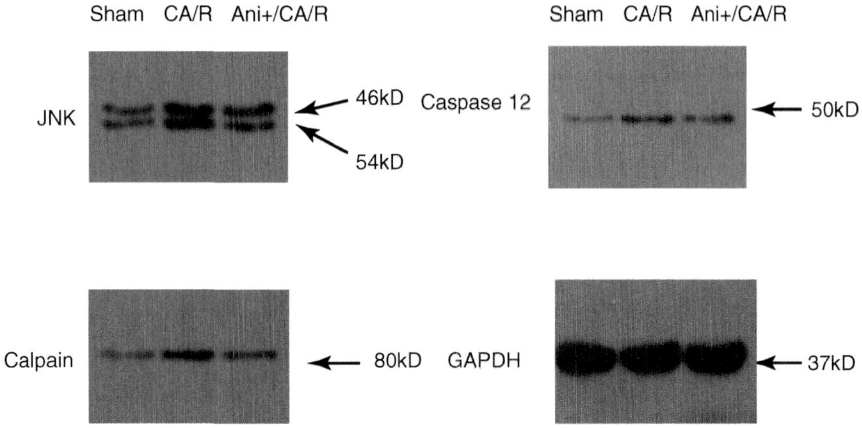


**Fig. 12.11** The expression of caspase 12, JNK, and calpain proteins in ROSC 24 h myocardia of each group

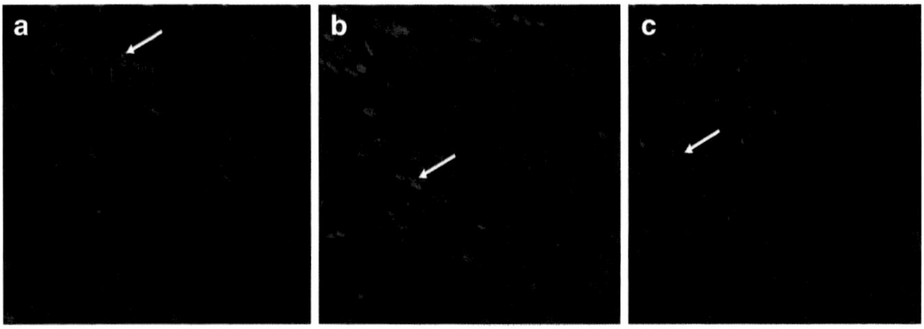


**Fig. 12.12** Apoptosis of cardiac myocytes in pigs 24 h after resuscitation after cardiac arrest. Hoechst 33258 staining fluorescence microscope photos: non-apoptotic cells and the nucleus of apoptotic cells can be stained to emit blue fluorescence, the nucleus of the non-apoptotic cells is large and stained evenly, but the nucleus of apoptotic cells shows nuclear concentration or fragmentation, and staining is not uniform, high brightness (**a**, control group; **b** adrenaline group; **c** anisodamine group)

## 12.6 Conclusions

Immediate and high-quality CPR remains the initial and primary treatment for both IHCA and OHCA patients. This article will introduce recent advances in cardiopulmonary resuscitation by integrating novel technologies and management strategies into clinical practice.

## References

1. Nair SU, Lundbye JB. The use of hypothermia therapy in cardiac arrest survivors. Ther Hypothermia Temp Manag. 2011;1:9–21. https://doi.org/10.1089/ther.2010.0002.

2. Neukamm J, Gräsner JT, Schewe JC, Breil M, Bahr J, Heister U, Wnent J, Bohn A, Heller G, Strickmann B, Fischer H, Kill C, Messelken M, Bein B, Lukas R, Meybohm P, Scholz J, Fischer M. The impact of response time reliability on CPR incidence and resuscitation success: a benchmark study from the German resuscitation registry. Crit Care. 2011;15(6):R282. Epub 2011 Nov 24. https://doi.org/10.1186/cc10566.
3. Do DH HJ, Tiecher RD, Bai Y, Hu X, Boyle NG. ECG changes on continuous telemetry preceding in-hospital cardiac arrests. J Electrocardiol. 2015;48(6):1062–8.
4. Hu Y, Xu J, Zhu H, Zhang G, Sun F, Zhang Y, Yu X. Profile and outcome of cardiopulmonary resuscitation after sudden cardiac arrests in the emergency department: a multicenter prospective observational study. Zhonghua Wei Zhong Bing Ji Jiu Yi Xue. 2018;30(3):234–9.
5. Soar J, Maconochie I, Wyckoff MH, et al. 2019 international consensus on cardiopulmonary resuscitation and emergency cardiovascular care science with treatment Recommendations. Circulation. 2019;140(24):e826–80. Epub 2019 Nov 14. https://doi.org/10.1161/CIR.0000000000000734.
6. Kouwenhoven WB, Jude JR, Knickerbocker GG. Landmark article July 9, 1960: closed-chest cardiac massage. By W. B. Kouwenhoven, James R. Jude, and G. guy Knickerbocker. JAMA. 1984;251(23):3133–6.
7. Patil KD, Halperin HR, Becker LB. Cardiac arrest: resuscitation and reperfusion. Circ Res. 2015;116(12):2041–9. https://doi.org/10.1161/CIRCRESAHA.116.304495.
8. Paradis NA, Martin GB, Rivers EP, Goetting MG, Appleton TJ, Feingold M, Nowak RM. Coronary perfusion pressure and the return of spontaneous circulation in human cardiopulmonary resuscitation. JAMA. 1990;263(8):1106–13.
9. Zhou MH, Ran QH, Liu YH, Li YH, Liu TY, Shen H. Effects of sustained abdominal aorta compression on coronary perfusion pressures and restoration of spontaneous circulation during cardiopulmonary resuscitation in swine. Resuscitation. 2011;82(8):1087–91.
10. Dai Z, Yu SJ, Shen H, et al. Assessment of the position of chest compressions in adults cardiopulmonary resuscitation by contrast-enhanced CT scan (CECT). Hong Kong J Emerg Med. 2012.
11. Idris AH, Guffey D, Aufderheide TP, et al. Relationship between chest compression rates and outcomes from cardiac arrest. Circulation. 2012;125:3004–12.
12. Edelson DP, Abella BS, Kramer-Johansen J, Wik L, Myklebust H, Barry AM, Merchant RM, Hoek TL, Steen PA, Becker LB. Effects of compression depth and pre-shock pauses predict defibrillation failure during cardiac arrest. Resuscitation. 2006;71(2):137–45.
13. Hellevuo H, Sainio M, Nevalainen R, Huhtala H, Olkkola KT, Tenhunen J, Hoppu S. Deeper chest compression—more complications for cardiac arrest patients? Resuscitation. 2013;84(6):760–5.
14. Poole K, Couper K, Smyth MA, Yeung J, Perkins GD. Mechanical CPR: who? when? how? Crit Care. 2018;22(1):140. https://doi.org/10.1186/s13054-018-2059-0.
15. Zhu N, Chen Q, Jiang Z, Liao F, Kou B, Tang H, Zhou M. A meta-analysis of the resuscitative effects of mechanical and manual chest compression in out-of-hospital cardiac arrest patients. Crit Care. 2019;23(1):100. https://doi.org/10.1186/s13054-019-2389-6.
16. Nichol G, Sayre MR, Guerra F, Poole J. Defibrillation for ventricular fibrillation: a shocking update. J Am Coll Cardiol. 2017;70(12):1496–509. https://doi.org/10.1016/j.jacc.2017.07.778.
17. Zoll PM, Linenthal AJ. Control of heart action by electrical and mechanical means. Dis Mon. 1966:2–25.
18. Weisfeldt ML, Becker LB. Resuscitation after cardiac arrest: a 3-phase time-sensitive model. JAMA. 2002;288(23):3035–8.
19. Coult J, Sherman L, Kwok H, Blackwood J, Kudenchuk PJ, Rea TD. Short ECG segments predict defibrillation outcome using quantitative waveform measures. Resuscitation. 2016;109:16–20.
20. Shen C, Nguyen D, Zhou Z, Jiang SB, Dong B, Jia X. An introduction to deep learning in medical physics: advantages, potential, and challenges. Phys Med Biol. 2020;65(5):05TR01. https://doi.org/10.1088/1361-6560/ab6f51.
21. Safar P. Recognition and management of airway obstruction. JAMA. 1969;208(6):1008–11.

22. Newell C, Grier S, Soar J. Airway and ventilation management during cardiopulmonary resuscitation and after successful resuscitation. Crit Care. 2018;22(1):190. https://doi.org/10.1186/s13054-018-2121-y.
23. Voss S, Rhys M, Coates D, Greenwood R, Nolan JP, Thomas M, Benger J. How do paramedics manage the airway during out of hospital cardiac arrest? Resuscitation. 2014;85(12):1662–6.
24. Nichol G, Leroux B, Wang H, Callaway CW, Sopko G, Weisfeldt M, Stiell I, Morrison LJ, Aufderheide TP, Cheskes S, Christenson J, Kudenchuk P, Vaillancourt C, Rea TD, Idris AH, Colella R, Isaacs M, Straight R, Stephens S, Richardson J, Condle J, Schmicker RH, Egan D, May S, Ornato JP, ROC Investigators. Trial of continuous or interrupted chest compressions during CPR. N Engl J Med. 2015;373(23):2203 14.
25. Wang HE, Prince DK, Stephens SW, Herren H, Daya M, Richmond N, Carlson J, Warden C, Colella MR, Brienza A, Aufderheide TP, Idris AH, Schmicker R, May S, Nichol G. Design and implementation of the Resuscitation Outcomes Consortium Pragmatic Airway Resuscitation Trial (PART). Resuscitation. 2016;101:57–64. https://doi.org/10.1016/j.resuscitation.2016.01.012. Epub 2016 Feb 2.
26. Min BC, Park JE, Lee GT, Kim TR, Yoon H, Cha WC, Shin TG, Song KJ, Park M, Han H, Hwang SY. C-MAC video laryngoscope versus conventional direct laryngoscopy for endotracheal intubation during cardiopulmonary resuscitation. Medicina (Kaunas). 2019;55(6):E225. https://doi.org/10.3390/medicina55060225.
27. Sandroni C, De Santis P, D'Arrigo S. Capnography during cardiac arrest. Resuscitation. 2018;132:73–7.
28. Gough CJR, Nolan JP. The role of adrenaline in cardiopulmonary resuscitation. Crit Care. 2018;22(1):139. https://doi.org/10.1186/s13054-018-2058-1.
29. Perkins GD, Ji C, Deakin CD, Quinn T, Nolan JP, Scomparin C, Regan S, Long J, Slowther A, Pocock H, Black JJM, Moore F, Fothergill RT, Rees N, O'Shea L, Docherty M, Gunson I, Han K, Charlton K, Finn J, Petrou S, Stallard N, Gates S, Lall R. A randomized trial of epinephrine in out-of-hospital cardiac arrest. N Engl J Med. 2018;379(8):711–21.
30. Lindner KH, Strohmenger HU, Prengel AW, Ensinger H, Goertz A, Weichel T. Hemodynamic and metabolic effects of epinephrine during cardiopulmonary resuscitation in a pig model. Crit Care Med. 1992;20(7):1020–6.
31. Ristagno G, Sun S, Tang W, Castillo C, Weil MH. Effects of epinephrine and vasopressin on cerebral microcirculatory flows during and after cardiopulmonary resuscitation. Crit Care Med. 2007;35(9):2145–9.
32. Ali MU, Fitzpatrick-Lewis D, Kenny M, Raina P, Atkins DL, Soar J, Nolan J, Ristagno G, Sherifali D. Effectiveness of antiarrhythmic drugs for shockable cardiac arrest: a systematic review. Resuscitation. 2018;132:63–72.
33. Poupko JM, Baskin SI, Moore E. The pharmacological properties of anisodamine. J Appl Toxicol. 2007;27(2):116–21.
34. Eisenkraft A, Falk A. Possible role for anisodamine in organophosphate poisoning. Br J Pharmacol. 2016;173:1719–27.
35. Jia LJ, Shen H. The application of Cytospaz in cardiopulmonary—cerebral resuscitation. Chin Gen Pract. 2007;10(8):644–5.
36. Xing K, Fu X, Jiang L, Wang Y, Li W, Gu X, et al. Cardioprotective effects of anisodamine against myocardial ischemia injury and its influence on cardiomyocyte apoptosis. Cell Biochem Biophys. 2015;73:707. https://doi.org/10.1007/s12013-015-0642-4.
37. Sun J, Chen W, Ji D, Shen H. Intervention of anisodamine on resuscitation of cardiac arrest rats and endothelial cell's injury. R331.3:R605.974.
38. Yin XL, Shen H, Zhang W, et al. Inhibition of endoplasm reticulum stress by anisodamine protects against myocardial injury after cardiac arrest and resuscitation in rats. Am J Chin Med. 2011;39(5):853–66.
39. Zhou MH. Effect of anisodamine on myocardial oxygen content and successful factors in resuscitation after cardiac arrest. Tianjin: Nankai University; 2012.
40. Yang Y. Study on the role of ANT and the protection mechanisms of Cytospa in post-cardiac arrest syndrome in rats. Beijing: Medical School of Chinese PLA; 2011.

41. Yin XL. Anisodamine inhibit endoplasmic reticulum stress induced myocardial injury after cardiac arrest and resuscitation in rats. Beijing: Medical School of Chinese PLA; 2011.
42. Dai Z. The protective effects of anisodamine on cerebral mitochondrial injury in cardiac arrest pig and measurement of cardiac compression position. Beijing: Medical School of Chinese PLA; 2012.
43. Zhang J, Liu YH, Shen H, et al. Protective effect and its mechanism of anisodamine on lung injury after CPR in pigs with sudden cardiac arrest. Pract J Cardiac Cerebral Pneumal Vasc Dis. 2015;23(10):40–4.
44. Chen W, Wang B, Shen H, et al. Effect of continuous adenosine infusion on mesentery microcirculation during cardiopulmonary resuscitation in rats with asphyxia. Med J Chin PLA. 2010;35(3):301–3.
45. Jia LJ. Intervention of anisodamine on cardiac pathology and microcirculation in rats during CPR. Beijing: Medical School of Chinese PLA; 2007.
46. Jia LJ, Meng FS, Shen H, et al. The effects of anisodamine on myocardial and brain tissues functions of cardiac arrest rats. Chin J Drug Appl Monit. 2017;14(2):84–7.
47. Liu YH. Effect of anisodamine on myocardial ultrastructure damage and intercellular signal transmission in cardiac arrest swine. Beijing: Medical School of Chinese PLA; 2012.

# Defibrillation in Sudden Cardiac Death 13

Miao Wu, Jie Wei, and Xiaowei Yan

**Abstract**

Ventricular fibrillation is one of the important causes of sudden cardiac death. Defibrillation is the most effective treatment for ventricular fibrillation. At present, there is no large-scale research report on the incidence of ventricular fibrillation in sudden cardiac death in China. Published studies have shown that the incidence of ventricular fibrillation in Chinese sudden cardiac death is not as high as in other countries. Patients with ventricular fibrillation often appear as unresponsive, with no normal breathing and no signs of circulation. For ventricular fibrillation, the initiating mechanisms include premature ventricular complexes or non-sustained VT. Defibrillation can improve prognosis of VT/VF, early defibrillation is vital, and rescuers should start pressing immediately after defibrillation. For nonmedical individuals, AED is safe, easy, and effective. Victims of OHCA should be initially treated with basic life support measures, including the immediate delivery of shocks by an AED. To improve the popularization of the knowledge of the first responders and promote the establishment of the awareness of the first aid, some expert consensus on cardiopulmonary resuscitation training in China were published. These consensuses combine with Chinese actual national conditions to provide guidance for the first responders and training, aiming to promote the development of first aid in China. In addition, China has also launched the "National Cardiopulmonary Resuscitation Popularization into 100 Million Precision Health Projects" – 525+ (I Love My Family) Project, aiming to popularize CPR to 200 million people in 5 years. By practicing "Healthy China 2030," Shenzhen launched "Public Defibrillation Project" in 2017, aiming to implement in public places with a high density and movement of citizens where trained CPR providers can get fast access to defibrillation. The most common medicine used in VF is amiodarone, and lidocaine has

M. Wu · J. Wei (✉) · X. Yan
Emergency Department, Renmin Hospital of Wuhan University, Wuhan, Hubei, China
e-mail: wu.miao@whu.edu.cn



H. Zhu (ed.), *Sudden Death*, https://doi.org/10.1007/978-981-15-7002-5_13

been suggested as first-line drug too. It requires more evidence to regulate the use of antiarrhythmic drugs in the process of adult defibrillation-refractory VF/pVT cardiac arrest patients or after ROSC. Defibrillation requirements for cardiac arrest during pregnancy are consistent with adult cardiopulmonary resuscitation guidelines. During cardiopulmonary resuscitation, attention should be paid to maternal recovery. It is not helpful to assess the condition of the fetus during this period. During pre-CA period, individual, family, community, healthcare system, and society should be regarded as a whole, and the composition of each element will become the key to determine the survival of CA. For high-risk groups with sudden cardiac death, effective measures should be taken to prevent ventricular fibrillation or to initiate CPR procedures as soon as possible.

**Keywords**

Ventricular fibrillation · Defibrillation · Cardiopulmonary resuscitation · Automatic external defibrillator · Public access defibrillation

## 13.1 Introduction of Sudden Cardiac Death and Ventricular Fibrillation

Cardiac arrest is defined as a sudden stop in cardiac activity, causing the victim to become unresponsive, without normal breathing and no signs of circulation. If proper treatment is not taken quickly, the victim may die suddenly. Cardiac arrest should be used to indicate the above events, usually reversed by CPR and/or defibrillation or cardioversion or cardiac pacing [1]. Sudden cardiac arrest and sudden cardiac death (SCD) are frequently used terms interchangeably. SCD was also defined as cardiac arrest caused by ventricular fibrillation (VF), a rhythm that can be shocked by a defibrillator, including automatic external defibrillator (AED), implantable cardioverter-defibrillator (ICD), or wearable cardioverter defibrillator (WCD) [2, 3]. Ventricular fibrillation is the most common type of cardiac arrest, accounting for 50% to 90% of arrhythmias at the onset of cardiac arrest. Data from seven Asian countries show that the incidence of VF/pVT in adults with out-of-hospital cardiac arrest (OHCA) is 4.1% to 19.8% [4]. According to statistics, the number of sudden cardiac deaths in China is as high as 550,000, and an average of about one person per minute dies from sudden cardiac death [5].

At present, the results of multicenter clinical trials of sudden cardiac death in China have not been published yet, so the actual incidence of sudden cardiac death and the proportion of ventricular fibrillation remain unclear. Previous research reported that more than 80% of sudden cardiac deaths are caused by ventricular fibrillation, but this data seems to be quite different from the actual situation in China. The emergency team of the Affiliated Beijing Chaoyang Hospital of Capital Medical University has conducted the first analysis of the prognosis of out-of-hospital cardiac arrest (OHCA) in Beijing, and the annual incidence of OHCA in Beijing urban area is 81/100,000 [6]. This incidence is similar to that reported by previous European and North American countries (from 87.4 to 96.5/100,000 population), but higher than other Asian countries (65.4/100,000 population), lower than Australia's report (108.9/100,000 population). The initial cardiac rhythm of patients with OHCA in Beijing urban area was mostly arrest (62.3%), and ventricular fibrillation only accounted for 11.1% of cases. A multicenter prospective observational study published in 2018 included data from 613 cardiac arrest patients in 13 hospitals from six provinces in China [7], and the results of this study showed that 20.7% of patients with cardiac arrest received defibrillation, but this defibrillation data included both in-hospital cardiac arrest (IHCA) and out-of-hospital cardiac arrest.

## 13.2 Clinical Features of Ventricular Fibrillation

Ventricular fibrillation is presented as a complete chaotic activity in the ventricle, which causes ineffective cardiac output and results in a cessation of cardiac contraction and cardiac arrest. The clinical manifestation of ventricular fibrillation usually refers to cardiac arrest. The patient had no signs of life, appeared unresponsive, had abnormal breathing, and was unable to palpate the carotid artery pulse certainly within 10 s. Ventricular fibrillation has no measurable heart rate and should never have a pulse, because the rhythm has no coordinated ventricular conduction or contraction. The ventricles are quivering with the presence of high frequency, usually more than 350 times per minute. Cardiac monitor or ECG displays a wavy baseline, but no clear identifiable QRS complexes and absence of P-waves and T-waves. PR interval is not measurable. The waves are irregular fibrillating undulations that are variable in both amplitude and periodicity. Frequently the VF waves range from coarse to fine in amplitude. They reflect the energy or signal of ventricular tissues. Coarse VF showing larger baseline undulations indicates a larger signal from a more extensive amount of tissue. When the lack of oxygen in heart persists, the myocardial cells become dysfunctional and fewer of them are able to depolarize, each time with less energy. The decreasing energy of myocardial cells causes smaller undulations, which are shown as fine VF.

## 13.3 Mechanism of Ventricular Fibrillation and Defibrillation

The trigger mechanism of VF includes premature ventricular complexes (PVCs) or non-sustained VT. They can originate from ventricular myocardium, Purkinje system, and infarcted and fibrotic areas. Early afterdepolarizations, delayed afterdepolarizations, or abnormal automaticity may cause PVCs. They may be unifocal or multifocal and may show a diurnal pattern. Myocardial ischemic areas may also induce rapid triggers. Ischemia lowers the resting threshold of cardiomyocytes, increases extracellular potassium, and reduces ATP-dependent potassium current. The above changes will lead to "injury current", which increases the abnormal automaticity, and the resulting rapid activations help to initiate VF. The transition mechanism is a dynamic process that occurs during rapid activation by a trigger, which can slow down conduction and block wavefront and promote the start of functional reentry through related processes. Then electrical rotors, focal activation, and multiwavelet reentry contributed in the maintenance of VF [8].

Nowadays, as well known, defibrillation can improve prognosis of VT/VF, and early defibrillation is vital. Defibrillation aims to stop arrhythmias in order to give a chance to the SA node taking over the rhythm again. Defibrillation refers to the depolarization of muscles in the myocardium by an electric current, which converts dysrhythmia back to normal sinus rhythm [9]. If an electric shock made enough cardiac tissue unexcitable temporarily, the uncoordinated wavefronts that excite permanent VF would be cleared, and then normal cardiac excitation and contraction would be resumed.

## 13.4 Precautions of Defibrillation

In the update of resuscitation guidelines, there is increasing emphasis on the importance of not delaying the first shock. If the ventricular fibrillation can be eliminated within 4 min, the survival rate of patients could reach more than 50%. Depending on the location of VF onset, defibrillation can either be performed using a manual defibrillator or an automated external defibrillator (AED). In recent years, the guidelines for resuscitation recommend that rescuers should not check the pulse immediately after defibrillation, but should start pressing immediately. This is because it takes time to check the pulse, and the long-term compression interruption is extremely harmful. Most patients only need to defibrillate once to terminate ventricular fibrillation. It is unreasonable to interrupt the compression to confirm ventricular fibrillation that may not exist. There is also no evidence that chest compressions after defibrillation can cause recurrence of ventricular fibrillation. Within a few minutes after the termination of ventricular fibrillation, the heart is not able to effectively pump blood, and immediate chest compressions are necessary [10, 11]. In addition, three consecutive defibrillations caused a longer interruption of chest compressions. In addition, the guidelines recommend that if there is a defibrillator on-site at the OHCA or IHCA, the chest compression should be started immediately when the defibrillator is prepared, and the defibrillator should be defibrillated as soon as it is ready. Because if the start of defibrillation after ventricular fibrillation is delayed by 1 min, the defibrillation success rate is reduced by 7% to 10% [12, 13]. Myocardial tissue is in a period of electrical activity within 4 min after the occurrence of ventricular fibrillation, so defibrillation should be given priority within 4 min before chest compression. After the ventricular fibrillation occurs for more than 4 min, the myocardial tissue is in the circulation phase, and the amplitude of the ventricular fibrillation becomes smaller. A graded inverse correlation between defibrillation time and neurological outcome was observed more than 3 min after cardiac arrest [14]. In hospitals with limited resources, the target time for defibrillation should be less than 3 min. Beyond this time, defibrillation is not easy to be successful, so chest compression should be performed first.

If the OHCA responder is not a prehospital emergency, the emergency responder can begin CPR first, use the AED or check the rhythm with an electrocardiogram, and prepare for defibrillation. In the above case, it is possible to consider a 2-min

CPR before attempting defibrillation. If two or three rescuers are on-site, CPR should be performed and a defibrillator should be taken at the same time. For IHCA, there is not sufficient evidence to support or oppose CPR prior to defibrillation. However, for patients with ECG monitoring, the time between VF and the shock should not exceed 3 min, and CPR should be started while waiting for the defibrillator to be ready [15–17]. Manual defibrillation is usually used in the hospital, because it requires the user to have an understanding of rhythm abnormalities. Medical professionals must ensure that the area is clear before charging the defibrillator and shocking the patient. If the defibrillators are monophasic, the energy should be set to 360 J for the shock. If the defibrillators are biphasic, the energy should usually be selected as 200 J. Always remember to apply gel pads if paddles are used.

For nonmedical individuals, AED is safe, easy to use, and effective. Victims of OHCA should be initially treated with basic life support measures, including the immediate delivery of shocks by an AED, if AED recognizes there is a shockable rhythm. AED machine has voice to guide the CPR provider on how to place the electrode pads on the patient, assure surrounding is clear, and deliver a shock. It analyzes the rhythm automatically. Only when VF is present, the machine will charge up and advises the CPR provider to shock (semiautomatic AED) or deliver the shock (fully automatic AED). Or it will suggest non-shockable rhythm and continue the CPR. During CPR, when the AED is available, the CPR provider switches on and follows instructions. It is important to expose the victim's chest bare and dry to attach the electrode pads firmly, so the hair may need to be shaved. The operator must ensure that no one touches the victim while the AED is analyzing the rhythm. If the shock is displayed, the voice prompt will require the operator to press the shock button. When a shock is delivered, immediate CPR should be restarted as the voice instruction will prompt. Children between 1 and 8 years old should have pediatric pads and attenuating energy.

## 13.5 Defibrillation Training

### 13.5.1 Expert Consensus on Cardiopulmonary Resuscitation Training in China

A key reason for the large difference in global OHCA discharge survival rates is the difference in public awareness, training, and implementation of CPR. CPR training involves social progress and human qualities. All participants from the government to the public and from the community to the EMSS, emergency department, and ICU are required. However, the CPR training rate in the Chinese public is less than 1%, so CPR training still has a long way to go. In order to promote the training and scientific popularization of cardiopulmonary resuscitation technology in China, the Cardiopulmonary Resuscitation Specialized Committee of Chinese Research Hospital Association and the Science Popularization Branch of the Chinese Medical Association jointly wrote "2018 National consensus on cardiopulmonary resuscitation training in China" [18]. The three skills involved in CPR training are standard skills, diverse skills, and individual skills.

It is mentioned in the consensus that for the public, the "professional" skills training is to acquire as much science and knowledge as possible, to cope with the occurrence of CA, and to start CPR according to the standard process. The basics of defibrillation and the use and operation of AEDs are an important part of standard skills. Standard skills are the premise and basis for other CPR skills training. Therefore, they are also compulsory and mandatory for all types of CPR training certification courses. For professionals (medical staff, professional rescue teams, etc.), we should gradually master diversified CPR and first-aid skills in order to improve the CPR rescue ability of medical teams and institutions. Implantable cardiac defibrillators (ICDs) have been widely recognized as the most effective preventive measures for high-risk patients in CA [19–21]. Knowledge and skills related to ICDs are also one of the diverse skills that require training and education [22, 23]. Individual skill means that the rescuer can comprehensively adopt targeted early intervention strategies according to the specific characteristics and morbidity of different patients and deal with relevant high-risk factors in CPR to ensure the success of CPR [24]. For example, the occurrence of ventricular fibrillation in athletes is often associated with genetic factors and sports injuries [25–30]. The timeliness of defibrillation is crucial.

To improve the popularization of the knowledge of the first responders and promote the establishment of the awareness of the first aid, First Aid Professional Committee of Chinese Aging Well Association formulated the Expert Consensus Group for First Responder on First Aid [31]. This consensus aims at the critical and weak link of emergency medical service system (EMSS) in China, providing the public with the first responder action guidance and guiding the public how to effectively rescue the "first scene", "first time" and "first responder" in the event of sudden injury or illness. It was mentioned in the consensus that the first-aid skills of the "first responder" should include AED. The best place, the best training method, and the best communication way to popularize the first aid knowledge and skills were also proposed, and the first responder action plan was jointly promoted from various social levels such as policy, law, science and technology, culture, and so on. This consensus combines with Chinese actual national conditions to provide guidance for the first responders' action and training, aiming to promote the development of first aid in China.

### 13.5.2 Public Access Defibrillation Programs

The trained social personnel are the best candidates for the first responders [32–35]. The greater the number of trainers, the higher the proportion of CPRs in the first responders [36–38]. In view of the fact that the CPR penetration rate in China is less than 1%, the ratio of medical personnel to CPR technology to family members is less than 1% [39], and the success rate of CA patients in the out-of-hospital CA is less than 1%. The Chinese Medical Association Science Popularization Branch and the Cardiopulmonary Resuscitation Specialized Committee of Chinese Research Hospital Association launched the "National Cardiopulmonary Resuscitation

Popularization into 100 Million Precision Health Projects" – 525+ (I Love My Family) Project [40, 41]. The aim of this project is to popularize CPR to 200 million people within 5 years, and each person trains five families. It has truly embarked on a path of accurate CPR popularization in line with China's national conditions, thereby enhancing the public awareness and skills of CPR.

The AED automatically recognizes defibrillation rhythms and is suitable for use by rescuers of all categories [42, 43]. In recent years, the success rate of OHCA patients in countries such as Europe, the United States, and Japan has improved rapidly, which is closely related to the wide prevalence of AED in these countries [44–46]. A study in Japan showed that in public locations, 29.3% of OHCA patients received PAD, which had notably better neurological outcomes when compared with patients without PAD [47]. Based on this, the 2016 National Consensus on Cardiopulmonary Resuscitation in China strongly recommends that public defibrillation should be implemented in public places where CA is highly developed, which is the public access defibrillation (PAD) program. The PAD program is to set up an AED in a public place that is likely to have eyewitnesses and a relatively high incidence of OHCA, so that the first responder can quickly obtain and implement defibrillation [47].

In developed countries such as the United States or in Europe, the application of the AED is very common. It is estimated that there are 317 AED per 100,000 people in the United States, 555 AEDs per 100,000 people in Japan, 695 AEDs per 100,000 people in the Netherlands, 544 AEDs per 100,000 people in Austria, 311 AEDs per 100,000 people in Norway, and 378 AEDs per 100,000 people in Denmark. In China, there are only a few regions and public places (airports) have improvised explosive devices. However, due to the lack of training and the lag of relevant laws, these devices failed to play their due role. By practicing "Healthy China 2030," Shenzhen, a city in south of China, launched "Public Defibrillation Project" in 2017, aiming to place AEDs in public places like airports, railway stations, bus terminals, sport facilities, and shopping malls where trained CPR providers can get fast access to defibrillation. Twenty times of using the AED after the project that made AEDs available in the public places has been a success, saving eight lives of victims of cardiac arrest, including two in airport, four in metro, one in sport stadium, and one in the shopping mall. Placing AEDs in public places has been evaluated for response time, not for survival benefit. We are expecting the survival of cardiac arrest will benefit from AED by conducting AEDs in public places.

## 13.6 Antiarrhythmic Drugs

Defibrillation has now become the first choice for resuscitation in patients with VF/pVT cardiac arrest. Antiarrhythmic drugs during resuscitation and after ROSC may be important factors in improving ROSC success rate and improving short-term prognosis [48, 49]. At present, antiarrhythmic drugs are still dominated by traditional drugs such as amiodarone, lidocaine, magnesium, and β-blockers. However, there was a large difference in the drug regimen and the recommended level. The clinical study requires more evidence to regulate the use of antiarrhythmic drugs in the process of adult defibrillation-refractory VF/pVT cardiac arrest patients or after ROSC.

The most common medicine used in VF is amiodarone. Currently, amiodarone may be used for VF which has no response to CPR, defibrillation, and vasopressor, as in the algorithm of advanced cardiovascular life support. Amiodarone is suggested to be administered after three shocks and administration of epinephrine. Some studies documented that amiodarone was associated with improvement in ROSC and survival to hospital admission, but not to discharge. An initial dose of 300 mg may be followed by a second dose of 150 mg. Lidocaine was considered as an alternative to amiodarone. In AHA 2018 guidelines focused updates for the use of antiarrhythmic drugs during resuscitation from adult VF, lidocaine has been suggested as first-line drug together with amiodarone. The initial dose is 1–1.5 mg/kg IV. If VF persists, second doses of 0.5–0.75 mg/kg IV push may be administered at 5–10-min intervals, up to a maximum dose of 3 mg/kg.

In clinical practice, there are still some confusions about the use of antiarrhythmic drugs in the defibrillation VF/pVT. Does the use of antiarrhythmic drugs improve the patient's long-term prognosis and improve the patient's nervous system function? What is the difference between these drugs in the application of VF/pVT in OHCA or IHCA? Is the combination of different antiarrhythmic drugs superior to single drug applications? What is the difference in efficacy between IV and IO administration during cardiopulmonary resuscitation? The timing of antiarrhythmia drugs after ROSC and the preventive application of antiarrhythmic drugs can improve the prognosis? These problems require clinicians to study and explore in practical work [50].

## 13.7 Defibrillation Treatment for Pregnant Women

Cardiac arrest during pregnancy is a rare, catastrophic event that can have serious consequences for maternal death [51]. Defibrillation requirements for cardiac arrest during pregnancy are consistent with adult cardiopulmonary resuscitation guidelines. As long as the electrical rhythm analysis prompts defibrillation, an automatic defibrillator should be provided promptly. When ventricular fibrillation and pulseless ventricular tachycardia occur in pregnant women, timely defibrillation is the key to maximizing survival. It is recommended that the anterior lateral position be the position of the defibrillation electrode piece and the lateral electrode piece position be under the breast. Adhesive impact pads are used to ensure that the pads are fixed. Electrical defibrillation is unlikely to cause an arc in the fetal monitor, and the presence of a fetal monitor should not prevent the rescuer from performing rapid electrical defibrillation. If the pregnant woman is prompted for electrical defibrillation, the physician should not hesitate to defibrillate quickly, and the risk of maternal delayed defibrillation will outweigh any potential concerns about defibrillation with a fetal monitor [52, 53].

Drug treatment during cardiac arrest in pregnant women is no different from nonpregnant women. For refractory ventricular fibrillation and tachycardia, AHA still prefers a rapid infusion of amiodarone 300 mg. If normal rhythm is not restored, a 150 mg rapid bolus is given after the shock. In the 2016 National Consensus on Cardiopulmonary Resuscitation in China, it is generally recommended that the total daily dose of amiodarone should not exceed 2 g [40]. Despite changes in drug distribution and clearance during pregnancy, there is little data available in the current recommendations to guide this change, so drug doses do not have to change due to physiological changes during pregnancy. In the case of cardiac arrest, you should not stop taking medicine for fear of fetal teratogenicity [54]. Physiological changes during pregnancy may affect the pharmacological effects of the drug, and there is no scientific basis in the current recommendations to guide these changes. Therefore, regular drugs and doses are recommended during advanced life support, and the use of other drugs is consistent with adult cardiopulmonary resuscitation.

In a positive cardiopulmonary resuscitation process, the focus should be taken on maternal recovery and recovery of the maternal pulse, blood pressure, and oxygenation index. It is not helpful to assess the condition of the fetus during this period, and there is only a risk of delaying maternal recovery and monitoring. Only when the mother's voluntary circulation is restored and the situation is stable, fetal heart monitoring can be performed at the appropriate time [53]. For pregnant women with severe trauma who are unable to recover, the resuscitation measures are obviously ineffective and cesarean section should be performed immediately (within 4 min). However, the decision-making for clinical emergency cesarean section is often complicated and should depend on the patient's factors (CA reasons, gestational age, etc.), the clinical ability of the rescue team, and system resources.

Maternal cardiac arrest is a rare emergency [55]. Due to the physiological changes of pregnant women and the need to manage two patients (pregnant women and fetuses), the clinical treatment is particularly complicated, and the obstetrician is slightly deficient in cardiopulmonary resuscitation. At this time, a professional first-aid team is needed to jointly manage the cardiac arrest of the pregnant woman [56, 57]. More and more evidence supports the use of simulation-based training in cardiopulmonary resuscitation to improve the first-aid technology of medicine staff [58, 59]. Medical institutions should establish a standardized training system for cardiopulmonary resuscitation in pregnant women and regularly organize multidisciplinary joint training and simulation exercises. Medical institutions should also establish a database of cardiac arrest and critical maternal data, including detailed records of treatment and prognosis and other resistance. Through continuous discussions with the emergency team in the hospital, corrective measures are proposed to continuously improve the medical safety system.

## 13.8 Early Prevention of Ventricular Fibrillation

The pre-CA period refers to the period before the patient has no heartbeat or respiratory arrest. A narrow sense of understanding of pre-CA refers to the very short period of aura symptoms before CA, often only a few minutes to hours. The pre-CA defined here should cover the entire time course before the patient actually appears CA. During this period, from individual to family, community, and healthcare system to society as a whole, the composition of each relevant element will become the key to determine the survival of CA patients [40, 60]. Pre-aware CA refers to the pre-recognition of high-risk patients for possible CA. If suspicious targets are found, timely interventions should be taken to prevent CAs or to initiate CPR processes early. High-risk groups of ventricular fibrillation include (1) patients with previous cardiac arrest due to ventricular arrhythmia and successful cardiopulmonary resuscitation, (2) patients with heart disease and rapid ventricular arrhythmia, (3) patients who have a myocardial infarction or decreased heart function, (4) patients who have other heart diseases and lower cardiac function, (5) people with special hereditary heart disease, and (6) people with sudden arrest in the family. Precautionary measures should be taken actively for these patients, and ICD can better prevent sudden cardiac death compared with other methods. The treatment of underlying diseases and the use of antiarrhythmic drugs (beta-blockers and amiodarone) are also important. In addition, patients with a family history of sudden cardiac death and previous history of CA should be highly valued and take necessary protective measures. As different individuals, the characteristics of the body that can predict the occurrence of VF are not the same. The results of familial sudden death suggest that genetic testing will become an important means of predicting VF. The predictors of hereditary arrhythmia are highly heterogeneous, with different types of hereditary arrhythmia predictors.

## 13.9 Conclusion

There is no large-scale research report on the incidence of sudden cardiac death or the proportion of ventricular fibrillation in China. For cardiac arrest caused by ventricular fibrillation, we should give timely defibrillation on the basis of understanding the basic knowledge of ventricular fibrillation and first-aid points. The rate of CPR training in the Chinese public is less than 1%, with the even lower prevalence of defibrillation. In order to promote the training and scientific popularization of cardiopulmonary resuscitation technology in China, the Cardiopulmonary Resuscitation Specialized Committee of Chinese Research Hospital Association and the Science Popularization Branch of the Chinese Medical Association jointly wrote "2018 National consensus on cardiopulmonary resuscitation training in China." The Chinese Medical Association Science Popularization Branch and the Cardiopulmonary Resuscitation Specialized Committee of Chinese Research Hospital Association launched the "National Cardiopulmonary Resuscitation Popularization into 100 Million Precision Health Projects" – 525+ (I Love My Family) Project. The public access defibrillation programs are also beginning to make progress in China. These measures have significantly increased the penetration rate of defibrillation and AED in China.

Defibrillation has now become the first choice for resuscitation in patients with VF/pVT cardiac arrest. Antiarrhythmic drugs during resuscitation and after ROSC may be important factors in improving ROSC success rate and improving short-term prognosis. Amiodarone and lidocaine are both recommended for antiarrhythmic treatment of ventricular fibrillation. Defibrillation for cardiac arrest during pregnancy is required to be consistent with adult cardiopulmonary resuscitation guidelines. Automatic defibrillators should be provided as soon as heart rhythm analysis indicates defibrillation. A pre-CA period was defined as the entire time course before the patient actually appears CA. During this period, individual, family, community, healthcare system, and society should connect into a whole, and the composition of each relevant element will become the key to determine the survival of CA. ICD can better prevent sudden cardiac death compared with other methods.

## References


1. Patel K, Hipskind JE. Cardiac arrest. In: StatPearls [Internet]. Treasure Island, FL: StatPearls; 2019.
2. Nichol G, Sayre MR, Guerra F, Poole J. Defibrillation for ventricular fibrillation: a shocking update. J Am Coll Cardiol. 2017;70(12):1496–509. https://doi.org/10.1016/j.jacc.2017.07.778.
3. Chieng D, Paul V, Denman R. Current device therapies for sudden cardiac death prevention—the ICD, subcutaneous ICD and wearable ICD. Heart Lung Circ. 2019;28(1):65–75. https://doi.org/10.1016/j.hlc.2018.09.011.
4. Ong ME, Shin SD, De Souza NN, Tanaka H, Nishiuchi T, Song KJ, Ko PC, Leong BS, Khunkhlai N, Naroo GY, Sarah AK, Ng YY, Li WY, Ma MH. Outcomes for out-of-hospital cardiac arrests across 7 countries in Asia: the Pan Asian resuscitation outcomes study (PAROS). Resuscitation. 2015;96:100–8. https://doi.org/10.1016/j.resuscitation.2015.07.026.
5. Shi HT, Ge JB. Improving public defibrillator use in China. Lancet (London, England). 2016;388(10050):1156–7. https://doi.org/10.1016/S0140-6736(16)31609-9.
6. Shao F, Li CS, Liang LR, Li D, Ma SK. Outcome of out-of-hospital cardiac arrests in Beijing, China. Resuscitation. 2014;85(11):1411–7. https://doi.org/10.1016/j.resuscitation.2014.08.008.
7. Hu Y, Xu J, Zhu H, Zhang G, Sun F, Zhang Y, Yu X. Profile and outcome of cardiopulmonary resuscitation after sudden cardiac arrests in the emergency department: a multicenter prospective observational study. Zhonghua wei zhong bing ji jiu yi xue. 2018;30(3):234–9. https://doi.org/10.3760/cma.j.issn.2095-4352.2018.03.009.
8. Krummen DE, Ho G, Villongco CT, Hayase J, Schricker AA. Ventricular fibrillation: triggers, mechanisms and therapies. Future Cardiol. 2016;12(3):373–90. https://doi.org/10.2217/fca-2016-0001.
9. Dosdall DJ, Fast VG, Ideker RE. Mechanisms of defibrillation. Annu Rev Biomed Eng. 2010;12:233–58. https://doi.org/10.1146/annurev-bioeng-070909-105305.
10. Bobrow BJ, Clark LL, Ewy GA, Chikani V, Sanders AB, Berg RA, Richman PB, Kern KB. Minimally interrupted cardiac resuscitation by emergency medical services for out-of-hospital cardiac arrest. JAMA. 2008;299(10):1158–65. https://doi.org/10.1001/jama.299.10.1158.
11. Rea TD, Helbock M, Perry S, Garcia M, Cloyd D, Becker L, Eisenberg M. Increasing use of cardiopulmonary resuscitation during out-of-hospital ventricular fibrillation arrest: survival implications of guideline changes. Circulation. 2006;114(25):2760–5. https://doi.org/10.1161/CIRCULATIONAHA.106.654715.
12. Larsen MP, Eisenberg MS, Cummins RO, Hallstrom AP. Predicting survival from out-of-hospital cardiac arrest: a graphic model. Ann Emerg Med. 1993;22(11):1652–8. https://doi.org/10.1016/s0196-0644(05)81302-2.
13. Eftestol T, Wik L, Sunde K, Steen PA. Effects of cardiopulmonary resuscitation on predictors of ventricular fibrillation defibrillation success during out-of-hospital cardiac arrest. Circulation. 2004;110(1):10–5. https://doi.org/10.1161/01.CIR.0000133323.15565.75.

14. Kang JY, Kim YJ, Shin YJ, Huh JW, Hong SB, Kim WY. Association between time to defibrillation and neurologic outcome in patients with in-hospital cardiac arrest. Am J Med Sci. 2019;358(2):143–8. https://doi.org/10.1016/j.amjms.2019.05.003.
15. Rea TD, Olsufka M, Bemis B, White L, Yin L, Becker L, Copass M, Eisenberg M, Cobb L. A population-based investigation of public access defibrillation: role of emergency medical services care. Resuscitation. 2010;81(2):163–7. https://doi.org/10.1016/j.resuscitation.2009.10.025.
16. Hanefeld C, Lichte C, Mentges-Schroter I, Sirtl C, Mugge A. Hospital-wide first-responder automated external defibrillator programme: 1 year experience. Resuscitation. 2005;66(2):167–70. https://doi.org/10.1016/j.resuscitation.2005.01.014.
17. Link MS, Berkow LC, Kudenchuk PJ, Halperin HR, Hess EP, Moitra VK, Neumar RW, O'Neil BJ, Paxton JH, Silvers SM, White RD, Yannopoulos D, Donnino MW. Part 7: adult advanced cardiovascular life support: 2015 American Heart Association guidelines update for cardiopulmonary resuscitation and emergency cardiovascular care. Circulation. 2015;132(18 Suppl 2):S444–64. https://doi.org/10.1161/CIR.0000000000000261.
18. Association SPBO, Association CPRP. 2018 National consensus on cardiopulmonary resuscitation training in China. [2018 National consensus on cardiopulmonary resuscitation training in China]. Chin Crit Care Med. 2018;30(5):385–400. https://doi.org/10.3760/cma.j.issn.2095-4352.2018.05.001.
19. Bauer A, Klemm M, Rizas KD, Hamm W, von Stulpnagel L, Dommasch M, Steger A, Lubinski A, Flevari P, Harden M, Friede T, Kaab S, Merkely B, Sticherling C, Willems R, Huikuri H, Malik M, Schmidt G, Zabel M. Prediction of mortality benefit based on periodic repolarisation dynamics in patients undergoing prophylactic implantation of a defibrillator: a prospective, controlled, multicentre cohort study. Lancet (London, England). 2019;394(10206):1344–51. https://doi.org/10.1016/S0140-6736(19)31996-8.
20. Kleemann T, Strauss M, Kouraki K, Lampropoulou E, Fendt A, Werner N, Zahn R. Contemporary benefit-harm profile over two decades in primary prophylactic ICD-therapy. Clin Cardiol. 2019;42(10):866–72. https://doi.org/10.1002/clc.23234.
21. Almqvist M, Mattsson G, Magnusson P. The wearable cardioverter defibrillator—temporary protection against sudden cardiac death. Lakartidningen. 2019;116:FIP4.
22. Zheng Z, Li S. Sudden death prevention. [sudden death prevention]. 2004.
23. Goldenberg I, Huang DT, Nielsen JC. The role of implantable cardioverter-defibrillators and sudden cardiac death prevention: indications, device selection, and outcome. Eur Heart J. 2019;41:2003. https://doi.org/10.1093/eurheartj/ehz788.
24. Drezner JA, Peterson DF, Siebert DM, Thomas LC, Lopez-Anderson M, Suchsland MZ, Harmon KG, Kucera KL. Survival after exercise-related sudden cardiac arrest in young athletes: can we do better? Sports Health. 2019;11(1):91–8. https://doi.org/10.1177/1941738118799084.
25. Behr ER, Dalageorgou C, Christiansen M, Syrris P, Hughes S, Tome EM, Rowland E, Jeffery S, McKenna WJ. Sudden arrhythmic death syndrome: familial evaluation identifies inheritable heart disease in the majority of families. Eur Heart J. 2008;29(13):1670–80. https://doi.org/10.1093/eurheartj/ehn219.
26. Harmon KG, Drezner JA, Maleszewski JJ, Lopez-Anderson M, Owens D, Prutkin JM, Asif IM, Klossner D, Ackerman MJ. Pathogenesis of sudden cardiac death in national collegiate athletic association athletes. Circ Arrhythm Electrophysiol. 2014;7(2):198–204. https://doi.org/10.1161/CIRCEP.113.001376.
27. Maron BJ, Gohman TE, Kyle SB, Estes NR, Link MS. Clinical profile and spectrum of commotio cordis. JAMA. 2002;287(9):1142–6. https://doi.org/10.1001/jama.287.9.1142.
28. Maron BJ, Haas TS, Ahluwalia A, Garberich RF, Estes NR, Link MS. Increasing survival rate from commotio cordis. Heart Rhythm. 2013;10(2):219–23. https://doi.org/10.1016/j.hrthm.2012.10.034.
29. Wisten A, Borjesson M, Krantz P, Stattin EL. Exercise related sudden cardiac death (SCD) in the young - pre-mortal characterization of a Swedish nationwide cohort, showing a decline in SCD among athletes. Resuscitation. 2019;144:99–105. https://doi.org/10.1016/j.resuscitation.2019.09.022.

30. DeFroda SF, McDonald C, Myers C, Cruz AI, Owens BD, Daniels AH. Sudden cardiac death in the adolescent athlete: history, diagnosis, and prevention. Am J Med. 2019;132:1374. https://doi.org/10.1016/j.amjmed.2019.05.025.
31. First APCO, Expert CGFF, Shi Z, Zhu Y. Expert consensus on the first responder of the first aid. Zhonghua wei zhong bing ji jiu yi xue. 2019;31(5):513–27. https://doi.org/10.3760/cma.j.issn.2095-4352.2019.05.001.
32. Barry T, Guerin S, Headon M, Bury G. GPs who volunteer to be first responders for out-of-hospital cardiac arrest: a qualitative study. Eur J Gen Pract. 2019;26:1–9. https://doi.org/10.1080/13814788.2019.1681194.
33. Kern KB, Colberg TP, Wunder CJ, Newton C, Slepian MJ. A local neighborhood volunteer network improves response times for simulated cardiac arrest. Resuscitation. 2019;144:131–6. https://doi.org/10.1016/j.resuscitation.2019.09.016.
34. Noel L, Jaeger D, Baert V, Debaty G, Genin M, Sadoune S, Bassand A, Tazarourte K, Gueugniaud PY, El KC, Hubert H, Chouihed T. Effect of bystander CPR initiated by a dispatch Centre following out-of-hospital cardiac arrest on 30-day survival: adjusted results from the French National Cardiac Arrest Registry. Resuscitation. 2019;144:91–8. https://doi.org/10.1016/j.resuscitation.2019.08.032.
35. Hedge SA, Gnugnoli DM. EMS, public access to defibrillation. Treasure Island, FL: StatPearls; 2019.
36. Gonzalez-Salvado V, Abelairas-Gomez C, Gude F, Pena-Gil C, Neiro-Rey C, Gonzalez-Juanatey JR, Rodriguez-Nunez A. Targeting relatives: impact of a cardiac rehabilitation programme including basic life support training on their skills and attitudes. Eur J Prev Cardiol. 2019;26(8):795–805. https://doi.org/10.1177/2047487319830190.
37. Kiyohara K, Sado J, Kitamura T, Ayusawa M, Nitta M, Iwami T, Nakata K, Sobue T, Kitamura Y. Public-access automated external defibrillation and bystander-initiated cardiopulmonary resuscitation in schools: a nationwide investigation in Japan. Europace. 2019;21(3):451–8. https://doi.org/10.1093/europace/euy261.
38. Barry T, Doheny MC, Masterson S, Conroy N, Klimas J, Segurado R, Codd M, Bury G. Community first responders for out-of-hospital cardiac arrest in adults and children. Cochrane Database Syst Rev. 2019;7:D12764. https://doi.org/10.1002/14651858.CD012764.pub2.
39. Wang L, Wang Y. Rethinking that the ratio of CPR taught to family members by medical practitioners is less than 1%. [rethinking that the ratio of CPR taught to family members by medical practitioners is less than 1%]. Chin J Crit Care Med. 2013;33(11):986–7. https://doi.org/10.3969/j.issn.1002-1949.2013.11.007.
40. Committee CRS. 2016 national consensus on cardiopulmonary resuscitation in China. [2016 national consensus on cardiopulmonary resuscitation in China]. Chin J Disaster Med. 2017;5(1):1–23. https://doi.org/10.13919/j.issn.2095-6274.2017.01.001.
41. Lixiang W, Faqiang W. The innovation practice of national CPR popularization and hundreds million of Health project. [the innovation practice of national CPR popularization and hundreds million of Health project]. J Chin Res Hosp. 2016;3(4):20–2. https://doi.org/10.19450/j.cnki.jcrh.2016.04.006.
42. Hallstrom AP, Ornato JP, Weisfeldt M, Travers A, Christenson J, McBurnie MA, Zalenski R, Becker LB, Schron EB, Proschan M. Public-access defibrillation and survival after out-of-hospital cardiac arrest. N Engl J Med. 2004;351(7):637–46. https://doi.org/10.1056/NEJMoa040566.
43. Wang TH, Lin HA, Kao WF, Chao CC. Locational effect on automated external defibrillator use and association of age with on-site return of spontaneous circulation. Am J Emerg Med. 2019;37(8):1446–9. https://doi.org/10.1016/j.ajem.2018.10.043.
44. Travers AH, Perkins GD, Berg RA, Castren M, Considine J, Escalante R, Gazmuri RJ, Koster RW, Lim SH, Nation KJ, Olasveengen TM, Sakamoto T, Sayre MR, Sierra A, Smyth MA, Stanton D, Vaillancourt C. Part 3: adult basic life support and automated external defibrillation: 2015 international consensus on cardiopulmonary resuscitation and emergency cardiovascular care science with treatment recommendations. Circulation. 2015;132(16 Suppl 1):S51–83. https://doi.org/10.1161/CIR.0000000000000272.

45. Delhomme C, Njeim M, Varlet E, Pechmajou L, Benameur N, Cassan P, Derkenne C, Jost D, Lamhaut L, Marijon E, Jouven X, Karam N. Automated external defibrillator use in out-of-hospital cardiac arrest: current limitations and solutions. Arch Cardiovasc Dis. 2019;112(3):217–22. https://doi.org/10.1016/j.acvd.2018.11.001.
46. Kobayashi D, Sado J, Kiyohara K, Kitamura T, Kiguchi T, Nishiyama C, Okabayashi S, Shimamoto T, Matsuyama T, Kawamura T, Iwami T. Public location and survival from out-of-hospital cardiac arrest in the public-access defibrillation era in Japan. J Cardiol. 2019;75:97. https://doi.org/10.1016/j.jjcc.2019.06.005.
47. Dicker B, Garrett N, Wong S, McKenzie H, McCarthy J, Jenkin G, Smith T, Skinner JR, Pegg T, Devlin G, Swain A, Scott T, Todd V. Relationship between socioeconomic factors, distribution of public access defibrillators and incidence of out-of-hospital cardiac arrest. Resuscitation. 2019;138:53–8. https://doi.org/10.1016/j.resuscitation.2019.02.022.
48. Kudenchuk PJ, Cobb LA, Copass MK, Cummins RO, Doherty AM, Fahrenbruch CE, Hallstrom AP, Murray WA, Olsufka M, Walsh T. Amiodarone for resuscitation after out-of-hospital cardiac arrest due to ventricular fibrillation. N Engl J Med. 1999;341(12):871–8. https://doi.org/10.1056/NEJM199909163411203.
49. Kudenchuk PJ, Brown SP, Daya M, Rea T, Nichol G, Morrison LJ, Leroux B, Vaillancourt C, Wittwer L, Callaway CW, Christenson J, Egan D, Ornato JP, Weisfeldt ML, Stiell IG, Idris AH, Aufderheide TP, Dunford JV, Colella MR, Vilke GM, Brienza AM, Desvigne-Nickens P, Gray PC, Gray R, Seals N, Straight R, Dorian P. Amiodarone, lidocaine, or placebo in out-of-hospital cardiac arrest. N Engl J Med. 2016;374(18):1711–22. https://doi.org/10.1056/NEJMoa1514204.
50. Na S, Rongbin Z. Interpretation of the updates in the use of antiarrhythmic drugs during resuscitation of patients with VF/pVT cardiac arrest or immediately after ROSC in 2018 International Consensus on Cardiopulmonary Resuscitation and Emergency Cardiovascular Care Science with Treatment Recommendations. [Interpretation of the updates in the use of antiarrhythmic drugs during resuscitation of patients with VF/pVT cardiac arrest or immediately after ROSC in 2018 International Consensus on Cardiopulmonary Resuscitation and Emergency Cardiovascular Care Science with Treatment Recommendations]. Chin Gen Pract. 2019;22(20):2393–7. https://doi.org/10.12114/j.issn.1007-9572.2019.00.296.
51. Chen D, Chen Y. Interpretation of the 2015 American Heart Association Guidelines on Cardiopulmonary Resuscitation in Pregnant Women. [Interpretation of the 2015 American Heart Association guidelines on cardiopulmonary resuscitation in pregnant women]. J Pract Obstet Gynecol. 2018;34(7):499–503.
52. Killion M. Cardiac arrest in pregnancy. MCN. Am J Matern Child Nurs. 2015;40(4):262. https://doi.org/10.1097/NMC.0000000000000155.
53. Jeejeebhoy FM, Zelop CM, Lipman S, Carvalho B, Joglar J, Mhyre JM, Katz VL, Lapinsky SE, Einav S, Warnes CA, Page RL, Griffin RE, Jain A, Dainty KN, Arafeh J, Windrim R, Koren G, Callaway CW. Cardiac arrest in pregnancy: a scientific statement from the American Heart Association. Circulation. 2015;132(18):1747–73. https://doi.org/10.1161/CIR.0000000000000300.
54. Pavek P, Ceckova M, Staud F. Variation of drug kinetics in pregnancy. Curr Drug Metab. 2009;10(5):520–9. https://doi.org/10.2174/138920009788897993.
55. Say L, Chou D, Gemmill A, Tuncalp O, Moller AB, Daniels J, Gulmezoglu AM, Temmerman M, Alkema L. Global causes of maternal death: a WHO systematic analysis. Lancet Glob Health. 2014;2(6):e323–33. https://doi.org/10.1016/S2214-109X(14)70227-X.
56. Lavonas EJ, Drennan IR, Gabrielli A, Heffner AC, Hoyte CO, Orkin AM, Sawyer KN, Donnino MW. Part 10: special circumstances of resuscitation: 2015 American Heart Association guidelines update for cardiopulmonary resuscitation and emergency cardiovascular care. Circulation. 2015;132(18 Suppl 2):S501–18. https://doi.org/10.1161/CIR.0000000000000264.
57. Lipman S, Cohen S, Einav S, Jeejeebhoy F, Mhyre JM, Morrison LJ, Katz V, Tsen LC, Daniels K, Halamek LP, Suresh MS, Arafeh J, Gauthier D, Carvalho JC, Druzin M, Carvalho B. The Society for Obstetric Anesthesia and Perinatology consensus statement on the management

of cardiac arrest in pregnancy. Anesth Analg. 2014;118(5):1003–16. https://doi.org/10.1213/ANE.0000000000000171.

58. Fisher N, Eisen LA, Bayya JV, Dulu A, Bernstein PS, Merkatz IR, Goffman D. Improved performance of maternal-fetal medicine staff after maternal cardiac arrest simulation-based training. Am J Obstet Gynecol. 2011;205(3):231–9. https://doi.org/10.1016/j.ajog.2011.06.012.
59. Wayne DB, Didwania A, Feinglass J, Fudala MJ, Barsuk JH, McGaghie WC. Simulation-based education improves quality of care during cardiac arrest team responses at an academic teaching hospital: a case-control study. Chest. 2008;133(1):56–61. https://doi.org/10.1378/chest.07-0131.
60. Berg DD, Bobrow BJ, Berg RA. Key components of a community response to out-of-hospital cardiac arrest. Nat Rev Cardiol. 2019;16(7):407–16. https://doi.org/10.1038/s41569-019-0175-4.

# Airway Management of Sudden Cardiac Death

# 14

Kui Jin, Feng Sun, and Jun Xu

**Abstract**

Sudden cardiac death is still one of the most common causes of death all over the world that is associated with great morbidity and mortality (Shao et al., Resuscitation 85(11):1411–7, 2014; Girotra et al., N Engl J Med 367(20):1912–20, 2012; Hasselqvist et al., N Engl J Med 372(24):2307–15, 2015). Oxygenation and ventilation are believed to be critical for successful resuscitation. A study from the USA showed that failure of first intubation attempt was associated with delayed return of spontaneous circulation (Kim et al., Resuscitation 85(5):623–7, 2014). However, optimal airway management strategy still is uncertain. Current guidelines and evidence are largely from observational studies. In this chapter, the authors try to provide a relatively simple practical way to manage airway during resuscitation of a patient who suffers sudden cardiac death. Procedures of airway evaluation, airway equipment, oxygenation, and ventilation targets are also reviewed.

**Keywords**

Airway management · Cardiopulmonary resuscitation · Intubation

K. Jin
Department of Emergency Medicine, Peking Union Medical College Hospital College Hospital, Beijing, China

Department of Emergency Intensive Care Medicine The First Affiliated Hospital of USTC, Division of Life Science and Medicine, University of Science and Technology of China, Hefei, Anhui, China

F. Sun
Department of Emergency Medicine, Peking Union Medical College Hospital College Hospital, Beijing, China

Department of Emergency Medicine, Jiang Su Provincial Hospital, NanJing, China

J. Xu (✉)
Department of Emergency Medicine, Peking Union Medical College Hospital College Hospital, Beijing, China



H. Zhu (ed.), *Sudden Death*, https://doi.org/10.1007/978-981-15-7002-5_14

## 14.1 Introduction

The best way to manage airway during sudden cardiac death (SCD) is still unknown. Current guidelines recommend that emergency physicians provide cardiopulmonary resuscitation (CPR) with manual breaths and chest compression with a ratio of 30:2 or uninterrupted chest compressions with no ventilations until a supraglottic airway or endotracheal tube (ET tube) is set up (strong recommendation), after which time continuous chest compressions and one breath every 5–6 s be performed [1]. However, the optimal solutions for airway management remain unclear (basic airway vs. advanced airway, bag mask ventilation vs. supraglottic airway devices or intubation). The best solutions for airway management among patients with cardiac arrest are debatable. Furthermore, characteristics of airway management in SCD in the departments of emergency medicine are different from either other circumstances or airway managements by anesthesiologists. The main characteristics of airway during SCD are time limited and unpredictable. First, under emergency conditions, history taking and physical examination are often inadequate. Second, airway management of SCD often is not fully prepared. Third, SCD patients have frequently poor oxygen reservation requiring artificial airway to be established in seconds to minutes. Therefore, special understanding and training are required for emergency physicians during airway management among cardiac arrest patients.

As is well known, the purpose of airway management is to assist with airway patency, oxygen delivery, and carbon dioxide excretion. Typically, airway management techniques can be classified into two categories: noninvasive airway and invasive airway. Noninvasive airway often refers to airways such as passive oxygenation, bag-valve-mask ventilation, supraglottic airways, and noninvasive positive-pressure ventilation, whereas invasive airway refers to endotracheal intubation and surgical airway (tracheostomy, cricothyroidotomy, and transcutaneous needle jet ventilation). Both invasive airway and noninvasive airway are commonly seen during cardiopulmonary resuscitation. In the following paragraph, we will review a common protocol that is specified in the field of emergency departments for cardiac arrest patients. It must be pointed out that this protocol is in part different from protocols used by an anesthetist that usually operates artificial airways in the operation room.

## 14.2 Open the Airway

When SCD occurs, a quick assessment of airway patency is critically important. Laboratory testing, history taking, or physical examination should not delay the decision to initiate chest compression and airway management strategies. Airway obstruction in SCD patients is often functional due to the decrease of muscle tone. Abnormal downward of tongue may be the most common cause leading to airway obstruction among SCD patients. When the lower jaw is moved forward, the tongue will be lift and the airway will be open.

There are two ways that were commonly used by emergency physicians to open the airway. Head tilt-chin lift maneuver can be used if a patient has no history of head or neck trauma. However, when there is risk of neck injury, head tilt-chin lift maneuver may cause further injury to the cervical cord, and jaw-thrust maneuver is chosen for airway opening.

### 14.2.1 **Head Tilt-Chin Lift Maneuver** (Fig. 14.1a)

In general, head tilt-chin lift was the most commonly used way to open the victim's airway in emergency departments (EDs). To accomplish this maneuver, a physician places one of their hands on the forehead of the patient, and backward pressure is applied with the physicians' palm to tilt the head back. The jaw is moved upward using the other hand. It will be easy to lift the jaw if physicians put fingers of the other hand under the bony part of the tip of the jaw near the chin. Furthermore, the chin will move forward when the jaw is pulled upward, and this maneuver will open the airway. Keep in mind that the soft tissue under the chin should not be pressed deeply because this might obstruct the airway.

### 14.2.2 **Jaw-Thrust Maneuver** (Fig. 14.1b)

If, for example, the victims of SCD are at high risk of neck or head injury, which in other words head tilt may not be safe, jaw-thrust maneuver may be appropriate. Jaw-thrust maneuver to open the airway should be mastered by all emergency physicians. The most important part of this useful maneuver is to open the airway without head tilt. The operator's hands should be placed on each side of the patient's head, with both elbows resting on the surface of resuscitation bed. Fingers are placed to grasp each side of the angles of the lower jaw, and then the fingers of both hands are lifted. This is an effective way to open the airway without moving the neck and head, but it requires education and practices for emergency physicians. It must be pointed out that this maneuver usually causes fatigue during clinical practices if not carried out appropriately.

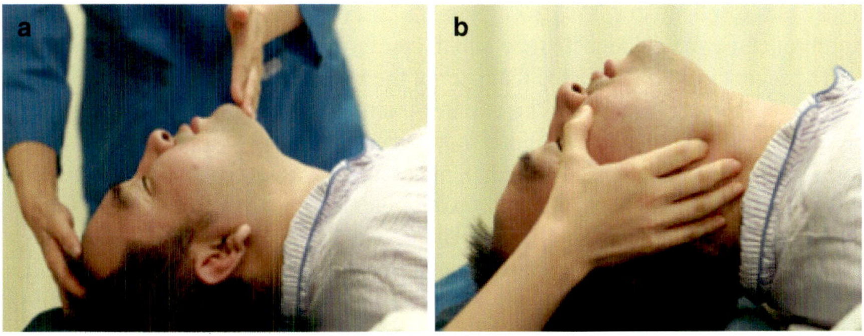

**Fig. 14.1** (**a**) Head tilt-chin lift maneuver: put one hand on the forehead of the patient and then move the forehead backward. Lift the jaw upward with fingers of the other hand. (**b**) Jaw-thrust maneuver: place one hand on each side of the victim's head and put the elbows on the beds. Catch the angles of the lower jaw and lift backward at the same time with both hands

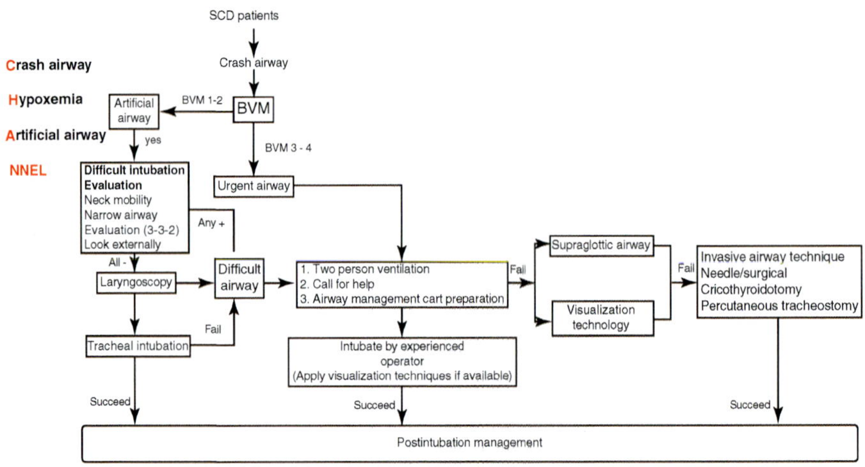


**Fig. 14.2** The CHANNEL principle for management of airway

### 14.2.3 Judgment of Difficult Emergency Airway Using "NNEL" Protocol

Difficult emergency airway is defined as an airway that is managed by well-trained emergency physicians who fail to maintain oxygenation with either bag-valve-mask (BVM) or intubation. Whether the airway is a difficult emergency airway should be determined before any attempt of intubation even in SCD patients. The NNEL principle is highly recommended to evaluate difficult airway in emergency departments (Fig. 14.2).

The first "N" is neck mobility which is critically important for the use of direct laryngoscopy. Use of direct laryngoscopy need to place tracheal intubation blade into the mouth of patients, and this required that the neck of the patients can be moved freely without fixation. Furthermore, as mentioned above, neck injury also makes placement of direct laryngoscopy dangerous with increased risk of further injury to the spinal cord. Visualization techniques such as video laryngoscopy and fibrobronchoscope guide technique may be preferred under these circumstances.

The second "N" is decreased diameter of the bronchus. Several factors may contribute to the narrowed bronchus. Extra-tracheal compression by tumor, local abscess, and hematoma is not uncommon; aspiration of foreign body, tracheal diseases, pulmonary radiotherapy, and healing of trachea wound may all cause narrowing of the trachea. This "N" definitely would increase the difficulty of intubation.

The third "E" represents evaluation. Use a "3-3-2" rule to evaluate the interaction of the three important landmark axes: the mouth axis, the pharynx axis, and the larynx axis. Each number of 3-3-2 was measured by the fingers of patients who receive intubation; a measurement less than the width of each "3-3-2" indicates a difficult airway. The first "3" represents the extent one can open the mouth should be more than "3" fingers, the second "3" represents the breadth between the tip of the chin and hyoid bone should be more than "3" fingers width, and the last "2" represents the distance of thyroid cartilage and hyoid bone should be more than "2" fingers.

The fourth "L" represents the outlook of the patients to evaluate whether there are signs of risk factors for difficult intubation. For example, extreme obesity, short neck, no teeth, long canine teeth, and face deformities caused by trauma may all lead to difficult airway management.

### 14.2.4 Decision-Making Strategies for SCD Patients: Two Steps and "CHANNEL" Principle

- Step 1: One must keep in mind that the one priority of airway management for SCD patients is keeping the patients from hypoxemia and maintaining $CO_2$ excretion or in other words ventilation and oxygenation. One should not only focus on intubation without keeping an eye on the monitoring of hypoxemia. Oxygenation and patients' safety are always more important than intubation itself.
- Step 2: Evaluate risk factors for difficult airway and administer an artificial airway. An airway management cart is extremely useful and recommended to ensure even the smallest piece of instruments necessary for airway management is available at any time conveniently. Furthermore, for SCD patients, rapid sequence intubation is not necessary, but as SCD patients have crash airway, experienced operator is required for airway management and visualization techniques is highly recommended if available. While determined by the physician as a difficult airway, one must follow the principle: "the priority is ventilation and oxygenation"; excessive unnecessary attempts must be avoided. The bible of airway management therefore should follow the "simplest and least injurious method of intubation" principle.

## 14.3 CHANNEL Principle of Airway Management for SCD Patients

*Crash airway* refers to patients who suffer SCD. With loss of consciousness, ventilation and oxygenation cannot be maintained, vital signs are not stable, and death may occur in a short period. A crash airway should be managed step by step following the flowsheet (i.e., bag-valve-mask (BVM) ventilation and rapidly moving to laryngoscopy).

### 14.3.1 Hypoxemia

In patients with SCD, the most important thing of airway management is to maintain oxygenation. In SCD patients, BVM ventilation is frequently required. There are two important things one must keep in mind when using BVM ventilation: avoid airway obstruction and minimize mask leaks when delivering positive pressure ventilation during inspiration. Risk factors associated with difficult BVM are age more than 55 years old, obesity with body mass index more than 26 $kg/m^2$, no teeth which make seal of the mask difficult, and beards that prevent the mask to attach firmly to the face. History of sleep apnea is often associated with larger tongue which is also a risk factor for difficult BVM ventilation. Grade system range from 1 to 4 of BVM is used to evaluate the difficulty of maintaining oxygenation with grade 1 having adequate ventilation in supine position and grade 4 not able to maintain $SpO_2 \geq 90\%$ even by two-person ventilation. Good ventilation refers to the following criteria: (1) no abnormal thoracoabdominal movement, (2) airway resistance ≤20 $cmH_2O$ at least three times during BVM ventilation, and (3) regular end-tidal carbon dioxide ($PetCO_2$) waveform. Unfit mask and large leakage of airflow must be excluded before defining good ventilation. Two-person ventilation method requires two well-trained physicians to maintain oxygenation using BVM. One physician opens the airway, and the other person presses the bag with enough pressure to ventilate. Usually, grades 1 to 2 can be well ventilated by a single person with BVM. Grades 3–4 often require two persons to ventilate together, with one person opening the airway and the other one squeezing the bag deeply to offer enough ventilation.

### 14.3.2 Artificial Airway

Noninvasive airways include intubation of endotracheal airway, supraglottic techniques, and so on. On the other hand, tracheotomy and needle or surgical cricothyroidotomy are often regarded as invasive airways. Intubation is the most often used way to set an artificial airway in clinical practices. One study evaluated the outcome of out-of-hospital cardiac arrest (OHCA) in patients receiving prehospital tracheal intubation vs. a supraglottic technique and indicated that for in-hospital cardiac arrest advanced airway techniques improved the quality of CPR as well as the survival rate. For OHCA, the supraglottic technique was reported to have a higher first-pass insertion success rate. Observational studies showed better outcome for intubation compared to the supraglottic technique, but those patients who received no advanced airway intervention showed the best outcome. One possible explanation for this observational study was that failed intubation attempts delay chest compression which is associated with the return of spontaneous circulation. However, there is no randomized trial to compare these airways, and well-designed, prospective, randomized trials are required to further address these issues.

### 14.3.3 Airway Management Cart

The most important characteristic of emergency airway management is that stabilizing the patients before intubation is often difficult. Moreover, physicians often failed to predict which patients may require intubation in the next few minutes or hours. Therefore, a well-prepared airway cart is essential when managing airway in emergency departments when facing SCD patients. A well-prepared airway management cart should be able to fulfill the requirement of devices to set artificial airway at different levels. Airway management cart should be equipped with the following: (1) laryngoscope equipped with full sizes of blades; (2) video laryngoscope with full sizes of blades; (3) endotracheal tubes of all sizes; (4) endotracheal catheter guide (common stylet, visualized tube stylet, lighted stylet, etc.); (5) supraglottic airway (laryngeal mask airway (LMA), intubating LMA); (6) fiberoptic device with protection sheath; (7) cricothyrotomy and (possibly) tracheotomy kits; (8) $PetCO_2$ monitoring devices; (9) suction equipment; and (10) noninvasive airways that can be used orally and nasally.

In general, crash airway, hypoxemia, airway type, neck morbidity, narrowing, evaluation, and look compose the principle of "CHANNEL" which are recommended for airway management of SCD. An SCD patient's airway is a typical "crash airway" with hypoxemia. The first goal is to maintain oxygen saturation using BVM. BVM grades 3–4 indicate difficulty of maintaining oxygen saturation. If possible, use a two-person method to ventilate, call other physicians for help, and prepare the airway management cart. Intubation should be performed by an experienced physician with visualization techniques as the first try choice if available. On the other hand, if BVM can maintain oxygen saturation, which is BVM grades 1–2, evaluation of NNEL will then be performed. Any positive findings indicate a difficult airway, and the management of difficult airway is the same as that of urgent airway. Invasive airway can be chosen if several attempts of intubation failed with even visualization techniques (Fig. 14.2).

### 14.3.4 Use of Impedance Threshold Device (ITD) for SCD Patients

Compression of the thoracic structure and increase of intrathoracic pressure are thought to be the mechanisms which make an anterograde blood flow. It has been thought that high quality of chest compression makes 30% of normal cardiac output. Venous return, however, is the main issue during standard CPR. Small passive pressure between venous system and right atrium is the only gradient for the venous return which is also the preload for cardiac ejection of next compression.

Passive vacuum is created mainly during decompression; the influx of gas into the thorax will decrease this negative pressure and therefore venous return during decompression phase. Recently, use of ITD was thought to block the entry of the inspiratory gas during the decompression phase and when combined with active compression decompression (ACD) may effectively increase venous return [2, 3]. ITD contains pressure sensitive valves and can impede the gas influx through the airway during chest wall decompression; theoretically, it will increase venous return. However, current evidence about the use of ITD is not clear. Studies failed to demonstrate improved outcomes with the use of ITD [4, 5], whereas other studies report a significantly improved survival rate when ITD and ACD are used together [2]. The main issue here, we believe, is the quality of chest compression. ITD is a device that relies on heart-lung interaction to increase blood flow; high quality of compression may be critically important for the effects of ITD during cardiopulmonary resuscitation. One new mode of mechanical ventilation has been designed by Department of Emergency Medicine, Peking Union Medical College, which combined ITD and mechanical ventilator, named "CPRV," and its use will be tested in the next 2–3 years.

## 14.4 Summary

Airway management is fundamental for successful CPR. It seems still unclear which type of airway can save life more than others. High quality of chest compression from the present evidence still is the priority of CPR, but heart-lung interaction and use of new devices such as ITD and ACD may add more information to current clinical practices of CPR. Determining rapidly whether the airway of SCD patients is difficult should be one of the primary goals of training for emergency physicians. Determining the types of airway and the equipment to be used for airway management is the key skill that is required for the safe and effective management of airway among SCD victims.

## References

1. Neumar RW, Shuster M, Callaway CW, et al. Part 1: executive summary: 2015 American Heart Association guidelines update for cardiopulmonary resuscitation and emergency cardiovascular care. Circulation. 2015;132(18 Suppl 2):S315–67.
2. Metzger AK, Herman M, Mcknite S, et al. Improved cerebral perfusion pressures and 24-hr neurological survival in a porcine model of cardiac arrest with active compression-decompression cardiopulmonary resuscitation and augmentation of negative intrathoracic pressure. Crit Care Med. 2012;40(6):1851–6.
3. Moore JC, Segal N, LicK MC, et al. Head and thorax elevation during active compression decompression cardiopulmonary resuscitation with an impedance threshold device improves cerebral perfusion in a swine model of prolonged cardiac arrest. Resuscitation. 2017;121:195–200.
4. Aufderheide TP, Nichol G, Rea TD, et al. A trial of an impedance threshold device in out-of-hospital cardiac arrest. N Engl J Med. 2011;365(9):798–806.
5. Jenkins C, Brinkley K, AlforD H, et al. Effects of the ResQPOD on kinetics, hemodynamics of vasopressin, and survivability in a porcine cardiac arrest model. Mil Med. 2015;180(9):1011–6.

## Suggested Reading

Shao F, Li CS, Liang LR, et al. Outcome of out-of-hospital cardiac arrests in Beijing, China. Resuscitation. 2014;85(11):1411–7.
Girotra S, Nallamothu BK, Spertus JA, et al. Trends in survival after in-hospital cardiac arrest. N Engl J Med. 2012;367(20):1912–20.
Hasselqvist-AX I, Riva G, Herlitz J, et al. Early cardiopulmonary resuscitation in out-of-hospital cardiac arrest. N Engl J Med. 2015;372(24):2307–15.
Kim J, Kim K, Kim T, et al. The clinical significance of a failed initial intubation attempt during emergency department resuscitation of out-of-hospital cardiac arrest patients. Resuscitation. 2014;85(5):623–7.

# Respiratory Support Strategy for Sudden Cardiac Death

# 15

Yingying Kong and Wei Guo

**Abstract**

Cardiopulmonary resuscitation (CPR), as the main treatment for sudden cardiac arrest, includes circulation, airway, breathing, and defibrillation; each of them is important for the overall success of CPR. Mechanical ventilation has been widely applied in the treatment of patients suffering from sudden cardiac death. However, current guidelines do not mention other ventilatory parameters other than respiratory frequency. Therefore, heterogeneity of ventilation practices may occur. The optimal mechanical ventilation strategy still remains highly controversial. Additionally, clinicians are often wondering how to wean from ventilator. In this review, we aimed to offer practical suggestion for clinicians based on the available published data. In the first half of this review, we discuss how to ventilate during CPR and after a return of spontaneous circulation (ROSC). In the second half, we discuss the principles of weaning from invasive mechanical ventilation. Because strong hemodynamic changes associated with evacuation of ventilation can lead to cardiac failure, we also describe the latest progress in diagnosis and treatment of weaning-induced cardiac failure and highlight the noninvasive mechanical ventilation.

**Keywords**

Ventilation during cardiopulmonary resuscitation · Ventilation after ROSC · Weaning · Cardiac dysfunction · Noninvasive mechanical ventilation

Y. Kong · W. Guo (✉)
Emergency Department, Beijing Tiantan Hospital, Capital Medical University, Beijing, China



H. Zhu (ed.), *Sudden Death*, https://doi.org/10.1007/978-981-15-7002-5_15

## 15.1 Introduction

Most cardiopulmonary resuscitation (CPR) research focused on optimizing chest compression quality over the recent years, but little research has focused on the role of ventilation. This may be because of the difficulty of measuring ventilation, especially during the early phases of CPR. We do not know the best way to ventilate the lungs during CPR nor do we know when and how much ventilation is necessary for successful resuscitation and good outcomes [1].

Patients suffering from sudden cardiac death often have poor prognosis because of postcardiac arrest syndrome (PCAS), which includes four components: (1) brain injury, (2) myocardial dysfunction, (3) systemic ischemia and reperfusion injury, and (4) persistent precipitating pathology. Previous studies mainly focused on myocardial and brain dysfunctions post-resuscitation; few studies mentioned respiratory dysfunction. Respiratory support strategy must take the potential pathophysiology causing the arrest, the effect of positive-pressure ventilation on hemodynamics, and the impact of oxygenation on the acute injured brain into account. The objective of our work is to understand the optimization of ventilation during CPR and post-return of spontaneous circulation (ROSC).

## 15.2 Ventilation During CPR

### 15.2.1 Chest Compression Only

Passive ventilation was first studied over two decades ago. Firstly, researchers favoring chest compression only believe that there is enough oxygen storage at the initial stage of cardiac arrest and extra oxygen is needed about 4 min later. Secondly, with an open airway, thorax rise and fall caused by chest compression produce passive ventilation for gas exchange and oxygen delivery. Thirdly, once cardiac arrest occurs, circulation relies mainly on chest compressions. Stopping compressions for any reason will immediately and rapidly reduce cardiac output and blood flow. The standard 30:2 strategy of stopping compressions for two ventilations may also lead to a significant reduction in blood flow, resulting in poor quality of CPR, especially when only one rescuer is present. The reason is that ventilation may increase the duration of the interruption of chest compression. Thus, resuscitation guidelines emphasize early defibrillation and high-quality chest compressions at early stage. Observational data confirm that early lay-bystander compression-only CPR improves survival after sudden cardiac arrest [2, 3].

But they did not take the duration of CPR into consideration. In patients suffering from cardiac arrest within 5 min, both clinical and animal studies have confirmed equivalent prognosis between chest compression-only CPR and standard CPR with ventilation [4–6]. And compression-only CPR resulted in poor resuscitation outcomes for untreated cardiac arrest beyond 6 min [7], which indicated that without additional oxygen, passive insufflation of oxygen provided by chest compression could not be sufficient in the late stage of cardiac arrest as chest resistance increases and lung compliance markedly decreases.

We have no idea whether chest compressions can generate enough tidal volume for gas exchange because the tidal volume may vary over time. Several researches [8, 9] revealed that the tidal volume of ventilation caused by compressions is between 41.5 ml and 156 ml, which is only enough to ventilate the lungs' dead space. Later study also showed these passive ventilations could not be adequate to prevent hypoxia and hypercarbia lasting 12 min or longer [5]. A recent survey in China showed that rescuers who advocated chest compression only did so for between less than 3 min and 9–12 min [10].

Therefore, chest compression-only CPR is recommended during the early stages of cardiac arrest or when an inexperienced bystander is unable to ventilate properly or unwilling to ventilate mouth to mouth. Ventilation is considered important when CPR is prolonged. At present, the specific range of prolonged untreated cardiac arrest remains unknown. The benefit of delaying ventilation for several minutes is worth exploring.

### 15.2.2 Passive Ventilation via CPAP

Passive ventilation such as continuous positive airway pressure (CPAP) with pure oxygen via a Boussignac device or CPAP plus pressure support ventilation might represent a promising alternative approach. The Boussignac endotracheal tube is a specific device capable of continuously and actively delivering oxygen to the lungs at a rate of 15 l/min through a multichannel cuffed endotracheal tube.

The advantage of CPAP during CPR is that it reduces peak airway pressure, thereby reducing the risk of lung injury and a potential enhancement in hemodynamics. However, it is rarely applied in clinical practice. An international survey from 54 countries on physician practices during CPR showed only 4% (18 of 490 respondents) applied CPAP via the Boussignac tube [11]. Furthermore, the optimal CPAP level to ensure sufficient tidal volumes has not yet been assessed in a patient. A recent study evaluated the tidal volumes and peak pressures generated by different ventilators, different CPAP levels, and different airway approaches during mechanical chest compression in a manikin model. They found that the average tidal volume during ventilation at 20 hPa CPAP via a tracheal tube varied from 125 ml to 309 ml. Passive tidal volume is not enough to provide adequate gas exchange [12, 13].

Thus, positive ventilation is still the gold standard during resuscitation in clinical practice.

### 15.2.3 Positive Ventilation

#### 15.2.3.1 Bag Mask

Bag-mask ventilation (BMV) with a self-inflating bag, often supplemented with an oropharyngeal or nasopharyngeal airway, is the most common initial approach used until advanced airway techniques are undertaken. During CPR, the bag mask is used to ventilate twice for every 30 compressions. BMV has advantages of being easier to implement and interfering less with chest compression. Large observational studies (including >100,000 patients) favor basic airway management (e.g., BMV) over tracheal intubation, which found that BMV had a better prognosis (return of spontaneous circulation [ROSC], 1-month survival, and neurological outcomes) [14]. However, these observational studies may have been prone to biases: patients who recover quickly from cardiac arrest may have better outcome without the need of advanced airway management. On the contrary, those who need advanced airway management are less likely to survive.

Available evidence challenges the view that basic interventions are better than advanced interventions during CPR. A large multicenter RCT randomly selected 2043 out-of-hospital cardiac arrest (OHCA) patients for early endotracheal intubation or bag-mask ventilation with delayed post-ROSC tracheal intubation. Bag mask showed no significant difference in 28-day survival with neurological function compared with tracheal tube [15]. The authors reported this as an "inconclusive result." Unexpectedly, airway complication (regurgitation of gastric contents) was more common in the bag-mask group than in the early tracheal intubation group.

Therefore, use of the BMV may be preferable for rescuers who are not highly skilled in tracheal intubation. The probability of regurgitation and aspiration cannot be underrated, which limits the application of BMV. Mechanical ventilation has been commonly applied to treat sudden cardiac death patients, especially for prolonged CPR.

### 15.2.3.2 Mechanical Ventilation

#### Ventilation Approaches

Although positive ventilation is widely used during CPR, the effect of positive-pressure ventilation on hemodynamics is still a great challenge: an increased pressure during inspiration may decrease venous blood flow into the right heart during the decompression period, sequentially reducing cardiac output during chest compressions. In order to increase blood flow to the heart and brain, new approaches during CPR are being explored, including chest compression synchronized ventilation (CCSV), CPR ventilation (CPRV), and ultra-low tidal volume ventilation [16].

##### Chest Compression Synchronized Ventilation (CCSV)

Chest compression synchronized ventilation was designed to deliver oxygen simultaneously with each chest compression. Oxygen is insufflated synchronized with the start of chest compressions, and these very short positive-pressure ventilations are terminated before the decompression period begins, which allows unhampered venous blood flow into the right heart and might increase the cardiopulmonary blood flow.

In animal model, CCSV resulted in superior arterial oxygenation and better maintenance of hemodynamics compared to intermittent positive-pressure ventilation (IPPV). Nevertheless, CCSV is still far from clinical application. First, compression-synchronized ventilation strategies provide sufficient oxygen, but inspiratory pressures of 60 mbar, which is required to provide adequate tidal volumes, put lung tissue at high risk of barotrauma during prolonged resuscitation [17]. In addition, all studies on CCSV were reported by Kill's research group; further research should be conducted to evaluate the safety and the efficacy of CCSV on the outcome of cardiac arrest in humans.

#### CPR Ventilation (CPRV)

Recently, a new simultaneous positive-pressure ventilation mode CPRV appears in China.

Positive-pressure ventilation during resuscitation is combined with an impedance threshold valve (ITV), which stops airflow into the lungs and reduces intrathoracic pressure during chest compression recoil, thus increasing the amount of blood flow returning to the heart and lungs. Further clinical studies are needed to confirm the effects of ventilation model on the outcomes of CPR.

#### Ultra-low Tidal Volume Ventilation (ULTVV)

A recent study is the first to evaluate whether normal minute ventilation values during CPR can be met by a novel ULTVV protocol (Respiratory Rate (RR), 50/min; Vt, 2–3 ml/kg; $FiO_2$, 1.0; positive end-expiratory pressure (PEEP), 5 mbar) in a prospective-randomized porcine CPR model. They found gas exchange equals standard intermittent positive-pressure ventilation. In addition, ULTVV has better pulmonary perfusion during CPR in early ROSC and less lung injury and brain inflammatory response. This method provides a feasible link between the circulatory benefits of passive oxygenation strategies and the need of adequate gas exchange provided by mechanical ventilation. Further study is needed to identify the innovative approach and its potential clinical application value [16].

In conclusion, devices or ventilator modes enhancing the blood returning to the heart might be advantageous, but no approach has been proven to be advantageous in survival of cardiac arrest so far. Positive-pressure ventilation remains the gold standard for ventilation during CPR.

### Ventilator Parameters During CPR

It is difficult to guarantee effective tidal volume using pressure control ventilation (PCV) mode because constant chest compression resulted in a great change of airway pressure. Thus, application of PCV is limited during CPR. Volume-controlled intermittent positive-pressure ventilation (IPPV) mode is recommended, which allows the ventilator to adjust the pressure level automatically according to the targeted tidal volume. After ventilator mode is selected, ventilator parameters will be set up; six key elements (inspiratory triggering, alarm, $FiO_2$, respiratory frequency, tidal volume, PEEP) need to be considered.

1. *Inspiratory Triggering Settings*: The IPPV mode in most ventilators works with patient-triggering systems to improve synchrony between patient and ventilators. In most common ventilators, pressure and flow-triggering systems cannot be turned off. In clinical practice, changes in airway pressure and airflow produced by chest compressions lead to abnormal inspiratory triggering, resulting in

significantly higher ventilation rates. Therefore, researchers suggest that the ventilator flow trigger function should be turned off during CPR, or the pressure trigger level should be adjusted to over 20 $cmH_2O$ if turned-off triggering is not available [18]

During CPR, decelerating wave is more reasonable than square wave because it can obviously reduce the peak airway pressure, the occurrence of barotrauma, and the probability of triggering high pressure ventilator alarm and improve the compliance of ventilator [19].

2. *Airway Pressure Alarm Threshold*: When chest compression and inspiration occur simultaneously, the peak airway pressure rise sharply. Ventilator will automatically switch to exhale when airway pressure exceed the alarm threshold. In this condition, sufficient tidal volume cannot be provided. Therefore, the airway pressure alarm threshold is suggested to be adjusted to 50 $cmH_2O$ during CPR [20].
3. *$FiO_2$ Oxygenation*: A lot of randomized controlled trials showed a linear increase in survival and good neurological outcome with increasing arterial oxygen tension ($PaO_2$). Tissue oxygen demand exceeds supply due to poor tissue perfusion, even with effective CPR during cardiac arrest. Human and animal researches indicated that brain tissue oxygenation remains low even with 100% oxygen; that is, CPR does not expose the brain to tissue hyperoxia. Thus, 100% oxygen is suggested by current guidelines during CPR [21].
4. *Respiratory Frequency*: Once an advanced airway is established, the latest guideline recommends ventilation at a frequency of 10 min and an inspiratory time of <1 s without interrupting chest compressions [21]. However, it is a very weak recommendation lacking high-quality evidence (predominantly on animal studies). Most previous studies focused on ventilation frequencies during CPR. But there is no strong evidence to confirm that a rate of 10/min improves survival or neurological outcome more than other frequencies. A systematic review including one human observational study with 67 patients and ten animal studies (234 pigs and 30 dogs) found no significant difference in ROSC between a ventilation rate of 10/min and other rate [22]. Recent human study also proved no improvement in survival to hospital discharge or 1-year survival with favorable neurological outcome [23]. The optimal ventilation frequency with a tracheal tube during CPR is still uncertain.
5. *Tidal Volume*: Interaction between ventilation and chest compressions to produce sufficient blood flow and oxygen delivery to vital organs is complicated. Excessive tidal volume during CPR, which increases intrathoracic pressure, reduces venous return to the heart, diminishes cardiac output and coronary perfusion pressure, and is strongly advised to be avoided in the current guidelines. The guidelines recommend tidal volumes of 6–7 ml/kg for $CO_2$ exhalation [21].

The duration of untreated cardiac arrest seems to affect respiratory requirements during CPR. Nevertheless, few studies revealed the influence of different tidal volume during different time on resuscitation outcome. Dingyu Tan et al. [24] are the first one to examine this problem in a pig model. Thirty-two pigs were divided into a ventricular fibrillation (VF)-4 min group and a VF-8 min group according to the duration of untreated VF (4 min or 8 min). They were randomly assigned to two different mechanical ventilation strategies during CPR. "Guideline" group's tidal volume was set at 7 ml/kg, and RR was set at 10/min, while "baseline" group received intervention ventilation (tidal volume 10 ml/kg, RR adjusted to maintain pulse oxygen saturation > 95%, an end-tidal $PCO_2$ ($P_{ET}CO_2$) between 35 and 40 mmHg). They found that in 8 min of VF, a higher tidal volume ventilation resulted in better oxygenation saturation, acid–base balance, aortic pressure, and coronary perfusion pressures after intravenous epinephrine and higher ROSC compared to the "guideline" group. However, for 4 min of VF, the guideline recommended ventilation strategy is appropriate for satisfactory outcomes.

This result can be explained by thoracic pump theory. Cardiac pump and thoracic pump work together during CPR [25]. In the early stage of CPR, cardiac pump plays a dominant role, while as CPR progresses, the thoracic pump may gradually become the main force pushing blood flow forward [26], especially when cardiac arrest goes untreated for a long time. Chest compression alone is not enough to keep thoracic pump working, especially when CPR is prolonged (positive and negative intrathoracic pressure variations decrease due to a reduction of lung volumes and chest wall resilience). Under this circumstance, higher tidal volume ventilation limited lung volume decline and leads to an increased positive intrathoracic pressures during compressions to amplify intrathoracic driving pressure while intrathoracic pressures remain negative during decompression. Greater positive and negative changes in intrathoracic pressures enhance the thoracic pump's ability to generate more forward blood flow through the heart and lungs in order to improve circulation.

With volume-controlled ventilation during CPR, approximately 75% of patient's peak airway pressures exceed 40 mbar [19]. Higher tidal volume ventilation can result in elevated peak airway pressures, which is deemed to be avoided in the previous research. However, in recent years, conflicting views challenge the adverse effects of high airway pressures during CPR. Higher mean airway pressure with a value of 42.5 mbar was reported to be related to higher ROSC in clinical practice [20].

6. *PEEP*: With continuous chest compression, a remarkable high intrathoracic pressure has an adverse effect on venous return to the heart. Thus, PEEP should be set to 0 $cmH_2O$ during CPR.

#### 15.2.3.3 A Gap Between Practices and Recommendation

The recommendations of popular guidelines and consensus statements lack detail in how to provide ventilations during CPR. Regarding practices, ventilation strategy during CPR is heterogeneous and varies widely around the world. And there is a gap between practices and recommendation in guidelines. Cordioli et al. [11] investigated physicians from several countries (54 countries) on their practices during CPR. They found more than a quarter of respondents adopt compression-only CPR, especially in the early stage of resuscitation performed by a single rescuer, highlighting chest compression over assisted ventilation. For non-intubated patient, 68%

of physicians always apply the 30:2 option to ventilate the patient with a bag-mask device when CPR was performed with an automated chest compression device. For intubated patient, 87% and 46% of physicians frequently use a bag mask and a ventilator, respectively. Ventilation differs when using an automatic mechanical chest compression device in comparison to manual chest compression. Both BMV and ventilator were often used when using automatic mechanical chest compression devices. Ventilatory problems with automatic chest compression devices seem to occur frequently, as most doctors declared experiencing major issues requiring adjustment of ventilator settings.

In China, there is also a considerable variation in CPR ventilation strategies. Liu [10] conducted a questionnaire-based survey including 438 tertiary hospitals from all 31 mainland Chinese provinces in order to assess the current state of ventilation strategies during CPR. They found physicians in most tertiary hospitals received CPR training based on the Chinese domestic consensus, about a quarter of them received AHA CPR training, and very few physicians received ECR CPR training. About 41.1% of respondents chose delayed or no ventilation during CPR within 12 min. In another international survey [11], 83.0% of respondents who provided ventilation chose to strictly follow the 30:2 strategy, while 17.0% chose ventilations concurrently with uninterrupted compressions. In terms of ventilator settings, the majority of respondents chose volume control (VC) mode (75.2%), a tidal volume of 6–7 ml/kg (72.1%), a PEEP of 0–5 $cmH_2O$ (69.9%), and an $FiO_2$ of 100% (66.9%). However, 62.0% of respondents had mistriggers after setting the ventilator, and 51.8% had high pressure alarms.

## 15.3 Post-resuscitation Neurological and Respiratory Dysfunction

### 15.3.1 Therapeutic Agent in Neurological Damaged Patient

Return of circulation after sudden cardiac death can lead to ischemia–reperfusion injury, especially to the brain and myocardium. Brain injury is the leading cause of death and disability after cardiac arrest. Therefore, post-resuscitation care focuses on how to reduce brain injury.

In animal models, helium has been demonstrated to reduce ischemia–reperfusion injury to the brain and myocardium [27–29], and helium can be delivered using regular ICU ventilators and can be used to reduce neurological injury in patients who experienced OHCA. However, until now, the accurate potential mechanisms of helium's organ protective effects are still unknown. Few studies in this field have been done so far. Brevoord et al. [30] were the first to confirm helium ventilation's safety and efficacy in a neurological damaged patient after OHCA. The study was an open-label single arm intervention study in a mixed-bed academic intensive care unit including 25 patients admitted after circulatory arrest. Helium was administrated in a 1:1 mix with oxygen for 3 h, and helium ventilation was started 4:59 ± 0:52 (mean ± SD) h after circulatory arrest; 64% of patients had a favorable neurological outcome. No adverse events related to the use of helium ventilation occurred during the 3 h of administration. This novel ventilation might provide new perspectives for treatment of brain injury after cardiac arrest.

Other noble gasses such as xenon also play a role of neuroprotective agents. Only animal studies have shown results regarding neuroprotective properties of xenon [31]. A randomized controlled trial that enrolled 110 patients found less white matter injury on magnetic resonance imaging (MRI), but no improvement in survival or neurological outcome using xenon [32]. The result is similar to another study [33]. Given xenon is scarce and requires a purposely designed ventilator and has no strong evidence improving neurological outcome, it is rarely applied in clinical care.

### 15.3.2 Respiratory Dysfunction

Previous studies mainly focused on myocardial and brain dysfunctions after resuscitation; few research has mentioned respiratory dysfunction. Multiple factors are involved in respiratory dysfunction post-CPR. First, the massive production of reactive oxygen species and the massive residual oxygen in the alveoli during post-cardiac arrest syndrome lead to oxidative lung damage. Second, both lungs receive the total cardiac output, so systemic inflammatory response may cause greater and more severe inflammation response in the lungs than in other organs. Third, pulmonary congestion due to chest trauma and cardiopulmonary resuscitation can also result in deterioration of lung compliance. Therefore, guidelines since 2010 have paid more attention to respiratory management in post-cardiac arrest care. However, it is unsatisfactory that there are no specific evidence-based recommendations for post-resuscitation respiratory care.

Yang et al. [34] investigated the changes in respiratory pathophysiology after ROSC by recording the ventilation, respiratory pressure, and neural respiratory drive (NRD) in a large animal model. First, the pulmonary pathophysiology after CPR includes deteriorated gas exchange, elevated NRD, increased inspiratory muscle activity and ventilation demand, and decreased dynamic pulmonary compliance and NRD efficiency. This suggests more inspiratory muscle effort is required to produce the same level of ventilation after ROSC. Second, abnormalities in respiratory mechanics, hypoxemia, and pulmonary edema can last for more than12 h even if spontaneous breathing resumes soon after ROSC. Therefore, respiratory care after resuscitation should be extended to a longer period after ROSC, especially for patients who have experienced prolonged cardiac arrest. Third, RR increased significantly, and tidal volume decreased in early stage after resuscitation, suggesting that the increase of ventilation after ROSC may be mainly realized by increasing the RR rather than tidal volume.

## 15.4 Ventilation Management After ROSC

The incidence of pulmonary complications following cardiac arrest is as high as 50%, including aspiration pneumonia, lung contusion, and cardiogenic pulmonary edema. In addition, improper mechanical ventilator parameters can be harmful to the lungs. The most common mechanisms of ventilator-associated lung injury (VALI) are as follows: (1) overstretching from high tidal volume (VT) and driving pressures, (2) repeated recruitment and de-recruitment of unstable lung units, (3) peripheral airway collapse at low end-expiratory lung volume and cyclic opening and closing of peripheral airway, and (4) bio-trauma, particularly in the extracellular matrix component during fluid-loading status.

### 15.4.1 Mode

Although different modes can control ventilation more precisely according to patients' pathology and pulmonary dynamics, there is no evidence of improved patient outcomes associated with the use of a specific invasive ventilation mode. In practical terms, there is no research on the effect of different modes on heart failure patients. Modes of ventilation that allow spontaneous respiratory activity have hemodynamic advantages over fully controlled modes of ventilation. The former generate lower mean airway pressure and intrapleural pressure within a given minute volume than the latter. Modes such as CPAP, SIMV, bilevel airway pressure, and pressure support ventilation allow for different degrees of spontaneous breaths, which can reduce the harmful effects of positive-pressure ventilation on cardiovascular physiology. On the contrary, in patients with severe cardiogenic shock, myocardial ischemia, or left ventricle dysfunction, full controlled ventilatory support may benefit more by eliminating the effect of increased myocardial oxygen consumption due to spontaneous breathing.

### 15.4.2 Oxygenation

Different from the hypoperfusion and hypoxia in the period of cardiac arrest, reperfusion and hyperemia are characteristics of the early period after ROSC. After reperfusion occurs, the reactive oxygen species (ROS) plays a dominant role in the aggravation of ischemic injury and worsening of brain injury by neuronal damage, mainly occurring 1 h after ROSC. Hyperoxemia can exacerbate ROS production and worsen cellular and mitochondrial function. In addition, hyperoxemia leads to vasoconstriction and induces myocardial ischemia, which is harmful to cerebral perfusion and promotes epileptic seizures.

Growing evidence has shown that hyperoxia may be associated with worse neurologic outcome after cardiac arrest. A recent meta-analysis, including six experimental studies in animals, found that the treatment with 100% oxygen had a poor neurological prognosis, namely, neurological deficit score and the presence of neuronal damage on histology as well as the indirect markers of cerebral metabolic function, compared with lower oxygen concentration. However, there is insufficient data on clinical outcome. A small randomized control trial revealed that there was no significant difference in survival between 100% and 30% oxygen administration at 1 h after out-of-hospital cardiac arrest (OHCA) with ROSC. In conclusion, it still seems feasible using 100% oxygen immediately on ROSC [35]. Once oxygenation can be reliably monitored with pulse oximetry, the inhaled oxygen should be titrated to achieve normal oxygen saturations (94–98%) [21].

### 15.4.3 Tidal Volume (TV)

Acute respiratory distress syndrome (ARDS) occurs in patients after cardiac arrest due to a variety of mechanisms: reperfusion injury, oxidative stress, pulmonary contusion from chest compressions, ventilator-induced lung injury, aspiration, and infection [36]. Higher tidal volume and higher plateau pressure (>30 $cmH_2O$) have shown a linear relation with mortality of cardiac arrest patients [37]. Lower tidal volume during the first 48 h of admission was associated with better neurocognitive outcome, earlier liberation from mechanical ventilation, and earlier release from circulatory shock after OHCA [38, 39]. The link between low tidal volume and good neurocognitive outcome may be explained by the following possible mechanisms: attenuation of lung injury–mediated systemic inflammation, pulmonary mechanotransduction, lung–brain crosstalk, differences in blood oxygen or carbon dioxide tension, and hemodynamic effects of lower mean airway pressures.

Hence, current guidelines for post-ROSC care recommend lung-protective ventilation with low tidal volumes (6–8 ml/kg of ideal body weight). At the same time, guidelines recommend that a constant temperature of comatose adult patients after ROSC should be maintained between 32 °C and 36 °C. However, how does temperature affect mechanical ventilation settings is unknown. A retrospective substudy of the multicenter, randomized, parallel-group, assessor-blinded target temperatures (TTM) trial firstly determined the effect of different target temperatures (TTM 33 °C versus TTM 36 °C) on ventilation settings. They found that TTM33 results in lower end-tidal $CO_2$ levels and a higher alveolar dead space fraction compared to TTM36. A possible reason for this result may be that increased vasoconstriction leads to decreased pulmonary perfusion at 33 °C. They assume that the demand for a minute volume ventilation decreased at 33 °C [37].

### 15.4.4 $CO_2$

There is an important and complex interaction between $PaCO_2$ and neurologic outcomes after cardiac arrest. (1) $PaCO_2$ plays a role in cerebral vasculature and cerebral blood flow regulation. A reduction of approximately 3% in cerebral blood flow for every 1 mmHg decrease in $PaCO_2$ has been reported in traumatic brain injury patients. (2) $CO_2$ may also regulate ischemia–reperfusion injury at the cellular level. Hypercapnic acidosis may reduce the production of superoxide catalyzed by xanthine oxidase, decreasing neuronal oxidative stress. In addition, high level of $PaCO_2$ may reduce the levels of detrimental amino acids like glutamate, thus reducing the excitotoxicity induced by high level of excitatory neurotransmitters. Therefore, arterial hypocarbia should be avoided as it is associated with worse neurologic prognosis after cardiac arrest.

In recent years, an experimental strategy of mild permissive hypercarbia after cardiac arrest has emerged. And, the relationship between hypercarbia and neurologic prognosis is contradictory, with previous studies revealing worsened [40], equivocal, and improved outcomes [41] compared with normocarbia. The reason for different conclusions is that the methods, definitions, and blood gas sampling intervals applied in each study are not uniform [42]. A recent multicenter RCT evaluated the feasibility of targeting low-normal (4.5–4.7 kPa) vs. high-normal (5.8–6.0 kPa) $PaCO_2$ during the first 36 h after ROSC in 123 comatose patients resuscitated from OHCA. There was no significant difference in the values of neuron-specific enolase (NSE), a biomarker of neurologic injury, at 48 h after ROSC [43]. Researchers found that the mild hypercapnia group had better arterial pressure and less neuronal degeneration in a porcine post-cardiac arrest model. However, there was no statistically significant difference in neurological recovery [44].

Thus, the recent guideline recommended maintaining the $PaCO_2$ within a normal physiological range (end-tidal $CO_2$ 30–40 mmHg or $PaCO_2$ 35–45 mmHg), taking into account any temperature correction [21]. Other $PaCO_2$ targets may be tolerated for specific patients. For example, mild hypocapnia may be a temporizing option in patient with cerebral edema. Permissive hypercapnia may be feasible in patients with acute lung injury or airway hypertension.

#### 15.4.4.1 When and How Frequently $PaCO_2$ Should Be Measured After ROSC?

The current guidelines recommend titrating minute ventilation (MV) to achieve a $PaCO_2$ of 40–45 mmHg in patients resuscitated from cardiac arrest. The recommended approach may result in delay in optimizing $PaCO_2$ (the time for initial available arterial blood gas (ABG) analysis and subsequent ventilation adjustments). So far, the initial prescribed relationship between MV and $PaCO_2$ in post-cardiac arrest syndrome has been rarely reported.

A prospectively compiled single-center study including 75 patients showed initial post-resuscitation prescribed MV had no obvious relationship with subsequent $PaCO_2$, revealing $PaCO_2$ is also affected by patient's other factors: etiology of cardiac arrest, use of neuromuscular blocking agents, lung compliance, intrinsic respiratory drive, lung injury, persistent post-resuscitation circulatory shock, body habitus, and dead space. Identifying these factors will facilitate the development of a volume-targeted ventilation strategy that focuses on adjusting initial prescribed MV by individual patient-related factors [45].

A recent study also showed the correlation between prescribed MV and $PaCO_2$ was poor at any time point (initial, 6, 12, 18, and 24 h after cardiac arrest), suggesting that setting the ventilator based on experience may lead to unexpected $PaCO_2$ values. Therefore, to achieve normocapnia during the initial post-ROSC period, early and multiple ABG analyses are necessary (considering the little correlation between end-tidal $CO_2$ measurements and $PaCO_2$ due to high dead space in the post-arrest patient; ABG should be monitored instead of end-tidal $CO_2$ measurements) [46].

### 15.4.5 PEEP

Pulmonary contusion, atelectasis, aspiration, and pulmonary edema due to chest compressions result in a low respiratory compliance in majority of patients after cardiac arrest. Thus, PEEP level should be set above 5 $cmH_2O$ and should be titrated to the target $SaO_2$ taking into account the hazards of excessive PEEP (such as reduced preload, barotrauma). Median PEEP was 7.7 $cmH_2O$ [37].

## 15.5 When and How to Wean from Invasive Mechanical Ventilation?

### 15.5.1 When Does the Weaning Start?

The American Thoracic Society guideline recommends liberation of patient from invasive mechanical ventilation after 24 h [47]. However, the specific time and steps to evacuate are not proposed.

Due to myocardial dysfunction peaks in the first 24 h following ROSC [48]. Some study suggested end-organ support and weaning post 72 h [49]. The weaning criteria include the following: (1) cardiac pathology leading to invasive mechanical ventilation(e.g., ischemia, cardiogenic shock, arrhythmia) has been improved; (2) hemodynamic stability, defined as systolic blood pressure between 90 and 160 mmHg and heart rate <140/min without vasopressors or with low doses of vasopressors; (3) respiratory stability (oxygen saturation > 90% with fraction of inspired oxygen [$FiO_2$] $\leq$0.4, RR < 35/min, spontaneous tidal volume > 5 ml/kg, ratio of RR to tidal volume < 100/min/l, and maximal inspiratory pressure > 15 $cmH_2O$); (4) the patient is conscious; and (5) the patient has little sputum.

### 15.5.2 The Reason of Weaning Failure: Weaning-Induced Pulmonary Edema

The withdrawal process can place a significant strain on the cardiovascular system particularly in patients with an underlying cardiac disease, aged >65 years, who is morbidly obese (body mass index $\geq$35 $kg/m^2$), resulting in weaning-induced pulmonary edema (WiPO), which is the main risk factor of weaning failure [50–52]. There are three triggering mechanisms. First, left ventricular preload and afterload increased, and left ventricular compliance decreased after removal of positive-pressure ventilation [53]. Second, the increased breathing work can result in the huge amounts of oxygen consumed by the respiratory muscles. Third, the emotional stress and potential hypercapnia or hypoxia lead to sympathetic excitability, which increases systemic arterial pressure and thus the LV afterload, the respiratory frequency, and the work of breathing.

### 15.5.3 Weaning Failure of Cardiovascular Origin: How to Suspect and Detect

Due to the above effects of removing positive-pressure ventilation on the cardiovascular system, weaning failure of cardiac origin usually occurs at the early stage of spontaneous breathing test (SBT) rather than later after extubation. Thus, weaning should be carried out in three steps: conducting the SBT, suspecting, and then evidencing weaning-induced cardiac failure.

#### 15.5.3.1 Performing the SBT

Pressure support ventilation (PSV, typically 5–8 $cmH_2O$ with or without a positive end-expiratory pressure of 5 $cmH_2O$), continuous positive airway pressure (CPAP), and the T-piece are often used in SBT. PS techniques provide pressure during inspiration to overcome endotracheal tube resistance. CPAP technique may improve respiratory mechanics or cardiac function and may overestimate patients' ability to breathe spontaneously after extubation. In contrast, the T-piece did not provide support and was thought to increase work of breathing, possibly underestimating patients' ability to breathe autonomously after extubation. Recently, high-flow oxygen therapy is firstly used for SBTs by connecting the device to the endotracheal tube during the SBT. It was demonstrated that high-flow nasal cannula (HFNC), like PSV, can shorten the time for patients receiving mechanical ventilation to pass the 2-h SBT [54]. In a previous report, the rate of successful extubation was significantly higher than T-piece SBTs [55], and PSV was recommended by the latest American Thoracic Society guidelines.

However, for post-cardiac death patient, the optimal SBT technique for diagnosing weaning-induced cardiac failure is still controversial. Physicians are concerned that patients who breathe comfortably with low levels of PSV during SBT could develop respiratory failure immediately after extubation [56]. Cabello et al. [57] assessed three types of SBTs performed in random order: T-piece trial, pressure support ventilation (7 $cmH_2O$) with low PEEP (5 $cmH_2O$), and pressure support ventilation (7 $cmH_2O$) without PEEP. All patients failed the T-piece trial, whereas 57% and 79% of them successfully passed the SBT using pressure support ventilation (7 $cmH_2O$) without PEEP and with low PEEP (5 $cmH_2O$), respectively. Another study also revealed that the T-piece trial induced the most significant reduction in intrathoracic pressure and the most marked increase in pulmonary artery occlusion pressure (PAOP), compared with pressure support with or without positive end-expiratory pressure [58]. A recent meta-analysis concluded that breathing through a T piece works just as well as breathing after extubation [59].

Taken together, T-piece trial better reflects the physiologic conditions after extubation and elicits the greatest burden on cardiocirculatory and respiratory functions during SBT. Because a patient with heart failure requires a higher extubation threshold, a successful T-piece trial seems to be more sensitive to assess patient's ability to tolerate spontaneous breathing [60] and may be more likely to stress the cardiorespiratory system to diagnose WiPO [61].

A failed SBT has the following signs: diaphoresis, alteration of consciousness, respiratory frequency more than 35 breaths/min or increase $\geq 50\%$, $PaO_2 \leq 50$ mmHg or $SpO_2 \leq 90\%$ (with $FiO_2 \geq 50\%$), heart rate ≥ 140 beats/min, systolic arterial pressure > 180 or < 90 mmHg, and new onset of supraventricular or ventricular arrhythmia [62]. A sudden onset of severe hypertension and respiratory distress after starting the SBT should be suspected of weaning-induced cardiac failure, but there is no documentary evidence to support this [63].

#### 15.5.3.2 Other Diagnostic Methods to Detect WiPO in Patients

If a patient is stable but fails to tolerate an initial SBT, we should be alert of the possibility of WiPO. The suspicious patients should be scheduled for a second SBT within 24 h after the first SBT, including a 2-h T-piece trial. At the same time, some approaches can be used to diagnose WiPO.

1. *Pulmonary Artery Catheterization*: Traditionally, the gold standard to diagnose WiPO relies on the monitoring of increased PAOP(≥18 mmHg) using a pulmonary artery catheter just before and at the end of the second SBT. However, pulmonary artery catheter is less used today due to its invasiveness and the lack of evidence of monitoring-related benefit [64]. Some noninvasive methods have been recently developed, such as echocardiography, cardiac biomarkers, biological signs of hemoconcentration, and extravascular pulmonary lung water. However, studies failed to assess and compare the respective diagnostic value of these different methods to identify WiPO.
2. *Echocardiography*: Transthoracic echocardiography (TTE) performed by trained operators is valuable in the diagnosis of WiPO during a second SBT. The combination of $E/A > 0.95$ and $E/e' > 8.5$ at the end of the SBT could detect a PAOP of at least 18 mmHg associated with LV diastolic dysfunction [65]. Remarkably, patients with impaired LV diastolic function, who were at high risk of a subsequent SBT failure, can be early detected by a sole TTE prior to SBT [53]. However, it is often difficult to perform echocardiography in patients with respiratory distress, so echocardiography is not the optimum technique to diagnose WiPO.
3. *Biochemical Indices of Weaning-Induced Cardiovascular Dysfunction*: B-type natriuretic peptide (BNP) and amino-terminal pro-brain natriuretic peptide (NT-proBNP), as biomarkers of the volume status and functional state of the heart, are collected before the end of second SBT. Numerous studies have shown that elevated basal levels of BNP or NT-proBNP and/or a BNP increase at SBT completion are helpful in the diagnosis of weaning-induced cardiac failure. Dres et al., using a pulmonary artery catheter as the reference method, revealed that an increase of BNP concentration more than 12% during SBT could predict WiPO with a sensitivity of 76% and a specificity of 78% [66]. Similar results were reported for NT-proBNP, but BNP performed better than NT-proBNP [67]. This may be attributed to the shorter half-life of BNP (22 min) compared with NT-proBNP (120 min).

   In summary, it is reasonable to consider that relative changes in BNP levels are helpful in the diagnosis of weaning-induced cardiac failure.
4. *Biological Signs of Hemoconcentration*: During the development of a hydrostatic pulmonary edema, the transfer of a hypooncotic fluid from the pulmonary

capillaries toward the interstitium often concerns an important volume so that it may result in a significant blood volume contraction. Anguel et al. [68] confirmed that an elevated plasma protein concentration exceeding 6% during SBT could predict WiPO with a sensitivity of 87% and a specificity of 95%. Dres [66] also found that an increase in the plasma protein or hemoglobin concentration more than 5% during SBT had a good sensitivity and specificity for predicting weaning-induced cardiac failure. In summary, biological signs of hemoconcentration collected before and at the end of a failing SBT are worthy, simple, and inexpensive to diagnose WiPO.

5. *Extravascular Lung Water*: Transpulmonary thermodilution can be particularly helpful to estimate pulmonary edema by measuring extravascular lung water (EVLW). An increase in EVLW exceeding 14% during an SBT predicted WiPO with a sensitivity of 67% and a specificity of 100% [66]. However, given the invasiveness and the cost, transpulmonary thermodilution devices are not commonly used during a weaning process.
6. *Passive Leg Raising*: Passive leg raising (PLR) by 45° is a dynamic test to evaluate cardiac preload status, which has been used to assess the risk of WiPO based on the expected increase in cardiac preload during transmission from mechanical ventilation to spontaneous breathing. A negative PLR test prior to SBT could predict weaning failure due to cardiovascular dysfunction with a sensitivity of 97% and a specificity of 81% [69].
7. *Critical Care Echocardiography*: Critical care echocardiography (CCE) is performed at bedside by a specially trained intensivist to establish diagnoses and guide therapeutic strategy, especially in patients with cardiopulmonary dysfunction. CCE is the only noninvasive approach which helps in identifying WiPO and its potential mechanism in real time. Therefore, CCE is well suited to detect high-risk patients of weaning failure during and after the SBT and to provide individualized treatment for those who failed.

#### 15.5.3.3 Definition of WiPO

Since the noninvasive consensual definition of WiPO has not yet been published, three criteria have been proposed in the recent literature: (1) echocardiographic signs of increased left atrial pressure at the end of the SBT: E/A ratio > 0.95 and E/e′ ratio > 8.5; (2) an increase of protein concentration (relative change >6%) during the SBT; and (3) an elevated BNP (absolute change ≥48 ng/l) or NT-proBNP (absolute change ≥21 ng/l) concentration during the SBT.

## 15.6 How to Prevent and Treat WiPO

In order to wean from mechanical ventilation successfully, the mechanisms which led to cardiac dysfunction have to be carefully analyzed to orientate the treatment, such as preload optimization guided by BNP, contractility improvement in severe systolic dysfunction, administration in excessive afterload and/or myocardial ischemia, as well as other reasonable treatment in specific indications. Among them, elective initiation of noninvasive ventilator (NIV) immediately after extubation has been demonstrated to reduce the incidence of WiPO.

### 15.6.1 Use of Noninvasive Ventilation in the Post-extubation Period as a Weaning Adjunct

Approximately 10–25% of patients require reintubation after successful SBT and extubation, and reintubation is associated with higher mortality rate [70]. The latest guidelines give noninvasive respiratory support a "strong recommendation" in high-risk patients, especially those with weaning-induced cardiac failure because it can increase intrathoracic pressure, reduces right ventricular and left ventricular (LV) preload and LV afterload, augments oxygenation, and improves dyspnea. If patients suffer from acute cardiogenic pulmonary edema with severe dyspnea (RR > 25 breaths/min, $SpO_2$ < 90%), NIV should be used immediately following extubation [71].

Noninvasive respiratory support encompasses strategies such as continuous positive airway pressure (CPAP), noninvasive pressure support ventilation (NIPSV), and HFNC.

#### 15.6.1.1 CPAP

CPAP is the simplest and cheapest technique, which includes applying a high flow in face mask leading to a continuous positive pressure into the lungs. It can be applied without the aid of a ventilator by using a source of air or oxygen and a mask equipped with PEEP valve or with the Boussignac system. CPAP has been most often used in hypoxemic patients in low-equipped areas. Early interest was sparked by observational and small randomized studies showing that CPAP improved oxygenation, reduced breathing work, and enhanced cardiac output in patients with cardiogenic pulmonary edema [21–23, 49, 50].

#### 15.6.1.2 NIPSV

NIPSV, also called noninvasive intermittent positive-pressure ventilation (NIPPV), is programmed with two levels of pressure: expiratory pressure (EPAP) or positive end-expiratory pressure (PEEP) and inspiratory pressure (IPAP). It requires a ventilator and it is preferred in patients with mild fatigue or significant hypercapnia [72]. The RR is not pre-set and is entirely dependent on the patient. Adequate synchrony is essential, so it requires some expertise to set the ventilator according to the changing demand of the patient.

#### 15.6.1.3 High-Flow Nasal Cannula

HFNC therapy, a recently developed oxygen therapy technology that has been widely accepted, provides a high flow rate of heated and humidified gas (up to 60–80 l/min, providing up to 7 $cmH_2O$ of PEEP) through a nasal cannula adjusted to the nostrils. It is increasingly used in patients with acute hypoxemic respiratory failure, improving comfort and reducing dryness of mouth and airway compared with conventional oxygen therapy [73]. A recent research reported HFNC therapy can reduce the reintubation rate, which may be attributable to several reasons. First, HFNC therapy provides a high flow of gas, leads to low levels of positive end-expiratory pressure, and increases the functional residual capacity and tidal volume, which in turn promotes ventilation. Second, the heating humidifier in the HFNC therapy device promotes the discharge of airway secretions and reduces the occurrence of respiratory obstruction [54].

Thus, it is considered in patients requiring prolonged ventilation or intolerant to other forms of NIPSV. However, HFNO requires closed mouth [74], which may be disadvantage for patients with severe dyspnea such as acute cardiogenic pulmonary edma (those patients generally breath by mouth).

### 15.6.2 Which One Is the Best?

Recently, considerable interest has been generated as to which therapy provides the most appropriate noninvasive support. But there are no trials or meta-analyses showing that one technique has a clear advantage over another one for important outcomes [75].

#### 15.6.2.1 NIPSV Versus CPAP

Theoretically NIPSV has an advantage over CPAP because it provides better breath inspiratory assistance, reducing work of breathing, increasing tidal volume more than CPAP, and therefore improving ventilation in patients with hypercarbia. The theory has been confirmed by a physiologic randomized crossover study revealing that NIPSV was more effective in terms of unloading respiratory muscles and improving cardiac function compared with CPAP. However, NIPSV has a higher incidence of myocardial ischemia than CPAP. The applicability of these findings is limited by the small size of studies included and wide variations in study populations and interventions. So far, Gray et al. performed the largest multicenter randomized controlled trial to evaluate the effect of noninvasive on acute cardiogenic pulmonary edema. The trial enrolled 1069 patients with acute cardiogenic pulmonary edema and evaluated the superiority of NIPSV over CPAP. There was no significant difference between CPAP (11.7%) and NIPSV (11.1% *P 5.81*) in the composite end point of short-term (within 7 days) mortality and intubation.

Recent guidelines from ERS/ATS suggested either NIPSV or CPAP for patients with acute cardiogenic pulmonary edema [76].

#### 15.6.2.2 High-Flow Nasal Cannula Versus NIPPV

There is no randomized controlled trial regarding HFNC's administration after extubation in patients at high risk of WiPO [77]. Only one small randomized study was published in 2017, which was the first to analyze the effect of HFNC and conventional oxygen therapy on acute cardiogenic pulmonary edema. There were no significant differences in the outcomes, but the study found a decrease in RR in patients with HFNC during the first 60 min [78].

### 15.6.3 How to Use NIV When Weaning-Induced Pulmonary Edema Occurs

For NIPSV, several different types of interfaces are available, including a total face mask (covering nose, mouth, and eyes), nasal mask, oronasal or full-face mask, and nasal pillows. Choosing an appropriate mask is important because adverse effects are mostly related to mask tolerance. To minimize air leakage, we have to cover both the nose and mouth with a mask and make sure the device is tightly sealed to the patient's face. Other interfaces such as nasal pillows, mouthpieces, or laryngeal masks are not considered in a patient with acute heart failure. Initial settings recommended are often low levels of pressure (IPAP, 10–12 $cmH_2O$/EPAP, 3–4 $cmH_2O$). IPAP is used to control ventilation ($PaCO_2$), and EPAP is generally titrated to oxygenation. It is necessary to increase IPAP progressively according to patient's adaptation in order to achieve the target tidal volumes >4–6 ml/kg. Increasing IPAP by 2–3 $cmH_2O$ can improve hypercapnia. High pressure can lead to excessive air leakage, asynchrony, and discomfort especially in patients with high RR. Thus, we should avoid IPAP >20 $cmH_2O$ to prevent aspiration caused by gastric insufflation. Initial $FiO_2$ can be set higher and then titrated to a target $SaO_2$ (e.g., 94–98%) while avoiding $SaO_2 > 98\%$.

When using CPAP, a general starting pressure is 5 $cmH_2O$ with titration by 2 $cmH_2O$ and is increased to 7.5 or 10 $cmH_2O$ according to the response.

When HFNC was used in critically ill patients, $FiO_2$ was set to 100% at the beginning and the maximum tolerated flow up to 50 l/min. Subsequently, $FiO_2$ and flow rate were titrated according to $SpO_2$ and patient's demand. In less severe cases, it is usually started with lower flow and $FiO_2$. During the application of NIV, RR (patient's effort), oxygen saturation (minimal required $FiO_2$), and pH/$PaCO_2$ (to assess efficacy) should be monitored in addition to standard physiologic parameters. The general recommendation is to reassess after 60 and/or 90–120 min.

The key issue is optimal synchronization with the ventilator. If NIPPV goes successfully, the patient's discomfort will be relieved generally within 1–2 h, with reduced RR, improved work of breathing, and improved gas exchange. Excessive leakage due to asynchrony can be prevented by adjusting the mask, shortening inspiration time, sedating, reducing PS, or changing inspiratory and expiratory triggers (when available). In general, leak less than 0.4 l/s (<25 l/min) is tolerable.

In nearly 20% of patients who show poor synchrony with NIV, mild sedation is required to decrease intolerance after nonpharmacological approaches have failed. Opioids (morphine, remifentanil), propofol, midazolam, and more recently dexmedetomidine have been commonly administrated in this condition. Minimal intermittent doses of a single drug are superior to continuous infusions or different drug combinations. NIV can be removed after patients recover satisfactorily (usually 2–5 h in patient with acute cardiogenic pulmonary edema).

## 15.7 Conclusion

Many controversies still exist in terms of the optimization of ventilation strategy during cardiopulmonary resuscitation and post-ROSC. Most of the current opinion is based on observational studies, animal trials, and expert opinion. Due to lack of reliable methods to detect and measure ventilation metrics, the relationship between ventilation quality and survival in patients with cardiac arrest is still unknown. Fortunately, techniques have been developed in recent years to detect lung inflation during CPR through the use of the thoracic impedance signal [79]. This may allow researchers to study ventilation metrics more accurately. More specific CPR ventilation recommendations should be made available to improve standardization among physicians.

## References

1. Chang MP, Idris AH. The past, present, and future of ventilation during cardiopulmonary resuscitation. Curr Opin Crit Care. 2017;23(3):188–92.
2. Ashoor HM, Lillie E, Zarin W, et al. Effectiveness of different compression-to-ventilation methods for cardiopulmonary resuscitation: a systematic review. Resuscitation. 2017;118:112–25.
3. Olasveengen TM, de Caen AR, Mancini ME, et al. 2017 international consensus on cardiopulmonary resuscitation and emergency cardiovascular care science with treatment recommendations summary. Resuscitation. 2017;121:201–14.
4. Hupfl M, Selig HF, Nagele P. Chest-compression-only versus standard cardiopulmonary resuscitation: a meta-analysis. Lancet. 2010;376(9752):1552–7.
5. Wang S, Li C, Ji X, et al. Effect of continuous compressions and 30:2 cardiopulmonary resuscitation on global ventilation/perfusion values during resuscitation in a porcine model. Crit Care Med. 2010;38(10):2024–30.
6. Ewy GA, Hilwig RW, Zuercher M, et al. Continuous chest compression resuscitation in arrested swine with upper airway inspiratory obstruction. Resuscitation. 2010;81(5):585–90.
7. Yannopoulos D, Matsuura T, McKnite S, et al. No assisted ventilation cardiopulmonary resuscitation and 24-hour neurological outcomes in a porcine model of cardiac arrest. Crit Care Med. 2010;38(1):254–60.
8. Deakin CD, O'Neill JF, Tabor T. Does compression-only cardiopulmonary resuscitation generate adequate passive ventilation during cardiac arrest? Resuscitation. 2007;75(1):53–9.
9. Safar P. Ventilation and circulation with closed-chest cardiac massage in man. JAMA. 1961;176(7):574.
10. Liu YC, Qi YM, Zhang H, et al. A survey of ventilation strategies during cardiopulmonary resuscitation. World J Emerg Med. 2019;10(4):222–7.
11. Cordioli RL, Brochard L, Suppan L, et al. How ventilation is delivered during cardiopulmonary resuscitation: an international survey. Respir Care. 2018;63(10):1293–301.
12. Winkler BE, Muellenbach RM, Wurmb T, et al. Passive continuous positive airway pressure ventilation during cardiopulmonary resuscitation: a randomized cross-over manikin simulation study. J Clin Monit Comput. 2017;31(1):93–101.
13. LeBlanc PA, Nadeau A. BET 1: continuous flow insufflation of oxygen in out-of-hospital cardiac arrest. Emerg Med J. 2018;35(1):65–6.

14. Fouche PF, Simpson PM, Bendall J, et al. Airways in out-of-hospital cardiac arrest: systematic review and meta-analysis. Prehosp Emerg Care. 2014;18(2):244–56.
15. Jabre P, Penaloza A, Pinero D, et al. Effect of bag-mask ventilation vs endotracheal intubation during cardiopulmonary resuscitation on neurological outcome after out-of-hospital cardiorespiratory arrest: a randomized clinical trial. JAMA. 2018;319(8):779–87.
16. Ruemmler R, Ziebart A, Moellmann C, et al. Ultra-low tidal volume ventilation—a novel and effective ventilation strategy during experimental cardiopulmonary resuscitation. Resuscitation. 2018;132:56–62.
17. Kill C, Galbas M, Neuhaus C, et al. Chest compression synchronized ventilation versus intermitted positive pressure ventilation during cardiopulmonary resuscitation in a pig model. PLoS One. 2015;10(5):e0127759.
18. Tan D, Xu J, Shao S, et al. Comparison of different inspiratory triggering settings in automated ventilators during cardiopulmonary resuscitation in a porcine model. PLoS One. 2017;12(2):e0171869.
19. Tian X, Fang W, Wu J. The effects of different mechanical ventilation flow model on the peak airway pressure during cardiopulmonary resuscitation. Zhonghua Wei Zhong Bing Ji Jiu Yi Xue. 2014;26(10):722–5.
20. Chalkias A, Pavlopoulos F, Koutsovasilis A, et al. Airway pressure and outcome of out-of-hospital cardiac arrest: a prospective observational study. Resuscitation. 2017;110:101–6.
21. Callaway CW, Donnino MW, Fink EL, Geocadin RG, Golan E, Kern KB, Leary M, Meurer WJ, Peberdy MA, Thompson TM, Zimmerman JL. Part 8: post-cardiac arrest care: 2015 American Heart Association guidelines update for cardiopulmonary resuscitation and emergency cardiovascular care. Circulation. 2015;132(18 Suppl 2):S465–82.
22. Vissers G, Soar J, Monsieurs KG. Ventilation rate in adults with a tracheal tube during cardiopulmonary resuscitation: a systematic review. Resuscitation. 2017;119:5–12.
23. Vissers G, Duchatelet C, Huybrechts SA, et al. The effect of ventilation rate on outcome in adults receiving cardiopulmonary resuscitation. Resuscitation. 2019;138:243–9.
24. Tan D, Sun J, Geng P. Duration of cardiac arrest requires different ventilation volumes during cardiopulmonary resuscitation in a pig model. J Clin Monit Comput. 2020;34(3):525–33.
25. Georgiou M, Papathanassoglou E, Xanthos T. Systematic review of the mechanisms driving effective blood flow during adult CPR. Resuscitation. 2014;85:1586–93.
26. Liu Y, Tian Z, Yu C, Walline J, Xu J, Zhu H, et al. Transesophageal echocardiography to assess mitral valve movement and flow during long term cardiopulmonary resuscitation: how cardiac effects fade with time. Int J Cardiol. 2016;223:693–8.
27. David HN, Haelewyn B, Chazalviel L, et al. Post-ischemic helium provides neuroprotection in rats subjected to middle cerebral artery occlusion-induced ischemia by producing hypothermia. J Cereb Blood Flow Metab. 2009;29(6):1159–65.
28. Liu Y, Xue F, Liu G, et al. Helium preconditioning attenuates hypoxia/ischemia-induced injury in the developing brain. Brain Res. 2011;1376:122–9.
29. Zhuang L, Yang T, Zhao H, et al. The protective profile of argon, helium, and xenonin a model of neonatal asphyxia in rats. Crit Care Med. 2012;40(6):1724–30.
30. Brevoord D, Beurskens CJ, van den Bergh WM. Helium ventilation for treatment of post-cardiac arrest syndrome: a safety and feasibility study. Resuscitation. 2016;107:145–9.
31. Fries M, Brücken A, Cizen A, et al. Combining xenon and mild therapeutic hypothermia preserves neurological function after prolonged cardiac arrest in pigs. Crit Care Med. 2012;40(4):1297–303.
32. Laitio R, Hynninen M, Arola O, et al. Effect of inhaled xenon on cerebral white matter damage in comatose survivors of out-of-hospital cardiac arrest: a randomized clinical trial. JAMA. 2016;315(11):1120–8.
33. Azzopardi D, Robertson NJ, Bainbridge A, et al. Moderate hypothermia within 6h of birth plus inhaled xenon versus moderate hypothermia alone after birth asphyxia (TOBY-Xe): a proof-of-concept, open-label, randomised controlled trial. Lancet Neurol. 2016;15(2):145–53.

34. Yang Z, Zheng H, Lin L, et al. Alterations in respiratory mechanics and neural respiratory drive after restoration of spontaneous circulation in a porcine model subjected to different downtimes of cardiac arrest. J Am Heart Assoc. 2019;8(19):e012441.
35. Nolan JP, Berg RA, Callaway CW, et al. The present and future of cardiac arrest care: international experts reach out to caregivers and healthcare authorities. Intensive Care Med. 2018;44(6):823–32.
36. Johnson NJ, Caldwell E, Carlbom DJ, et al. The acute respiratory distress syndrome after out-of-hospital cardiac arrest: incidence, risk factors, and outcomes. Resuscitation. 2019;135:37–44.
37. Harmon MBA, van Meenen DMP, van der Veen ALIP, Binnekade JM, Dankiewicz J, Ebner F, Nielsen N, Pelosi P, Schultz MJ, Horn J, Friberg H, Juffermans NP, TTM trial investigators. Practice of mechanical ventilation in cardiac arrest patients and effects of targeted temperature management: a substudy of the targeted temperature management trial. Resuscitation. 2018;129:29–36.
38. Beitler JR, Ghafouri TB, Jinadasa SP, Mueller A, Hsu L, Anderson RJ, Joshua J, Tyagi S, Malhotra A, Sell RE, Talmor D. Favorable neurocognitive outcome with low tidal volume ventilation after cardiac arrest. Am J Respir Crit Care Med. 2017;195(9):1198–206.
39. Johnson NJ, Carlbom DJ, Gaieski DF. Ventilator management and respiratory care after cardiac arrest. Chest. 2018;153(6):1466–77.
40. Wang HE, Prince DK, Drennan IR, Grunau B, Carlbom DJ, Johnson N, Hansen M, Elmer J, Christenson J, Kudenchuk P, Aufderheide T, Weisfeldt M, Idris A, Trzeciak S, Kurz M, Rittenberger JC, Griffiths D, Jasti J, May S, Resuscitation Outcomes Consortium (ROC) Investigators. Post-resuscitation arterial oxygen and carbon dioxide and outcomes after out-of-hospital cardiac arrest. Resuscitation. 2017;120:113–8.
41. Eastwood GM, Schneider AG, Suzuki S, Peck L, Young H, Tanaka A, Mårtensson J, Warrillow S, McGuinness S, Parke R, Gilder E, Mccarthy L, Galt P, Taori G, Eliott S, Lamac T, Bailey M, Harley N, Barge D, Hodgson CL, Morganti-Kossmann MC, Pébay A, Conquest A, Archer JS, Bernard S, Stub D, Hart GK, Bellomo R. Targeted therapeutic mild hypercapnia after cardiac arrest: a phase II multi-centre randomized controlled trial (the CCC trial). Resuscitation. 2016;104:83–90.
42. Vaahersalo J, Bendel S, Reinikainen M, Kurola J, Tiainen M, Raj R, Pettilä V, Varpula T, Skrifvars MB, FINNRESUSCI Study Group. Arterial blood gas tensions afterresuscitation from out-of-hospital cardiac arrest: associations with long-term neurological outcome. Crit Care Med. 2014;42(6):1463–70.
43. Jakkula P, Reinikainen M, Hastbacka J, Loisa P, Tiainen M, Pettila V, Toppila J, Lahde M, Backlund M, Okkonen M, Bendel S, Birkelund T, Pulkkinen A, Heinonen J, Tikka T, Skrifvars MB, COMACARE study group. Targeting two different levels of both arterial carbon dioxide and arterial oxygen after cardiac arrest and resuscitation: a randomised pilot trial. Intensive Care Med. 2018;44(12):2112–21.
44. Babini G, Ristagno G, Boccardo A, De Giorgio D, De Maglie M, Affatato R, Ceriani S, Zani D, Novelli D, Staszewsky L, Masson S, Pravettoni D, Latini R, Belloli A, Scanziani E, Skrifvars M. Effect of mild hypercapnia on outcome and histological injury in a porcine post cardiac arrest model. Resuscitation. 2019;135:110–7.
45. Roberts BW, Kilgannon JH, Chansky ME, Trzeciak S. Association between initial prescribed minute ventilation and post-resuscitation partial pressure of arterial carbon dioxide in patients with post-cardiac arrest syndrome. Ann Intensive Care. 2014;4(1):9.
46. Tolins ML, Henning DJ, Gaieski DF, Grossestreuer AV, Jaworski A, Johnson NJ. Initial arterial carbon dioxide tension is associated with neurological outcome after resuscitation from cardiac arrest. Resuscitation. 2017;114:53–8.
47. Schmidt GA, Girard TD, Kress JP, Morris PE, Ouellette DR, Alhazzani W, Burns SM, Epstein SK, Esteban A, Fan E, Ferrer M, Fraser GL, Gong MN, Hough CL, Mehta S, Nanchal R, Patel S, Pawlik AJ, Schweickert WD, Sessler CN, Strøm T, Wilson KC, Truwit JD. Liberation from mechanical ventilation in critically III adults: executive summary of an official American college of chest physicians/American thoracic society clinical practice guideline. Chest. 2017;151(1):160–5.

48. Topjian AA, Berg RA, Taccone FS. Haemodynamic and ventilator management in patients following cardiac arrest. Curr Opin Crit Care. 2015;21(3):195–201.
49. Randhawa VK, Grunau BE, Debicki DB, Zhou J, Hegazy AF, McPherson T, Nagpal AD. Cardiac intensive care unit management of patients after cardiac arrest: now the real work begins. Can J Cardiol. 2018;34(2):156–67.
50. Frutos-Vivar F, Esteban A. Our paper 20 years later: how has withdrawal from mechanical ventilation changed? Intensive Care Med. 2014;40(10):1449–59.
51. Liu J, Shen F, Teboul JL, Anguel N, Beurton A, Bezaz N, Richard C, Monnet X. Cardiac dysfunction induced by weaning from mechanical ventilation: incidence, risk factors, and effects of fluid removal. Crit Care. 2016;20(1):369.
52. Roche-Campo F, Bedet A, Vivier E, Brochard L, Mekontso DA. Cardiac function during weaning failure: the role of diastolic dysfunction. Ann Intensive Care. 2018;8(1):2.
53. Konomi I, Tasoulis A, Kaltsi I, Karatzanos E, Vasileiadis I, Temperikidis P, Nanas S, Routsi CI. Left ventricular diastolic dysfunction—an independent risk factor for weaning failure from mechanical ventilation. Anaesth Intensive Care. 2016;44(4):466–73.
54. Liu F, Shao Q, Jiang R, Zeng Z, Liu Y, Li Y, Liu Q, Ding C, Zhao N, Peng Z. Qian K high-flow oxygen therapy to speed weaning from mechanical ventilation: a prospective randomized study. Am J Crit Care. 2019;28(5):370–6.
55. Subirà C, Hernández G, Vázquez A, Rodríguez-García R, González-Castro A, García C, Rubio O, Ventura L, López A, de la Torre MC, Keough E, Arauzo V, Hermosa C, Sánchez C, Tizón A, Tenza E, Laborda C, Cabañes S, Lacueva V, Del Mar Fernández M, Arnau A, Fernández R. Effect of pressure support vs t-piece ventilation strategies during spontaneous breathing trials on successful extubation among patients receiving mechanical ventilation a randomized clinical trial. JAMA. 2019;321(22):2175–82.
56. Tobin MJ. Extubation and themyth of "minimal ventilator settings". Am J Respir Crit Care Med. 2012;185(4):349–50.
57. Cabello B, Thille AW, Roche-Campo F, Brochard L, Gómez FJ, Mancebo J. Physiological comparison of three spontaneous breathing trials in difficult-to-wean patients. Intensive Care Med. 2010;36(7):1171–9.
58. Thille AW, Cortés-Puch I, Esteban A. Weaning from the ventilator and extubation in ICU. Curr Opin Crit Care. 2013;19(1):57–64.
59. Sklar MC, Burns K, Rittayamai N, Lanys A, Rauseo M, Chen L, Dres M, Chen GQ, Goligher EC, Adhikari NKJ, Brochard L, Friedrich JO. Effort to breathe with various spontaneous breathing trial techniques: a physiologic meta-analysis. Am J Respir Crit Care Med. 2017;195(11):1477–85.
60. Kuhn BT, Bradley LA, Dempsey TM, Puro AC, Adams JY. Management of mechanical ventilation in decompensated heart failure. J Cardiovasc Dev Dis. 2016;3(4):pii: E33.
61. Burns KEA, Soliman I, Adhikari NKJ, Zwein A, Wong JTY, Gomez-Builes C, Pellegrini JA, Chen L, Rittayamai N, Sklar M, Brochard LJ, Friedrich JO. Trials directly comparing alternative spontaneous breathing trial techniques: a systematic review and meta-analysis. Crit Care. 2017;21(1):127.
62. Quintard H, l'Her E, Pottecher J, Adnet F, Constantin JM, De Jong A, Diemunsch P, Fesseau R, Freynet A, Girault C, Guitton C, Hamonic Y, Maury E, Mekontso-Dessap A, Michel F, Nolent P, Perbet S, Prat G, Roquilly A, Tazarourte K, Terzi N, Thille AW, Alves M, Gayat E, Donetti L. Experts' guidelines of intubation and extubation of the ICU patient of French Society of Anaesthesia and Intensive Care Medicine (SFAR) and French-speaking Intensive Care Society (SRLF) : In collaboration with the pediatric Association of French-speaking Anaesthetists and Intensivists (ADARPEF), French-speaking Group of Intensive Care and Paediatric emergencies (GFRUP) and Intensive Care physiotherapy society (SKR). Ann Intensive Care. 2019;9(1):13.
63. Teboul JL. Weaning-induced cardiac dysfunction: where are we today? Intensive Care Med. 2014;40(8):1069–79.
64. Harvey S, Harrison DA, Singer M, Ashcroft J, Jones CM, Elbourne D, Brampton W, Williams D, Young D, Rowan K, PAC-Man study collaboration. Assessment of the clinical effectiveness

of pulmonary artery catheters in management of patients in intensive care (PAC-man): a randomized controlled trial. Lancet. 2005;366(9484):472–7.
65. Lamia B, Maizel J, Ochagavia A, Chemla D, Osman D, Richard C, Teboul JL. Echocardiographic diagnosis of pulmonary artery occlusion pressure elevation during weaning from mechanical ventilation. Crit Care Med. 2009;37(5):1696–701.
66. Dres M, Teboul JL, Anguel N, Guerin L, Richard C, Monnet X. Extravascular lung water, B-type natriuretic peptide and blood volume contraction enable diagnosis of weaning-induced pulmonary edema. Crit Care Med. 2014;42(8):1882–9.
67. Zapata L, Vera P, Roglan A, Gich I, Ordonez-Llanos J, Betbesé AJ. B-type natriuretic peptides for prediction and diagnosis of weaning failure from cardiac origin. Intensive Care Med. 2011;37(3):477–85.
68. Anguel N, Monnet X, Osman D, Castelain V, Richard C, Teboul JL. Increase in plasma protein concentration for diagnosing weaning-induced pulmonary oedema. Intensive Care Med. 2008;34(7):1231–8.
69. Dres M, Teboul JL, Anguel N, Guerin L, Richard C, Monnet X. Passive leg raising performed before a spontaneous breathing trial predicts weaning-induced cardiac dysfunction. Intensive Care Med. 2015;41:487–94.
70. Jaber S, Quintard H, Cinotti R, Asehnoune K, Arnal JM, Guitton C, Paugam-Burtz C, Abback P, Mekontso Dessap A, Lakhal K, Lasocki S, Plantefeve G, Claud B, Pottecher J, Corne P, Ichai C, Hajjej Z, Molinari N, Chanques G, Papazian L, Azoulay E, De Jong A. Risk factors and outcomes for airway failure versus non-airway failure in the intensive care unit: a multicenter observational study of 1514 extubation procedures. Crit Care. 2018;22(1):236.
71. Ponikowski P, Voors AA, Anker SD, Bueno H, Cleland JGF, Coats AJS, Falk V, González-Juanatey JR, Harjola VP, Jankowska EA, Jessup M, Linde C, Nihoyannopoulos P, Parissis JT, Pieske B, Riley JP, Rosano GMC, Ruilope LM, Ruschitzka F, Rutten FH, van der Meer P. ESC guidelines for the diagnosis and treatment of acute and chronic heart failure. Rev Esp Cardiol. 2016;69(12):1167.
72. Nava S, Carbone G, DiBattista N, Bellone A, Baiardi P, Cosentini R, Marenco M, Giostra F, Borasi G, Groff P. Noninvasive ventilation in cardiogenic pulmonary edema: a multicenter randomized trial. Am J Respir Crit Care Med. 2003;168(12):1432–7.
73. Rittayamai N, Tscheikuna J, Rujiwit P. High-flow nasal cannula versus conventional oxygen therapy after endotracheal extubation: a randomized crossover physiologic study. Respir Care. 2014;59(4):485–90.
74. Luo JC, Lu MS, Zhao ZH, Jiang W, Xu B, Weng L, Li T, Du B. Positive end-expiratory pressure effect of 3 high-flow nasal cannula devices. Respir Care. 2017;62(7):888–95.
75. Liesching T, Nelson DL, Cormier KL, Sucov A, Short K, Warburton R, Hill NS. Randomized trial of bilevel versus continuous positive airway pressure for acute pulmonary edema. J Emerg Med. 2014;46(1):130–40.
76. Rochwerg B, Brochard L, Elliott MW, Hess D, Hill NS, Nava S, Navalesi P, Members of the Steering Committee, Antonelli M, Brozek J, Conti G, Ferrer M, Guntupalli K, Jaber S, Keenan S, Mancebo J, Mehta S, Raoof S, Members of the Task Force. Official ERS/ATS clinical practice guidelines: noninvasive ventilation for acute respiratory failure. Eur Respir J. 2017;50(2):pii: 1602426.
77. Alviar CL, Miller PE, McAreavey D, Katz JN, Lee B, Moriyama B, Soble J, van Diepen S, Solomon MA, Morrow DA, ACC Critical Care Cardiology Working Group. Positive pressure ventilation in the cardiac intensive care unit. J Am Coll Cardiol. 2018;72(13):1532–53.
78. Makdee O, Monsomboon A, Surabenjawong U, Praphruetkit N, Chaisirin W, Chakorn T, Permpikul C, Thiravit P, Nakornchai T. High-flow nasal cannula versus conventional oxygen therapy in emergency department patients with cardiogenic pulmonary edema: a randomized controlled trial. Ann Emerg Med. 2017;70(4):465.e2–72.e2.
79. Aramendi E, Lu Y, Chang MP, Elola A, Irusta U, Owens P, Idris AH. A novel technique to assess the quality of ventilation during pre-hospital cardiopulmonary resuscitation. Resuscitation. 2018;132:41–6.

# The Use of Extracorporeal Life Support (ECLS) in Sudden Cardiac Death

16

Simon Wai Ching Sin and Pauline Pui Ning Yeung

**Abstract**

The survival of refractory cardiac arrest is dismal. The use of extracorporeal life support (ECLS), in particular venoarterial type of ECLS, has gained attention in the last decade, which aims at improving the outcome of such disease entity. The implementation of an ECLS-assisted resuscitation (ECPR) programme is a multidisciplinary effort involving extensive collaboration and training. Currently, robust evidence and scientific data on ECPR are pending, and generalized use of such technology cannot be recommended. However, the ongoing high-quality studies will give us a better insight on the impact of ECPR on the outcome of refractory cardiac arrest.

**Keywords**

Outcome · Refractory cardiac arrest · Extracorporeal life support (ECLS) Venoarterial ECLS · ECPR

## 16.1 Introduction

The rates of success with conventional cardiopulmonary resuscitation (CPR) for cardiac arrest is modest. The use of extracorporeal resuscitation in cardiac arrest was first reported in the 1990s [1, 2]. The idea and principle originated from the technique of

S. W. C. Sin
Department of Adult Intensive Care, Queen Mary Hospital, The University of Hong Kong, Pokfulam, Hong Kong, China

Department of Anaesthesiology, The University of Hong Kong, Pokfulam, Hong Kong, China

P. P. N. Yeung
Department of Adult Intensive Care, Queen Mary Hospital, The University of Hong Kong, Pokfulam, Hong Kong, China

Department of Medicine, The University of Hong Kong, Pokfulam, Hong Kong, China



H. Zhu (ed.), *Sudden Death*, https://doi.org/10.1007/978-981-15-7002-5_16

cardiopulmonary bypass in cardiothoracic surgery. The postulated benefit is in maintaining better oxygen delivery during and after cardiac arrest in patients failing to respond to conventional resuscitation. In the last decade, advancing extracorporeal technology has enabled widespread adoption of a modified cardiopulmonary bypass system known as extracorporeal life support (ECLS) outside the setting of an operating theatre, to support refractory respiratory and/or circulatory failure. Taken one step further, such systems have been applied to resuscitate patients who do not respond to conventional cardiopulmonary resuscitation. There is growing data to guide the use of extracorporeal CPR (ECPR) and identify factors associated with its success.

In this chapter, we will begin by describing the current state of ECLS. We will then discuss its application in sudden circulatory collapse.

## 16.2 The ECLS Circuit

ECLS is a temporary measure to support failing cardiopulmonary function of critically ill patients. It is not a treatment by itself but serves as a bridge to recovery of disease or other forms of long-term support. ECLS can be broadly classified into venoarterial (V-A) and veno-venous (V-V). The discussion of hybrid modes of ECLS, such as veno-arterial-venous (V-AV), is beyond the scope of this chapter.

The basic ECLS circuit consists of drainage cannula, blood pump, membrane oxygenator and return cannula. The venous drainage cannula is inserted into central veins (internal jugular, femoral or subclavian), and venous blood is drained by the blood pump (most commonly a centrifugal pump) into a membrane oxygenator. A gas line connected to the oxygenator supplies oxygen and removes carbon dioxide. Oxygenated and decarboxylated blood will then be returned to the systemic circulation via the return cannula, inserted into either central veins or arteries (aorta, subclavian or femoral artery). After blood flow is established in the ECLS circuit, patients usually receive systemic anticoagulation unless contraindicated to prevent thrombosis. Figure 16.1a, b illustrates the basic setup and the basic principle of an ECLS circuit.

When the return cannula is inserted into the venous system, the ECLS is known as veno-venous (V-V) ECLS and mainly provides respiratory support. The presence of an extracorporeal route of gaseous exchange reduces demand on mechanical ventilation and reduces ventilator-induced lung injury to severely diseased lungs.

In the case of venoarterial (V-A) ECLS, the return cannula is inserted into the arterial system, and both circulatory and respiratory support is provided. During V-A ECLS, cerebral perfusion and systemic oxygen delivery are maintained to facilitate definitive interventions (e.g. percutaneous coronary intervention), bridge to recovery (e.g. fulminant myocarditis) or bridge to destination therapy (e.g. ventricular assist device, heart transplant).

## 16.3 General Indications and Contraindications of ECLS

Indications for ECLS cover a broad spectrum of diseases causing cardiorespiratory failure. In principle, when considering ECLS, the disease while not responding to conventional methods of support, e.g. advanced ventilatory support or high dose

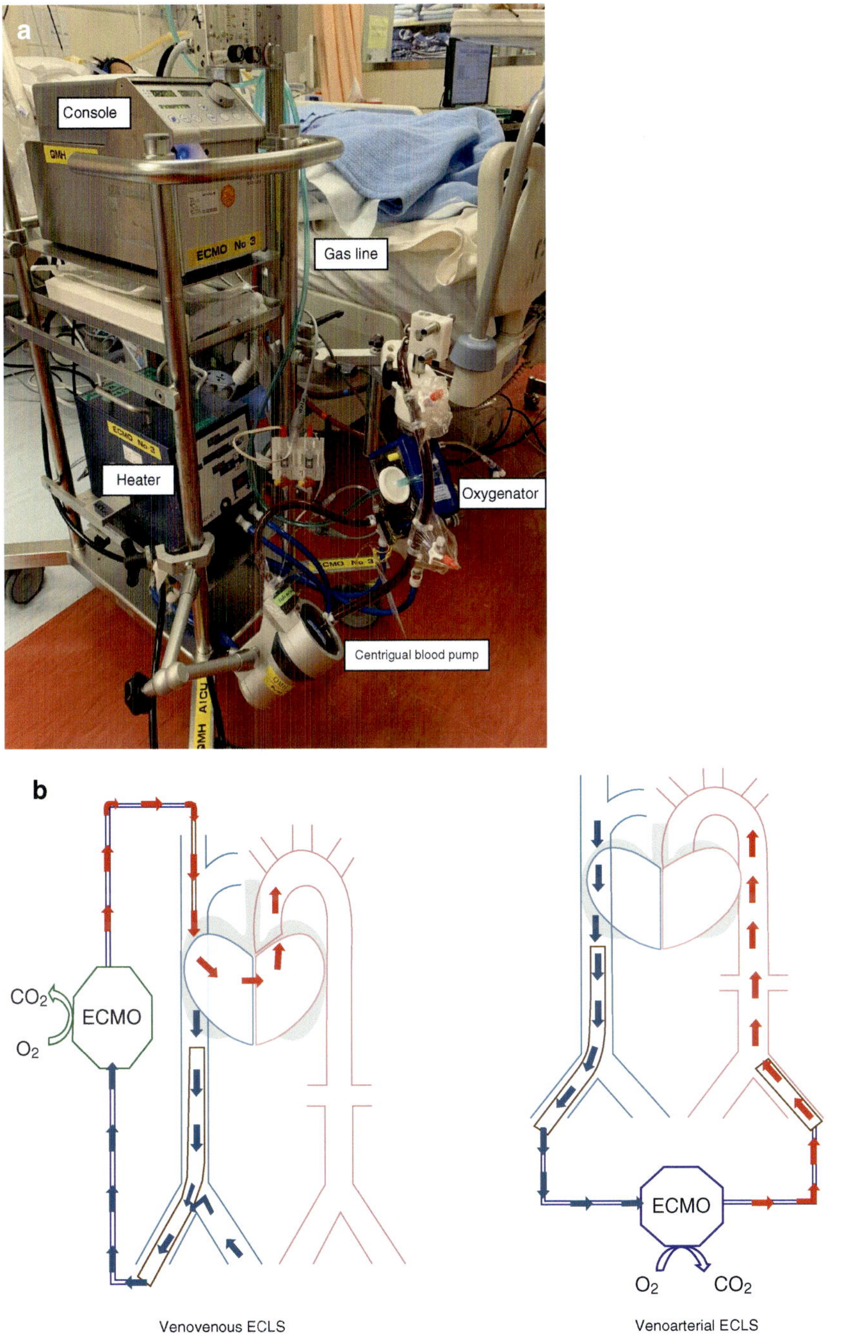


**Fig. 16.1** (**a**) Basic setup of an ECLS circuit. (**b**) The principle of two main modes of ECLS. Left panel: Veno-venous ECLS, where deoxygenated blood is drained from the central vein to the oxygenator, and oxygenated blood returns to the venous circulation. Right panel: Venoarterial ECLS, where deoxygenated blood is drained from the central vein to the oxygenator, and oxygenated blood returns to the arterial circulation

**Table 16.1** Common indications of ECLS

| Veno-venous ECLS | Venoarterial ECLS |
|---|---|
| Acute respiratory distress syndrome due to various causes (infection, aspiration, inhalation injury, etc.) | Cardiogenic shock due to various causes (acute coronary syndrome, refractory malignant arrhythmia, myocarditis, cardiodepressant overdose, etc.) |
| Pulmonary contusion, lung trauma | Chronic cardiomyopathy as a bridge to transplant or ventricular assist device |
| Major airway injury or obstruction | Massive pulmonary embolism |
| Status asthmaticus | Post-cardiotomy syndrome |
| Bridge to lung transplant, e.g. cystic fibrosis | Periprocedural support for high-risk percutaneous intervention, e.g. complex coronary anatomy |
| Congenital diaphragmatic hernia (neonate) | Extracorporeal cardiopulmonary resuscitation |

inotropes, should be potentially reversible. The premorbid condition of the patient including the physiological age should be factored into determining the chance of gaining meaningful recovery. At the same time, there should be a plan for bridging the condition to a longer-term support (ventricular assist device) or transplantation. The common indications for ECLS are listed in Table 16.1.

Contraindications to ECLS include terminal malignancy, irreversible brain injury, end-stage cardiac or pulmonary failure without chance of transplant or ventricular assist device (VAD), and aortic dissection and severe aortic regurgitation (for V-A ECLS). Nevertheless, with evolving technology and growing experience in the management of patients on ECLS, successful ECLS runs have been reported in patients who were previously considered absolutely contraindicated to ECLS, e.g. patients with advanced age, immunocompromised status and active bleeding [3]. In these circumstances, the decision should be individualized with consideration of the risk and benefit after initiation of support. Moreover, institutional guidelines and agreement have to be developed based on centre experience, resources and infrastructure.

## 16.4 What Is ECPR?

ECPR refers to the use of extracorporeal technology, specifically V-A ECLS, to support the circulation of patients with refractory cardiac arrest. It represents an adjunct to conventional CPR that may help to sustain adequate oxygen delivery while awaiting return of spontaneous circulation (ROSC). It has to be distinguished from the use of V-A ECLS in patients with cardiogenic shock, in whom the management and prognosis are significantly different. For the purposes of this chapter, we will focus the discussion on the use of ECLS in out-of-hospital cardiac arrest (OHCA).

### 16.4.1 Implementation of ECPR

#### 16.4.1.1 Patient Selection

Generally speaking, all patients with cardiac arrest presumed to be cardiac in origin who fail to achieve ROSC with conventional CPR are eligible candidates for

ECPR. However, as the overall prognosis for patients with cardiac arrest is poor and ECPR is resource intensive, patient selection becomes an important consideration to ensure the sustainability and cost-effectiveness of an ECPR programme.

It is important to define "refractoriness" to conventional CPR for both clinical and research purposes. Premature initiation of ECPR may put patients at unnecessary risk for an invasive procedure. On the contrary, delay in activation of ECPR jeopardizes the outcome for patients who may benefit from ECPR. Earlier studies described a period ranging from 10 to 30 min of conventional resuscitation prior to initiating the ECPR process [4]. However, recent studies showed that 20 min may be a more reasonable cut-off time for activation of ECPR. Reynold et al. showed that when there is no ROSC after 16 min of conventional CPR, the rate of survival with good neurological outcome drops significantly to 1% [5]. Kim et al. also reported similar findings that the optimal time for transition of conventional CPR to ECPR for good neurological outcome is 21 min [6]. Recently, the Extracorporeal Life Support Organization (ELSO) Position Paper suggested adopting 20 min as optimal cut-off [7].

Learning from the experience in basic life support, one of the most important determinants of favourable outcome would be the "no flow time", which refers to the time from cardiac arrest to start of basic life support (BLS), either by bystander or emergency medical service (EMS). As a result, almost all ECPR protocols include the presence of bystander CPR or no flow time less than 5 min as an important inclusion criterion [4]. Table 16.2 summarizes the favourable prognostic factors in patient selection for ECPR [8–10].

Nevertheless, it is necessary to point out that there are no absolute predictors for survival after ECPR. Despite stringent selection criteria in some studies, patient mortality remains high [11]. At the same time, there are also case reports of survivors despite poor prognostic factors upon ECPR initiation [12, 13]. This highlights the importance of ongoing research in patient selection.

#### 16.4.1.2 The ECPR Team

Once the decision of ECPR initiation is made, all effort should be focused on delivering ECPR timely and safely. A "low flow time", defined as the duration from commencing CPR to established ECLS, of less than 60 min has been persistently reported as a favourable survival factor in ECPR for OHCA [14, 15]. A recent study suggested that every 1 min delay in establishing ECLS translates to a 3% decrease in survival [16]. Depending on the staffing pattern of the hospital, the ECPR team

**Table 16.2** Favourable prognostic factors in ECPR

| |
|---|
| Presence of bystander CPR or no flow time < 5 min |
| Signs of life, e.g. breathing, gasping, pupillary reflex, movement |
| Shockable rhythm |
| Intermittent ROSC before ECLS |
| End-tidal carbon dioxide ($ETCO_2$) > 10 mmHg |
| Lower baseline lactate level |
| Higher baseline pH value |

may be made up of emergency physicians, intensivists, critical care physicians, vascular or cardiothoracic surgeons, cardiologists, perfusionists and nurse specialists. The presence of multiple disciplines working in a highly intense environment requires precise role delegation and interdisciplinary communication. Most ECPR teams are further subdivided into resuscitation, cannulation and circuit priming teams.

The primary responsibility of the resuscitation team is to ensure that good quality CPR is being conducted. During ECPR and amidst multiple competing priorities, it is essential to maintain consistent and high-quality chest compressions. Mechanical chest compression devices may be considered to reduce the requirement on manpower, but it should be noted that current evidence does not suggest the superiority of mechanical devices over manual chest compression [17].

Cannulation during CPR is the most challenging part of the ECPR. Most typically, 21–23 French-sized venous and 15–17 French-sized arterial cannulas are inserted via the femoral vein and artery, respectively. Depending on the expertise of the cannulation team, surgical cutdown, percutaneous Seldinger and semi-Seldinger techniques may be used. Blood vessels are not uncommonly difficult to be localized in view of intense vasoconstriction and continuous motion during CPR. To improve the rate of success and reduce complications from cannulation, imaging modalities including transthoracic/transoesophageal echocardiography or fluoroscopy should be used to confirm the site and position of guidewires and cannula. Moreover, the resuscitation team has to coordinate closely with the cannulation team to coordinate the timing of defibrillation to minimize interruption during cannulation [18]. To the author's knowledge, many ECLS centres withhold defibrillation and adrenaline injection once the cardiac arrest is considered refractory. Typically, a well-trained cannulation team would complete cannulation in 15 min [19, 20]. Once blood flow in the ECLS circuit has been established, chest compressions can be stopped.

The circuit priming team is usually lead by nurses or perfusionists. They are responsible for circuit priming and operating the ECLS machine. Many high case volume ECLS centres have pre-primed ECLS circuits to reduce manpower tension during ECPR. It has been shown that wet-primed ECLS circuits can remain sterile for 2 months [21], and current recommendations from the ELSO Infectious Disease Task Force state that pre-primed circuits can be maintained for 30 days. Figure 16.2 describes the organization of the ECPR team and the role of individual members (courtesy of Dr. Tomoyuki Endo).

#### 16.4.1.3 Team Training

A rapid response multidisciplinary team is essential for ECPR implementation. Team members are often required to perform under stressful and complex clinical contexts, and a high level of interprofessional cooperation is needed. As a result, simulation training [22], focusing on psychomotor and behavioural skills, has gained interest by ECLS educators for its supplementary role to traditional education modalities, namely didactic lectures and water drills [23, 24]. Allan et al. has shown that simulation training shortened the cannulation time for the paediatric ECPR team [25]. Another study showed that by incorporating simulation training

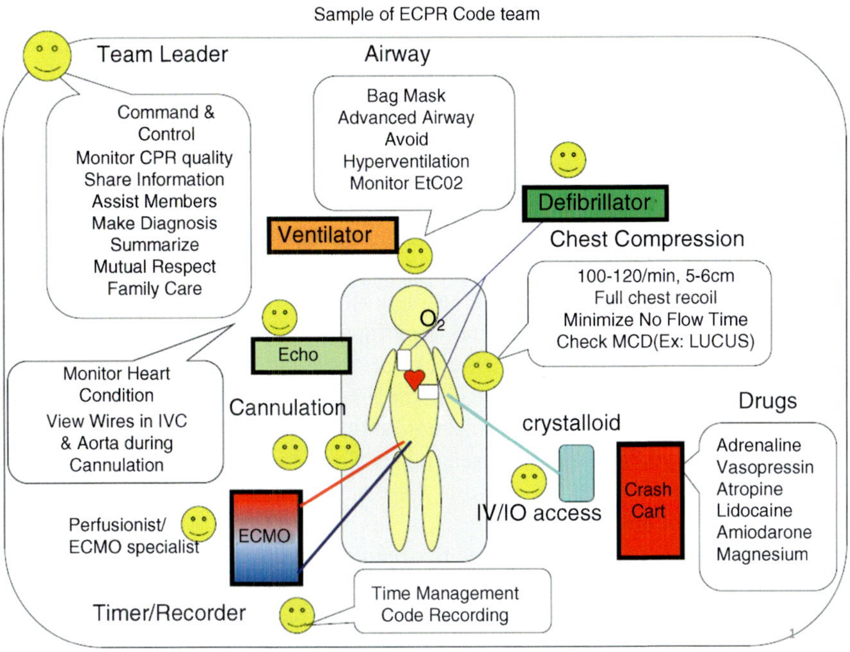


**Fig. 16.2** The organization of the ECPR team and the role of individual members

**Table 16.3** Common scenarios for ECPR simulation training

| |
|---|
| Patient selection |
| Deployment of mechanical chest compression device and its troubleshooting |
| Cannulation during CPR |
| Team dynamics during ECPR (ACLS, cannulation and circuit priming) |
| Low blood flow after ECLS initiation |
| Persistent ventricular arrhythmia after establishing ECLS |
| ECLS transport for further procedure, e.g. cardiac catheterization |

into existing training curriculum, time required for cannulation, circuit priming and to establish full ECLS support was shortened immediately and 3 months after training [26]. Many ECLS centres have incorporated simulation training into an essential part of their ECLS training and credentialing programme [23, 24]. The question of whether such improvements in team performance with simulation training translate to better patient outcomes remains to be answered. Table 16.3 lists the common scenarios used for ECPR simulation training.

#### 16.4.1.4 Post-resuscitation Care

After restoration of organ perfusion by the ECLS circuit, it is important to identify and treat the underlying cause of cardiac arrest. Given that ischaemic heart disease is the most common cause of cardiac arrest, input from interventional cardiologists is frequently needed. Kagawa et al. had shown that ECPR patients who received primary coronary intervention had a better prognosis [27]. Massive pulmonary embolism, after stabilization by ECPR, should be tackled with systemic thrombolytic, catheter-based embolectomy or surgical embolectomy [28, 29]. Despite mortality remaining high and the lack of high-grade evidence on the best treatment approach, the role of ECPR for pulmonary embolism has been incorporated into the guidelines from the European Society of Cardiology [30].

Targeted temperature management (TTM) is another potentially important intervention after ECPR that may improve the neurological outcome [31, 32]. Clinical practice of TTM in post-ECPR patients is extrapolated from cardiac arrest patient without ECPR [33]. Currently, robust evidence for TTM in patients who received ECPR has yet to be established, and the precise temperature targets await to be determined. The benefit of neuroprotection should be balanced against the side effects of TTM, especially the increased risk of bleeding [34].

#### 16.4.1.5 Complications

Complications in ECPR may be related to cannulation or the ECLS circuit.

Cannulation during ECPR is difficult and has been associated with devastating vascular complications such as vessel perforation, dissection and major bleeding. The use of image guidance by echocardiography and/or fluoroscopy may decrease these occurrences. Limb ischaemia is another important complication with reported incidence up to 10% [35]. After cannulation of the common femoral artery, the antegrade blood flow to the ipsilateral distal lower limb is potentially obstructed by the cannula occupying the vessel lumen, especially under intense vasoconstriction during cardiac arrest. Distal limb circulation should be monitored closely by physical examination, Doppler ultrasound or near-infrared spectroscopy (NIRS) [36]. A distal perfusion cannula may be inserted in the superficial femoral artery in an antegrade manner (Fig. 16.3) or in the posterior tibial artery [37] in a retrograde manner to perfuse the lower limb. Some institutions routinely insert distal perfusion cannula whilst others adopt an initial conservative approach.

Acute mechanical failure and circuit complications can account for 14% of technical complications during ECLS [38]. Since ECLS patients' native cardiopulmonary function is severely impaired and most patients are ECLS dependent, any mechanical or circuit complications resulting in system malfunction can cause rapid clinical deterioration. Amongst all, failure of the mechanical blood pump or oxygen supply, massive circuit air embolism and accidental decannulation are particularly disastrous. A systematic approach to tackling these emergencies should be established and continually reviewed with all ECLS providers.

Bleeding is another major complication. Intracranial bleeding is the most devastating and results in high patient mortality. Other sites of bleeding include the site of cannulation, gastrointestinal bleeding, retroperitoneal bleeding and pulmonary haemorrhage. The coagulopathy that may be present after ECPR [34] may augment the effect of routine anticoagulation. Hence, some institutions do not routinely heparinize patients after ECPR [39]. Table 16.4 summarizes some of the complications of ECLS.

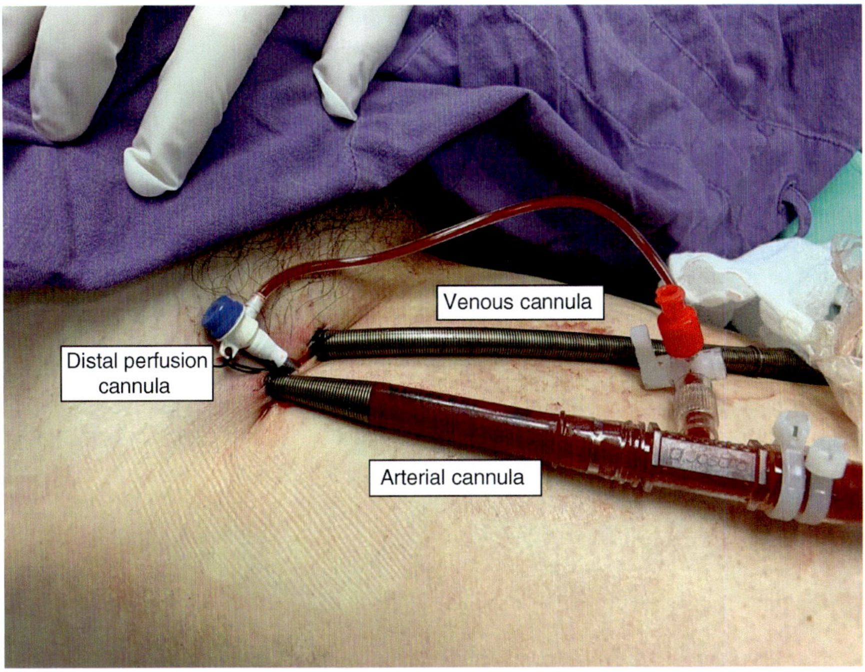


**Fig. 16.3** Femoro-femoral V-A ECLS configuration and distal perfusion cannula (inserted in an antegrade manner into superficial femoral artery)

**Table 16.4** Complications of ECLS

| Cannulation related | Mechanical/circuit related | General to ECLS |
|---|---|---|
| Selection of wrong vessels, major vessel injury, dissection, perforation | Machine/blood pump failure | Bleeding complications including intracranial, cannulation site, gastrointestinal, retroperitoneal and pulmonary |
| Myocardial injury with cardiac tamponade | Oxygen supply failure | Cannula-related bloodstream infection |
| Cannula malposition | Massive circuit air embolism | Cannulation site infection |
| Limb ischaemia | Accidental decannulation | Thromboembolism, e.g. deep vein thrombosis |
| | Oxygenator thrombosis | Heparin-induced thrombocytopenia (HIT) |
| | Haemolysis and disseminated intravascular coagulopathy | |

#### 16.4.1.6 Current Evidence and Recommendation

Current ECPR protocols remain highly variable among centres, and study designs on OHCA ECPR are heterogenous and non-randomized. As a result, the reported survival and neurological outcomes in the literature are inconsistent and at high risk of bias. For instance, reported survival with good neurological recovery ranges from 4% to 42% [11]. It is worthy to highlight that a novel approach of enlisting emergency medical service (EMS) to transport patients in ventricular tachycardia or ventricular fibrillation directly to the cardiac catheterization laboratory together with early ECPR and immediate coronary angiography with intervention as needed was shown to produce good patient outcomes [40]. Table 16.5 lists the key findings of recent studies on ECPR for OHCA.

A multicentre, prospective, randomized clinical trial examining a "hyperinvasive" approach for the management of OHCA is underway. This approach, comprising of prehospital intra-arrest hypothermia, mechanical chest compression device, ECLS and early invasive investigation and treatment (coronary angiography/percutaneous coronary intervention, pulmonary angiography/percutaneous embolectomy and aortography) in all patients with OHCA of presumed cardiac origin, will be compared to standard of care [41].

The recently published 2019 American Heart Association Focused Update on Advanced Cardiovascular Life Support suggested that there is insufficient evidence to recommend the routine use of ECPR for patients with cardiac arrest, but that ECPR may be considered for selected patients as rescue therapy when conventional CPR efforts are failing, in settings in which it can be expeditiously implemented and supported by skilled providers (Class 2b; Level of Evidence C) [42].

## 16.5 Future Directions

It is well-established that the time interval between cardiac arrest and restoration of adequate blood flow is inversely proportional to patient outcome after ECPR. Hence, a lot of efforts have been concentrated on minimizing this duration. Well-trained ECPR teams nowadays perform consistently in establishing ECLS after patient arrival to hospital, and the room to further shorten this time interval is minimal. Therefore, a new concept targeted at shortening the duration of prehospital CPR attempts to examine the feasibility and outcomes of performing ECPR in the prehospital stage [8]. Most of the available data on prehospital ECPR are limited to case studies and case series [49]. Further research is required to delineate the patient selection, logistic and resource implications.

## 16.6 Conclusion

ECPR is a cumulation of extracorporeal technology and multidisciplinary expertise teamwork to support a highly selected patient subset with refractory cardiac arrest. Although promising, it is a complex and resource-demanding technology and

**Table 16.5** Description and key findings of recent studies on ECPR for OHCA

| Author | Study nature and sample size | Inclusion/exclusion criteria | Outcomes |
|---|---|---|---|
| Cesana (2018) [43] | Retrospective analysis<br>$N = 63$ | *Inclusion criteria*<br>Age 18–75 years, witnessed cardiac arrest, no ROSC after 15 min of CCPR, no flow time ≤ 6 min, low flow time ≤ 45 min, $ETCO_2 > 10$ mmHg<br>*Exclusion criteria*<br>Terminal malignancy, aortic dissection, severe peripheral vascular disease, severe cardiac failure without indication of heart transplantation | Hospital discharge survival 21%<br>CPC 1 at 6 month 92% |
| Choi (2016) [44] | Observational from prospective registry<br>$N = 10$ | *Inclusion criteria*<br>Age ≤ 75 years, witnessed cardiac arrest, bystander administration of CPR or no flow time ≤ 5 min, prehospital low flow time ≤ 30 min and refractory arrest >10 min of CCPR at the emergency department (ED)<br>*Exclusion criteria*<br>Do-not-resuscitate order, severe comorbidities that preclude admission to the intensive care unit, poor performance status or terminal illness (malignancy or neurologic disease, trauma, intracranial haemorrhage, acute aortic dissection with pericardial effusion observed by echocardiography), sustained return of spontaneous circulation within 10 min after ED arrival | 1-month survival 30%<br>CPC 1–2 at 1 month 30% |
| Maekawa (2013) [45] | Post hoc analysis of data from a prospective observational cohort<br>$N = 24$ | *Inclusion criteria*<br>Patient received CPR for longer than 20 min after witnessed arrest of presumed cardiac origin<br>*Exclusion criteria*<br>Patient who had previously signed “do-not-resuscitate” orders and who are pronounced dead before hospital arrival | 3-month survival 37.5%<br>CPC 1 29.2% |
| Schober (2017) [46] | Retrospective cohort analysis based on a prospectively designed and conducted registry<br>$N = 7$ | *Inclusion criteria*<br>Refractory arrest was defined as 30 min of ongoing resuscitation, without occurrence of return of spontaneous circulation<br>Other criteria not specifically mentioned | 6-month survival with good neurological outcome 14% |

(continued)

**Table 16.5** (continued)

| Author | Study nature and sample size | Inclusion/exclusion criteria | Outcomes |
|---|---|---|---|
| Siao (2015) [47] | Retrospective chart review study<br>$N = 20$ | *Inclusion criteria*<br>Age 18–75 years, cardiac arrest with initial ventricular fibrillation and CCPR initiated within 5 min (no flow duration <5 min), refractory ventricular fibrillation defined as ventricular fibrillation resistant to at least three defibrillations, 3 mg of epinephrine, 300 mg of amiodarone, no ROSC achieved after CPR for more than 10 min<br>*Exclusion criteria*<br>Severe head trauma or severe acute active bleeding, severe sepsis, ventricular fibrillation that developed during resuscitation for initial asystole or pulseless electrical activity, terminal stage of malignancy, any history of severe neurological deficits (including dementia, intracranial haemorrhage, or ischemic stroke and bedridden state) | Discharge and 1-year survival 50%<br>CPC 1–2 at discharge and 1 year 40% |
| Sakamoto (2014) [32] | Multicentre, prospective, observational study<br>$N = 260$ | *Inclusion criteria*<br>VF/VT on the initial ECG, cardiac arrest on hospital arrival with or without prehospital ROSC, within 45 min from reception of the emergency call or the onset of cardiac arrest to the hospital arrival, no ROSC at least during the 15 min after hospital arrival (or after contact with a doctor) even though conventional CPR was performed<br>*Exclusion criteria*<br>Age 20–75 years, poor level of activities of daily living before the onset of cardiac arrest, non-cardiac origin (e.g. external factors such as trauma and drug intoxication, primary cerebral disorders, acute aortic dissection diagnosed prior to the introduction of PCPS and terminal phase of cancer), core body temperature of less than 30 °C, no informed consent from the individuals representing patients | Hospital discharge: not mentioned<br>CPC 1–2 at 1 month 12.3%<br>CPC 1–2 at 6 month 11.2% |
| Yannopoulos (2016) [48] | Retrospective analysis<br>$N = 18$ | *Inclusion criteria*<br>Age 18–75 years, body habitus accommodating automated Lund University Cardiopulmonary Assist System (LUCAS) cardiopulmonary resuscitation (CPR) and estimated transfer time from the scene to the cardiac catheterization laboratory of ≤30 min<br>Refractory VF/VT arrest was defined as failure to achieve sustained return of spontaneous circulation after treatment with three direct current shocks and administration of 300 mg of intravenous/intraosseous amiodarone<br>*Exclusion criteria*<br>Known terminal illness, “do not resuscitate/do not intubate” status, traumatic arrest and significant bleeding | Hospital discharge survival 55%<br>CPC 1–2 at 1 month 50% |

| | | | |
|---|---|---|---|
| Yannopoulos (2017) [40] | Retrospective analysis<br>$N = 62$ | *Inclusion criteria*<br>Age 18–75 years, OHCA of presumed cardiac origin, VF/VT as first presenting rhythm, no ROSC despite 3 EMS delivered direct current shocks and 300 mg amiodarone, estimate transfer time from scene to CCL of <30 min<br>*Minnesota protocol*<br>Continuous mechanical chest compression, early emergency medical service to transport VT/VF patient directly to the cardiac catheterization laboratory, early ECLS for patient without ROSC and immediate coronary angiography with intervention as needed<br>*Exclusion criteria*<br>CCL resuscitation discontinuation and declared death when $ETCO_2 < 10$ mmHg in CCL arrival, $PaO_2 < 50$ mmHg or $O_2$ sat < 85%, serum lactate >18 mmol/L | Twenty-six (42%) survival to discharged with CPC 1–2 |
| Kim (2014) [6] | Retrospective analysis<br>$N = 55$ | *Inclusion criteria*<br>Age ≥ 18 years, sudden cardiac arrest with presumed correctable causes, witnessed cardiac arrest with or without bystander CPR, no flow time (time interval from presumed arrest to CPR started by the EMS provider) was expected to be short, even for unwitnessed arrests.<br>Prolonged CPR more than 10 min as in-hospital CPR duration or recurrently arrested in the ED after achievement of ROSC (≥20 min)<br>The initial cardiac arrest rhythm documented pre-hospitalization was not considered as an indication for ECPR<br>*Exclusion criteria*<br>Cardiac arrest due to a clearly uncorrectable cause, presence of a terminal illness or malignancy, suspected or confirmed traumatic origin of arrest, no informed consent from the family | Survival at 3 months 14.3%<br>CPC 1–2 at 3 months 14.3% |

*ROSC* return of spontaneous circulation, *CCPR* conventional cardiopulmonary resuscitation, *$ETCO_2$* end-tidal carbon dioxide, *CPC* cerebral performance category, *VT* ventricular tachycardia, *VF* ventricular fibrillation, *EMS* emergency medical service carries the risk of life-threatening complications. Existing evidence drawn from heterogenous studies is still inadequate to provide definitive practice recommendations. Further large randomized studies are needed to define its role in refractory cardiac arrest.

## References


1. Martin GB, Rivers EP, Paradis NA, Goetting MG, Morris DC, Nowak RM. Emergency department cardiopulmonary bypass in the treatment of human cardiac arrest. Chest. 1998;113(3):743–51.
2. Younger JG, Schreiner RJ, Swaniker F, Hirschl RB, Chapman RA, Bartlett RH. Extracorporeal resuscitation of cardiac arrest. Acad Emerg Med. 1999;6(7):700–7.
3. Swol J, Belohlavek J, Brodie D, Bellezzo J, Weingart SD, Shinar Z, et al. Extracorporeal life support in the emergency department: a narrative review for the emergency physician. Resuscitation. 2018;133:108–17.
4. Ortega-Deballon I, Hornby L, Shemie SD, Bhanji F, Guadagno E. Extracorporeal resuscitation for refractory out-of-hospital cardiac arrest in adults: a systematic review of international practices and outcomes. Resuscitation. 2016;101:12–20.
5. Reynolds JC, Frisch A, Rittenberger JC, Callaway CW. Duration of resuscitation efforts and functional outcome after out-of-hospital cardiac arrest: when should we change to novel therapies? Circulation. 2013;128(23):2488–94.
6. Kim SJ, Jung JS, Park JH, Park JS, Hong YS, Lee SW. An optimal transition time to extracorporeal cardiopulmonary resuscitation for predicting good neurological outcome in patients with out-of-hospital cardiac arrest: a propensity-matched study. Crit Care. 2014;18(5):535.
7. Conrad SA, Broman LM, Taccone FS, Lorusso R, Malfertheiner MV, Pappalardo F, et al. The extracorporeal life support organization maastricht treaty for nomenclature in extracorporeal life support. A position paper of the extracorporeal life support organization. Am J Respir Crit Care Med. 2018;198(4):447–51.
8. Lamhaut L, Hutin A, Puymirat E, Jouan J, Raphalen JH, Jouffroy R, et al. A pre-hospital extracorporeal cardio pulmonary resuscitation (ECPR) strategy for treatment of refractory out hospital cardiac arrest: an observational study and propensity analysis. Resuscitation. 2017;117:109–17.
9. Wang J, Ma Q, Zhang H, Liu S, Zheng Y. Predictors of survival and neurologic outcome for adults with extracorporeal cardiopulmonary resuscitation: a systemic review and meta-analysis. Medicine (Baltimore). 2018;97(48):e13257.
10. Debaty G, Babaz V, Durand M, Gaide-Chevronnay L, Fournel E, Blancher M, et al. Prognostic factors for extracorporeal cardiopulmonary resuscitation recipients following out-of-hospital refractory cardiac arrest. A systematic review and meta-analysis. Resuscitation. 2017;112:1–10.
11. Le Guen M, Nicolas-Robin A, Carreira S, Raux M, Leprince P, Riou B, et al. Extracorporeal life support following out-of-hospital refractory cardiac arrest. Crit Care. 2011;15(1):R29.
12. Shin JS, Lee SW, Han GS, Jo WM, Choi SH, Hong YS. Successful extracorporeal life support in cardiac arrest with recurrent ventricular fibrillation unresponsive to standard cardiopulmonary resuscitation. Resuscitation. 2007;73(2):309–13.
13. Pabst D, Brehm CE. Is pulseless electrical activity a reason to refuse cardiopulmonary resuscitation with ECMO support? Am J Emerg Med. 2018;36(4):637–40.
14. Wang CH, Chou NK, Becker LB, Lin JW, Yu HY, Chi NH, et al. Improved outcome of extracorporeal cardiopulmonary resuscitation for out-of-hospital cardiac arrest—a comparison with that for extracorporeal rescue for in-hospital cardiac arrest. Resuscitation. 2014;85(9):1219–24.
15. Wengenmayer T, Rombach S, Ramshorn F, Biever P, Bode C, Duerschmied D, et al. Influence of low-flow time on survival after extracorporeal cardiopulmonary resuscitation (eCPR). Crit Care. 2017;21(1):157.
16. Park JH, Song KJ, Shin SD, Ro YS, Hong KJ. Time from arrest to extracorporeal cardiopulmonary resuscitation and survival after out-of-hospital cardiac arrest. Emerg Med Australas. 2019;31(6):1073–81.

17. Liu M, Shuai Z, Ai J, Tang K, Liu H, Zheng J, et al. Mechanical chest compression with LUCAS device does not improve clinical outcome in out-of-hospital cardiac arrest patients: a systematic review and meta-analysis. Medicine (Baltimore). 2019;98(44):e17550.
18. Hutin A, Abu-Habsa M, Burns B, Bernard S, Bellezzo J, Shinar Z, et al. Early ECPR for out-of-hospital cardiac arrest: best practice in 2018. Resuscitation. 2018;130:44–8.
19. Stub D, Bernard S, Pellegrino V, Smith K, Walker T, Sheldrake J, et al. Refractory cardiac arrest treated with mechanical CPR, hypothermia, ECMO and early reperfusion (the CHEER trial). Resuscitation. 2015;86:88–94.
20. Otani T, Sawano H, Natsukawa T, Nakashima T, Oku H, Gon C, et al. Low-flow time is associated with a favorable neurological outcome in out-of-hospital cardiac arrest patients resuscitated with extracorporeal cardiopulmonary resuscitation. J Crit Care. 2018;48:15–20.
21. Tan VE, Evangelista AT, Carella DM, Marino D, Moore WS, Gilliam N, et al. Sterility duration of preprimed extracorporeal membrane oxygenation circuits. J Pediatr Pharmacol Ther. 2018;23(4):311–4.
22. Sin SWC, Ng PY, Ngai WCW, Lai PCK, Mok AYT, Chan RWK. Simulation training for crises during venoarterial extracorporeal membrane oxygenation. J Thorac Dis. 2019;11(5):2144–52.
23. Cook MR, Badulak J, Coruh B, Kiraly LN, Zonies D, Cuschieri J, et al. Fellowship training in extracorporeal life support: characterization and educational needs assessment. J Crit Care. 2018;46:159–61.
24. Muratore S, Beilman G, John R, Brunsvold M. Extracorporeal membrane oxygenation credentialing: where do we stand? Am J Surg. 2015;210(4):655–60.e2.
25. Allan CK, Pigula F, Bacha EA, Emani S, Fynn-Thompson F, Thiagarajan RR, et al. An extracorporeal membrane oxygenation cannulation curriculum featuring a novel integrated skills trainer leads to improved performance among pediatric cardiac surgery trainees. Simul Healthc. 2013;8(4):221–8.
26. Whitmore SP, Gunnerson KJ, Haft JW, Lynch WR, VanDyck T, Hebert C, et al. Simulation training enables emergency medicine providers to rapidly and safely initiate extracorporeal cardiopulmonary resuscitation (ECPR) in a simulated cardiac arrest scenario. Resuscitation. 2019;138:68–73.
27. Kagawa E, Dote K, Kato M, Sasaki S, Nakano Y, Kajikawa M, et al. Should we emergently revascularize occluded coronaries for cardiac arrest?: rapid-response extracorporeal membrane oxygenation and intra-arrest percutaneous coronary intervention. Circulation. 2012;126(13):1605–13.
28. Meneveau N, Guillon B, Planquette B, Piton G, Kimmoun A, Gaide-Chevronnay L, et al. Outcomes after extracorporeal membrane oxygenation for the treatment of high-risk pulmonary embolism: a multicentre series of 52 cases. Eur Heart J. 2018;39(47):4196–204.
29. Corsi F, Lebreton G, Brechot N, Hekimian G, Nieszkowska A, Trouillet JL, et al. Life-threatening massive pulmonary embolism rescued by venoarterial-extracorporeal membrane oxygenation. Crit Care. 2017;21(1):76.
30. Task Force M, Konstantinides SV, Meyer G, Becattini C, Bueno H, Geersing GJ, et al. ESC guidelines for the diagnosis and management of acute pulmonary embolism developed in collaboration with the European Respiratory Society (ERS): the Task Force for the diagnosis and management of acute pulmonary embolism of the European Society of Cardiology (ESC). Eur Respir J. 2019;54(3):1901647.
31. Choi DS, Kim T, Ro YS, Ahn KO, Lee EJ, Hwang SS, et al. Extracorporeal life support and survival after out-of-hospital cardiac arrest in a nationwide registry: a propensity score-matched analysis. Resuscitation. 2016;99:26–32.
32. Sakamoto T, Morimura N, Nagao K, Asai Y, Yokota H, Nara S, et al. Extracorporeal cardiopulmonary resuscitation versus conventional cardiopulmonary resuscitation in adults with out-of-hospital cardiac arrest: a prospective observational study. Resuscitation. 2014;85(6):762–8.
33. Nielsen N, Wetterslev J, Cronberg T, Erlinge D, Gasche Y, Hassager C, et al. Targeted temperature management at 33 degrees C versus 36 degrees C after cardiac arrest. N Engl J Med. 2013;369(23):2197–206.
34. Ruggeri L, Franco A, Alba AC, Lembo R, Frassoni S, Scandroglio AM, et al. Coagulation derangements in patients with refractory cardiac arrest treated with extracorporeal cardiopulmonary resuscitation. J Cardiothorac Vasc Anesth. 2019;33(7):1877–82.

35. Bonicolini E, Martucci G, Simons J, Raffa GM, Spina C, Coco VL, et al. Limb ischemia in peripheral veno-arterial extracorporeal membrane oxygenation: a narrative review of incidence, prevention, monitoring, and treatment. Crit Care. 2019;23(1):266.
36. Patton-Rivera K, Beck J, Fung K, Chan C, Beck M, Takayama H, et al. Using near-infrared reflectance spectroscopy (NIRS) to assess distal-limb perfusion on venoarterial (V-A) extracorporeal membrane oxygenation (ECMO) patients with femoral cannulation. Perfusion. 2018;33(8):618–23.
37. Spurlock DJ, Toomasian JM, Romano MA, Cooley E, Bartlett RH, Haft JW. A simple technique to prevent limb ischemia during veno-arterial ECMO using the femoral artery: the posterior tibial approach. Perfusion. 2012;27(2):141–5.
38. Lubnow M, Philipp A, Foltan M, Bull Enger T, Lunz D, Bein T, et al. Technical complications during veno-venous extracorporeal membrane oxygenation and their relevance predicting a system-exchange—retrospective analysis of 265 cases. PLoS One. 2014;9(12):e112316.
39. Wood KL, Ayers B, Gosev I, Kumar N, Melvin AL, Barrus B, et al. Venoarterial ECMO without routine systemic anticoagulation decreases adverse events. Ann Thorac Surg. 2020;109(5):P1458–66.
40. Yannopoulos D, Bartos JA, Raveendran G, Conterato M, Frascone RJ, Trembley A, et al. Coronary artery disease in patients with out-of-hospital refractory ventricular fibrillation cardiac arrest. J Am Coll Cardiol. 2017;70(9):1109–17.
41. Belohlavek J, Kucera K, Jarkovsky J, Franek O, Pokorna M, Danda J, et al. Hyperinvasive approach to out-of hospital cardiac arrest using mechanical chest compression device, prehospital intraarrest cooling, extracorporeal life support and early invasive assessment compared to standard of care. A randomized parallel groups comparative study proposal. "Prague OHCA study". J Transl Med. 2012;10:163.
42. Panchal AR, Berg KM, Hirsch KG, Kudenchuk PJ, Del Rios M, Cabanas JG, et al. 2019 American Heart Association focused update on advanced cardiovascular life support: use of advanced airways, vasopressors, and extracorporeal cardiopulmonary resuscitation during cardiac arrest: an update to the American heart association guidelines for cardiopulmonary resuscitation and emergency cardiovascular care. Circulation. 2019;140(24):e881–e94.
43. Cesana F, Avalli L, Garatti L, Coppo A, Righetti S, Calchera I, et al. Effects of extracorporeal cardiopulmonary resuscitation on neurological and cardiac outcome after ischaemic refractory cardiac arrest. Eur Heart J Acute Cardiovasc Care. 2018;7(5):432–41.
44. Choi DH, Kim YJ, Ryoo SM, Sohn CH, Ahn S, Seo DW, et al. Extracorporeal cardiopulmonary resuscitation among patients with out-of-hospital cardiac arrest. Clin Exp Emerg Med. 2016;3(3):132–8.
45. Maekawa K, Tanno K, Hase M, Mori K, Asai Y. Extracorporeal cardiopulmonary resuscitation for patients with out-of-hospital cardiac arrest of cardiac origin: a propensity-matched study and predictor analysis. Crit Care Med. 2013;41(5):1186–96.
46. Schober A, Sterz F, Herkner H, Wallmueller C, Weiser C, Hubner P, et al. Emergency extracorporeal life support and ongoing resuscitation: a retrospective comparison for refractory out-of-hospital cardiac arrest. Emerg Med J. 2017;34(5):277–81.
47. Siao FY, Chiu CC, Chiu CW, Chen YC, Chen YL, Hsieh YK, et al. Managing cardiac arrest with refractory ventricular fibrillation in the emergency department: conventional cardiopulmonary resuscitation versus extracorporeal cardiopulmonary resuscitation. Resuscitation. 2015;92:70–6.
48. Yannopoulos D, Bartos JA, Martin C, Raveendran G, Missov E, Conterato M, et al. Minnesota resuscitation consortium's advanced perfusion and reperfusion cardiac life support strategy for out-of-hospital refractory ventricular fibrillation. J Am Heart Assoc. 2016;5(6):e003732.
49. Pozzi M, Dubien PY, Cesareo E, Pinero D, Obadia JF, Richard JC. Pre-hospital extracorporeal cardiopulmonary resuscitation. J Cardiothorac Vasc Anesth. 2020;34(2):571–2.

# Hypothermia Therapy in Sudden Death

17

Alan Araiza and Joseph Varon

**Abstract**

Therapeutic hypothermia has been used for millennia, but more recently, targeted temperature management has caught physician's interest as the main neuroprotective strategy for cardiac arrest patients who remain comatose after return of spontaneous circulation. Randomized clinical trials have shown benefits in neurologic and mortality outcomes when lowering body's core temperature to mild-to-moderate ranges of hypothermia, in conjunction with strict hyperthermia prevention measurements. The *International Liaison Committee on Resuscitation* recommends in their current guidelines to use a target temperature between 32 °C and 36 °C, for at least 24 h, in post-cardiac arrest patients, regardless of their initial rhythm (shockable vs. non-shockable). Therapeutic hypothermia consists of three well-defined phases: induction, maintenance, and rewarming. Each of these phases has very specific physiologic and clinical considerations for optimal patient management. The optimal dose, the induction and maintenance method, and the temperature monitoring technique remain unclear and are the focus of future research. Despite the overwhelmingly positive data regarding the benefits of therapeutic hypothermia, this technique remains underused. Clinicians should be familiar with this therapeutic intervention.

A. Araiza
Dorrington Medical Associates, Houston, TX, USA

Universidad Autónoma de Baja California, Tijuana, Mexico

United Memorial Medical Center, Houston, TX, USA

J. Varon (✉)
Dorrington Medical Associates, Houston, TX, USA

United Memorial Medical Center, Houston, TX, USA
e-mail: Joseph.varon@uth.tmc.edu


H. Zhu (ed.), *Sudden Death*, https://doi.org/10.1007/978-981-15-7002-5_17

**Keywords**

Therapeutic hypothermia · Targeted temperature management · Cardiac arrest · Reperfusion injury · Induced hypothermia

## 17.1 Overview

Cardiac arrest (CA) remains as one of the main causes of death, accounting for over 500,000 deaths per year just in North America [1]. Overall, CA survival seems to be improving due to advances in cardiopulmonary resuscitation and post-cardiac arrest care. Targeted temperature management (TTM) or therapeutic hypothermia (TH) has demonstrated to improve survival and neurologic outcome when used as a postresuscitation technique in patients with postanoxic/hypoxic encephalopathy [2–5]. For its utilization in CA, support came from the results of two multicenter randomized controlled trials (RCTs) in 2002 and 45 nonrandomized studies. The American Heart Association and the European Resuscitation Council recommend TTM use since 2003, and despite the overwhelming positive results, the implementation rate of TTM in many countries remains low [6].

Nielsen and coworkers in 2013 reported results from a large randomized clinical trial in 2013, in which they cooled down CA patients to either 33 °C or 36 °C and found no survival or neurological outcome difference. This trial remains highly controversial with people accepting Nielsen's study results and others remaining convinced that 32–34 °C are adequate target temperatures. The TTM Trial by Nielsen has been criticized for its possible selection bias, delays in cooling initiation of up to 4 h, up to 10 h to reach a target temperature of 33 °C, and excessively fast rewarming rate, among other issues [7].

Following Nielsen's findings, a leading center in CA conducted a retrospective cohort study after changing their TTM approach from 33 °C to 36 °C, and they found their fever rates increased (0% vs 19%), and there was a decrease in alive discharges (71% vs 58%) and home discharge with good neurological outcome (71% vs 56%) [8].

In this chapter, the authors will review the history of TH, pathophysiology of ischemic-reperfusion injury, protective mechanisms of TTM, physiology of cooling, current indications for TH, controversies, and future directions.

## 17.2 Historical Aspects of Therapeutic Hypothermia

Therapeutic hypothermia dates back millennia. Hippocrates recommended the use of snow and ice packing to diminish blood loss in the injured [9]. The modern clinical use has been documented for the last 217 years [10]. In 1803, the "Russian method of resuscitation" was described as burying in snow CA patients in an attempt to resuscitate them [11]. The surgeon Baron Dominique-Jean Larrey was intrigued by how injured soldiers could sustain the pain in cold temperatures and described how injuries exposed to either ice or cold temperatures bled less when compared to those in warmer weather. In 1812, Baron Larrey, as Napoleon's chief surgeon, during the Russian campaign, used TH to better preserve wounded limbs and as an anesthesia method prior to amputations [12].

Dr. Temple Fay, the head of the Neurosurgery Department at Philadelphia's Temple University Hospital, is attributed as having introduced TH, both localized and whole body, to the modern medical setting. Fay conducted a series of experiments in the 1990s to assess the effects of varying temperatures on tissue growth of both normal and cancerous cells. He reported that cellular differentiation in chicks practically stopped at 32.2 °C. With these findings, he felt confident applying his knowledge at the bedside, thus beginning the largest series of hypothermia experiments in humans of its time, which would eventually end up catalyzing hypothermia usage in mainstream modern medicine [9, 13, 14].

Fay's first hypothermia patient was a woman with metastatic breast cancer and neoplasm-related pain. He started his therapy by applying cold locally to the breast tumor area for weeks. After repeat biopsies, regression was noted, and the local infection seemed cured. With this evidence at hand and concerned of the persistent generalized pain, he decided to attempt to reach deeper structures. In 1938, Fay "cooled" this lady to 32 °C for 24 h, utilizing what he called "generalized refrigeration" (ice packs), and successfully rewarmed her. He reported a reduction in pain symptoms in 95.7% of surviving patients with a mortality rate of 10% [14, 15].

Bigelow and McBirnie found a possible use for TH during cardiac surgery in an animal model. They reported that during deep hypothermia (<25 °C), the area of neurological injury had less bleeding, cerebral edema, and inflammatory response [16]. One year later, in 1954, Rosomoff and collaborators demonstrated a direct relationship between core body temperature and intracranial pressure. These researchers proved that hypothermia decreased the cerebral blood flow and the metabolic rate in dogs as they were cooled from 35 °C to 26 °C [17, 18].

Benson, a professor of anesthesia at Johns Hopkins, conducted in 1958 the first clinical trial of TH outside the operating room, specifically in comatose post-cardiac arrest patients. This therapeutic measure showed 50% survival in the hypothermia group (33 °C) vs. 14% in the normothermic group [19].

Although studies in the 1970s showed promising results, between the 1960s and 1990s, TH research slowed down due to the recognition of clinical complications (mainly cold-induced coagulopathies). True resurgence of interest for TH occurred until the late 1980s, with advances in management of coagulopathies [14, 20].

It was not until 2002 that the American Heart Association (AHA), followed by the European Resuscitation Council in 2003, recommended TH as a post-resuscitative measure for out-of-hospital cardiac arrest patients that remained comatose after return of spontaneous circulation (ROSC). This recommendation was based on the results from two multicenter, prospective, randomized, controlled, clinical trials published in 2002 [21, 22]. One of the studies was conducted in Europe, in which 275 patients with cardiac arrest secondary to ventricular fibrillation were enrolled; 137 patients were managed at mild hypothermic ranges (32–34 °C) for 24 h, and 138 were normothermic control patients. The hypothermia group showed improved favorable outcomes in 55% of patients vs. 39% in the normothermic group [3].

The other 2002 study was done by Bernard and colleagues in Australia, in which they enrolled 77 patients, all of which had an initial rhythm of ventricular fibrillation. They were divided into two groups: a hypothermia group (a target temperature of 33 °C for 12 h) with 43 patients and a normothermia control group with 34 patients. Forty-nine percent of patients in the hypothermia group had a favorable neurological outcome vs. 26% in the normothermia group [2].

These two randomized, clinical trials once again sparked physician's interest in TH, not only inside the operating room, or in post-cardiac arrest patients, but also in many other instances. However, before talking about present-day indications, it is imperative to review the pathophysiology of ischemic/reperfusion injury and the physiologic rationale behind the beneficial effects that hypothermia confers when used promptly in postanoxic/hypoxic patients.

## 17.3 Pathophysiology of Ischemic Insult and Reperfusion Injury

The return of spontaneous circulation after a CA in which the patient was subject to prolonged whole-body ischemia will give place to a complex pathophysiological state, originally coined *postresuscitation disease* by Dr. Vladimir Negovsky in 1970 [23]. Although appropriate for its time, "postresuscitation" implies that resuscitation has been achieved, due to which in 2008 the term was changed to *post-cardiac arrest syndrome* (PCAS) [24].

Even though prolonged whole-body ischemia will cause global tissue and organ damage, there will be additional insult during and after ROSC due to reperfusion injury. Ischemia/reperfusion response, post-cardiac arrest brain injury, post-cardiac arrest myocardial stunning, and persistent damage by the underlying pathology precipitating the cardiac arrest are the main components of PCAS [24–26]. The clinical presentation of PCAS resembles a systemic inflammatory response syndrome (SIRS)/sepsis-like state which will vary individually depending on the severity of the ischemic injury, the underlying cause of the CA, and the patient's comorbidities [27–29]. Making this even more complex, determining the exact incidence and prevalence of this phenomenon is a challenging task, as there is no simple diagnostic test; hypotension, reduced cardiac output, usage of vasopressors, and laboratory abnormalities, among others, have been used as screening methods for PCAS but have failed to be reliable [28, 30, 31].

A pathophysiological approach to PCAS would be to define the phases according to time. The *immediate post-arrest phase* occurs in the first 20 min after ROSC. *Early post-arrest phase* lasts from 20 min to the first 12 h after ROSC, a period in which early therapeutic interventions might be the most beneficial. The *intermediate phase* is between 12 h and 72 h post-ROSC, during which ischemia/reperfusion injuries are still ongoing and aggressive treatment can still be initiated. Lastly, the *recovery phase* extends beyond 3 days, when prognostication is easier and outcome is more predictable [24, 25]. Understanding the pathophysiology behind the ischemia/reperfusion injury that occurs during the CA and afterward during PCAS will be the deciding factor for adequate individualized treatment for patients.

The ischemic injury starts seconds after the arrest even if the patient experiencing the CA is lucky enough to have a bystander who can initiate cardiopulmonary resuscitation (CPR) in an early fashion. Under perfect conditions, CPR generates 1.3 l/min of forward flow (15–25% of normal cardiac output), which can only maintain about 30% of the baseline cerebral blood flow (CBF). This flow rate usually is not able to generate a coronary flow that keeps up with the demands of a dysfunctional heart [32–34]. Due to this, brain injury and myocardial instability management have proved to be the main survival determinants after a CA [35]. In 2005, Laver and company identified that two-thirds of post-cardiac arrest patients admitted to the intensive care units died due to neurological injury [36].

The central nervous system (CNS) receives about 30% of total cardiac output [37]. During CA, the CBF stops completely, reducing the delivery of oxygen and glucose. Consciousness is lost within the first 10 s, and by 20 s, the neurological oxygen reserve is depleted, followed by isoelectric electroencephalographic activity in the next couple of seconds [20, 34]. As previously mentioned, even with CPR, the CBF is only 15–30% of the baseline [37]. The CNS is only suited to tolerate brief periods of ischemia as glucose and adenosine triphosphate (ATP) stores are completely lost by 5 min of circulatory arrest, making this a critical period during which tissue can still be salvaged [19, 38, 39]. Energy depletion enhances anaerobic metabolism increasing lactate, hydrogen, and phosphate production, promoting tissue acidosis [34, 40]. The pathological mechanisms that ensue after cardiac arrest will lead to cell death by both necrosis and apoptosis.

During ischemia, due to the depletion of oxygen and glucose, there will be a rapid reduction/depletion of ATP production and ATP reserves. By not having enough oxygen available to be used as the final electron acceptor in the mitochondria, there is a REDOX shift toward reduction, causing an increase of electron-rich metabolites which cannot follow the regular mitochondrial cytochrome oxidase pathway. This begins an electron "leakage" within the mitochondria, thus starting the production of reactive oxygen species (ROS), also known as free radicals, during the ischemia phase [41–43]. At the same time, ATP deficiency generates a disruption of ion homeostasis by affecting the transmembrane transport structures like $Na^+/K^+$-ATPase and $Ca^{2+}$-ATPase pumps. Inhibition of these pumps leads to an ion gradient shift, which causes an increase in interstitial $K^+$ and intracellular $Ca^{2+}$, giving rise to an excitotoxic release of extracellular glutamate from presynaptic nerve terminals and astrocytes [44–46].

Even in the subacute phase of ischemic/reperfusion insult, after restoration of circulation and replenishment of energy reserves, tissue injury will persist. The damage will come from nocive pathways that started during the acute ischemia phase, plus secondary reperfusion mechanisms, all happening simultaneously [47].

N-Methyl-D-aspartate (NMDA) receptors are activated by the, previously described, increase of extracellular glutamate, as well as the increase of body temperature that occurs after ROSC [19, 20]. Activation of NMDA receptors further increases intracellular $Ca^{2+}$ levels via glutamate receptor-gated ion channels [48]. By activating NMDA receptors, the postsynaptic cells will have an influx of $Na^+$ and $Cl^-$, thus generating an intracellular hyperosmolar state with consequent influx of water to the cell. The end result of this influx will be a decrease of the inhibitory effect that $Mg^{2+}$ has on NMDA receptors, thus making them more sensitive to glutamate levels, which allows more $Ca^{2+}$ entrance, promoting cellular edema and eventual neuronal necrosis [40, 49]. It's important to understand that this increase in intracellular $Ca^{2+}$ creates a harmful positive feedback loop that dictates glutamate release, all of which is completely dependent on the severity of the ischemia [50]. Overall, the elevation of intracellular $Ca^{2+}$ will activate a cascade of calcium-dependent enzymatic pathways (proteases, nucleases, and lipases) that contribute to cell membrane disintegration and eventual tissue necrosis [37, 48].

In normal conditions, the endoplasmic reticulum and the mitochondria can sequester $Ca^{2+}$ if the intracellular levels increase, but during anoxia and ischemia, this regulatory mechanism is impaired [40]. Calcium regulation by the mitochondria is ATP and oxygen dependent, and as explained, within seconds to minutes after the $CA^{2+}$, the ATP and oxygen reserves are completely depleted [19, 20, 34]. During ischemia, as $Ca^{2+}$ influx is first happening, the mitochondria are able to buffer some of it by sequestering some of the $Ca^{2+}$, which leads to mitochondrial depolarization and overall mitochondrial dysfunction [9, 40].

The mitochondrial dysfunction is mainly caused by an increase in the permeability of the inner mitochondrial membrane (IMM) that occurs due to both the electron leakage and the opening of permeability transition pores (PTPs) [42, 49]. These pores are multiprotein complexes that create nonselective pores in the IMM that contribute to the IMM depolarization, which transforms the mitochondria from an ATP producer organelle to an ATP consumer by reversing the ATP synthase pump action, in an attempt to maintain the membrane potential [51]. Mitochondrial PTPs appear to be sensitive to $Ca^{2+}$, pH, voltage changes, and REDOX reactions. With reperfusion, mitochondria are at high risk of PTP opening due to the increase of intracellular $Ca^{2+}$ levels, the alkalosis seen as the acidosis is washed away, and the increase of ROS that first started with the electron leakage and the synthesis of nitric oxide due to glutamate excess [9, 50, 52, 53].

After ROSC, due to the sudden oxidative stress experienced with reperfusion and reoxygenation, there will be a secondary rapid increase of ROS, mainly in highly metabolically active organs, like the brain and heart [43, 41, 54]. These free radicals are a result of different pathways, mainly mitochondrial dysfunction, uncoupled nitric oxide synthase, glutamate and consequent activation of NMDA receptors, arachidonic acid, and catecholamines [40, 41, 54, 55].

Since 1995, Globus and colleagues demonstrated that ROS production and glutamate release into extracellular space are temperature dependent [40, 56]. This becomes clinically relevant when we take into consideration the pyrexia that patients experience post-ROSC, as this pyrexia enhances the damaging effects of free radicals, when patient's temperature increase by >0.5 °C over 37 °C [19, 20]. Free radicals will cause oxidative damage, post-ROSC, by acting in DNA, lipid membranes, proteins, and enzymes, eventually leading to cell death [40, 41, 54].

Both ischemia and reperfusion mechanisms play a big role in the cell's fate. Ischemia primes mitochondria for PTP opening, and reperfusion triggers PTP opening. Depending on the severity of PTP opening, the mitochondrial membrane depolarization will be either transient or sustained. If the depolarization is severe, cytochrome C, along with other apoptogenic factors (apoptosis-inducing factor, Smac/DIABLO, and Apa-1), can leak from the intermembrane space into the cytosol, activating both caspase-dependent and caspase-independent pathways which culminate in mitochondrial-mediated apoptosis days to weeks after the ischemia episode [40, 51, 52, 54, 57].

The combination of elevation of intracellular $Ca^{2+}$ and production of ROS due to ischemia/reperfusion mechanisms contributes to cell membrane disintegration and eventual neuronal death by either necrosis or apoptosis, mainly observed in neurologic and myocardial tissue [19, 20, 43, 58].

Due to the nature of the pathophysiology described in PCAS, the main goals of treatment in post-cardiac arrest patients should be identifying and treating the precipitating cause of the cardiac arrest, minimizing the brain injury, controlling the cardiovascular dysfunction, and managing any metabolic issues that arise from the ischemic/reperfusion insult [24]. One therapeutic approach that allows healthcare providers to address multiple of these potential issues is TH, as it has proven to have beneficial effects in multiple of the damaging pathways of the ischemic/reperfusion insult.

## 17.4 Protective Mechanisms and Effects of Therapeutic Hypothermia

Therapeutic hypothermia was first used under the rationale that its protective mechanism was completely due to slowing the metabolic rate, specifically the cerebral metabolism [59]. Cerebral oxygen consumption, glucose utilization, and lactate production are all temperature-dependent processes which benefit from hypothermia induction [19]. Cerebral metabolic rate is estimated to decrease 6–7% for each 1 °C below a body core temperature of 37 °C [60].

During the ischemic episode, CBF has either completely stopped or is significantly reduced. As circulation is restored (ROSC), hyperemia occurs in cerebral vessels, followed by a steady decline of blood flow over a period of hours. Therapeutic hypothermia has shown to blunt the hyperemia episode seen in the immediate post-ROSC phase. Avoiding this increase of blood flow allows the brain to preserve its energy reserves of ATP and to maintain the pH [50].

As previously explained, ATP is needed to maintain ion gradients, and when reserves are depleted, as it happens during ischemia, there is a rapid calcium influx which leads to the increased release of glutamate and other excitotoxic amino acids. Hypothermia plays a role in preventing this excitotoxic cascade by limiting the calcium influx by multiple mechanisms. Preserving ATP levels minimizes ion pump malfunction, reducing intracellular calcium entrance. One study showed that hypothermia decreases the ischemia-induced downregulation of the glutamate receptor 2 (GluR2) subunit of the AMPA receptor, which is thought to play a role in limiting calcium influx [61]. Hypothermia further prevents calcium influx by affecting NMDA receptors. N-Methyl-D-aspartate receptors are temperature dependent, so as patients are cooled down, these receptors are inhibited [20, 48]. Also, hypothermia reduces brain glycine levels which makes NMDA receptors more responsive to glutamate levels, so by reducing glycine levels, the NMDA-glutamate pathway is blunted [40].

The protection TH confers to post-cardiac arrest patients cannot be fully explained by the prevention of ATP depletion or blunting of the excitotoxic cascade due to a decrease of intracellular calcium influx and glutamate release. Still during the acute ischemic phase, TH affects early gene expression. Expression of 70-kDa inducible heat shock protein (HSP70) increases during hypothermia, thus enhancing its neuroprotective properties [50].

During the subacute phase of PCAS (1–7 days post-ischemia), reperfusion pathways in conjunction with the ischemic mechanisms can widen the tissue injury [47]. Free radical formation is the main pathway by which reperfusion injures organs [41]. Therapeutic hypothermia is useful in this subacute phase as ROS production is another temperature-dependent process which slows down from cooling the patient [19]. Additionally, inflammatory responses activate during this period, which lead to cell death by both necrosis and apoptosis. Hypothermia affects these cell death pathways in a way that favors cell survival [4].

In an ischemia setting, necrosis is caused because of the intracellular swelling due to the ion pump malfunction. By allowing ion pumps to work, hypothermia decreases cellular necrosis. The other cell death pathway is apoptosis, which consists of two main pathways. The intrinsic pathway is found at mitochondrial level and is initiated in response to "death signals" (DNA damage, hypoxia, and mitochondrial membrane instability). This pathway is highly regulated by antiapoptotic molecules, such as those of BCL-2 family; apoptotic signals lead to a release of cytochrome c from within the mitochondria to the cytosol, where it will activate the caspase 9, which in turn activates caspase 3, eventually leading to apoptosis [40, 50]. Cooling can interfere with the intrinsic pathway by modifying the expression of BCL-2 family members, decreasing cytochrome c release by the mitochondria and decreasing caspase activation [62].

The extrinsic pathway starts outside the cell, by the activation of death receptors, the FAS (apoptosis-inducing receptor) and FASL (ligand) being the most studied extrinsic signaling pathway. Activation of death receptors leads to caspase 8 activation, which, same as in the intrinsic pathway, activates caspase 3, leading to apoptosis. Apoptosis has shown to suppress the expression of both FAS and FASL, thus decreasing activation of the extrinsic pathway [50].

At the same time, while blunting cell death pathways, hypothermia has shown to promote neuronal growth. Brain-derived neurotrophic factor (BDNF), glial cell-derived neurotrophic factor (GDNF), and neurotrophin all help preserve neuronal integrity, and hypothermia significantly increases its levels[40, 50]. The synergy between hypothermia and BDNF has been reported to decrease neuronal damage and reduce infarction size up to 40% [63].

In a way, TH decreases the magnitude of the damaging pathways that ensue during and after a CA. The protective mechanisms come from preventing or decreasing the energy depletion, thus diminishing the overall metabolic malfunction that develops afterward. In addition, TH promotes cell survival while blunting the cell death pathways. Each of the three separate phases of injury seen in PCAS can potentially benefit from TTM. The therapeutic usefulness will vary accordingly to the severity of the ischemia, the cause of the CA, and the baseline comorbidities of different patients, but overall, TTM will allow the body's metabolism to slow down, preventing further tissue damage and allowing, to some extent, the injured cells to heal and regain function [64].

## 17.5 Physiology of Cooling and Clinical Considerations

As core body temperature decreases, for each 1 °C below 37 °C, the cerebral metabolism decreases 6–7%, along with brain oxygen and glucose consumption [60]. Therapeutic hypothermia improves the oxygen delivery to the ischemic areas of the brain. Intracranial pressure (ICP) is reduced with TH because of a hypothermia-induced vasoconstriction that decreases cerebral blood flow, thus decreasing ICP and providing an anticonvulsant effect on the patient (which can be used to treat refractory status epilepticus) [40].

The main physiologic responses to mild-to-moderate TH in the cardiovascular system are a decrease in heart rate and an increase of the systemic vascular resistance [65]. Recent studies have associated bradycardia during TH with better outcome [66, 67]. This bradycardia is attributed to a prolonged action potential, as well as less spontaneous repolarization of the cardiomyocyte [68]. In 2002, Lewis and associates analyzed heart contractility of 10 patients who were under hypothermia, at 33 °C, and reported that patients had an impaired contractility when the heart rate was "artificially" sustained during hypothermia, thus demonstrating that the heart's contractility is directly related to a low heart rate [69]. Hypothermia will be accompanied by a release of catecholamine, which will cause an increase of the stroke volume and initially an increase in cardiac output. As core temperature continues to decrease, the effect over cardiac output will shift, but the mean arterial pressure will be preserved due to the increase of the peripheral vascular resistance [58].

The catecholamine surge will also cause coronary artery vasodilation, improving myocardial perfusion and oxygenation. This is clinically important, as TH not only diminishes the overall metabolic rate and the oxygen demand but also increases oxygen delivery to both brain and heart [50, 70].

When core temperature is 32 °C, the metabolic rate is 50–60% of baseline. The oxygen consumption and carbon dioxide production shift in a parallel manner, giving rise to important respiratory considerations. Mechanical ventilation settings need to be adjusted frequently because if left unchanged, patients are at risk of hyperventilating [19], which could in turn cause cerebral vasoconstriction and affect the oxygen delivery to an already injured brain. To manage ventilator settings appropriately, blood gases should be taken frequently, especially during the induction phase [4].

Therapeutic hypothermia causes increased renal blood flow, which in turn causes what is known as "cold diuresis." This diuresis is especially relevant during induction phase, as the diuresis can cause hypovolemia, manifesting as hypotension. During this same phase, potassium will shift intracellularly, leading to hypokalemia. Correction of the hypokalemia during induction phase can be harmful later on during the maintenance and rewarming phases as the potassium will exit the cell and cause rebound hyperkalemia. From an acid-base perspective, for every 1 °C below 37 °C, the intracellular pH increases 0.016 points [65].

The ischemic injury in conjunction with hypothermia causes intestinal dysfunction. Patients will have a delayed gastric emptying due to a decrease of peristalsis [71]. Traditionally, enteral feeding has been deferred until rewarming phase, but recent studies have shown that enteral nutrition is feasible in patients undergoing TH. It is important to keep in mind that predictive equations will most likely overestimate the patient's nutritional needs due to the decrease in metabolic rate. Further research is needed to define optimal feeding rates [72, 73].

Some associations between hypothermia and coagulopathies have been reported [74]. At temperatures ≤35 °C, there will be mild platelet dysfunction, with some inhibition of the coagulation cascade, prolonging both prothrombin and partial thromboplastin times [75]. At the same time, with hypothermia, there is an increased incidence of neutropenia, being pneumonia a common infection seen during TH [47].

## 17.6 Applications and Indications of Targeted Temperature Management

In the past decades, CA research has focused on methods to obtain more easily and at a higher rate ROSC [24]. Cardiopulmonary resuscitation continues being the treatment of choice to counteract CA, and despite the huge effort put into promoting early initiation of CPR, mortality and neurologic morbidity remain high in post-cardiac arrest patients with ROSC [46]. So, how do we manage post-cardiac arrest patients? Therapeutic hypothermia with TTM is a therapeutic intervention that has been implemented in an attempt to minimize the mortality and the neurologic damage experienced in the PCAS. The initial rationale behind the clinical implementation of TTM was that it decreases the metabolic rate, thus allowing the injured brain to heal [64].

In 2002, two multicenter, prospective, controlled RCTs showed a favorable neurological outcome in post-cardiac arrest patients with ROSC who underwent hypothermia vs. those who were managed with a normothermia approach [2, 3]. One year after these clinical trials, the *Advanced Life Support Task Force of the International Liaison Committee on Resuscitation* (ILCOR) wrote an advisory statement, recommending for the first time that comatose adult patients with ROSC after out-of-hospital cardiac arrest (OHCA) should undergo TH with TTM (32–34 °C for 12–24 h) when initial rhythm, during the arrest, was ventricular fibrillation [21].

Nielsen and colleagues, in 2013, published an RCT that compares TTM at 33 °C with TTM at 36 °C in OHCA patients, focusing in survival and neurological outcomes [76]. The results showed no difference in either outcome between both target temperature groups, leading to a debate regarding expanding target temperature to 36 °C instead of 32 °C–34 °C, as the 2010 guidelines recommended. Many centers understood Nielsen's results as TTM no longer being required or that fever control would suffice post-cardiac arrest management, which is not at all the case [6, 59].

The ILCOR does not take part in the debate regarding ideal target temperature that sparked after Nielsen's TTM Trial. Instead, they continue to recommend TTM use and expanded their previous temperature range recommendation of 32–34 °C to a constant target temperature between 32 °C and 36 °C [77]. Specific information about the ideal duration of TTM is lacking [59], due to which current recommendation is temperature control for at least 24 h since achievement of selected target temperature, as it was done in the two largest randomized clinical trials in 2002 [77].

Traditionally, TTM had been reserved only for patients who remained comatose after OHCA with an initial shockable rhythm [21, 64, 78, 79]. In 2015, the *Advanced Life Support Task Force of the International Liaison Committee on Resuscitation* and the *American Heart Association Emergency Cardiovascular Care Committee* and the *Council on Cardiopulmonary, Critical Care, Perioperative and Resuscitation* published an advisory statement with the most recent and current recommendations for TH with TTM in post-cardiac arrest patients [77]. Between 2010 and 2015, clinical trials showed a neurological benefit when TTM was used for both OHCA with initial non-shockable rhythm and in-hospital cardiac arrest (IHCA) regardless of initial rhythm [80–84], which prompted a change to prior guidelines. Current guidelines recommend to:

- Initiate TTM for adult patients who remain comatose after ROSC in OHCA which initially had a *shockable* rhythm.
- Initiate TTM for adult patients who remain comatose after ROSC in OHCA which initially had a *non-shockable* rhythm.
- Initiate TTM for adult patients who remain comatose after ROSC in IHCA, *regardless of initial rhythm.*

By making these strong recommendations, the task force group is stating that essentially there are no patients in whom temperature control between 32 °C and 36 °C is contraindicated [85]. After 24 h of temperature control in between that range, slow rewarming is recommended (≤0.25 °C/h), followed by strict hyperthermia management [6, 77, 85]. This way, the ILCOR supports TTM as a protective intervention from a neurologic and cardiovascular standpoint [77, 86].

There is conflicting data on benefit and risk of cooling induction in a prehospital setting [87–92]. Current guidelines recommend against usage of large volumes of cold fluid in a prehospital setting for induction of TH right after ROSC and make no comment on other prehospital cooling techniques [85].

One year after the release of the current guidelines, in 2016, Schenone et al. presented a meta-analysis and systematic review in which they reviewed the mortality and neurologic outcome when utilizing expanded criteria for targeted temperature in OHCA survivors [93]. Fifty-one percent of the patients included in the meta-analysis had initially a shockable rhythm, with arrest times ranging from 20 to 34.6 min (a mean of 24.6) [93], which compares with the downtimes in the TTM trial, which excluded patients with downtimes of more than 20 min [76]. Schenone showed that the use of TH correlates with a higher survival rate and a better neurological outcome after OHCA, regardless of initial rhythm and with a more flexible downtime window. These results seem to help elucidate the questions regarding TTM usage, favoring TTM use in all cardiac arrest patients, even when patients had a longer downtime or a delay in initiation of therapy [94].

Despite the overwhelming positive evidence of TTM in post-cardiac arrest patients, TTM remains underutilized [86, 95–99]. It is our opinion that we should initiate TTM in all cardiac arrest patients with ROSC, regardless of their downtime and initial rhythm, when feasible.

Success utilizing TH in cardiac arrest's RCTs, coupled with physiologic knowledge on the hypothermia topic, has motivated physicians on expanding the utilization of TH to other pathologies apart from PCAS [64]. There is data of benefit in diseases like ischemic stroke [100–102], traumatic brain injury [103], near-drowning [104], neonatal hypoxic-ischemic encephalopathy [105], hepatic encephalopathy [106–108], and acute respiratory distress syndrome [109], among others. Therapeutic hypothermia protocols might differ in target temperature and duration of TTM in these other clinical indications.

## 17.7 Time Window and Timing

The extent of neurologic damage seen in post-cardiac arrest patients is primarily related to the duration of ischemia [20]. The first 5 min after the circulatory arrest delimits the classic threshold in which brain tissue can still be completely salvaged [38, 39]. For this reason, reaching the selected target temperature (32–36 °C) as quickly as possible after ROSC is the main goal in post-cardiac arrest care [19]. Laboratory analysis has shown that the therapeutic window for hypothermia is initiation in less than 6 h after ROSC; however, clinical trials do not support this finding, and currently, we remain without a defined therapeutic window [110].

Animal studies have shown neurologic benefit with very early initiation of TTM after ROSC [111, 112]. However, human studies have failed to provide definitive data regarding prehospital induction of TH [47, 113]. Physicians have even looked into initiating hypothermia during the intra-arrest phase, utilizing different techniques, with inconclusive results [88, 114]. Nonetheless, clinical studies have shown a remarkable therapeutic benefit from TTM even when cooling initiation was delayed for several hours [93, 104]. Taking all this into consideration, the reality is that TTM remains being a neuroprotective intervention, which ideally should be started as early as possible, in a hospital environment. The traditional time window to achieve target temperature after obtaining ROSC is 4 h, but patients with delayed induction of hypothermia can still benefit from being cooled down [94].

The ideal duration of TTM in order to obtain a good neurological outcome remains unknown. The ILCOR originally had recommended 12–24 h of TTM at 32–34 °C [21, 78, 79]. A recent multicenter RCT, in 2017, compared TTM use for 48 h with TTM use for 24 h and reported no significant differences between both groups in neurologic outcome or survival rate at 6-month follow-up [115]. Current resuscitation guidelines recommend at least 24 h of TTM between 32 °C and 36 °C [85]. However, a clinical trial has yet to prove benefit from TTM for durations longer than 24 h [115]. Then again, dose-finding RCTs cannot assume there is an optimal fixed duration that can be applied to all the post-cardiac arrest patient population [116].

## 17.8 Cooling Techniques

There are multiple techniques to induce TH [60, 117]. Current recommendations do not specify the optimal method for initiating and/or maintaining TH, as the ideal cooling device has yet to be developed, and there is insufficient evidence to recommend a specific cooling method [85, 118]. The ideal cooling device would have a high cooling rate with short induction times, preferentially would be directed toward target organs (brain and heart), would be easy to transport (lightweight, portable, and durable), and could be used in a prehospital setting, maybe even during cardiopulmonary resuscitation. The main modalities used nowadays are surface and invasive cooling [47, 119].

Surface cooling methods are relatively easy to use but take a longer time to cool down patients to the desired target temperature (2–8 h). They include circulating cold-water blankets, cold air-forced blankets, self-adhesive hydrogen-coated pads, and less sophisticated methods like ice packs and cold-water immersion.

Immersing patients in cold water is an option but should be avoided as it compromises monitoring temperature, and it is troublesome to defibrillate patients, as it takes time to dry them off [47]. Ice-pack usage remains a viable cost-effective option that can be used in conjunction with more advanced cooling techniques. Main disadvantages of ice packs, other than being labor intensive, are that unintentional overcooling past target temperature is common and if applied directly to the skin, they can cause skin necrosis [117]. One of the major drawbacks from surface techniques is that the shivering response seen during the induction phase is increased [20]. Due to this, appropriate prevention and/or treatment of the shivering is needed as the increased oxygen consumption could mitigate the protective mechanisms that TH confers [4].

Invasive endovascular cooling methods were developed mainly because of the major drawbacks of surface cooling [47]. Methods included in this modality are infusion of cold intravenous fluid (4 °C), cold carotid infusions, single-carotid artery perfusion with extracorporeal cooled blood circulation, ice water nasal lavage, cardiopulmonary bypass, cold peritoneal lavage, nasogastric and rectal lavage, and esophageal cold-water circulating device [47, 120]. Cold intravenous fluid infusion has shown to be easily available and cost-effective in inducing hypothermia, but not in maintaining it. Up to two liters of cold intravenous fluid is safe to administer in post-cardiac arrest patients [117].

Overall, endovascular cooling methods have shown to have faster cooling rates and, more importantly, more time within target temperature with less temperature fluctuations. Tight temperature control, limiting temperature fluctuations, might become more important with the newer recommendations to manage patients at temperatures up to 36 °C, as a shivering episode could lead to a 1.5 °C increase in temperature, placing the patient in the febrile territory [121].

A newer method is through an esophageal device. This device maintains standard orogastric tube functions while cooling down patients at a rate of 1.3 °C/h, with minimal temperature fluctuations [120].

In many cases, a combination of hypothermia induction methods is used to reach target temperature in a faster manner [4]. Maintenance of TH is usually done based on the characteristics of the patient, in conjunction with the physician's expertise with different devices, as well as the availability of different methods [120].

## 17.9 Monitoring Temperature

Therapeutic hypothermia levels are classically divided into four: mild, 34–36 °C; moderate, 28–32 °C; deep, 17–27 °C; and profound, 4–16 °C [19]. Induced TH is currently recommended in a mild-to-moderate (32–36 °C) fashion, as in between this temperature range the protective mechanisms have shown to outweigh the possible complications [85].

Regardless of the hypothermia induction method and the TTM maintenance technique, reliable continuous temperature monitoring is imperative for adequate neuroprotection [110]. Even though the brain is the main end-organ target of TTM, core temperature is usually the one measured in order to have tight temperature control [122]. Despite it being more than 15 years since the release of the first TTM recommendations, current guidelines do not recommend a specific site for temperature measurement [21, 85].

Monitoring can be done with a variety of invasive or noninvasive probes, including pulmonary artery catheter, nasopharyngeal, esophageal, tympanic membrane, bladder, and rectal [19]. Blood in the pulmonary artery catheter is considered the "gold standard" of core temperature measurement, as it has a higher accuracy and precision than other monitoring methods [123], but its use in an emergency setting can be impractical.

Physicians need to take into consideration that the devices used to measure temperature during a hypothermia regimen were not designed to detect quick shifts in temperature. Inevitably, these temperature monitoring devices will be "lagging" behind in time when compared to "true" core temperature. This time lag will be greater when cooling is being done at fast rates (as seen in newer cooling devices). Due to this, during the induction phase, the measured temperature will be constantly behind the actual core temperature. It means that the cooling device will keep cooling down the patient even if the target core temperature has been achieved, and by the time the measured temperature reflects the target temperature, the patient's core temperature may be significantly below the therapeutic range [71].

Nasopharyngeal and esophageal temperatures have shown to correlate better with brain temperature than other body site temperatures further away from the brain, during TH [124, 125]. Tympanic membrane temperature is readily available in a noninvasive manner and seems to correlate well with brain temperature [75]; however, measurement can be impaired when there is an ear canal obstruction (i.e., ear wax). If tympanic temperature is the choice, cooling of the head should be avoided to reduce the chance of "false" readings [126–128]. Rectal probes are not ideal, as fecal impaction can disrupt measurements when compared to intracranial temperature [47]. Bladder probe is another option that seems to correlate well with pulmonary artery temperatures, making it an easy-to-use option [20].

## 17.10 Therapeutic Hypothermia Phases

A TH cycle is clinically divided into three phases [60]:

1. *Induction phase*, defined as the period since the patient is first being cooled down until reaching the selected target temperature. The aim is to get the patient's core temperature to a desired target temperature between 32 °C and 36 °C as quickly as possible.
2. *Maintenance phase* starts as soon as target temperature has been reached. The main goal is to manage core temperature strictly, with minimal or no fluctuation in body core temperature (maximum fluctuation of 0.2–0.5 °C).
3. *Rewarming phase* occurs after at least 24 h of TH. Rewarming should be done at a slow rate, ranging from 0.25 °C to 0.5 °C/h.

Each phase has their own clinical considerations that need to be kept in mind. When attempting to cool down a patient, counter-thermoregulatory mechanisms will activate [71]. At a core temperature of 36.5 °C, there will be vasoconstriction of the skin in an attempt to decrease the body's heat loss. In this case, the vasoconstriction of skin vessels makes more difficult inducing hypothermia, especially when using surface cooling methods. In addition, about 1 °C below skin vessels vasoconstriction, shivering will kick in attempting to maintain body temperature by increasing heat production [129]. If left untreated, shivering will increase the systemic oxygen consumption, decrease the neurologic oxygenation, increase the ICP, and will interfere with the cooling rate, prolonging induction's phase duration [110, 130].

Patient's shivering while inducing hypothermia can be treated with sedatives, anesthetics, opiates, magnesium, neuromuscular blockade, etc. Despite neuromuscular paralytic agents being an option, they should probably be avoided, if possible [130]. First, when utilizing paralytic agents, there will be muscular blunting, but centrally, there won't be any effect. Second, paralytic agents can mask seizure activity. Third, sedatives in conjunction with anesthetics can usually manage the shivering and can help with the cooling rate as they can cause vasodilation. Lastly, paralysis may mask insufficient sedation [4].

Short-term paralysis seems appropriate as a first-line option to treat shivering in patients in whom hemodynamic stability is a concern (in whom sedatives and/or analgesics could cause hypotension) [131]. It appears reasonable that paralysis should be used only when appropriate sedation and analgesia failed to manage shivering. But, even then, shivering response decreases past the 33.5 °C mark. For this reason, the sedation strategy should aim for a high bolus dose during the induction phase, continued by a relatively low dose during maintenance phase, as there will be a decreased drug clearance [71].

The induction phase represents the period during which the patient is at highest risk for short-term side effects like hypovolemia, electrolyte imbalances, and hyperglycemia [65]. Hypovolemia can develop due to hypothermia-induced "cold-diuresis" or a fluid shift toward the extravascular space. Electrolyte disorders occur by a combination of an increased renal excretion (by both cold diuresis and tubular dysfunction) and an intracellular shift. Magnesium and $K^+$ depletion are especially important [4]. The recommendation is to keep $K^+$ at a level between 3.0 and 3.5 mmol/l during the induction phase (and maintenance phase) to avoid the risk of rebound hyperkalemia during rewarming phase (see later) [110]. Magnesium supplementation is important, as several studies have shown a relationship between hypomagnesemia and increased mortality in the intensive care unit (ICU) [132, 133]. Giving $Mg^{2+}$ to these patients is also useful as $Mg^{2+}$ happens to be an NMDA receptor antagonist that increases the shivering threshold [60]. Hyperglycemia happens due to the decrease in insulin sensitivity and a reduction of insulin secretion by the pancreatic islet cells, caused by the hypothermia [47].

Management during the induction phase is critical for the patient's outcome, with frequent adjustments to ventilator settings, sedation, insulin and vasopressor dosage, and fluids and electrolyte management. A way to minimize these side effects is by shortening the induction phase duration by reaching the maintenance phase as quickly as possible, which can be obtained by combining cooling techniques [4].

The maintenance phase is characterized by patient "stability" when compared to the induction phase. The shivering response diminishes past the 33.5 °C mark [71]. The risk for hypovolemia or electrolyte imbalance is less of a concern during this phase. Attention should be given to the prevention of infections, pressure ulcers, and deep venous thrombosis prophylaxis [71].

After completing at least 24 h of TH, the best approach for rewarming and continuing temperature management remains unknown [85]. Rewarming after TH should be done at a slow rate, between 0.25 °C and 0.5 °C/h, as plasma electrolytes, intravascular volume, and metabolic rate can shift quickly during rewarming [60, 134]. Studies have shown that a fast rewarming rate is associated with a worse outcome [135, 136].

During the rewarming phase, it is common for patients to present shivering and hypotension [20]. Shivering should be controlled as it can eliminate the protective effects of TH by increasing the overall metabolic rate. Hypotension is caused by a redistribution of intravascular fluid, as skin vessels dilate with the temperature going up [137].

In patients in whom intracranial hypertension is being controlled with TH, the rewarming rate should be even slower; recommended rewarming rate is 0.5–1 °C/day [47]. After achieving normothermia, in the post-therapeutic hypothermia phase, studies have noted that hyperthermia presents in a considerable amount of patients [138, 139]. Rebound hyperthermia management is key in the post-rewarming period, as it also is associated with worse neurological outcome [140]. Further research is required to define a maximum safe target temperature post-rewarming and the duration of hyperthermia prevention post-cardiac arrest [118].

## 17.11 Complications

Hypothermia causes physiologic changes in all the organs of the body [141]. It is important to differentiate between these physiologic changes that occur and the true side effects and complications of TH. But, even after making this distinction, some of these normal physiologic changes are unwanted in critically ill patients, requiring prompt medical management. Other side effects are expected but will not endanger patient's lives [71]. The most important complications of TH will be discussed below.

Bradycardia is the most common heart dysrhythmia during TH. However, it is important to remember that myocardial contractility is highly related with a low heart rate (at least in this temperature setting), due to which patients should not receive chronotropic medications in order to keep the heart rate up. Forty beats per minute can be considered a normal heart rate for patients being managed at 32 °C. Overall, the risk of developing life-threatening dysrhythmias is very low at temperatures above 30 °C [58]. In a more profound hypothermia regimen, patients usually start with atrial fibrillation, which can shift to any dysrhythmia, most commonly being to either ventricular fibrillation or ventricular tachycardia. A major clinical consideration to keep in mind is that at profound hypothermia levels, dysrhythmias are harder to manage with anti-arrhythmic drugs because myocardial tissue is less responsive [71]. Appropriate care involves constant reliable temperature monitoring not only to diminish temperature fluctuations but also to prevent going below the recommended therapeutic range [110].

A major concern with hypothermia is the supposed predisposition for bleeding. Hypothermia causes some degree of platelet dysfunction, decreases platelet count, and affects kinetics within the coagulation cascade, affecting both prothrombin and partial thromboplastin times [20, 47]. Clinically, this does not represent a major concern in patients who are not actively bleeding when hypothermia is induced. However, the situation changes when patients are actively bleeding prior to cooling them down. In this case, the bleeding should be stopped prior to initiating temperature management. When bleeding is a concern, it is worth knowing that platelet dysfunction does not happen until the temperature is ≤35 °C and the coagulation cascade is not blunted until the temperature is ≤33 °C [4, 142]. These temperature levels are the basis for some authors recommending higher temperatures of TH for patients in whom bleeding is a concern, but this bleeding risk is not a reason to not initiate TH [110].

One of the major protective attributes of TH is the inhibition of various inflammatory pathways [40]. With this inhibitory effect, its inherent that there will also be impairment of the immune system response. Inhibition of proinflammatory cytokines, leukocyte migration, and phagocytosis make the body more susceptible to infections [71]. Other factor that further enables infection development is the hypothermia-induced hyperglycemia, caused by both increased insulin resistance and diminished insulin secretion [142].

The most common infection seen in TH patients is pneumonia. Information regarding what aspect of TH (duration, temperature, method, etc.) causes the increased risk for infection remains unknown. An increased incidence of infection during hypothermia opens up the debate regarding prophylactic administration of antibiotics, but guidelines remain neutral on the topic [143]. Even if antibiotics are used prophylactically or not, prevention of pressure ulcers during hypothermia should be a big priority as hypothermia increases the risk of wound infection. Special attention should be given to surgical wounds or catheter insertion sites [71, 144].

A clinical tie-in with the increased risk of wound infection is the possibility of skin necrosis if direct cold injury occurs. As previously explained, hypothermia induction can be done through multiple methods. If surface cooling is the option selected, one possibility is that if cold substances (i.e., ice, pads with hydrogel) are applied directly on top of the skin, there will be severe peripheral vasoconstriction which can lead to skin necrosis [145]. Again, wound prevention is very important during TH.

## 17.12 Controversies

In 2013, Nielsen and colleagues published the TTM Trial. This international RCT reported that TTM at 33 °C conferred no benefit regarding survival rate and neurologic outcome when compared to a target temperature of 36 °C [76]. This publication sparked a debate within the hypothermia community that threatened TTM usage.

The results from the Nielsen's TTM Trial are usually interpreted as if TH only confers protective mechanisms by controlling/preventing fever in post-cardiac arrest patients. This hypothesis is partially true in the sense that fever in post-cardiac arrest patients has been shown to be harmful in those who had an ischemic event [146]. For years authors have stated the detrimental effect that hyperthermia has on prognosis, but hyperthermia prevention is not the only mechanism by which TH confers beneficial effects [118]. The question that Nielsen was seeking to answer with this trial is very valid, but the execution of the study was probably suboptimal.

The study design was an international RCT, which involved 36 intensive care units (ICUs) in Europe and Australia. During 26 months, patients 18 years or older, who suffered an OHCA, who remained comatose at least 20 min after

ROSC were screened to form part of the trial. The main exclusion criteria were that more than 240 min had passed since ROSC until screening and asystole as initial rhythm [76].

Between November 2010 and January 2010, 950 patients were enrolled in the TTM Trial (476 assigned to 33 °C and 474 assigned to 36 °C). These numbers mean that on average each center was enrolling only one patient per month into the trial. Were all post-cardiac arrest patients with ROSC screened for this study? We believe physicians were subconsciously preselecting patients who they thought could benefit from TH [146].

Additionally, a major concern within the design of this study is the time allowance for screening of up to 4 h [147]. Animal studies and pathophysiologic knowledge support that early induction of hypothermia correlates with better protective effectiveness [111, 112]. Thus, with the design of the study, patients could go up to 4 h, before initiating the cooling process, with some patients not reaching target temperature after up to 10 h post-ROSC. This skews their proposed analysis and results, as medical literature states that the time window to reach target temperature to have the greatest effectiveness is 4 h [7].

Clinical data and patient characteristics play a big role when comparing both groups (33 °C vs. 36 °C). The patients in the 33 °C group were already hypothermic upon admission, which in this setting means a more severe brain injury. This alone might define the study patient population as heterogeneous, thus affecting the interpretation of results [76].

Rewarming rate has shown to affect the outcome of patients. Studies have shown that fast rewarming is associated with poorer outcomes and that fast rewarming can even negate the benefits that TH provides. In the TTM Trial, patients were rewarmed at a rate of 0.5 °C/h, which could translate to a mitigation of the beneficial effects of patients cooled down to either 33 °C or 36 °C [148]. Literature has stress that rewarming should be slow, and guidelines state that the rate of 0.5 °C/h was based on clinical surveys, rather than a scientifically proven benefit [60].

After the release of the TTM Trial, some major medical centers in the world stopped inducing TH on their post-cardiac arrest patients or changed target temperature to 36 °C [6]. This has become one of the major concerns after Nielsen's trial; due to the misunderstanding that strict normothermia and hyperthermia avoidance would apparently yield the same results as a hypothermia regimen, there has been some trend to stop using hypothermia, between the mild-to-moderate range, in the post-cardiac arrest patient population. Temperature control at 36 °C is harder as the shivering response is increased and a single shivering episode could increase temperature to 37.5 °C, putting the patient in the febrile territory, and more importantly, brain temperature is usually 0.34–2.0 °C above body core temperature, and avoiding brain hyperthermia is one of the main post-cardiac arrest goals [121]. It is imperative to debunk the misinterpreted results from the TTM Trial that can lead to more harm than good.

There is no doubt that the TTM Trial shows the benefits from strict hyperthermia control in diminishing postanoxic brain injury in cardiac arrest patients. But, is this information sufficient to state that TH confers no additional benefit than strict fever prevention? We believe that the study has shown the importance of strict hyperthermia control after a TH regimen, but that does not mean that fever control is the only method by which TH confers benefits to CA patients. The results from the TTM Trial show that fever control could suffice, to some extent, in some CA patients, but we do not believe 36 °C should become the new ideal target temperature. This trial raises important questions regarding ideal target temperature to specific patient population [7].

Recently, an open-label RCT, which included 25 French ICUs, compared moderate TH at 33 °C for 24 h with targeted normothermia at 37 °C for 48 h. The study included 581 patients, 284 in the hypothermia group and 297 in the normothermia group. They assessed neurological and mortality outcome on day 90 after randomization. Lascarrou and colleagues reported that 10.2% of patients in hypothermia group had a favorable neurologic outcome, compared to the normothermia group which had a good neurologic outcome in 5.7% of patients. Mortality at 90 days after randomization did not differ in both groups [149].

This RCT has some important limitations. First, the primary outcome was assessed through a phone interview. Second, an important proportion of patients were hyperthermic, despite the TTM, especially those in the normothermia group. Third, patients in the hypothermia group had TTM for up to 64 h, compared to only 48 h in the normothermia group. Lastly, as stated in the paper, an outcome change in one patient would make a difference in dictating if hypothermia was statistically significant, compared to normothermia, regarding the primary outcome [149].

Despite the important limitations of this study, it demonstrates the importance of TH in post-cardiac arrest patient. Patients in the normothermia group had a much higher incidence of hyperthermia, which correlates with the data that states that normothermia is more difficult to maintain than hypothermia [7]. Many questions remain unanswered, which should be the focus on future research.

## 17.13 Future Directions

Despite the overwhelmingly positive evidence regarding TTM, this therapy remains underused [95–98]. Focus should be put into promoting and educating healthcare providers in the usage of TH. Standardization of guidelines and recommendations is required to achieve a higher adequate usage of this beneficial therapy. The ILCOR has attempted to standardize TH usage through their recommendations which are updated every 5 years [21, 78, 60, 85]. Despite all the research in the TH field, many questions remain unanswered. As it has been explained, there still is confusion on the target temperature during induced hypothermia, remaining as one of the main challenges that researchers have: How low should we go in temperature for the optimal protection? We know that mild-to-moderate hypothermia confers organic protection in patients with ischemic events, but an ideal temperature has yet to be defined [59].

Traditionally, hypothermia is maintained for at least 24 h in post-cardiac arrest patients, but this time duration needs to be looked into, as the recommendation stems from the time used in the major RCTs. Research is required to identify if certain patient population could benefit from a longer or shorter hypothermia regimen [115].

A major area of interest is the post-rewarming period. It is known that a slower rewarming rate is better than a fast one, but there is no definite study that shows what should be the optimal target temperature in the post-rewarming phase and for how long should patients have strict hyperthermia avoidance. This aspect is very relevant, as there is evidence that fast rewarming and/or poor temperature control after rewarming can mitigate the beneficial effects of TH [135, 150].

Studies have shown that early hypothermia induction is associated with better outcomes in post-cardiac arrest patients [88, 113]. But, how early can we start cooling down patients? Data has shown that the initiation of hypothermia during the intra-arrest phase is possible and might be feasible. Cooling down patients this way would not only shorten the time until the desired target temperature is reached but would also promote TTM usage [151].

Targeted temperature management could expand to other clinical scenarios in the next couple of years. Study after study has shown the positive effects of hypothermia in the body. Healthcare providers need to acknowledge the beneficial effects of induced hypothermia for certain patient populations and start integrating it as part of their therapeutic options [19, 20].

## References

1. Benjamin EJ, Muntner P, Alonso A, Bittencourt MS, Callaway CW, Carson AP, et al. Heart disease and stroke statistics-2019 update: a report from the American Heart Association. Circulation. 2019;139(10):e56–e528. https://doi.org/10.1161/CIR.0000000000000659.
2. Bernard SA, Gray TW, Buist MD, Jones BM, Silvester W, Gutteridge G, et al. Treatment of comatose survivors of out-of-hospital cardiac arrest with induced hypothermia. N Engl J Med. 2002;346(8):557–63. https://doi.org/10.1056/NEJMoa003289.
3. Hypothermia after Cardiac Arrest Study G. Mild therapeutic hypothermia to improve the neurologic outcome after cardiac arrest. N Engl J Med. 2002;346(8):549–56. https://doi.org/10.1056/NEJMoa012689.
4. Polderman KH. Mechanisms of action, physiological effects, and complications of hypothermia. Crit Care Med. 2009;37(7 Suppl):S186–202. https://doi.org/10.1097/CCM.0b013e3181aa5241.
5. Girotra S, Chan PS, Bradley SM. Post-resuscitation care following out-of-hospital and in-hospital cardiac arrest. Heart. 2015;101(24):1943–9. https://doi.org/10.1136/heartjnl-2015-307450.
6. Polderman KH, Varon J. Confusion around therapeutic temperature management hypothermia after in-hospital cardiac arrest? Circulation. 2018;137(3):219–21. https://doi.org/10.1161/circulationaha.117.029656.
7. Polderman KH, Varon J. How low should we go? Hypothermia or strict normothermia after cardiac arrest? Circulation. 2015;131(7):669–75. https://doi.org/10.1161/circulationaha.114.012165.
8. Bray JE, Stub D, Bloom JE, Segan L, Mitra B, Smith K, et al. Changing target temperature from 33 degrees C to 36 degrees C in the ICU management of out-of-hospital cardiac arrest: a before and after study. Resuscitation. 2017;113:39–43. https://doi.org/10.1016/j.resuscitation.2017.01.016.

9. Karnatovskaia LV, Wartenberg KE, Freeman WD. Therapeutic hypothermia for neuroprotection: history, mechanisms, risks, and clinical applications. Neurohospitalist. 2014;4(3):153–63. https://doi.org/10.1177/1941874413519802.
10. Varon J. Therapeutic hypothermia in cardiac arrest: 206 years later! Resuscitation. 2009;80(12):1335. https://doi.org/10.1016/j.resuscitation.2009.08.021.
11. Liss HP. A history of resuscitation. Ann Emerg Med. 1986;15(1):65–72. https://doi.org/10.1016/s0196-0644(86)80490-5.
12. Remba SJ, Varon J, Rivera A, Sternbach GL. Dominique-Jean Larrey: the effects of therapeutic hypothermia and the first ambulance. Resuscitation. 2010;81(3):268–71. https://doi.org/10.1016/j.resuscitation.2009.11.010.
13. Alzaga AG, Salazar GA, Varon J. Resuscitation great. Breaking the thermal barrier: Dr. Temple Fay. Resuscitation. 2006;69(3):359–64. https://doi.org/10.1016/j.resuscitation.2006.02.014.
14. Bohl MA, Martirosyan NL, Killeen ZW, Belykh E, Zabramski JM, Spetzler RF, et al. The history of therapeutic hypothermia and its use in neurosurgery. J Neurosurg. 2018:1–15. https://doi.org/10.3171/2017.10.JNS171282.
15. Fay T. Observations on prolonged human refrigeration. NY State J Med. 1941;2(3):347.
16. Bigelow WG, McBirnie JE. Further experiences with hypothermia for intracardiac surgery in monkeys and groundhogs. Ann Surg. 1953;137(3):361–5. https://doi.org/10.1097/00000658-195303000-00010.
17. Rosomoff HL, Holaday DA. Cerebral blood flow and cerebral oxygen consumption during hypothermia. Am J Phys. 1954;179(1):85–8. https://doi.org/10.1152/ajplegacy.1954.179.1.85.
18. Bonaventura J, Alan D, Vejvoda J, Honek J, Veselka J. History and current use of mild therapeutic hypothermia after cardiac arrest. Arch Med Sci. 2016;12(5):1135–41. https://doi.org/10.5114/aoms.2016.61917.
19. Alzaga AG, Cerdan M, Varon J. Therapeutic hypothermia. Resuscitation. 2006;70(3):369–80. https://doi.org/10.1016/j.resuscitation.2006.01.017.
20. Varon J, Acosta P. Therapeutic hypothermia: past, present, and future. Chest. 2008;133(5):1267–74. https://doi.org/10.1378/chest.07-2190.
21. Nolan JP, Morley PT, Vanden Hoek TL, Hickey RW, Kloeck WG, Billi J, et al. Therapeutic hypothermia after cardiac arrest: an advisory statement by the advanced life support task force of the International Liaison Committee on Resuscitation. Circulation. 2003;108(1):118–21. https://doi.org/10.1161/01.Cir.0000079019.02601.90.
22. Nolan JP, Hazinski MF, Steen PA, Becker LB. Controversial Topics from the 2005 International Consensus Conference on cardiopulmonary resuscitation and emergency cardiovascular care science with treatment recommendations. Resuscitation. 2005;67(2–3):175–9. https://doi.org/10.1016/j.resuscitation.2005.09.008.
23. Negovsky VA. The second step in resuscitation—the treatment of the 'post-resuscitation disease'. Resuscitation. 1972;1(1):1–7.
24. Nolan JP, Neumar RW, Adrie C, Aibiki M, Berg RA, Bottiger BW, et al. Post-cardiac arrest syndrome: epidemiology, pathophysiology, treatment, and prognostication. A Scientific Statement from the International Liaison Committee on Resuscitation; the American Heart Association Emergency Cardiovascular Care Committee; the Council on Cardiovascular Surgery and Anesthesia; the Council on Cardiopulmonary, Perioperative, and Critical Care; the Council on Clinical Cardiology; the Council on Stroke. Resuscitation. 2008;79(3):350–79. https://doi.org/10.1016/j.resuscitation.2008.09.017.
25. Binks A, Nolan JP. Post-cardiac arrest syndrome. Minerva Anestesiol. 2010;76(5):362–8.
26. Madder RD, Reynolds JC. Multidisciplinary management of the post-cardiac arrest patient. Cardiol Clin. 2018;36(1):85–101. https://doi.org/10.1016/j.ccl.2017.08.005.
27. Bougouin W, Cariou A. Management of postcardiac arrest myocardial dysfunction. Curr Opin Crit Care. 2013;19(3):195–201. https://doi.org/10.1097/MCC.0b013e3283607740.
28. Polderman KH, Varon J. Cool hemodynamics—the intricate interplay between therapeutic hypothermia and the post-cardiac arrest syndrome. Resuscitation. 2014;85(8):975–6. https://doi.org/10.1016/j.resuscitation.2014.06.002.

29. Oksanen T, Skrifvars M, Wilkman E, Tierala I, Pettila V, Varpula T. Postresuscitation hemodynamics during therapeutic hypothermia after out-of-hospital cardiac arrest with ventricular fibrillation: a retrospective study. Resuscitation. 2014;85(8):1018–24. https://doi.org/10.1016/j.resuscitation.2014.04.026.
30. Kleinman ME, Perkins GD, Bhanji F, Billi JE, Bray JE, Callaway CW, et al. ILCOR scientific knowledge gaps and clinical research priorities for cardiopulmonary resuscitation and emergency cardiovascular care: a consensus statement. Resuscitation. 2018;127:132–46. https://doi.org/10.1016/j.resuscitation.2018.03.021.
31. Jones AE, Shapiro NI, Kilgannon JH, Trzeciak S. Emergency medicine shock research network I. Goal-directed hemodynamic optimization in the post-cardiac arrest syndrome: a systematic review. Resuscitation. 2008;77(1):26–9. https://doi.org/10.1016/j.resuscitation.2007.10.021.
32. Lurie KG, Nemergut EC, Yannopoulos D, Sweeney M. The physiology of cardiopulmonary resuscitation. Anesth Analg. 2016;122(3):767–83. https://doi.org/10.1213/ANE.0000000000000926.
33. Lewis LM, Stothert JC Jr, Gomez CR, Ruoff BE, Hall IS, Chandel B, et al. A noninvasive method for monitoring cerebral perfusion during cardiopulmonary resuscitation. J Crit Care. 1994;9(3):169–74.
34. Maramattom BV, Wijdicks EF. Postresuscitation encephalopathy. Current views, management, and prognostication. Neurologist. 2005;11(4):234–43. https://doi.org/10.1097/01.nrl.0000159985.07242.22.
35. Ferreira Da Silva IR, Frontera JA. Targeted temperature management in survivors of cardiac arrest. Cardiol Clin. 2013;31(4):637–55. https://doi.org/10.1016/j.ccl.2013.07.010. ix
36. Laver S, Farrow C, Turner D, Nolan J. Mode of death after admission to an intensive care unit following cardiac arrest. Intensive Care Med. 2004;30(11):2126–8. https://doi.org/10.1007/s00134-004-2425-z.
37. Tahsili-Fahadan P, Farrokh S, Geocadin RG. Hypothermia and brain inflammation after cardiac arrest. Brain Circ. 2018;4(1):1–13. https://doi.org/10.4103/bc.bc_4_18.
38. Holzer M. Targeted temperature management for comatose survivors of cardiac arrest. N Engl J Med. 2010;363(13):1256–64. https://doi.org/10.1056/NEJMct1002402.
39. Eleff SM, Maruki Y, Monsein LH, Traystman RJ, Bryan RN, Koehler RC. Sodium, ATP, and intracellular pH transients during reversible complete ischemia of dog cerebrum. Stroke. 1991;22(2):233–41. https://doi.org/10.1161/01.str.22.2.233.
40. Gonzalez-Ibarra FP, Varon J, Lopez-Meza EG. Therapeutic hypothermia: critical review of the molecular mechanisms of action. Front Neurol. 2011;2:4. https://doi.org/10.3389/fneur.2011.00004.
41. Granger DN, Kvietys PR. Reperfusion injury and reactive oxygen species: the evolution of a concept. Redox Biol. 2015;6:524–51. https://doi.org/10.1016/j.redox.2015.08.020.
42. Han F, Da T, Riobo NA, Becker LB. Early mitochondrial dysfunction in electron transfer activity and reactive oxygen species generation after cardiac arrest. Crit Care Med. 2008;36(11 Suppl):S447–53. https://doi.org/10.1097/ccm.0b013e31818a8a51.
43. Patil KD, Halperin HR, Becker LB. Cardiac arrest: resuscitation and reperfusion. Circ Res. 2015;116(12):2041–9. https://doi.org/10.1161/CIRCRESAHA.116.304495.
44. Vaagenes P, Ginsberg M, Ebmeyer U, Ernster L, Fischer M, Gisvold SE, et al. Cerebral resuscitation from cardiac arrest: pathophysiologic mechanisms. Crit Care Med. 1996;24(2 Suppl):S57–68.
45. Kuffler DP. Maximizing neuroprotection: where do we stand? Ther Clin Risk Manag. 2012;8:185–94. https://doi.org/10.2147/TCRM.S16196.
46. Kuschner CE, Becker LB. Recent advances in personalizing cardiac arrest resuscitation. F1000Res. 2019;8:F1000 Faculty Rev-915. https://doi.org/10.12688/f1000research.17554.1.
47. Varon J, Marik PE, Einav S. Therapeutic hypothermia: a state-of-the-art emergency medicine perspective. Am J Emerg Med. 2012;30(5):800–10. https://doi.org/10.1016/j.ajem.2011.03.007.

48. Zipfel GJ, Babcock DJ, Lee JM, Choi DW. Neuronal apoptosis after CNS injury: the roles of glutamate and calcium. J Neurotrauma. 2000;17(10):857–69. https://doi.org/10.1089/neu.2000.17.857.
49. Small DL, Morley P, Buchan AM. Biology of ischemic cerebral cell death. Prog Cardiovasc Dis. 1999;42(3):185–207.
50. Yenari MA, Han HS. Neuroprotective mechanisms of hypothermia in brain ischaemia. Nat Rev Neurosci. 2012;13(4):267–78. https://doi.org/10.1038/nrn3174.
51. Hurst S, Hoek J, Sheu SS. Mitochondrial Ca(2+) and regulation of the permeability transition pore. J Bioenerg Biomembr. 2017;49(1):27–47. https://doi.org/10.1007/s10863-016-9672-x.
52. Honda HM, Korge P, Weiss JN. Mitochondria and ischemia/reperfusion injury. Ann N Y Acad Sci. 2005;1047:248–58. https://doi.org/10.1196/annals.1341.022.
53. Arun S, Liu L, Donmez G. Mitochondrial biology and neurological diseases. Curr Neuropharmacol. 2016;14(2):143–54.
54. Jung JE, Kim GS, Chen H, Maier CM, Narasimhan P, Song YS, et al. Reperfusion and neurovascular dysfunction in stroke: from basic mechanisms to potential strategies for neuroprotection. Mol Neurobiol. 2010;41(2–3):172–9. https://doi.org/10.1007/s12035-010-8102-z.
55. Brennan AM, Suh SW, Won SJ, Narasimhan P, Kauppinen TM, Lee H, et al. NADPH oxidase is the primary source of superoxide induced by NMDA receptor activation. Nat Neurosci. 2009;12(7):857–63. https://doi.org/10.1038/nn.2334.
56. Globus MY, Busto R, Lin B, Schnippering H, Ginsberg MD. Detection of free radical activity during transient global ischemia and recirculation: effects of intraischemic brain temperature modulation. J Neurochem. 1995;65(3):1250–6. https://doi.org/10.1046/j.1471-4159.1995.65031250.x.
57. Li Y, Tang Q, Wang P, Qin J, Wu H, Lin J, et al. Dynamic changes of mitochondrial fusion and fission in brain injury after cardiac arrest in rats. Biomed Res Int. 2017;2017:1948070. https://doi.org/10.1155/2017/1948070.
58. Chavez LO, Leon M, Einav S, Varon J. Editor's choice- inside the cold heart: a review of therapeutic hypothermia cardioprotection. Eur Heart J Acute Cardiovasc Care. 2017;6(2):130–41. https://doi.org/10.1177/2048872615624242.
59. Walker AC, Johnson NJ. Targeted temperature management and postcardiac arrest care. Emerg Med Clin North Am. 2019;37(3):381–93. https://doi.org/10.1016/j.emc.2019.03.002.
60. Deakin CD, Nolan JP, Soar J, Sunde K, Koster RW, Smith GB, et al. European Resuscitation Council Guidelines for Resuscitation 2010 Section 4. Adult advanced life support. Resuscitation. 2010;81(10):1305–52. https://doi.org/10.1016/j.resuscitation.2010.08.017.
61. Colbourne F, Grooms SY, Zukin RS, Buchan AM, Bennett MV. Hypothermia rescues hippocampal CA1 neurons and attenuates down-regulation of the AMPA receptor GluR2 subunit after forebrain ischemia. Proc Natl Acad Sci U S A. 2003;100(5):2906–10. https://doi.org/10.1073/pnas.2628027100.
62. Liu L, Yenari MA. Therapeutic hypothermia: neuroprotective mechanisms. Front Biosci. 2007;12:816–25. https://doi.org/10.2741/2104.
63. Berger C, Schabitz WR, Wolf M, Mueller H, Sommer C, Schwab S. Hypothermia and brain-derived neurotrophic factor reduce glutamate synergistically in acute stroke. Exp Neurol. 2004;185(2):305–12. https://doi.org/10.1016/j.expneurol.2003.10.008.
64. Perman SM, Goyal M, Neumar RW, Topjian AA, Gaieski DF. Clinical applications of targeted temperature management. Chest. 2014;145(2):386–93. https://doi.org/10.1378/chest.12-3025.
65. Varon J. Therapeutic hypothermia: implications for acute care practitioners. Postgrad Med. 2010;122(1):19–27. https://doi.org/10.3810/pgm.2010.01.2095.
66. Staer-Jensen H, Sunde K, Olasveengen TM, Jacobsen D, Draegni T, Nakstad ER, et al. Bradycardia during therapeutic hypothermia is associated with good neurologic outcome in comatose survivors of out-of-hospital cardiac arrest. Crit Care Med. 2014;42(11):2401–8. https://doi.org/10.1097/CCM.0000000000000515.
67. Thomsen JH, Hassager C, Bro-Jeppesen J, Soholm H, Nielsen N, Wanscher M, et al. Sinus bradycardia during hypothermia in comatose survivors of out-of-hospital cardiac arrest—

a new early marker of favorable outcome? Resuscitation. 2015;89:36–42. https://doi.org/10.1016/j.resuscitation.2014.12.031.

68. Kiyosue T, Arita M, Muramatsu H, Spindler AJ, Noble D. Ionic mechanisms of action potential prolongation at low temperature in guinea-pig ventricular myocytes. J Physiol. 1993;468:85–106. https://doi.org/10.1113/jphysiol.1993.sp019761.
69. Lewis ME, Al-Khalidi AH, Townend JN, Coote J, Bonser RS. The effects of hypothermia on human left ventricular contractile function during cardiac surgery. J Am Coll Cardiol. 2002;39(1):102–8. https://doi.org/10.1016/s0735-1097(01)01694-1.
70. Frank SM, Satitpunwaycha P, Bruce SR, Herscovitch P, Goldstein DS. Increased myocardial perfusion and sympathoadrenal activation during mild core hypothermia in awake humans. Clin Sci (Lond). 2003;104(5):503–8. https://doi.org/10.1042/CS20020256.
71. Polderman KH, Herold I. Therapeutic hypothermia and controlled normothermia in the intensive care unit: practical considerations, side effects, and cooling methods. Crit Care Med. 2009;37(3):1101–20. https://doi.org/10.1097/CCM.0b013e3181962ad5.
72. Dobak S, Rincon F. "Cool" topic: feeding during moderate hypothermia after intracranial hemorrhage. JPEN J Parenter Enteral Nutr. 2017;41(7):1125–30. https://doi.org/10.1177/0148607116655448.
73. Williams ML, Nolan JP. Is enteral feeding tolerated during therapeutic hypothermia? Resuscitation. 2014;85(11):1469–72. https://doi.org/10.1016/j.resuscitation.2014.08.018.
74. Varon J, Acosta P. Coagulopathy during therapeutic hypothermia: where are the data? Resuscitation. 2009;80(7):726–7. https://doi.org/10.1016/j.resuscitation.2009.04.036.
75. Zeiner A, Holzer M, Sterz F, Behringer W, Schorkhuber W, Mullner M, et al. Mild resuscitative hypothermia to improve neurological outcome after cardiac arrest. A clinical feasibility trial. Hypothermia After Cardiac Arrest (HACA) Study Group. Stroke. 2000;31(1):86–94. https://doi.org/10.1161/01.str.31.1.86.
76. Nielsen N, Wetterslev J, Cronberg T, Erlinge D, Gasche Y, Hassager C, et al. Targeted temperature management at 33 degrees C versus 36 degrees C after cardiac arrest. N Engl J Med. 2013;369(23):2197–206. https://doi.org/10.1056/NEJMoa1310519.
77. Donnino MW, Andersen LW, Berg KM, Reynolds JC, Nolan JP, Morley PT, et al. Temperature management after cardiac arrest: an advisory statement by the advanced life support task force of the international liaison committee on resuscitation and the American heart association emergency cardiovascular care committee and the council on cardiopulmonary, critical care, perioperative and resuscitation. Circulation. 2015;132(25):2448–56. https://doi.org/10.1161/CIR.0000000000000313.
78. Part 7.5: postresuscitation support. Circulation. 2005;112(24_supplement):IV-84–IV-8. https://doi.org/10.1161/circulationaha.105.166560.
79. Morrison Laurie J, Deakin Charles D, Morley Peter T, Callaway Clifton W, Kerber Richard E, Kronick Steven L, et al. Part 8: advanced life support. Circulation. 2010;122(16_suppl_2):S345–421. https://doi.org/10.1161/circulationaha.110.971051.
80. Nichol G, Huszti E, Kim F, Fly D, Parnia S, Donnino M, et al. Does induction of hypothermia improve outcomes after in-hospital cardiac arrest? Resuscitation. 2013;84(5):620–5. https://doi.org/10.1016/j.resuscitation.2012.12.009.
81. Testori C, Sterz F, Behringer W, Haugk M, Uray T, Zeiner A, et al. Mild therapeutic hypothermia is associated with favourable outcome in patients after cardiac arrest with non-shockable rhythms. Resuscitation. 2011;82(9):1162–7. https://doi.org/10.1016/j.resuscitation.2011.05.022.
82. Dumas F, Grimaldi D, Zuber B, Fichet J, Charpentier J, Pene F, et al. Is hypothermia after cardiac arrest effective in both shockable and nonshockable patients?: insights from a large registry. Circulation. 2011;123(8):877–86. https://doi.org/10.1161/circulationaha.110.987347.
83. Vaahersalo J, Hiltunen P, Tiainen M, Oksanen T, Kaukonen KM, Kurola J, et al. Therapeutic hypothermia after out-of-hospital cardiac arrest in Finnish intensive care units: the FINNRESUSCI study. Intensive Care Med. 2013;39(5):826–37. https://doi.org/10.1007/s00134-013-2868-1.

84. Mader TJ, Nathanson BH, Soares WE 3rd, Coute RA, McNally BF. Comparative effectiveness of therapeutic hypothermia after out-of-hospital cardiac arrest: insight from a large data registry. Ther Hypothermia Temp Manag. 2014;4(1):21–31. https://doi.org/10.1089/ther.2013.0018.
85. Callaway CW, Donnino MW, Fink EL, Geocadin RG, Golan E, Kern KB, et al. Part 8: post-cardiac arrest care: 2015 American heart association guidelines update for cardiopulmonary resuscitation and emergency cardiovascular care. Circulation. 2015;132(18 Suppl 2):S465–82. https://doi.org/10.1161/CIR.0000000000000262.
86. Guterman EL, Kim AS, Josephson SA. Neurologic consultation and use of therapeutic hypothermia for cardiac arrest. Resuscitation. 2017;118:43–8. https://doi.org/10.1016/j.resuscitation.2017.06.025.
87. Kim F, Nichol G, Maynard C, Hallstrom A, Kudenchuk PJ, Rea T, et al. Effect of prehospital induction of mild hypothermia on survival and neurological status among adults with cardiac arrest: a randomized clinical trial. JAMA. 2014;311(1):45–52. https://doi.org/10.1001/jama.2013.282173.
88. Lyon RM, Van Antwerp J, Henderson C, Weaver A, Davies G, Lockey D. Prehospital intranasal evaporative cooling for out-of-hospital cardiac arrest: a pilot, feasibility study. Eur J Emerg Med. 2014;21(5):368–70. https://doi.org/10.1097/mej.0000000000000100.
89. Nie C, Dong J, Zhang P, Liu X, Han F. Prehospital therapeutic hypothermia after out-of-hospital cardiac arrest: a systematic review and meta-analysis. Am J Emerg Med. 2016;34(11):2209–16. https://doi.org/10.1016/j.ajem.2016.09.007.
90. Scales DC, Cheskes S, Verbeek PR, Pinto R, Austin D, Brooks SC, et al. Prehospital cooling to improve successful targeted temperature management after cardiac arrest: a randomized controlled trial. Resuscitation. 2017;121:187–94. https://doi.org/10.1016/j.resuscitation.2017.10.002.
91. Schenfeld EM, Studnek J, Heffner AC, Nussbaum M, Kraft K, Pearson DA. Effect of prehospital initiation of therapeutic hypothermia in adults with cardiac arrest on time-to-target temperature. CJEM. 2015;17(3):240–7. https://doi.org/10.2310/8000.2014.141307.
92. Uray T, Mayr FB, Stratil P, Aschauer S, Testori C, Sterz F, et al. Prehospital surface cooling is safe and can reduce time to target temperature after cardiac arrest. Resuscitation. 2015;87:51–6. https://doi.org/10.1016/j.resuscitation.2014.10.026.
93. Schenone AL, Cohen A, Patarroyo G, Harper L, Wang X, Shishehbor MH, et al. Therapeutic hypothermia after cardiac arrest: a systematic review/meta-analysis exploring the impact of expanded criteria and targeted temperature. Resuscitation. 2016;108:102–10. https://doi.org/10.1016/j.resuscitation.2016.07.238.
94. Surani S, Varon J. The expanded use of targeted temperature management: time for reappraisal. Resuscitation. 2016;108:A8–9. https://doi.org/10.1016/j.resuscitation.2016.09.002.
95. Patel PV, John S, Garg RK, Temes RE, Bleck TP, Prabhakaran S. Therapeutic hypothermia after cardiac arrest is underutilized in the United States. Ther Hypothermia Temp Manag. 2011;1(4):199–203. https://doi.org/10.1089/ther.2011.0015.
96. Jena AB, Romley JA, Newton-Cheh C, Noseworthy P. Therapeutic hypothermia for cardiac arrest: real-world utilization trends and hospital mortality. J Hosp Med. 2012;7(9):684–9. https://doi.org/10.1002/jhm.1974.
97. Dresden SM, O'Connor LM, Pearce CG, Courtney DM, Powell ES. National trends in the use of postcardiac arrest therapeutic hypothermia and hospital factors influencing its use. Ther Hypothermia Temp Manag. 2015;5(1):48–54. https://doi.org/10.1089/ther.2014.0023.
98. Morrison LJ, Brooks SC, Dainty KN, Dorian P, Needham DM, Ferguson ND, et al. Improving use of targeted temperature management after out-of-hospital cardiac arrest: a stepped wedge cluster randomized controlled trial. Crit Care Med. 2015;43(5):954–64. https://doi.org/10.1097/CCM.0000000000000864.
99. Varon J, Acosta P. Therapeutic hypothermia use among health care providers in 2 developing countries. Am J Emerg Med. 2008;26(2):244. https://doi.org/10.1016/j.ajem.2007.05.025.

100. Guluma KZ, Hemmen TM, Olsen SE, Rapp KS, Lyden PD. A trial of therapeutic hypothermia via endovascular approach in awake patients with acute ischemic stroke: methodology. Acad Emerg Med. 2006;13(8):820–7. https://doi.org/10.1197/j.aem.2006.03.559.
101. Geurts M, Petersson J, Brizzi M, Olsson-Hau S, Luijckx GJ, Algra A, et al. COOLIST (cooling for ischemic stroke trial): a multicenter, open, randomized, phase II. Clin Trial Strok. 2017;48(1):219–21. https://doi.org/10.1161/STROKEAHA.116.014757.
102. Kurisu K, Yenari MA. Therapeutic hypothermia for ischemic stroke; pathophysiology and future promise. Neuropharmacology. 2018;134(Pt B):302–9. https://doi.org/10.1016/j.neuropharm.2017.08.025.
103. Fox JL, Vu EN, Doyle-Waters M, Brubacher JR, Abu-Laban R, Hu Z. Prophylactic hypothermia for traumatic brain injury: a quantitative systematic review. CJEM. 2010;12(4):355–64.
104. Varon J, Marik PE. Complete neurological recovery following delayed initiation of hypothermia in a victim of warm water near-drowning. Resuscitation. 2006;68(3):421–3. https://doi.org/10.1016/j.resuscitation.2005.07.020.
105. Jacobs SE, Berg M, Hunt R, Tarnow-Mordi WO, Inder TE, Davis PG. Cooling for newborns with hypoxic ischaemic encephalopathy. Cochrane Database Syst Rev. 2013;(1):CD003311. https://doi.org/10.1002/14651858.CD003311.pub3.
106. Rose C, Michalak A, Pannunzio M, Chatauret N, Rambaldi A, Butterworth RF. Mild hypothermia delays the onset of coma and prevents brain edema and extracellular brain glutamate accumulation in rats with acute liver failure. Hepatology. 2000;31(4):872–7. https://doi.org/10.1053/he.2000.5923.
107. Vaquero J, Rose C, Butterworth RF. Keeping cool in acute liver failure: rationale for the use of mild hypothermia. J Hepatol. 2005;43(6):1067–77. https://doi.org/10.1016/j.jhep.2005.05.039.
108. Stravitz RT, Lee WM, Kramer AH, Kramer DJ, Hynan L, Blei AT. Therapeutic hypothermia for acute liver failure: toward a randomized, controlled trial in patients with advanced hepatic encephalopathy. Neurocrit Care. 2008;9(1):90–6. https://doi.org/10.1007/s12028-008-9090-y.
109. Villar J, Slutsky AS. Effects of induced hypothermia in patients with septic adult respiratory distress syndrome. Resuscitation. 1993;26(2):183–92. https://doi.org/10.1016/0300-9572(93)90178-s.
110. Madden LK, Hill M, May TL, Human T, Guanci MM, Jacobi J, et al. The implementation of targeted temperature management: an evidence-based guideline from the neurocritical care society. Neurocrit Care. 2017;27(3):468–87. https://doi.org/10.1007/s12028-017-0469-5.
111. Che D, Li L, Kopil CM, Liu Z, Guo W, Neumar RW. Impact of therapeutic hypothermia onset and duration on survival, neurologic function, and neurodegeneration after cardiac arrest. Crit Care Med. 2011;39(6):1423–30. https://doi.org/10.1097/CCM.0b013e318212020a.
112. Kuboyama K, Safar P, Radovsky A, Tisherman SA, Stezoski SW, Alexander H. Delay in cooling negates the beneficial effect of mild resuscitative cerebral hypothermia after cardiac arrest in dogs: a prospective, randomized study. Crit Care Med. 1993;21(9):1348–58. https://doi.org/10.1097/00003246-199309000-00019.
113. Cabanas JG, Brice JH, De Maio VJ, Myers B, Hinchey PR. Field-induced therapeutic hypothermia for neuroprotection after out-of hospital cardiac arrest: a systematic review of the literature. J Emerg Med. 2011;40(4):400–9. https://doi.org/10.1016/j.jemermed.2010.07.002.
114. Bernard SA, Smith K, Finn J, Hein C, Grantham H, Bray JE, et al. Induction of therapeutic hypothermia during out-of-hospital cardiac arrest using a rapid infusion of cold saline: the RINSE Trial (Rapid Infusion of Cold Normal Saline). Circulation. 2016;134(11):797–805. https://doi.org/10.1161/circulationaha.116.021989.
115. Kirkegaard H, Soreide E, de Haas I, Pettila V, Taccone FS, Arus U, et al. Targeted temperature management for 48 vs 24 hours and neurologic outcome after out-of-hospital cardiac arrest: a randomized clinical trial. JAMA. 2017;318(4):341–50. https://doi.org/10.1001/jama.2017.8978.

116. Callaway CW. Targeted temperature management after cardiac arrest: finding the right dose for critical care interventions. JAMA. 2017;318(4):334–6. https://doi.org/10.1001/jama.2017.8977.
117. Vaity C, Al-Subaie N, Cecconi M. Cooling techniques for targeted temperature management post-cardiac arrest. Crit Care. 2015;19:103. https://doi.org/10.1186/s13054-015-0804-1.
118. Fukuda T. Targeted temperature management for adult out-of-hospital cardiac arrest: current concepts and clinical applications. J Intensive Care. 2016;4:30. https://doi.org/10.1186/s40560-016-0139-2.
119. Glover GW, Thomas RM, Vamvakas G, Al-Subaie N, Cranshaw J, Walden A, et al. Intravascular versus surface cooling for targeted temperature management after out-of-hospital cardiac arrest—an analysis of the TTM trial data. Crit Care. 2016;20(1):381. https://doi.org/10.1186/s13054-016-1552-6.
120. Tommasi E, Lazzeri C, Bernardo P, Sori A, Chiostri M, Gensini GF, et al. Cooling techniques in mild hypothermia after cardiac arrest. J Cardiovasc Med (Hagerstown). 2017;18(7):459–66. https://doi.org/10.2459/JCM.0000000000000130.
121. Sonder P, Janssens GN, Beishuizen A, Henry CL, Rittenberger JC, Callaway CW, et al. Efficacy of different cooling technologies for therapeutic temperature management: a prospective intervention study. Resuscitation. 2018;124:14–20. https://doi.org/10.1016/j.resuscitation.2017.12.026.
122. Coppler PJ, Marill KA, Okonkwo DO, Shutter LA, Dezfulian C, Rittenberger JC, et al. Concordance of brain and core temperature in comatose patients after cardiac arrest. Ther Hypothermia Temp Manag. 2016;6(4):194–7. https://doi.org/10.1089/ther.2016.0010.
123. Akata T, Setoguchi H, Shirozu K, Yoshino J. Reliability of temperatures measured at standard monitoring sites as an index of brain temperature during deep hypothermic cardiopulmonary bypass conducted for thoracic aortic reconstruction. J Thorac Cardiovasc Surg. 2007;133(6):1559–65. https://doi.org/10.1016/j.jtcvs.2006.11.031.
124. Stone JG, Young WL, Smith CR, Solomon RA, Wald A, Ostapkovich N, et al. Do standard monitoring sites reflect true brain temperature when profound hypothermia is rapidly induced and reversed? Anesthesiology. 1995;82(2):344–51. https://doi.org/10.1097/00000542-199502000-00004.
125. Markota A, Palfy M, Stozer A, Sinkovic A. Difference between bladder and esophageal temperatures in mild induced hypothermia. J Emerg Med. 2015;49(1):98–103. https://doi.org/10.1016/j.jemermed.2014.12.059.
126. Zweifler RM, Voorhees ME, Mahmood MA, Parnell M. Rectal temperature reflects tympanic temperature during mild induced hypothermia in nonintubated subjects. J Neurosurg Anesthesiol. 2004;16(3):232–5.
127. McIlvoy L. Comparison of brain temperature to core temperature: a review of the literature. J Neurosci Nurs. 2004;36(1):23–31.
128. Cabanac M, Germain M, Brinnel H. Tympanic temperatures during hemiface cooling. Eur J Appl Physiol Occup Physiol. 1987;56(5):534–9. https://doi.org/10.1007/bf00635366.
129. Lopez M, Sessler DI, Walter K, Emerick T, Ozaki M. Rate and gender dependence of the sweating, vasoconstriction, and shivering thresholds in humans. Anesthesiology. 1994;80(4):780–8. https://doi.org/10.1097/00000542-199404000-00009.
130. Choi HA, Ko SB, Presciutti M, Fernandez L, Carpenter AM, Lesch C, et al. Prevention of shivering during therapeutic temperature modulation: the Columbia anti-shivering protocol. Neurocrit Care. 2011;14(3):389–94. https://doi.org/10.1007/s12028-010-9474-7.
131. Howes D, Gray SH, Brooks SC, Boyd JG, Djogovic D, Golan E, et al. Canadian Guidelines for the use of targeted temperature management (therapeutic hypothermia) after cardiac arrest: a joint statement from The Canadian Critical Care Society (CCCS), Canadian Neurocritical Care Society (CNCCS), and the Canadian Critical Care Trials Group (CCCTG). Resuscitation. 2016;98:48–63. https://doi.org/10.1016/j.resuscitation.2015.07.052.

132. Rubeiz GJ, Thill-Baharozian M, Hardie D, Carlson RW. Association of hypomagnesemia and mortality in acutely ill medical patients. Crit Care Med. 1993;21(2):203–9. https://doi.org/10.1097/00003246-199302000-00010.
133. Chernow B, Bamberger S, Stoiko M, Vadnais M, Mills S, Hoellerich V, et al. Hypomagnesemia in patients in postoperative intensive care. Chest. 1989;95(2):391–7. https://doi.org/10.1378/chest.95.2.391.
134. Arrich J, European Resuscitation Council Hypothermia After Cardiac Arrest Registry Study G. Clinical application of mild therapeutic hypothermia after cardiac arrest. Crit Care Med. 2007;35(4):1041–7. https://doi.org/10.1097/01.CCM.0000259383.48324.35.
135. Zhu SZ, Gu Y, Wu Z, Hu YF, Pan SY. Hypothermia followed by rapid rewarming exacerbates ischemia-induced brain injury and augments inflammatory response in rats. Biochem Biophys Res Commun. 2016;474(1):175–81. https://doi.org/10.1016/j.bbrc.2016.04.095.
136. Naito H, Isotani E, Callaway CW, Hagioka S, Morimoto N. Intracranial pressure increases during rewarming period after mild therapeutic hypothermia in postcardiac arrest patients. Ther Hypothermia Temp Manag. 2016;6(4):189–93. https://doi.org/10.1089/ther.2016.0009.
137. Bro-Jeppesen J, Annborn M, Hassager C, Wise MP, Pelosi P, Nielsen N, et al. Hemodynamics and vasopressor support during targeted temperature management at 33 degrees C Versus 36 degrees C after out-of-hospital cardiac arrest: a post hoc study of the target temperature management trial*. Crit Care Med. 2015;43(2):318–27. https://doi.org/10.1097/CCM.0000000000000691.
138. Bro-Jeppesen J, Hassager C, Wanscher M, Soholm H, Thomsen JH, Lippert FK, et al. Post-hypothermia fever is associated with increased mortality after out-of-hospital cardiac arrest. Resuscitation. 2013;84(12):1734–40. https://doi.org/10.1016/j.resuscitation.2013.07.023.
139. Winters SA, Wolf KH, Kettinger SA, Seif EK, Jones JS, Bacon-Baguley T. Assessment of risk factors for post-rewarming "rebound hyperthermia" in cardiac arrest patients undergoing therapeutic hypothermia. Resuscitation. 2013;84(9):1245–9. https://doi.org/10.1016/j.resuscitation.2013.03.027.
140. Monsieurs KG, Nolan JP, Bossaert LL, Greif R, Maconochie IK, Nikolaou NI, et al. European Resuscitation Council Guidelines for Resuscitation 2015: section 1. Executive summary. Resuscitation. 2015;95:1–80. https://doi.org/10.1016/j.resuscitation.2015.07.038.
141. Karcioglu O, Topacoglu H, Dikme O, Dikme O. A systematic review of safety and adverse effects in the practice of therapeutic hypothermia. Am J Emerg Med. 2018;36(10):1886–94. https://doi.org/10.1016/j.ajem.2018.07.024.
142. Saigal S, Sharma JP, Dhurwe R, Kumar S, Gurjar M. Targeted temperature management: current evidence and practices in critical care. Indian J Crit Care Med. 2015;19(9):537–46. https://doi.org/10.4103/0972-5229.164806.
143. Geurts M, Macleod MR, Kollmar R, Kremer PH, van der Worp HB. Therapeutic hypothermia and the risk of infection: a systematic review and meta-analysis. Crit Care Med. 2014;42(2):231–42. https://doi.org/10.1097/CCM.0b013e3182a276e8.
144. Kurz A, Sessler DI, Lenhardt R. Perioperative normothermia to reduce the incidence of surgical-wound infection and shorten hospitalization. Study of Wound Infection and Temperature Group. N Engl J Med. 1996;334(19):1209–15. https://doi.org/10.1056/nejm199605093341901.
145. Liu YM, Ibrahim A, Jan T, Chang P, Fagan S, Goverman J. Skin necrosis as a complication of therapeutic hypothermia. J Burn Care Res. 2014;35(3):e184–e6. https://doi.org/10.1097/BCR.0b013e3182a22730.
146. Polderman KH, Varon J. Interpreting the results of the targeted temperature management trial in cardiac arrest. Ther Hypothermia Temp Manag. 2015;5(2):73–6. https://doi.org/10.1089/ther.2014.0031.
147. Stub D. Targeted temperature management after cardiac arrest. N Engl J Med. 2014;370(14):1358. https://doi.org/10.1056/NEJMc1401250.
148. Varon J, Polderman K. Targeted temperature management after cardiac arrest. N Engl J Med. 2014;370(14):1358–9. https://doi.org/10.1056/NEJMc1401250.

149. Lascarrou J-B, Merdji H, Le Gouge A, Colin G, Grillet G, Girardie P, et al. Targeted temperature management for cardiac arrest with nonshockable rhythm. N Engl J Med. 2019;381(24):2327–37. https://doi.org/10.1056/NEJMoa1906661.
150. Cariou A, Payen JF, Asehnoune K, Audibert G, Botte A, Brissaud O, et al. Targeted temperature management in the ICU: guidelines from a French expert panel. Ann Intensive Care. 2017;7(1):70. https://doi.org/10.1186/s13613-017-0294-1.
151. Stratil P, Holzer M. Is hypothermia indicated during cardiopulmonary resuscitation and after restoration of spontaneous circulation? Curr Opin Crit Care. 2016;22(3):212–7. https://doi.org/10.1097/mcc.0000000000000299.

# 18 Progress in Clinical Application of Subcutaneous Implantable Cardioverter Defibrillator in Patients Who Suffer Sudden Cardiac Death

Wei Hua, Yiran Hu, Nixiao Zhang, Xi Liu, and Minsi Cai


**Abstract**

Subcutaneous implantable cardioverter defibrillator (S-ICD) is an important alternative treatment for traditional implantable cardioverter defibrillator (ICD) patients, especially for those who are not suitable for intravenous access (such as patients with venous anatomical abnormalities and with high risk of infection and those who underwent mechanical tricuspid valve replacement). In addition, it has obvious advantages for young patients with a long-expected survival time who may need to replace the defibrillation lead repeatedly. So, its status in prevention of sudden cardiac death (SCD) continues to rise. At present, the number of implantation of S-ICD in European and American countries has exceeded 60,000, while in China, there are less than 100, which shows a huge gap. As the results of IDE and EFFORTLESS studies revealed, the effectiveness and safety of S-ICD have been proved. Nowadays, the clinical studies of S-ICD mainly focus on primary prevention of SCD. However, the inability to provide long-term pacing function and a relative short battery life are still the major disadvantages restricting the further expansion of the clinical application of S-ICD. With the rapid development of science and technology, the fourth generation of S-ICD compatible with the leadless pacemaker is being rapidly developed, which is expected to solve the above problems. It is believed that in the near future, S-ICD with small size, long life span, and stable pacing function will show great clinical value in preventing sudden cardiac death.



W. Hua (✉) · Y. Hu · N. Zhang · X. Liu · M. Cai
The Cardiac Arrhythmia Center, State Key Laboratory of Cardiovascular Disease, National Clinical Research Center of Cardiovascular Diseases, Fuwai Hospital, National Center for Cardiovascular Diseases, Chinese Academy of Medical Sciences and Peking Union Medical College, Beijing, China
e-mail: drhua@vip.sina.com





H. Zhu (ed.), *Sudden Death*, https://doi.org/10.1007/978-981-15-7002-5_18

**Keywords**

Subcutaneous implantable cardioverter defibrillator · Sudden cardiac death · Progress

The application of implantable cardioverter defibrillator (ICD) has gained great breakthroughs in primary and secondary prevention for sudden cardiac death (SCD) patients, which is better than drug therapy especially in treating malignant ventricular arrhythmia, showing a great reduction in mortality [1–4]. However, clinical application of ICD with intravenous access has been found to face a series of intractable problems, such as anatomical abnormalities of the subclavian vein or superior vena cava, abrasion and fracture of defibrillation leads, lead-related infection, and thrombosis [5–7]. Although implanting electrode by epicardial access or pericardial window treatment can avoid the complications caused by intravenous access, it is still limited due to the big trauma and low success rate [4]. So, subcutaneous implantable cardioverter defibrillator (S-ICD) arises at this moment, for its defibrillation leads and pulse generator are buried in subcutaneous pocket, not directly in contact with the heart and related vein, which can effectively avoid the lead-related complications [1]. This chapter introduces the latest development of subcutaneous implantable cardioverter defibrillator in the clinical application of sudden cardiac death.

## 18.1 Real-World Applications

The S-ICD (Fig. 18.1) consists of a pulse generator and electrodes with defibrillation coils. Pulse generator is buried under the junction between the fifth rib and the midaxillary line; by establishing a connection to the pocket horizontal tunnel with the longitudinal tunnel located near the sternum, the defibrillation electrode is implanted, which is solid and can tolerate external pressure [1, 7]. The proximal electrode is always located near the xiphoid, while the distal electrode is usually located close to the supraclavicular fossa. Under general or local anesthesia, S-ICD can be implanted only according to the anatomical landmarks on the body surface, and no X-ray fluoroscopy is needed during the implantation process, thus avoiding X-ray damage and lead-related complications [5, 6, 8].

The first attempt of S-ICD in human was in 2002. Clinical trials of S-ICD were subsequently approved in 2008 and certified by the European Union in 2009 [1]. The application of S-ICD was approved by the Food and Drug Administration (FDA) in 2012 [4]. The first-generation S-ICD (SQ-RX™) has a volume of 69 cc and a thickness of 15.7 mm. The pulse generator is expected to have a life span of 5.1 years. In 2015, the second-generation S-ICD (EMBLEM™ model: A209) came to the market with a further reduction in volume and thickness (12.7 mm), an increase in the expected life span of the pulse generation to 7.3 years (real world LATITUDE™ data showed an average life span of 8.7 years), an increase in

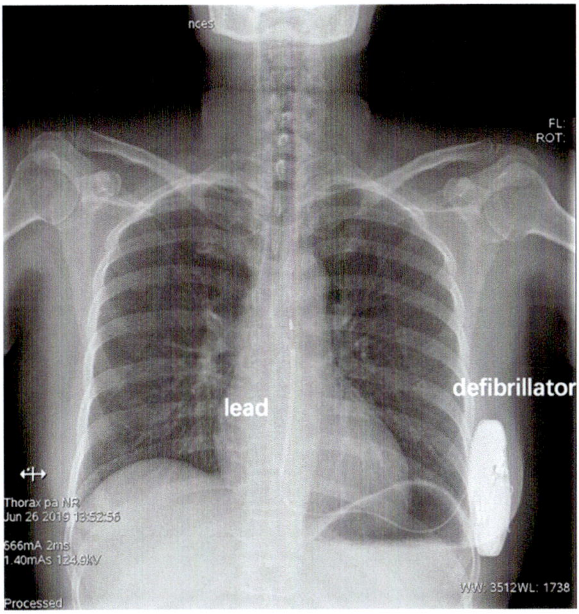


**Fig. 18.1** X-ray of S-ICD

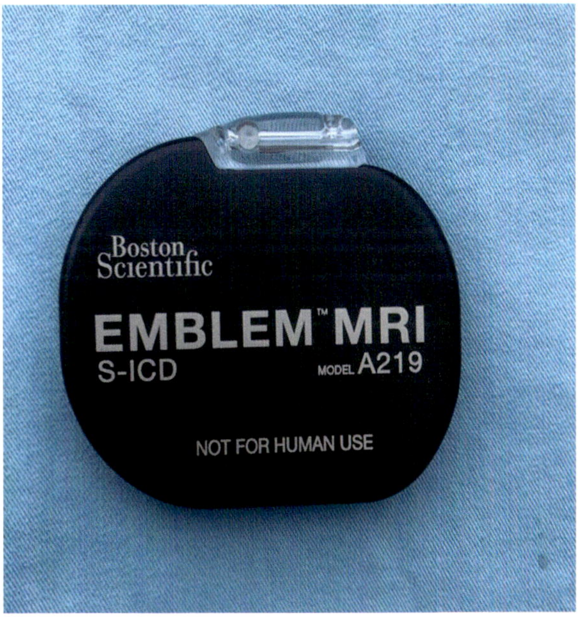


**Fig. 18.2** The third generation of S-ICD (model: A219)

ImageReady™ technology which is full body compatible w1.5T MRI, and an increase in SMART Pass™ technology which reduces 82% T wave oversensing [9, 10]. The third-generation S-ICD (EMBLEM™ model: A219) (Fig. 18.2) added AF Monitor™ monitoring function on the basis of the second generation. At present, the clinical application of the third-generation S-ICD has been carried out in Europe,

America, and other countries, while China's CFDA has not approved it, only allowing its application in Hainan Boao Medical Pilot Zone.

Currently, America and Europe hold the lead in the number of S-ICD implantation, with more than 60,000 [1, 11]. In China, the application is relatively late. On December 23, 2014, Professor Wei Hua and Professor Shu Zhang completed the first implantation of the first-generation S-ICD in China. By July 2019, 95 S-ICDs have been implanted in China.

## 18.2 The Latest Clinical Research on S-ICD

### 18.2.1 The UNTOUCHED Study

The UNTOUCHED Study: the effect of S-ICD for primary prevention in patients with low left ventricular ejection fraction (LVEF) heart failure [12].

The therapeutic effect of S-ICD for primary prevention in patients with low LVEF heart failure was presented at the 2019 Heart Rhythm Society Annual Scientific Sessions. The UNTOUCHED Study is a global, multi-site, prospective, nonrandomized study. The inclusion criteria were the following: (1) patients had LVEF of 35% or less and were indicated for an ICD for primary prevention of sudden cardiac death (SCD), and (2) patients passed the screening for S-ICD. The exclusion criteria included: (1) patients had prior sustained ventricular tachycardia (VT) or ventricular fibrillation (VF); (2) patients had indications for cardiac pacing; and (3) patients had advanced heart failure (HF) and renal failure. The primary endpoints were the efficacy of defibrillation and the complications within 30 days post-operation.

From June 2015 to April 2018, a total of 1173 patients at 110 sites were enrolled, of whom 1103 patients were finally followed up and included in the final analysis. The UNTOUCHED study showed that the mean implant time was 55.8 min, and the S-ICD therapy had a 95.8% complication-free rate at 30 days post-operation, with most complications occurring either during the operation or in the first 24 h, and had an up to 99.2% conversion efficacy of induced VF. The S-ICD terminated VF with a successful defibrillation testing (DFT) at ≤65 joule (J) shock in over 90% of the patients, and a >65 J shock was successful in 52 patients (5.7%). Lower body mass index (BMI) (OR, 0.94, 95% CI 0.91–0.98, $P = 0.002$) and presence of diabetes (OR, 2.4, 95% CI 1.1–5.2, $P = 0.03$) were predictors of DFT success ≤65 J.

Therefore, S-ICD therapy has low perioperative complication rates and high conversion efficacy of induced VT/VF in DFT for low LVEF patients. This established the application of S-ICD in the primary prevention of SCD in such kind of patients.

### 18.2.2 The PRAETORIAN Score Study

The PRAETORIAN Score Study: a novel tool to evaluate the implant position and predict defibrillation success of the S-ICD [13].

The PRAETORIAN score which is recently published in the *HeartRhythm* journal is based on clinical and computer modeling knowledge of factors affecting the DF: sub-coil fat, sub-generator fat, and anterior positioning of the S-ICD generator.

The score has three categories: 30–89 points presenting a low risk, 90–149 points presenting an intermediate risk, and ≥ 150 points representing a high risk of defibrillation failure. The scoring model consisted of 181 S-ICD subjects, and the validation cohort included 321 patients. The results showed that the negative predictive value of patients with low PRAETORIAN score was 99.8%, and the positive predictive value of patients with an intermediate or high PRAETORIAN score was 51%.

The PRAETORIAN score allows to identify patients at high risk of high threshold value by routine chest X-ray examination as well as to provide feedback on which element of the implant contributes to the high risk of DF failure. However, it should be validated by further RCT studies.

### 18.2.3 MADIT S-ICD Trial

In post-myocardial infarction (MI), diabetes patients with a relatively preserved EF of 36–50%, will S-ICD benefit the survival? [14].

Post-MI patients with diabetes have significant risk for SCD even with a relatively preserved LVEF. Therefore, this study allows to determine whether S-ICD in these patients will significantly reduce all-cause mortality in comparison with conventional medical treatment. The inclusion criteria were (1) age ≥ 65 years, (2) diabetes mellitus, (3) an LVEF of 36–50%, and (4) one or more clinically documented, enzyme-positive MIs more than 3 months. The eligible patients were randomized to receive conventional medical therapy plus an S-ICD or conventional medical therapy alone in a 2:1 ratio. The primary endpoint was death.

A total of 1800 subjects will be recruited, and the first patient was enrolled on April 17, 2017. The research is ongoing and the results are expected to be published.

### 18.2.4 The Preliminary Clinical Application of S-ICD in China

From December 23, 2014, to December 31, 2016, 12 patients with successful S-ICD implants at nine centers in China were continuously enrolled. There were nine males (75%) aged 35–78 (51.9 ± 15.5) years. The implant time was 70–120 (93.3 ± 18.7) min, the shock impedance was 57–103 (70 ± 15.4) Ω, and the time from diagnosis to therapy was 12–30 (16.4 ± 5.0) s. Moreover, no severe complications occurred during the operation. This study is the first to present the experience and clinical data of the initial application of S-ICD in the mainland of China as well as to provide the evidence-based concept for further popularizing the clinical performance of S-ICD in the future.

### 18.2.5 The Study of "Prospective S-ICD Register in an Asian Population"

This study, led by professor Hung-Fat Tse of Queen Mary Hospital, The University of Hong Kong, which is the latest research on S-ICD in Asia, aims to explore the long-term safety and feasibility of S-ICD in an Asian population with smaller body build. Professor Wei Hua from China participated as a co-researcher. This study was initiated in May 2017 and is actively in progress.

## 18.3 Updated S-ICD Recommendations

S-ICD was first mentioned in the 2015 ESC Guidelines to be an alternative treatment for intravenous ICD, and it was considered as Class I recommendation in 2017 AHA/ACC/HRS guidelines [11, 15]. The S-ICD recommendations were listed in Table 18.1.

## 18.4 Limitations of S-ICD in Clinical Practice

### 18.4.1 The Lack of Function for Pacing and Antitachycardia Pacing (ATP)

Devices with traditional transvenous approach implantation have functions of defibrillation which can prevent sudden cardiac death, pacing, and cardiac resynchronization therapy. S-ICD lacks the latter two, limiting the application of ATP among patients who need pacing [16, 17]. Compared with ATP, shock will predispose to higher mortality and lower quality of life of patients. The PainFREE Rx II study found that ATP treatment for rapid ventricular tachycardia based on experience is as

**Table 18.1** Updated recommendations for S-ICD

| Recommendations | Class | Level |
|---|---|---|
| *2015 ESC guidelines for the management of patients with ventricular arrhythmia and the prevention of SCD* | | |
| S-ICD should be considered as an alternative to transvenous defibrillators in patients with an indication for an ICD when pacing therapy for bradycardia support, cardiac resynchronization, or antitachycardia pacing is not needed | IIa | C |
| S-ICD may be considered as a useful alternative to the transvenous ICD system when venous access is difficult, after the removal of a transvenous ICD for infections or in young patients with a long-term need for ICD therapy | IIb | C |
| *2017 AHA/ACC/HRS guidelines for the management of patients with ventricular arrhythmia and the prevention of SCD* | | |
| In patients who meet the criteria for an ICD who have inadequate vascular access or are at high risk for infection, and in whom pacing for bradycardia or VT termination or as part of CRT is neither needed nor anticipated, an S-ICD is recommended | I | B-NR |
| In patients who meet indications for an ICD, implantation of an S-ICD is reasonable if pacing for bradycardia or VT termination or as part of CRT is neither needed nor anticipated | IIa | B-NR |

*S-ICD* subcutaneous implantable cardioverter defibrillator, *SCD* sudden cardiac death, *CRT* cardiac resynchronization therapy, *VT* ventricular tachycardia, *B-NR* moderate-quality evidence from 1 or more well-designed, well-executed nonrandomized studies, observational studies, or registry studies, from meta-analyses of such studies safe and efficacious as shock therapy [18]. Other studies have shown that a significant proportion of patients with ventricular tachycardia can return to sinus rhythm spontaneously before ATP and only 72% of them receive successful ATP [17]. The evidence indicates that a part of ATP treatment may not be necessary. Although S-ICD lacks ATP at the moment, there is no limitation on its use. Avoiding the implantation of S-ICD in patients with recurrent episodes of persistent monomorphic ventricular tachycardia can improve application effectiveness and security of S-ICD [2, 7].

### 18.4.2 Longevity

The replacement of implanted devices will increase the infection rate and the incidence of complications, so the longevity of pulse generator is an important issue to consider at implantation [1, 4]. The expected longevity of the first-generation S-ICD is about 5 years, and it is about 7.3 years for the second-generation S-ICD, which has not been confirmed in clinical practice. S-ICD will need more pulse generator replacement than traditional ICDs due to battery exhaustion, and future upgradation in prolonged longevity will hopefully improve this situation.

### 18.4.3 Prolonged Time to Shock

Extending detection time to wait for spontaneous termination of ventricular tachycardia or ventricular fibrillation will reduce unnecessary shock treatment and mortality as well [19]. The detection and charging time of S-ICD are longer than ICD, resulting in significant prolonged time to shock treatment (7.1 ± 1.6s vs. 14.6 ± 2.9s). The MADIT-RIT study also demonstrates that delayed treatment in detection zone with high rate ventricular tachycardia can significantly reduce inappropriate treatments and all-cause mortality [7, 11]. However, the prolonged time to shock treatment of S-ICD means a high risk of syncope or failure to terminate ventricular tachycardia in time via shock treatment, the pros and cons of which are still widely disputed [20].

## 18.5 Challenges from Extravascular ICD

In 2016, SPACE study has provided a new and feasible mechanism for S-ICD with pacing function by placing ICD electrodes underneath the sternum of 26 patients through non-venous approach [15]. Non-intravenous ICD (Extravascular ICD, EV-ICD)-related clinical trials have been highly valued by physicians for the device ability of avoiding complications from intravenous implantation, as well as the advantages of smaller size, longer battery life, and lower defibrillation thresholds.

The latest clinical findings of EV-ICD were presented at the 2019 HRS Annual Meeting. The EV-ICD study is the first long-term, prosperous, nonrandomized clinical trial in humans who meet the guideline Class I or IIa recommendations for ICD implantation. The defibrillation electrode was buried underneath the sternum under X-ray via an electrode insertion tool used for tunneling and pulse generator at the left midaxillary line. Defibrillation effectiveness was tested by defibrillation threshold test (DFT), and the energy of shock treatment is normally 20 J per single time or 30 J twice in a row. Follow-up is carried out at 2 weeks, 4–6 weeks, and 3 months after operation, including imaging data, outpatient interrogation data, ICD intracardiac electrogram, and pacing or sensing data. The primary endpoint of safety is surgical or device-related complications 3 months after surgery.

A total of 26 patients were included in the study, and 20 cases were successfully implanted with EV-ICD. The proportion of male patients was 81%, with an average LVEF of 43 ± 18%. There were 11 cases of nonischemic cardiomyopathy (52%) and six cases of hypertrophic cardiomyopathy. DFT for 17 patients (89.5%) successfully terminated the ventricular tachycardia with 30 J energy, and the median energy is 15 J (one patient with failed DFT during operation). In addition, the average pacing threshold was 5.1 ± 1.9 V, and the average R wave sensing was 3.2 ± 1.7 mV. No patients had surgery-related complications. Three-month follow-up shows that one patient has received inappropriate treatment, considering that it was related to P-wave oversensing due to improper position of the lead. Five patients with adverse events (two cases of incision swelling, one case of incision epidermal infection, two cases of respiratory-related pain) were given proper treatment.

EV-ICD study has proven the feasibility of ICD electrode implantation underneath the sternum and the efficacy of pacing and defibrillation treatment. Although limitation on sample size and short term follow-up exists, it provides new insight to improve S-ICD and conduct clinical trials with larger sample size.

## 18.6 Prospect of Clinical Application

S-ICD is an important alternative treatment for traditional SCD patients, especially for those who are not suitable for intravenous defibrillation leads [1, 21]. In addition, there are also many significant advantages for young people who need to replace leads repeatedly. However, the inability to provide long-term pacing function remains a major disadvantage limiting the further expansion of S-ICD [7]. It is believed that in the near future, S-ICD with small size, long life span, and stable pacing function will show great clinical value in preventing sudden cardiac death.

## References

1. Lewis GF, Gold MR. Clinical experience with subcutaneous implantable cardioverter-defibrillators. Nat Rev Cardiol. 2015;12:398–405.
2. Burke MC, Gold MR, Knight BP, et al. Safety and efficacy of the totally subcutaneous implantable defibrillator: 2-year results from a pooled analysis of the IDE study and effortless registry. J Am Coll Cardiol. 2015;65:1605–15.

3. Providência R, Kramer DB, Pimenta D, et al. Transvenous implantable cardioverter-defibrillator (ICD) lead performance: a meta-analysis of observational studies. J Am Heart Assoc. 2015;4:e002418.
4. Moss A, Zareba W, Hall W, et al. Multicenter automatic defibrillator implantation trial II investigators. Prophylactic implantation of a defibrillator in patients with myocardial infarction and reduced ejection fraction. N Engl J Med. 2002;346:877–83.
5. Knops RE, Brouwer TF, Barr CS, et al., IDE and EFFORTLESS investigators. The learning curve associated with the introduction of the subcutaneous implantable defibrillator. Europace. 2016;18:1010–1015.
6. Ellenbogen KA, Wood MA, Shepard RK, et al. Detection and management of an implantable cardioverter defibrillator lead failure: incidence and clinical implications. J Am Coll Cardiol. 2003;41:73–80.
7. Weiss R, Knight BP, Gold MR, et al. Safety and efficacy of a totally subcutaneous implantable-cardioverter defibrillator. Circulation. 2013;128:944–53.
8. Knops RE, Olde Nordkamp LR, de Groot JR, et al. Two-incision technique for implantation of the subcutaneous implantable cardioverter-defibrillator. Heart Rhythm. 2013;10:1240–3.
9. Theuns D, Brouwer TF, Jones PW, et al. Prospective blinded evaluation of a novel sensing methodology designed to reduce inappropriate shocks by the subcutaneous implantable cardioverter-defibrillator. Heart Rhythm. 2018;15:1515–22.
10. Stiles MK, Fauchier L, Morillo CA, Wilkoff BL. 2019 HRS/EHRA/APHRS/LAHRS focused update to 2015 expert consensus statement on optimal implantable cardioverter-defibrillator programming and testing. Heart Rhythm. 2020;17(1):E220–8. https://doi.org/10.1002/joa3.12178.
11. Priori SG, Blomstrom-Lundqvist C, Mazzanti A, et al. 2015 ESC Guidelines for the management of patients with ventricular arrhythmias and the prevention of sudden cardiac death: the Task Force for the management of patients with ventricular arrhythmias and the prevention of sudden cardiac death of the European Society of Cardiology (ESC)endorsed by: Association for European Paediatric and Congenital Cardiology (AEPC). Europace. 2015;17:1601–87.
12. Gold MR, Knops R, Burke MC, et al. The design of the understanding outcomes with the S-ICD in primary prevention patients with low EF study (UNTOUCHED). Pacing Clin Electrophysiol. 2017;40:1–8.
13. Quast ABE, Baalman SWE, Brouwer TF, et al. A novel tool to evaluate the implant position and predict defibrillation success of the subcutaneous implantable cardioverter-defibrillator: the PRAETORIAN score. Heart Rhythm. 2019;16:403–10.
14. Kutyifa V, Beck C, Brown MW, et al. Multicenter automatic defibrillator implantation trial-subcutaneous implantable cardioverter defibrillator (MADIT S-ICD): design and clinical protocol. Am Heart J. 2017;189:158–66.
15. Al-Khatib SM, Stevenson WG, Ackerman MJ, et al. 2017 AHA/ACC/HRS guideline for management of patients with ventricular arrhythmias and the prevention of sudden cardiac death: executive summary: a report of the American College of Cardiology/American Heart Association Task Force on Clinical Practice Guidelines and the Heart Rhythm Society. Heart Rhythm. 2018;15:e190–252.
16. Gold MR, Aasbo JD, El-Chami MF, et al. Subcutaneous implantable cardioverter-defibrillator post-approval study: clinical characteristics and perioperative results. Heart Rhythm. 2017;14:1456–63.
17. Boersma L, Barr C, Knops R, et al. Implant and midterm outcomes of the subcutaneous implantable cardioverter-defibrillator registry: the EFFORTLESS study. J Am Coll Cardiol. 2017;70:830–41.
18. Wathen MS, DeGroot PJ, Sweeney MO, et al., PainFREE Rx II Investigators. Prospective randomized multicenter trial of empirical anti-tachycardia pacing versus shocks for spontaneous rapid ventricular tachycardia in patients with implantable cardioverter-defibrillators: pacing fast ventricular tachycardia reduces shock therapies (PainFREE Rx II) trial results. Circulation. 2004;110:2591–2596.

19. Kirkfeldt RE, Johansen JB, Nohr EA, et al. Complications after cardiac implantable electronic device implantations: an analysis of a complete, nationwide cohort in Denmark. Eur Heart J. 2014;35:1186–94.
20. Olde Nordkamp LR, Brouwer TF, Barr C, et al. Inappropriate shocks in the subcutaneous ICD: incidence, predictors and management. Int J Cardiol. 2015;195:126–33.
21. Bardy GH, Smith WM, Hood MA, et al. An entirely subcutaneous implantable cardioverter-defibrillator. N Engl J Med. 2010;363:36–44.

# Part IV

# Sudden Non-cardiac Death

# Progress in Diagnosis and Treatment of Sudden Death Caused by Respiratory Diseases

19

Junfeng Chen, Yi Xu, Jiang Wang, and Guo Xin Mo

**Abstract**

Sudden death (SD) is the most serious condition in humans. The World Health Organization defined it as follows: "In an unexpectedly short period of time, a sudden death as a result of a natural illness is a sudden death in a patient who is usually in good health or appears to be in good health." Sudden death is mainly caused by cardiovascular diseases; because of the sudden onset, most of them occur outside the hospital. Respiratory diseases that cause sudden death occur from time to time. Common diseases include acute pulmonary embolism, asthma, acute respiratory distress syndrome (ARDS), etc. These diseases have the characteristics of rapid progress and rapid death, which pose a serious threat to human health. This chapter mainly describes the analysis of the sudden death caused by respiratory diseases and studies the latest progress in diagnosis and treatment. Early identification and treatment are of great significance to reduce mortality and thus save lives.

**Keywords**

Acute pulmonary embolism · Bronchial asthma · Respiratory diseases · Sudden death · Diagnosis and treatment

## 19.1 Bronchial Asthma and Sudden Death

### 19.1.1 Overview

Bronchial asthma is a heterogeneous disease characterized by chronic airway inflammation. This chronic inflammation leads to the occurrence and

J. Chen · Y. Xu · J. Wang · G. X. Mo (✉)
Department of Pulmonary & Critical Care Medicine, General Hospital of Chinese People's Liberation Army, Beijing, People's Republic of China





H. Zhu (ed.), *Sudden Death*, https://doi.org/10.1007/978-981-15-7002-5_19

development of airway hyperresponsiveness (AHR). A limitation of air flow is usually characterized by reversibility. The clinical manifestations are recurrent wheezing, shortness of breath, chest tightness, cough, and other symptoms. Symptoms and airflow limits vary with time and intensity. Exercise, allergen or irritant exposure, weather changes, or viral respiratory tract infection can be triggered. Sudden death from bronchial asthma is an important cause of death in patients with asthma. There are many risk factors, and acute severe attack of asthma threatens the lives of patients. There are refractory severe asthma, airway mucus embolism, depression, inappropriate drug use, and so on.

### 19.1.2 Epidemiology

In recent years, the prevalence rate of asthma has been increasing year by year all over the world, and the prevalence rate of asthma has increased year by year in various parts of the world. According to relevant reports [1], more than 300 million people worldwide suffer from asthma. The prevalence of asthma increased by 12.6% between 1990 and 2015 [2]. The latest survey data on asthma published in the *Lancet* led by Academician Wang Chen shows that the prevalence rate of asthma in Chinese adults aged ≥20 years old is 4.2%, and the prevalence rate of asthma increases with age [3]. Due to the continuous update of the "Global Asthma Prevention and Control Strategy Initiative" (GINA) program every year and the improvement of diagnosis and treatment methods and standardized treatment of asthma, the disease control and quality of life of patients with asthma were significantly improved. There are few longitudinal data on the incidence of asthma and the overall risk of death caused by asthma in young people [4]. But there are still cases of death from asthma, and some tragedies could not have happened. Of course, the reasons are complex and multifaceted. In the late 1980s, the number of asthma deaths in the United States was 4000 a year. In a Danish study [5], 625 sudden deaths were found in people aged 1–35 years old in Denmark between 2000 and 2006. Among them, 49 patients suffered from uncontrollable asthma, and in 31 cases (63%), the cause of death was sudden cardiac death, while 13 cases (27%) had fatal asthma attacks. In the past [6], it has been reported that of the 214 cases who died of asthma, except 30 cases who died within 1 hour of arriving at the hospital, the rest died within 1 h of arriving at the hospital, suggesting death caused by asthma. Most of them died suddenly after acute attack of asthma [7]. In a retrospective study of 19 patients who died of asthma in China, 16 cases died of acute attack of asthma at night, but because there was no systematic autopsy in sudden death cases, the direct or indirect cause of death of asthma was ignored. Understanding the various causes of death related to asthma can help to better understand the physiological and pathological mechanism of asthma. For patients with asthma-related death risk factors, they should go to the hospital as soon as possible, and we need to pay great attention to these patients.

### 19.1.3 Fatal Asthma

The death from fatal asthma occurs not only in patients with severe asthma but also in patients with mild and moderate asthma. Some patients with asthma may have an increased risk of sudden death during acute exacerbation. These patients are generally referred to as fatal asthma or near-fatal asthma patients [8]. Sudden death from asthma has the following characteristics: (1) endotracheal intubation and mechanical ventilation for respiratory failure caused by acute attack of asthma; (2) sudden acute attack or accompanied by hypoxemia, respiratory acidosis, and low respiratory peak flow rate; (3) under the control of long-term oral corticosteroids, with more than two or more emergency visits or hospitalization; (4) two times of asthma with mediastinal pneumothorax or pneumothorax; (5) excessive dependence on available β2 receptor agonists, especially in patients who use more than one dose of salbutamol (or equivalent drug) per month [9]; (6) presence of mental illness or psychosocial problems, including the use of sedatives; and (7) a history of noncompliance with asthma treatment plans and use of three or more types of asthma treatment measures.

### 19.1.4 Causes of Sudden Death from Asthma

#### 19.1.4.1 Severe Refractory Asthma (SRA)

In recent years, studies have found that the incidence, disability, and mortality of asthma are increasing year by year. According to ERS and ATS reports [10], severe refractory asthma accounts for 5–10% of patients with asthma. According to related reports, up to 60% of patients have increased tissue eosinophils and persistent severe eosinophil inflammation. Through the release of allergic mediators increased mucus secretion, release of interleukin-5 and leukotriene, etc., despite inhalation of high doses of glucocorticoid, symptoms could not be improved [11]. According to Mohamed et al. [12], vascular endothelial growth factor (VEGF) is considered to be the most important angiogenic factor, which induces the proliferation of vascular endothelial cells, forms tubules, and increases microvascular permeability. In the study, serum levels of angiopoietin-2 and VEGF were higher in patients with SRA than in healthy subjects, both of whom were involved in remodeling and angiogenesis in SRA, leading to resistance to inhaled steroids. After treatment, the symptoms cannot be effectively relieved.

#### 19.1.4.2 Increased Airway Responsiveness

Airway hyperresponsiveness and airway inflammation are the main pathophysiological features of asthma [13]. Mast cells, IgE, and TNF can induce allergic airway inflammation. When the patient receives the stimulator, the airway appears to contract too strongly or prematurely. In the provocation test of this kind of patients, the dose response curve of histamine $<0.1$ μmol was extremely steep and straight, and the significant decrease of FEV1 and the decrease of peak expiratory flow rate (PEFR) were observed [14].

#### 19.1.4.3 Diffuse Airway Mucus Embolism Caused by Coinfection

Airway inflammation and mucus hypersecretion are important characteristics of asthma. Due to abnormal airway mucus secretion and eosinophil infiltration, the probability of infection is increased. Edema and inflammatory cell infiltration lead to significant thickening of the basement membrane of the bronchial mucosa [15]. The airway stenosis caused by smooth muscle contraction is enhanced, which seriously leads to respiratory airflow limitation, insufficient ventilation, or airway occlusion [16], which aggravates the severity of asthma attack and sudden death [17]. Asthma mucus hypersecretion is produced by goblet cells and submucosal glands distributed along airway epithelium. The mechanisms include the proliferation and degranulation of secretory mucous cells, the microvascular remodeling and leakage, and the chemical attraction of inflammatory cells, especially the increase of goblet cells, which leads to a significant increase in mucus production [18]. The probability of infection is increased because of abnormal airway mucus secretion and eosinophil infiltration.

#### 19.1.4.4 Mental Depression

According to relevant reports, many patients often have depressive symptoms before their death as a result of repeated treatment without control, financial burden, and mental stress [19]. Anxiety and depression are the most common adverse emotions associated with asthma [20]. A multivariate analysis of 566 patients with asthma showed that more than one-third of the patients (202 cases, 35.69%) had combined anxiety and depressive disorders [21]. A study of more than 20,000 people in 41 states suggests that asthma patients have anxiety (23.5%) and depression (19.4%), compared with normal controls. The combined rates of anxiety and depression were 10.2% and 7.7%, respectively. In a life-threatening controlled study of asthma [22], 77 patients with severe life-threatening asthma (SLTA) were admitted to intensive care units. Two hundred thirty-nine patients in the control group were admitted to the general ward of asthma. Hospitalized patients with acute asthma (SLTA and hospital control) had higher prevalence of anxiety and depression and higher incidence of total life events. In these patients, the number of cholinergic receptors in fibroblasts increased, and the amount of cholinergic receptor protein also increased, which meant that cholinergic activity increased, which promoted asthma and sudden death. Patients with fatal asthma have a strong tendency to deny the disease. Denial emotion may pose a serious obstacle to inappropriate self-management strategies. Patients with a higher level of denial may show non-symptoms gradually aggravated, but a sudden attack.

#### 19.1.4.5 Inappropriate Medication History: An Inappropriate History of Drug Use

According to recent research, such as those about aminophylline poisoning [23, 24], intravenous injection of aminophylline, especially when its blood concentration is >404 g/ml, can cause sudden death if the concentration is too high or the injection is too fast. In addition, theophylline can stimulate the release of endogenous catecholamine and produce a series of cardiovascular effects. The blood concentration of aminophylline is affected by many factors and drugs. Even if the dosage of aminophylline remains unchanged, if combined with some drugs, the plasma concentration of aminophylline can be increased to a dangerous level. In previous studies, asthma has been associated with increased cardiovascular risk in patients with long QT syndrome (LQTS); however, the use of beta agonists is one of the treatments for asthma. In a study of 3287 patients with LQTS, it was reported that there were significant differences in baseline ECG, baseline QTc, and heart rate in the beta-agonist treatment group. The risk of cardiovascular events tripled [25]. In a national cohort study of asthma in Sweden, the risk of oral corticosteroid (OCS)-related diseases and mortality was assessed. Data on 217,993 patients with asthma (age $\geq$ 6 years) were determined using the Swedish National Health Registration system between 2007 and 2014. Recent studies have also shown that OCS-related morbidity and all-cause mortality are higher [26].

#### 19.1.4.6 Other

The main causes of sudden death caused by bronchial asthma are complex and multifaceted. According to the recent research, the analysis of different angles, the reasons are also lack of consistency. There are also reports in the literature:

1. Asphyxia: due to severe airway spasm, resulting in atresia/bronchial obstruction, resulting in asphyxial death.
2. Arrhythmia: type I respiratory failure caused by severe hypoxia, hypercapnia caused by carbon dioxide retention, and severe acid-base and electrolyte balance disorder are the main causes of arrhythmia. There are various types of arrhythmias, and reports show that patients with asthma have a higher risk of atrial fibrillation and ventricular fibrillation [27]. If ventricular arrhythmia occurs, the prognosis is extremely poor, and the mortality rate can be as high as 54% [28].
3. Secondary pulmonary hypertension and/or acute right heart failure: on the one hand, pulmonary vasoconstriction was caused by hypoxemia in patients with asthma. On the other hand, when hyperinflation occurred, the intra-alveolar pressure increased, and the driving pressure of pulmonary blood flow also increased, resulting in pulmonary hypertension and even right heart hypertrophy and failure [29], which in turn increased the risk of sudden death in patients with asthma.
4. Obesity: obesity increases the severity of asthma because excessive abdominal fat reduces lung volume, thus affecting the function of the diaphragm, and the diaphragm is prone to fatigue during stressful activity. The average body mass index can increase the severity of asthma in patients, thereby increasing their mortality [30, 31].
5. Increased tension of vagus nerve: The time of sudden death in some patients with asthma mostly occurred in the early morning. Due to the increase of vagus nerve tension at night, the level of catecholamine in the body was in the trough stage, and bronchoconstriction and spasm occur, resulting in increased airway resistance and decreased compliance, thus promoting sudden death in patients with

asthma [32]. The cause of death of some people is difficult to determine; even autopsy cannot explain the cause.

### 19.1.5 Causes and Seizures of Sudden Death from Asthma: Induction and Attack Pattern

Asthma inducing factors refer to the factors that can induce acute attack and aggravate asthma symptoms in patients with asthma. A variety of inducing factors have seasonal characteristics, which are related to respiratory tract infection, allergen inhalation, and weather changes. And according to a survey of sudden death from asthma, common causes of severe seizures are the following: the rescue group's lack of understanding of asthma (63%), wrong grading of symptoms (49%), improper personality and treatment (45%), inadequate education for patients (43%), frequent medical visits, non-scheduled time visits, etc. [33]. There are reports of 90 deaths [34] from fatal asthma attacks. Of the 90 patients, ten were seriously ill and had frequent episodes for a long time, and death was considered inevitable due to the cause of the illness. Of the 77 patients who were not hospitalized, 23 had rapid seizures that lasted less than an hour. Sixty-seven (77%) delayed medical treatment because they did not realize the severity of the asthma attack. Of the 13 patients who were hospitalized, three believed that the attending doctor had failed to understand the severity of the illness. The symptoms of asthma attack can be divided into mild, moderate, severe, and extremely severe. However, most of the sudden death cases of asthma occurred outside the hospital, and most of the patients died at home or on the way to the hospital, while some of the patients with acute severe attacks had out-of-hospital treatment before arriving at the hospital, but the specific treatment was not clear [35]. There are three types of fatal severe seizures: sudden onset, unstable type (from mild to moderate attack to severe attack), and intermittent type. According to the investigation results of the investigation team and the lethal asthma group of the Japanese Allergy Society, it was found that the unstable mutants were more common in the lethal group and the successful rescue group.

### 19.1.6 Early Identification and Evaluation of Acute Attack of Asthma

Early symptom recognition improves the need for early self-identification of acute asthma symptoms, such as cough, chest tightness, shortness of breath, and decreased activity endurance; most asthma has early signs before acute attack. According to the multicenter cross-sectional study conducted by Lin Jiangtao et al. [36], in a survey of outpatients with asthma in 30 Grade A hospitals in China from October 2015 to May 2016, occurrences of symptoms of acute asthma attacks less than 1 h accounted for 39.6%, and those occurring less than 24 h accounted for 24.4%. If it is not dealt with in time after onset, the risk of sudden death will be increased. The severity of asthma attacks varies, and so does the rate of development of the disease, which can occur within hours or days and can occasionally be life-threatening within minutes. It is worth noting that severe asthma attacks can also be seen in patients with mild or well-controlled asthma.

For any acute attack of asthma, in addition to the symptoms of patients, careful observation and dynamic blood gas analysis to evaluate the condition, especially for refractory asthma, and the need for mechanical ventilation are necessary. Acute severe attacks of asthma are characterized by persistent wheezing and rapid exacerbation, limited speech and extreme intolerance of physical activity, rapid cyanosis, increased heart rate and respiration, chest and abdominal contradictory breathing, three concave signs, and extensive wheezing, which can be heard in the lungs. Some patients have abnormal consciousness, such as eosinophilia, coma, and so on. Blood gas analysis indicates severe acidosis and severe ventilation, which can be life-threatening. Severe fatal respiratory failure, or even respiratory and cardiac arrest could occur at any time.

### 19.1.7 Treatment of Acute Asthma Attacks

#### 19.1.7.1 Routine Treatment

The treatment of acute attacks of asthma depends on the severity of the attack and the response to the treatment. The purpose of treatment is to relieve symptoms, airflow restriction, and hypoxemia as soon as possible. At the same time, long-term treatment programs need to be developed to prevent recurrent acute attacks.

1. Carry on the asthma health education to the patients, improve the compliance of the asthma patients in the long run, and master the methods on how to operate the inhalation device skillfully so as to improve the self-management level of the patients.
2. It is necessary to avoid exposure to allergens, dust, and harmful gases in the environment.
3. Improve the understanding of the disease and appropriate psychological treatment, and reduce mental anxiety and depression. The drugs mainly include glucocorticoids, β2 receptor agonists, anticholinergic drugs, leukotriene regulators, theophyllines, immunosuppressants, and so on. In recent years, biological targeted drugs (such as omalizumab and mepolizumab) and bronchoplasty have also been used in the clinic.

#### 19.1.7.2 Treatment of Critical Asthma

In the event of an acute attack of asthma, especially severe asthma, the risk of sudden death is extremely high. Patients with acute severe attacks can die within a few minutes, and sudden death can occur without timely treatment. Sudden death is the most serious complication of acute asthma attacks. Often without obvious aura symptoms, the condition of a patient suddenly deteriorates in a rapid manner, and it is often too late to save the patient's life. Therefore, it is very important to identify patients with high risk factors of asthma-related death. These patients should first deal with themselves in the event of acute attack and then go to medical institutions as soon as possible. They should receive methods for rapid relief of bronchospasm and control of respiratory inflammation, to correct hypoxemia and respiratory failure. And the complications should be managed. Treatment measures should be timely use of bronchodilators and systemic hormones, oxygen therapy (need to maintain arterial oxygen saturation above 93%), and respiratory support therapy. At this time, endotracheal intubation to establish artificial airway and timely mechanical ventilation treatment are inevitable and necessary rescue means, and reasonable selection of ventilation methods and parameters, monitoring of blood gas and electrolytes in the course of treatment, and timely judgment of curative effect and disease evolution are important. It is helpful to reduce complications and sudden death rate.

**Noninvasive Positive-Pressure Ventilation (NPPV)** [37]
Studies have shown that NPPV can improve blood gas analysis and lung function. In recent years, epidemiological data in the United States have found that the proportion of patients with fatal asthma using noninvasive ventilation has increased significantly. A study analysis showed [38]that 112 patients with asthma had respiratory distress and hypercapnia in addition to routine use of glucocorticoids and bronchial relaxants. The intubation rate decreased after the application of noninvasive ventilation. According to the relevant guidelines, this can be applied if there is no indication of emergency intubation or noninvasive contraindications.

**Invasive Positive-Pressure Ventilation** [39, 40]
The first choice is to intubate through the oral tube and place the large tube diameter catheter to avoid tracheotomy leading to tracheal stenosis. The indication of intubation includes: (1) cardiac arrest; (2) chronic respiratory slowdown or stop; (3) disturbance of consciousness; (4) silent lung; (5) pure oxygen mask oxygen $PO_2 < 60$ mmHg, or PH < 7.2; (6) respiration ≥40 times. It is recommended that volume control ventilation (VCV) mode be used at the initial stage of ventilation, which can obtain higher driving pressure and maintain ventilation. High minute ventilation can lead to pulmonary hyperinflation. The low tidal volume should be 6–8 ml/kg, the respiratory rate should be controlled at 10–15 times/min, and the inspiratory time should be controlled at 0.8–1.2 s. The airway pressure adjustment parameters should be monitored according to the results of blood gas analysis. For positive end-expiratory pressure (PEEP) setting, there is no PEEPi at the beginning of ventilation, and administration of PEEP at this time may increase the end-expiratory lung volume and aggravate the condition. It is recommended that you set up a low level of PEEP (usually $\leq 5cmH_2O$). Low tidal volume may lead to insufficient ventilation and carbon dioxide retention. Hypercapnia can be allowed and $PaCO_2$ can be reduced properly (no less than 7.20–7.25). When using a ventilator, patients have irritability, delirium, man-machine confrontation, or severe airway spasm; sedatives and/or muscle relaxants can be properly selected. Sedatives can be diazepam or propofol and fentanyl. Vecuronium 0.08 mg and 0.10 mg were commonly used as muscle relaxants, which were injected intravenously and maintained at 0.01–0.015 mg/kg.

#### 19.1.7.3 Correction of Water and Electrolyte and Acid-Base Imbalance

Along with heat-related water loss during asthma attack, we should actively correct dehydration, humidify the airway, and prevent excess mucus production. The daily infusion volume was controlled at 2500–4000 ml, and the daily urine volume was above 1000 ml. For large amounts of mucus leading to severe airway obstruction, affecting the therapeutic effect, ventilation cannot be improved; bronchoalveolar lavage can be performed to remove mucus in the airway [41]. There is a need to prevent sudden death, monitor blood gas analysis and electrolytes, and timely detect and correct acid-base imbalance and electrolyte disorders. Hypercapnia can be allowed only in the case of respiratory acidosis. When pH is $<7.20$, alkali (5% sodium bicarbonate) can be supplemented to reach pH $> 7.20$.

#### 19.1.7.4 Research Progress in the Treatment of Severe Asthma

Tezepelumab is a human monoclonal antibody against epithelial cytokine thymic stromal lymphopoietin (TSLP), which can block the interaction between TSLP and receptor complex and prevent the release of proinflammatory cytokines from immune cells targeted by TSLP. To prevent asthma attacks and improve symptom control, it can be used in a wide range of patients with severe refractory asthma. Related clinical studies have shown that [42] tezepelumab can reduce the annual incidence of acute exacerbation in patients with refractory asthma by 71% and can significantly improve lung function, improve asthma control, and reduce the incidence of sudden death.

Eosinophilia is associated with the deterioration of asthma severity and the decrease of pulmonary function, and the frequency of aggravation increases. Benralizumab is a monoclonal antibody against interleukin-5 receptor alpha [43]. According to a study from 374 regions in 17 countries [44], benralizumab is effective and safe in patients with severe asthma and eosinophil elevation, who are not controlled by high doses of inhaled corticosteroids (ICS) plus long acting β agonist (LABA). Benralizumab is also supported as an additional option for the treatment of the disease in this group of patients.

### 19.1.8 Prevention and Management of Sudden Death Caused by Asthma

Early detection of the risk signs of sudden death asthma, early identification and diagnosis once found, and rapid and effective treatment measures are the key to prevent sudden death caused by asthma.

From the point of view of the risk factors of fatal asthma attack, due to the lack of education of the patients and the lack of understanding of asthma, the doctors do not pay enough attention to asthma and cannot distinguish and identify the risk degree of asthma. It is necessary to strengthen the communication between doctors and patients and their families, and the doctors in charge should have a full grasp of the patient's condition.

The incidence of sudden death from asthma was high from night to early morning. Due to the increase of vagus nerve excitability at night, the level of intracellular cyclic adenosine monophosphate (CAMP) decreased, which could not prevent the release of bioactive substances, and the level of adrenocortical hormone was low, resulting in a decrease in effective blood concentration. Therefore, the maintenance of nocturnal serum effective plasma concentration in patients with severe asthma is helpful to reduce the occurrence of sudden death asthma.

Self-management of asthma peak expiratory flow (PEF) monitoring is necessary. According to related reports [45], PEF often fluctuates the day and night before fatal asthma attacks leading to death. Therefore, strengthening PEF self-monitoring can also reduce the number of acute asthma attacks. According to a prospective, randomized parallel study, Group 1 was given routine treatment, and the other group was monitored by self-PEF on the basis of routine treatment. The results showed that the number of acute exacerbation in PEF self-monitoring group was better than that in routine treatment group.

The monitoring of exhaled nitric oxide can help in determining the compliance of inhaled glucocorticoid (ICS) therapy, evaluating the level of airway inflammation, evaluating the level of asthma control, and predicting the risk of acute attack of asthma. Cohort Analysis based on the Refractory Asthma (Hi-CARAT) study in Hokkaido, Japan [46], evaluates the clinical indicators and acute attack status of 105 patients with severe asthma. Multivariate analysis was performed on three groups of subjects (persistent non-acute onset, persistent frequent acute onset, and intermittent acute onset). Of the several biomarkers associated with Th2, only FeNO is associated with aggravation of the disease. The results showed that the effect of FeNO on predicting the deterioration of the disease in the future was still significant.

·Studies on sudden death from asthma show that some patients do not pay enough attention to asthma and do not strengthen education on asthma. To be able to judge the severity of acute asthma and to skillfully master the use of all kinds of asthma drugs are the basis for the prevention of acute exacerbation of asthma and the effective measures to prevent sudden death from asthma.

### 19.1.9 Conclusion

For sudden death from asthma, the onset of the disease is very rapid and can quickly progress to death. To identify the risk signs of sudden death early, make diagnosis as soon as possible, and take effective treatment and monitoring measures in time to reduce or prevent sudden death from asthma. Cardiopulmonary resuscitation and invasive ventilator support for endotracheal intubation are the key measures to improve the success rate of sudden death from asthma. Targeted treatment of severe asthma attacks caused by different causes is beneficial. During the attack of asthma, targeted treatment can prevent asphyxia caused by severe hypoxia or sputum obstruction. It is necessary to avoid all kinds of stimulating factors as far as possible and systematically use adrenocortical hormone to prevent the serious attack of asthma. However, for patients with long course of disease and frequent episodes, resulting in unstable mental stress and mood fluctuations, and patients with serious psychological disorders, psychological counseling is given to advise them to treat the disease correctly. Good mental state plays an active role in reducing attacks and symptoms during attacks and in reducing the rate of sudden death. Since most of the sudden deaths from asthma occur at night, preventing the attack of asthma at night is an important link to reduce the mortality rate. In addition, reasonable and correct use of drugs and avoiding overuse of bronchodilators, glucocorticoids, and sympathetic drugs are also effective ways to reduce sudden death from asthma. There is a certain relationship between sudden death from asthma and critical asthma. Sudden asthma with protuberance within a few minutes to hours can lead to sudden death without timely treatment. Therefore, improving the rescue success rate of critical asthma and standardizing the prevention and treatment of asthma have important clinical significance to reduce the mortality of bronchial asthma. With the rapid development of health care, there is a need to expand the future research on the potential treatment of asthma, improve the level of asthma control, enhance the study of new asthma treatment, develop accurate medical programs, and reduce the incidence of severe asthma and acute asthma attacks to lower the sudden death rate from asthma.

## 19.2 Acute Pulmonary Embolism

### 19.2.1 Overview and Epidemiology

Acute pulmonary embolism is a common venous thromboembolism, second only to myocardial infarction and stroke. The clinical manifestations of pulmonary embolism are variable and usually nonspecific, making it difficult to diagnose. In the United States, pulmonary embolism causes approximately 100,000 to 300,000 deaths per year [47, 48]. In Europe, pulmonary embolism causes 300,000 deaths per year, one-third of which are due to sudden fatal pulmonary embolism. About 34% of pulmonary embolism leads to sudden death [49]. Seven percent of patients were diagnosed before dying, and the rest were diagnosed after death; but many causes of sudden cardiac death are secondary to pulmonary embolism, so the actual mortality caused by pulmonary embolism is difficult to estimate.

### 19.2.2 Classification

Pulmonary embolism can be divided into acute, subacute, and chronic onset according to the course of the disease. Patients with acute pulmonary embolism usually have symptoms and signs immediately after pulmonary vascular occlusion. Some patients with pulmonary embolism may also present symptoms within a few days or weeks after the initial event. Chronic pulmonary embolism patients have symptoms of pulmonary hypertension slowly over the years, which is called chronic thromboembolic pulmonary hypertension. We will mainly discuss sudden death caused by acute and subacute pulmonary embolism.

According to the stable classification of hemodynamics, pulmonary embolism can be divided into high-risk, intermediate-risk, and low-risk pulmonary embolism. The definition of hemodynamic instability includes (1) cardiac arrest, requiring cardiopulmonary resuscitation; (2) obstructive shock, systolic blood pressure < 90 mmHg or the need of sufficient vasopressor to maintain blood pressure ≥ 90 mmHg, and end-perfusion insufficiency (mental state changes; cold, moist skin; oliguria/no urine; increased serum lactic acid); and (3) sustained hypotension systolic blood pressure < 90 mmHg or systolic blood pressure decreased ≥40 mmHg for more than 15 min and not caused by new arrhythmia, hypovolemia, or sepsis. Although hemodynamically unstable, pulmonary embolism is usually caused by a large pulmonary embolism; sometimes a small block of pulmonary embolism can cause this condition in patients with underlying cardiopulmonary disease.

It is important to distinguish between hemodynamically stable and hemodynamically unstable pulmonary embolism, as patients with hemodynamically unstable pulmonary embolism are more likely to die from obstructive shock (i.e., severe right ventricular failure). Death from unstable pulmonary embolism usually occurs within the first 2 h, and the risk remains high for up to 72 h after onset.

### 19.2.3 Risk Factor

Factors that cause venous stasis, vascular endothelial damage, and hypercoagulability (Virchow's three factors) are risk factors for venous thromboembolism (VTE), including hereditary and acquired.

#### 19.2.3.1 Hereditary Factors

These include factor V Leiden mutation and prothrombin gene mutation (20210-A) [49], often with repeated arterial and venous thromboses as the main clinical manifestations. Patients <50 years old have no risk factor of recurrent VTE. It is a familial morbidity and needs to be alerted due to the presence of thrombophilia.

#### 19.2.3.2 Acquired Factors

Acquired risk factors refer to a variety of pathophysiological abnormalities that are acquired after birth, which are often temporary or reversible, such as surgery, trauma, acute medical diseases (such as heart failure, respiratory failure, and infection), and some chronic diseases (such as antiphospholipid syndrome, nephrotic syndrome, inflammatory bowel disease, and myeloproliferative diseases); malignant tumors are important risk factors for VTE, but different types of tumors have different VTE risks. Pancreatic, cranial, pulmonary, ovarian, and hematological malignancies are considered to have the highest risk of VTE, while VTE risk increases during malignant activity.

VTE has common risk factors for certain arterial diseases, especially atherosclerosis, such as smoking, obesity, hypercholesterolemia, hypertension, and diabetes. Myocardial infarction and heart failure can also increase the risk of VTE. Sexual risk factors can be caused by disease alone or simultaneously and synergistic effect.

Age is an independent risk factor. As the age increases, the incidence of VTE increases gradually.

Some VTE patients cannot identify the risk factors by more complete testing methods, called idiopathic VTE. Some patients with idiopathic VTE have occult malignant tumors, which should be screened and followed up.

### 19.2.4 Pathophysiology

The embolism of pulmonary embolism can be derived from the superior and inferior vena cava or right heart cavity. Most of the emboli are derived from the veins of the lower extremities, including femoral vein and iliac vein. About 70% of patients with pulmonary embolism can find deep vein thrombosis (DVT) in the lower extremities, and pulmonary embolism exists in 50% of patients with proximal DVT. With the prolonged internal jugular vein and subclavian vein catheterization and intravenous chemotherapy, thrombosis from the superior vena cava also appears to increase. Pulmonary embolism can cause a series of pathophysiological reactions that can be divided into two aspects: impaired circulatory function and impaired respiratory function.

#### 19.2.4.1 Impaired Circulatory Function

Vascular bed obstruction, which increases pulmonary vascular resistance and decreases arterial compliance in patients with pulmonary embolism, can be caused by pulmonary embolism, thromboxane A2 or serotonin release, and hypoxic vasoconstriction of pulmonary artery system. The obstruction can lead to increased right ventricular afterload and pulmonary artery pressure, causing right ventricular dilatation and left ventricular septal shift, affecting left ventricular preload, thereby reducing cardiac output. At last, hypotension occurs.

#### 19.2.4.2 Impaired Respiratory Function

Pulmonary embolism obstructs blood vessels, and inflammation leads to alveolar surfactant dysfunction and atelectasis, which makes the proportion of ventilated blood flow imbalanced. The distal small embolism can cause local alveolar hemorrhage, and pleurisy and chest cavity can occur. The effusion further affects the gas exchange. In some patients, because the right atrial pressure is increased, the foramen ovale opens again, resulting in a right-to-left shunt, leading to severe hypoxemia and increasing the risk of sudden death.

### 19.2.5 Clinical Manifestation

Pulmonary embolism has a variety of onset characteristics, ranging from no symptoms to shock or sudden death [50, 51]. The most common complaints are dyspnea, followed by chest pain, cough, and DVT symptoms. Hemoptysis is an uncommon complaint. Very few patients have shock, arrhythmia, or syncope. Many patients (including some patients with massive pulmonary embolism) have no symptoms or have mild or nonspecific symptoms. Therefore, it is essential to maintain a high degree of suspicion of the disease to avoid missing clinically relevant cases.

Pulmonary embolism is a common cause of sudden death, especially in patients <65 years of age. Ninety-one percent of these patients have dyspnea or hypopnea. Large pulmonary embolism (PE) may be associated with acute right ventricular failure, manifested as elevated jugular venous pressure, right third heart sound, parasternal lift pulsation, cyanosis, and obstructive shock. But small PE patients with severe basal pulmonary hypertension may also experience shock. A change from tachycardia to bradycardia, or from narrow QRS tachycardia to wide QRS tachycardia (i.e., right bundle branch block), is a bad sign of right ventricular strain and impending shock [52].

### 19.2.6 Diagnosis

Any branch of the pulmonary artery (backbone, leaf, segment, subsegment) has a marked filling defect after contrast enhancement, i.e., a diagnosis of PE. When a filling defect is not clearly observed (e.g., the embolus is in a small peripheral pulmonary artery), poor contrast enhancement and patient movement or metallic beam hardening artifacts lead to poor imagery, and scan results are reported as uncertain or nondiagnostic.

Pulmonary embolism can be diagnosed by pulmonary segment or subsegment perfusion defect, with normal ventilation. When the image is interpreted, the probability of classification as PE is high, medium, or low or normal. In the case of low clinical probability of PE, the scan result is normal, and the probability of showing PE as low is enough to rule out the PE. V/Q scan shows a high probability of PE and a high clinical probability of PE, confirming all other combinations of PE. V/Q results and clinical probability are not diagnostic.

Transcatheter pulmonary angiography revealed filling defects or sudden truncation of blood vessels, diagnosed as emboli. Echocardiography rarely diagnoses PE, but patients with hemodynamic instability can use this method to make a presumptive diagnosis, which can be given life-saving treatment. Proximal vein compression of the lower extremity confirmed that DVT could not be diagnosed as PE, but it may indicate that it is suitable for treatment. Sometimes, PE is found when standard contrast-enhanced computed tomography (CT) is used for other reasons, or pathological examination is performed on the resected lung lobe. It was found that in these cases, special pulmonary or leg vein imaging may be required to diagnose residual PE or DVT.

#### 19.2.6.1 Arterial Blood Gas

If the chest X-ray is normal, but there is an unexplained hypoxemia, the possibility of PE should be considered and should suggest further evaluation. However, although the results of arterial blood gas (ABG) analysis of patients with suspected PE are often abnormal, many ABG results were normal in 18% of PE patients.

However, abnormal gas exchange may be caused by and/or worsened by basal cardiopulmonary disease [53]. Common abnormalities in ABG analysis include one or more of the following: hypoxemia (74%), alveolar-arterial oxygen partial pressure difference (62–86%), respiratory alkalosis, and hypocapnia (41%). Hypercapnia, respiratory acidosis, and lactic acidosis are not common. However, these conditions may occur in patients with massive PE with obstructive shock and respiratory arrest. Oxygenation abnormalities may have prognostic value. For example, patients with hypoxemia at diagnosis or pulse oximetry readings at room air <95% have an increased risk of complications including respiratory failure, obstructive shock, and death.

#### 19.2.6.2 Electrocardiogram

Abnormal electrocardiograms are common in suspected PE patients, but they are not specific [54]. The most common findings are tachycardia and nonspecific ST segment and T wave changes (70%). Previously considered to be abnormal for PE (S1Q3T3 waveform, right ventricular strain), new incomplete right bundle branch block is not common (<10%). Among patients diagnosed with PE, ECG abnormalities associated with poor prognosis include atrial arrhythmia (e.g., atrial fibrillation), bradycardia (<50 beats/min) or tachycardia (>100 beats/min), new right bundle branch block, Q wave (II, III, and aVF leads) in the inferior leads, anterior wall ST segment change and T wave inversion, and S1Q3T3 waveform.

#### 19.2.6.3 CTPA

CT pulmonary angiography (CTPA), also known as chest contrast-enhanced CT angiography, is the preferred method for diagnostic imaging studies in most patients with suspected PE because of its sensitivity and specificity (especially when integrated into the diagnostic pathway) [55]. Other diseases can be found by this method. The imaging technique is widely used, and in most cases, the examination can be carried out as soon as possible or in an emergency. If there is a contraindication to CTPA in some cases, it is easy to resolve the problem(e.g., premedication when allergic to contrast agents), and if imaging (e.g., V/Q scan) is not feasible, CTPA can also be performed after a short delay (e.g., 8–12 h).

For patients with a history of moderate to severe iodine-containing contrast agents or renal insufficiency [eGFR<30 ml/(min·1.73 $m^2$)], CTPA may be relatively banned. The risk of these contraindications must be weighed against two factors: the clinical importance of CTPA examination and the availability of other imaging methods (e.g., V/Q scan) [56].

Most studies report that CTPA diagnosis of PE has >90% sensitivity and specificity, especially when the clinical risk is low and moderate [57]. It is reported that when the clinical probability of CTPA combined with PE is moderate to high, the sensitivity is highest (≥96%), but the sensitivity was lower in patients with low suspicion. However, many cohort studies using advanced technology scanners and specific CTPA programs consistently show that PE occurs in patients with low clinical suspicions and normal CTPA results. The rate is low (<2%) [58, 59]. However, patients with normal CTPA results and with clinically highly suspected PE [60] have a risk of PE (up to 5% when using MDCT with ≤64 rows of probes).

#### 19.2.6.4 Ventilation/Perfusion Scan

V/Q scans are basically only used for patients with uncertain outcomes and when CTPA is banned or when additional tests are required. Chest radiographs are usually required before V/Q scans. Scanning patients with abnormal chest X-rays is more likely to be false-positive because the images of such patients are rarely normal or have a low probability of PE. Patients will be required to sit for 30–60 min for V/Q scan. The approximate effective radiation dose is <2 mSv. Most patients scan for uncertainty. This is the main limitation of V/Q scanning because the uncertain scan results are not enough to confirm the diagnosis of PE, nor is it sufficient to exclude PE, requiring additional examination. A systematic review analyzed more than 7000 cases from 25 prospective studies [54, 61]. In three patients, after 3 months of follow-up, three diagnostic strategies were found to safely exclude PE patients: in patients with low clinical probability of PE and exclusion of PE based on normal D-dimer levels, the incidence of PE was <3%. Among patients with clinical probabilities combined with D-dimer assessment, conventional perfusion scans (Q scans) can safely exclude PE. In patients with a high probability of PE on V/Q scans, the next step is performed (e.g., catheter pulmonary angiography or continuous lower extremity venous ultrasound) safely.

### 19.2.7 Resuscitation and Treatment Principles

Initial support for pulmonary embolism should focus on restoring tissue perfusion [62, 63], for example, venous fluid resuscitation, vasopressor support, and oxygenation, as well as intubation and mechanical ventilation to stabilize the airway.

For most patients with hemodynamically stable resuscitation but with highly suspected pulmonary embolism, unfractionated heparin is used immediately for anticoagulation, and rapid imaging studies are performed to confirm the diagnosis. For patients with high clinically suspected pulmonary embolism, hemodynamic instability, and metastasis confirmed by the radiology department for whom CTPA is considered unsafe, bedside echocardiography is performed empirically before systemic thrombolytic therapy (i.e., reperfusion therapy). If the cardiogram is delayed or not possible, thrombolytic therapy should be used as a life-saving measure according to the patient's specific conditions; if thrombolytic therapy is not available, the patient should be treated with empirical anticoagulant therapy. Anticoagulant therapy should not be delayed. For patients with known pulmonary embolism, if antihypertensive therapy is accompanied by hypotension and anticoagulant therapy is still highly suspected of pulmonary embolism recurrence, we recommend a similar approach.

For patients with low or moderate suspicion of pulmonary embolism and hemodynamic instability, the empirical anticoagulation method should be the same as that of hemodynamically stable patients; empirical thrombolytic therapy should not be performed in this patient population.

#### 19.2.7.1 Transcatheter Pulmonary Angiography

Pulmonary angiography is the injection of contrast agent through the catheter into the right heart under fluoroscopy. It used to be the gold standard for diagnosis of PE. With the popularity of CTPA, this operation has been rarely used, only for rare cases, i.e., the patient's PE. The clinical probability is high, but the CTPA or V/Q scan is not diagnostic, and the diagnosis will determine important clinical decisions (e.g., intervention). Pulmonary angiography does not appear to be as accurate as CTPA, and diagnostic performance varies widely and depends on the operator's experience. Therefore, transcatheter pulmonary angiography is most commonly used in patients scheduled for concurrent treatment because it combines diagnostics with therapeutic interventions designed to dissolve blood clots (e.g., catheter-guided thrombectomy and/or thrombolytic therapy). The application of this method in this case is also influenced by local professionalism.

Transcatheter pulmonary angiography as a previous gold standard has not been formally evaluated for its sensitivity and specificity for the diagnosis of PE. However, a retrospective analysis of 20 patients showed that the sensitivity of detecting small embolism may be low. However, in patients with negative angiographic results, the risk of subsequent symptomatic embolization was lower (<2%).

#### 19.2.7.2 Respiratory Support

The target oxygen saturation is ≥90% after intubation and mechanical ventilation. Patients with right ventricular failure are prone to hypotension after intubation. Therefore, for this patient group, it may be prudent to consult with cardiovascular anesthesiologists. High platform pressure should be avoided. Extracorporeal membrane oxygenation may also be considered (successful use in patients with severe refractory hypoxemia and/or hypotension).

#### 19.2.7.3 Hemodynamic Support

The exact threshold for hemodynamic support is determined by the patient's baseline blood pressure and whether there is clinical evidence of hypoperfusion (e.g., altered consciousness, decreased urine output). In general, we tend to give a small amount of intravenous rehydration, usually 500–1000 ml saline, if the patient's perfusion status does not change after intravenous rehydration, followed by vasopressor treatment.

Intravenous rehydration is a first-line treatment for patients with hypotension. However, for patients with right ventricular dysfunction, limited data suggest that active fluid resuscitation is not beneficial or even harmful [64]. The rationale for limiting intravenous rehydration comes from preclinical studies. And a small observational study in humans reported that a small amount of intravenous rehydration would increase the heart index of patients with pulmonary embolism, while excessive intravenous rehydration would lead to excessive expansion of the right ventricle (i.e., right ventricular overload), right ventricular ischemia and right heart failure increase.

The best vasopressor for patients with shock caused by acute pulmonary embolism is usually preferred to norepinephrine.

#### 19.2.7.4 Empirical Anticoagulant Therapy

The application of empirical anticoagulant therapy depends on the risk of bleeding, the degree of clinical suspicion of pulmonary embolism, and the estimated time of the diagnostic test [65]. For most patients with hemodynamically stable resuscitation but with highly suspected pulmonary embolism, we tend to use ordinary heparin for immediate anticoagulation. There is no best predictive tool for assessing the risk of bleeding in patients with pulmonary embolism [66].

If patients presents with absolute contraindications to anticoagulation therapy (e.g., recent surgery, hemorrhagic stroke, active bleeding) or if physicians have assessed an unacceptably high risk of bleeding (e.g., aortic dissection, intracranial tumor, or spinal cord tumor), empirical anticoagulant therapy should not be used. Diagnostic assessment should be expedited so that alternative treatments can be initiated when a diagnosis of pulmonary embolism is initiated, such as inferior vena cava (IVC) filter placement, thrombectomy, and surgery.

#### 19.2.7.5 Thrombolytic Therapy and Catheter-Assisted Thrombectomy

Systemic thrombolysis is a widely accepted treatment for patients with pulmonary embolism after recovery from sudden death. For specific patients, catheter thrombectomy (with or without thrombolytic therapy) may also be used, especially in patients with a higher risk of bleeding [67, 68]. For patients who have failed systemic thrombolysis, the best treatment is not clear. Alternative treatments include repeated systemic thrombolysis, catheter thrombolysis, and catheter or surgical thrombectomy, depending on available resources and local expertise.

For patients with hemodynamically unstable pulmonary embolism who are contraindicated with thrombolytic therapy, thrombectomy is required. Thrombectomy is also a treatment option for patients with failed thrombolysis. The embolus can be removed by surgery or using a catheter. The choice depends on the expertise, whether the pulmonary embolism has been diagnosed, and the patient's response to these treatments. One of the advantages of this method is that it can be used for both diagnostic and therapeutic interventions. Selective thrombectomy techniques include ultrasound-assisted thrombolysis, flow decompression, rotary thrombectomy and suction thrombectomy [69].

Catheter-assisted thrombectomy has the risk of pulmonary perforation; although rare, it can lead to pericardial tamponade and life-threatening hemoptysis, with very serious consequences. Other complications include venous puncture site bleeding and infection, cardiac arrest and death, as well as equipment-specific adverse reactions. Combined application of thrombolytic therapy can aggravate hemorrhagic side effects.

#### 19.2.7.6 Surgical Thrombectomy

Routine indications for surgical thrombectomy are hemodynamic instability due to acute pulmonary embolism and contraindications to thrombolytic therapy (systemic or catheterization), which is also an option for patients with failed thrombolysis [70]. It may include echocardiography showing that the embolus is trapped in the patent foramen ovale, or in the right atrium or right ventricle. Surgical thrombectomy is usually performed only in large medical centers because an experienced surgeon is required to perform the procedure. Surgical thrombectomy has a higher mortality rate, especially in the elderly. The proximal embolus (i.e., the right ventricle, the main pulmonary artery, and the embolus in the extrapulmonary branches of the pulmonary artery) is easily removed by surgery, but far-end thrombosis (e.g., a thrombus in a branch of the pulmonary artery) is usually not surgically removed.

A retrospective database study comparing 257 patients with pulmonary embolism undergoing surgical thrombectomy with 1854 patients with pulmonary embolism undergoing thrombolysis showed no significant difference in mortality on the 30th day (15% vs 13%) [71]. The observational study included 40 patients with pulmonary embolism who failed systemic thrombolysis, and the rate of pulmonary embolism was lower in patients undergoing surgical thrombectomy compared with patients receiving repeated thrombolysis (0 vs 35%) [72]. In addition, there were fewer deaths and severe bleeding complications in the surgical thrombectomy group, but the difference in these data was not statistically significant. Another case series included 115 patients who underwent surgical thrombectomy. Patients with unstable pulmonary embolism were found to have higher operative mortality (10% vs 4%) and lower survival rates (75% vs 93%) compared with patients with stable pulmonary embolism [73].

Transesophageal echocardiography (TEE) should be performed before or during thrombectomy to determine the presence of extrapulmonary thrombosis (e.g., thrombus in the right atrium, right ventricle, or vena cava). A series of 50 patients with pulmonary embolism were included in the study. TEE detected 13 patients (26%) with extrapulmonary thrombosis, which resulted in changes in surgical treatment in five patients (10%) [74].

#### 19.2.7.7 Shock and Right Ventricular Dysfunction

Echocardiography or CTPA assessment showed that right ventricular dysfunction was associated with increased mortality [75]. A meta-analysis included 3395 patients with normotensive and hypotensive pulmonary embolism in seven studies and found that right ventricular dysfunction was associated with pulmonary embolism in the hospital [76]. There was a twofold increase in the mortality rate. However, a subgroup analysis of patients with normal blood pressure found that the correlation between right ventricular dysfunction and mortality found by echocardiography or CT was weak, indicating that the symptom that can predict death is right ventricular dysfunction. A study enrolled 1950 patients with a diagnosis of PE who underwent a corresponding treatment in a prospective multicenter trial and found that CTPA showed a larger diameter of the pulmonary trunk and a higher duration of treatment for 3–6 months [77]. Mortality (OR, 2.8, 95% CI 1.3–5.7) was associated with mortality at 1 year of treatment (OR, 2.3, 95% CI 1.4–4.0). There was no correlation with right ventricular dysfunction.

#### 19.2.7.8 Right Ventricular Thrombus

Echocardiography or CT examination found that approximately 4% of patients with pulmonary embolism had active right heart thrombosis, which was higher in patients with severe disease (up to 18%) [78]. Several studies have shown that right heart thrombus and right ventricle insufficiency are associated with higher early mortality. For example, data from the International Registry of Patients with Pulmonary Embolism shows 14-day mortality in patients with right ventricular thrombosis (21% vs 11%) compared with patients without right ventricular thrombosis and 3-month mortality (29% vs 16%) is higher [79].

## References

1. Becker AB, Abrams EM. Asthma guidelines: the global initiative for asthma in relation to national guidelines. Curr Opin Allerg Clin Immunol. 2017;17(2):99.
2. Collaborators G B D M M. Global, regional, and national levels of maternal mortality, 1990-2015: a systematic analysis for the global burden of disease study 2015. Lancet. 2016;388(10053):1775–812.
3. Huang K, Yang T, Xu J, et al. Prevalence, risk factors, and management of asthma in China: a national cross-sectional study. Lancet. 2019;394(10196):407–18.
4. Marco RD, Locatelli F, Cazzoletti L, et al. Incidence of asthma and mortality in a cohort of young adults: a 7-year prospective study. Respiratory Res. 2005;6(1):95.
5. Gullach AJ, Risgaard B, Lynge TH, et al. Sudden death in young persons with uncontrolled asthma—a nationwide cohort study in Denmark. BMC Pulm Med. 2015;15:35.
6. Xu Z. Respiratory diseases and sudden death. Chinese Emerg Med. 1994;01:47–50.
7. Shen Z. 19 clinical analysis of sudden death caused by bronchial asthma. Chinese J Modern Med. 2007;17(14):1780.
8. Chuntao L, Yulin F. Fatal asthma and its special types. Med J New Knowled. (1):4–5.
9. Tieying Z. Effect of irregular use of β 2 receptor agonists on acute attack of bronchial asthma. Chinese Ethnic Folk Med. 2010;19(4):31.
10. Reddel HK, Taylor DR, Bateman ED, et al. An official American thoracic society/European respiratory society statement: asthma control and exacerbations: standardizing endpoints for clinical asthma trials and clinical practice. Am J Respir Crit Care Med. 2009;180(1):59–99.
11. Menzella F, Lusuardi M, Galeone C, et al. Profile of anti-IL-5 mAb mepolizumab in the treatment of severe refractory asthma and hypereosinophilic diseases. J Asthma Allergy. 2015;8:105–14.
12. Hantera M, El-Hafiz HA, Abdelnaby AY, et al. Serum levels of angiopoietin-2 and vascular endothelial growth factor in severe refractory asthma. Egypt J Chest Dis Tuberc. 2014;63(4):751–4.
13. Susumu N, Ho LH, Mang Y, et al. Mast cell-derived TNF contributes to airway hyperreactivity, inflammation, and TH2 cytokine production in an asthma model in mice. J Allergy Clin Immunol. 2007;120(1):48–55.
14. Brannan JD, Lougheed MD. Airway hyperresponsiveness in asthma: mechanisms, clinical significance, and treatment. Front Physiol. 2012;3:460.
15. Jatakanon A, Uasuf C, Maziak W, et al. Neutrophilic inflammation in severe persistent asthma. Am J Respir Crit Care Med. 1999;160(5 Pt 1):1532–9.

16. Jeffery PK. Proceedings of the American Thoracic Society. Remodeling and inflammation of bronchi in asthma and chronic obstructive pulmonary disease. Proc Am Thorac Soc. 2004;1(3):176–83.
17. Lai HY, Rogers DF. New pharmacotherapy for airway mucus hypersecretion in asthma and COPD: targeting intracellular signaling pathways. J Aerosol Med Pulm Drug Deliv. 2010;23(4):219–31.
18. Fahy JV. Goblet cell and mucin gene abnormalities in asthma*. Chest. 2002;122(6):320S–6S.
19. Scott KM, Lim C, Al-Hamzawi A, et al. Association of mental disorders with subsequent chronic physical conditions: world mental health surveys from 17 countries. JAMA Psychiat. 2016;73(2):150–8.
20. Haining L, Ma Q, Wang C, et al. Multivariate analysis of anxiety/depression in patients with bronchial asthma. Int Resp Magazine. 2017;37(23):1761–5.
21. Strine T, Mokdad A, Balluz L, et al. Impact of depression and anxiety on quality of life, health behaviors, and asthma control among adults in the United States with asthma, 2006. J Asthma. 2008;45(2):123–33.
22. Kolbe JJT. Case-control study of severe life threatening asthma (SLTA) in adults: psychological factors. Thorax. 2002;57(4):317–22.
23. Yihu Z, Li Z, Jun H, et al. Toxicity of aminophylline: a cause of death of medical negligence that has not been paid attention to. Evidence Sci. 2000;7(2):64–5.
24. Juan. Combination of epinephrine and aminophylline in the treatment of fatal asthma. Chinese Gerontol. 2014;(16):4678–4679.
25. Thottathil P, Acharya J, Moss AJ, et al. Risk of cardiac events in patients with asthma and long-QT syndrome treated with beta(2) agonists. Am J Cardiol. 2008;102(7):871–4.
26. Ekström M, Nwaru BI, Hasvold P, et al. Oral corticosteroid use, morbidity, and mortality in asthma: a nationwide prospective cohort study in Sweden. Allergy. 2019;74(11):2181–90.
27. Bozkurt Yilmaz HE, Yilmaz M, Şen N, et al. Assessment of atrial fibrillation and ventricular arrhythmia risk in patients with asthma by P wave/corrected QT interval dispersion. Eur Rev Med Pharmacol Sci. 2018;22(3):756.
28. Herlitz J, Ekström L, Wennerblom B, et al. Hospital mortality after out-of-hospital cardiac arrest among patients found in ventricular fibrillation. Resuscitation. 1995;29(1):11–21.
29. Wang H, Yonghong Z, Mingxia L. Advances in the pathogenesis of hypoxic pulmonary hypertension. Chinese J Pract Pediatr. 2009;03:74–7.
30. Xiaohong J, Jinbo Z, Jianhua C, et al. Clinical study on the relationship between obesity and the severity and prognosis of severe asthma. Modern Pract Med. 2013;025(004):385–6.
31. Cluley S, Cochrane GM. Psychological disorder in asthma is associated with poor control and poor adherence to inhaled steroids. Respir Med. 2001;95(1):37–9.
32. Steyn E, Mohamed Z, Husselman C. Non-invasive vagus nerve stimulation for the treatment of acute asthma exacerbations—results from an initial case series. Int J Emerg Med. 2013;6(1):7.
33. Suteng S, Wan X. Current situation and countermeasures of fatal asthma. Japan Med Introd. 1999;1:7–9.
34. Johnson AJ, Nunn AJ, Somner AR, et al. Circumstances of death from asthma. Br Med J. 1984;288:1870–2.
35. Hannaway PJ. Demographic characteristics of patients experiencing near-fatal and fatal asthma: results of a regional survey of 400 asthma specialists. Ann Allergy Asthma Immunol. 2000;84(6):587–93.
36. Investigation and analysis of disease severity and complications of patients with bronchial asthma in urban outpatient clinics in China. Chinese J Respir Crit Care. 2019;18(01):57, 59–62.
37. Huang-Yang HE, Hui C. Efficacy of BiPAP respiratory therapy in patients with exacerbations of acute severe bronchial asthma. J Trop Med. 2009;9(11):1278–9.
38. Liang D. Application value of non-invasive mechanical ventilation in emergency rescue of patients with severe asthma complicated with type II respiratory failure. Chinese Dis Med. 2015;000(010):118–119,120.

39. Asthma Group, Respiratory Association of Chinese Medical Association, China Asthma Alliance. Evaluation and management of acute attack of bronchial asthma by Chinese experts. Clin Med Res Pract. 2018;3(06):207.
40. Rowe BH, Bretzlaff JA, Bourdon C, et al. Magnesium sulfate for treating exacerbations of acute asthma in the emergency department. Cochrane Database Syst Rev. 2000;(2):CD001490.
41. Jinguo X, Jinsong J, Zaiqing L. Application of fiberoptic bronchoscope in the rescue of patients with critical asthma. Med Clin Res. 2007;24(3):463–5.
42. Corren J, Parnes JR, Wang L, et al. Tezepelumab in adults with uncontrolled asthma. N Engl J Med. 2017;377(10):936–46.
43. Pham TH, Damera G, Newbold P, et al. Reductions in eosinophil biomarkers by benralizumab in patients with asthma. Respir Med. 2016;111(21):9.
44. Ferguson GT, Fitzgerald JM, Bleecker ER, et al. Benralizumab for patients with mild to moderate, persistent asthma (BISE): a randomised, double-blind, placebo-controlled, phase 3 trial. Lancet Respir Med. 2017;5(7):568–76.
45. Milenkovi BA, Stankovi IJ, Ili AM, et al. Peak expiratory flow-guided self-management treatment of asthma in Serbia. J Asthma. 2007;44(9):699–704.
46. Kimura H, Konno S, Makita H, et al. Prospective predictors of exacerbation status in severe asthma over a 3-year follow-up. Clin Exp Allergy. 2018;48(9):1137–46.
47. Wiener RS, Schwartz LM, Woloshin S. Time trends in pulmonary embolism in the United States: evidence of over diagnosis. Arch Intern Med. 2011;171(9):831–7.
48. Konstantinides SV. Trends in incidence versus case fatality rates of pulmonary embolism: good news or bad news? Thromb Haemost. 2016;115(2):233–5.
49. Cohen AT, Agnelli G, Anderson FA, et al. Venous thromboembolism (VTE) in Europe. The number of VTE events and associated morbidity and mortality. Thromb Haemost. 2007;98(4):756–64.
50. Investigators P. Value of the ventilation/perfusion scan in acute pulmonary embolism. Results of the prospective investigation of pulmonary embolism diagnosis (PIOPED). JAMA. 1990;263(20):2753–9.
51. Stein PD, Beemath A, Matta F, et al. Clinical characteristics of patients with acute pulmonary embolism: data from PIOPED II. Am J Med. 2007;120(10):871–9.
52. Kucher N, Goldhaber SZ. Management of massive pulmonary embolism. Circulation. 2005;112(2):e28–32.
53. Rodger MA, Carrier M, Jones GN, et al. Diagnostic value of arterial blood gas measurement in suspected pulmonary embolism. Am J Respir Crit Care Med. 2000;162(6):2105–8.
54. Geibel A, Zehender M, Kasper W, et al. Prognostic value of the ECG on admission in patients with acute major pulmonary embolism. Eur Respir J. 2005;25(5):843–8.
55. Remy-Jardin M, Pistolesi M, Goodman LR, et al. Management of suspected acute pulmonary embolism in the era of CT angiography: a statement from the Fleischner Society. Radiology. 2007;245(2):315–29.
56. Raja AS, Greenberg JO, Qaseem A, et al. Evaluation of patients with suspected acute pulmonary embolism: best practice advice from the clinical guidelines committee of the American college of physicians. Ann Intern Med. 2015;163(9):701–11.
57. Courtney DM, Miller C, Smithline H, et al. Prospective multicenter assessment of interobserver agreement for radiologist interpretation of multidetector computerized tomographic angiography for pulmonary embolism. J Thromb Haemost. 2010;8(3):533–9.
58. Wang L, Kang W, Zu M, et al. Application of 128-slice spiral CT combination scanning in the diagnosis of embolisms in pulmonary arteries and lower extremity veins. Exp Ther Med. 2014;7(2):401–4.
59. Kligerman SJ, Lahiji K, Galvin JR, et al. Missed pulmonary emboli on CT angiography: assessment with pulmonary embolism-computer-aided detection. AJR Am J Roentgenol. 2014;202(1):65–73.
60. Musset D, Parent F, Meyer G, et al. Diagnostic strategy for patients with suspected pulmonary embolism: a prospective multicentre outcome study. Lancet. 2002;360(9349):1914–20.

61. Kruip MJ, Leclercq MG, Van Der Heul C, et al. Diagnostic strategies for excluding pulmonary embolism in clinical outcome studies. A systematic review. Ann Intern Med. 2003;138(12):941–51.
62. Yoo HH, Nunes-Nogueira VS, Fortes Villas Boas PJ, et al. Outpatient versus inpatient treatment for acute pulmonary embolism . Cochrane Database Syst Rev. 2019;(3):CD010019.
63. Roy PM, Corsi DJ, Carrier M, et al. Net clinical benefit of hospitalization versus outpatient management of patients with acute pulmonary embolism. J Thromb Haemost. 2017;15(4):685–94.
64. Konstantinides SV, Torbicki A, Agnelli G, et al. ESC guidelines on the diagnosis and management of acute pulmonary embolism. Eur Heart J. 2014;35(43):3033–69, 69a-69k
65. Kearon C, Akl EA, Comerota AJ, et al. Antithrombotic therapy for VTE disease: antithrombotic therapy and prevention of thrombosis, 9th ed: American college of chest physicians evidence-based clinical practice guidelines. Chest. 2012;141(2 Suppl):e419S–e96S.
66. Yoo H H, Queluz TH, El Dib R. Anticoagulant treatment for subsegmental pulmonary embolism. Cochrane Database Syst Rev. 2016;(1):CD010222.
67. Chechi T, Vecchio S, Spaziani G, et al. Rheolytic thrombectomy in patients with massive and submassive acute pulmonary embolism. Catheter Cardiovasc Interv. 2009;73(4):506–13.
68. Nassiri N, Jain A, Mcphee D, et al. Massive and submassive pulmonary embolism: experience with an algorithm for catheter-directed mechanical thrombectomy. Ann Vasc Surg. 2012;26(1):18–24.
69. Stein PD, Goodman LR, Hull RD, et al. Diagnosis and management of isolated subsegmental pulmonary embolism: review and assessment of the options. Clin Appl Thromb Hemost. 2012;18(1):20–6.
70. Osborne ZJ, Rossi P, Aucar J, et al. Surgical pulmonary embolectomy in a community hospital. Am J Surg. 2014;207(3):337–41. discussion 40-1
71. Lee T, Itagaki S, Chiang YP, et al. Survival and recurrence after acute pulmonary embolism treated with pulmonary embolectomy or thrombolysis in New York State, 1999 to 2013. J Thorac Cardiovasc Surg. 2018;155(3):1084–90.e12.
72. Meneveau N, Seronde MF, Blonde MC, et al. Management of unsuccessful thrombolysis in acute massive pulmonary embolism. Chest. 2006;129(4):1043–50.
73. Neely RC, Byrne JG, Gosev I, et al. Surgical embolectomy for acute massive and submassive pulmonary embolism in a series of 115 patients. Ann Thorac Surg. 2015;100(4):1245–51. discussion 51-2
74. Rosenberger P, Shernan SK, Mihaljevic T, et al. Transesophageal echocardiography for detecting extrapulmonary thrombi during pulmonary embolectomy. Ann Thorac Surg. 2004;78(3):862–6. discussion 6
75. Becattini C, Casazza F, Forgione C, et al. Acute pulmonary embolism: external validation of an integrated risk stratification model. Chest. 2013;144(5):1539–45.
76. Ten Wolde M, Sohne M, Quak E, et al. Prognostic value of echocardiographically assessed right ventricular dysfunction in patients with pulmonary embolism. Arch Intern Med. 2004;164(15):1685–9.
77. Beenen LFM, Bossuyt PMM, Stoker J, et al. Prognostic value of cardiovascular parameters in computed tomography pulmonary angiography in patients with acute pulmonary embolism. Eur Respir J. 2018;52(1):1702611.
78. Casazza F, Bongarzoni A, Centonze F, et al. Prevalence and prognostic significance of right-sided cardiac mobile thrombi in acute massive pulmonary embolism. Am J Cardiol. 1997;79(10):1433–5.
79. Torbicki A, Galie N, Covezzoli A, et al. Right heart thrombi in pulmonary embolism: results from the International Cooperative Pulmonary Embolism Registry. J Am Coll Cardiol. 2003;41(12):2245–51.

# Sudden Unexpected Death in Endocrine Diseases

# 20

Zhaojun Wang, Hanyi Zhang, and Wei Chong

**Abstract**

Sudden unexpected death (SUD) refers to the sudden (usually occurs within 24 h from the onset of the initial symptoms) and unexpected (not caused by obvious reasons like trauma, poisoning, violent asphyxia, etc.) death of a person. It may be the result of one or several serious underlying diseases, while the initial symptoms may be totally different from the common manifestations of those diseases. Disorders of many endocrine organs can cause SUD, and some of these conditions are reviewed in this article.

**Keywords**

Sudden unexpected death · Endocrine disease · Pheochromocytoma · Hyperthyroidism

## 20.1 Diseases of the Pituitary Gland

The pituitary gland (i.e., hypophysis) underlies the base of the hypothalamus within the sella turcica ("Turkish saddle") of the sphenoid bone. It is a delicate protective bony structure that is attached to the brain by blood vessels and nerve cell axons. Two major parts are found in the human pituitary gland: the adenohypophysis and

Z. Wang · W. Chong (✉)
Emergency Department, First Affiliated Hospital, China Medical University, Shenyang, Liaoning, China
e-mail: wchong@cmu.edu.cn

H. Zhang
Radiology Department, First Affiliated Hospital, China Medical University, Shenyang, Liaoning, China



H. Zhu (ed.), *Sudden Death*, https://doi.org/10.1007/978-981-15-7002-5_20

the neurohypophysis. It is made up of several cell types that receive sensory and hormonal inputs from the hypothalamic neurosecretory cells to maintain hormonal homeostasis, which is indispensable for survival via downstream control of the thyroid through thyroid-stimulating hormone (TSH), control of the adrenal cortex through adrenocorticotropic hormone (ACTH), and control of the gonads through follicle-stimulating hormone (FSH) and luteinizing hormone (LH).

In many circumstances, the pituitary gland may be damaged, which leads to insufficient hormone release by the pituitary gland [1]. Its common manifestations include:

1. Adrenocorticotropic hormone deficiency → weakness, tiredness, fatigue, anorexia, gastrointestinal disorders, weight loss, hyperpigmentation, hypotension, hyponatremia, hyperkalemia, azotemia, anemia, etc.
2. Thyroid-stimulating hormone deficiency → myxedematous, decreased pulse pressure and blood flow caused by hypodynamia of myocardium and pericardial effusion, anemia, impaired intellectual functions, etc.
3. Luteinizing and follicle-stimulating hormone deficiency → depends on the time point of the onset, causing a variety of syndromes.
4. Growth hormone deficiency → hypoglycemia.
5. Antidiuretic hormone deficiency → polyuria and hyponatremia.

ACTH deficiency can cause adrenal crises: hypoglycemia, hypotension, hyponatremia, etc. TSH deficiency can cause bradycardia and hypotension. In severe cases, these can be life-threatening [2]. Despite congenital disorders or space-occupying lesions, there are several conditions commonly seen in emergency that can cause acquired pituitary insufficiency.

### 20.1.1 Traumatic Brain Injury

Traumatic brain injury (TBI) has an annual incidence rate of 295 per 100,000 worldwide [3]. In Schneider's systematic review, a pooled prevalence of anterior pituitary hormone deficiency due to TBI of 27.5% was reported. Besides, approximately 5% of all hypopituitarism cases were caused by TBI [4]. Bevenga et al. found that pituitary dysfunction and necrosis existed in at least 30% of TBI fatalities reported in literatures from 1970 through 1998 [5]. Systematic imaging studies by Schneider et al. have shown that there is a high incidence of undiagnosed post-traumatic anterior pituitary abnormalities, which may lead to potentially fatal endocrine crises [6].

The causes of post-traumatic hypopituitarism may include direct mechanical trauma, vascular disorder of the hypothalamus or the pituitary gland, hypoxia, hypotension, increased intracranial pressure [7] etc. Several recent studies have revealed the role of Apolipoprotein E3 in the development of TBI-induced hypopituitarism [8–11]. Since trauma patients may have similar clinical manifestations to those of pituitary failure [12] (for example, increased cortisol due to systemic inflammatory response syndrome, SIRS; fatigue; concentration difficulties; and depression due to post-traumatic stress disorder, PTSD), diagnosis of hypopituitarism is often missed until it becomes serious or even sometimes life-threatening [13].

Recommendations assembled by the Defense Centers of Excellence (DCoE) for Psychological Health and Traumatic Brain Injury were released in December 2012 [14]. As the commonly used Glasgow Coma Scale (GCS) cannot tell whether a patient's pituitary gland is involved or not, this guideline encouraged primary care providers to consider screening patients with persistent symptoms after TBI and even up to 36 months post injury. Advanced age, basal skull fracture, focal cortical contusion, intracranial or petechial brain hemorrhage, diffuse axonal injury, increased intracranial pressure, seizure, and sustained coma or intubation are the factors that have been found to correlate with post-traumatic hypopituitarism [14–17].

Although hormone replacement therapy (HRT) is essential in many other causes of hypopituitarism, whether a patient with post-traumatic hypopituitarism will benefit from HRT or not may depend on whether the disorder is permanent or transient [14]. Nevertheless, most studies show a positive effect of HRT on TBI-induced hypopituitarism [18–24].

### 20.1.2 Hantavirus Infection

Hantaviruses are a group of viruses that are most commonly found in America, Europe, and Asia. In humans, they cause two classical syndromes: Hantavirus cardiopulmonary syndrome (HCPS) and hemorrhagic fever with renal syndrome (HFRS) [25, 26]. Patients usually suffer from hemorrhagic fevers with either acute respiratory distress syndrome (in HCPS) or renal failure (in HFRS).

Interestingly, some patients with Hantavirus infection develop hypopituitarism. Several studies have found pituitary gland atrophy, hemorrhage and necrosis in HFRS patients, which is possibly caused by hemorrhagic complications (thrombocytopenia, endothelial cell dysfunction, disseminated intravascular coagulation, etc.) [27–29]. However, there is no clear proof that pituitary hemorrhage is directly correlated with hypopituitarism, as some studies observed an exacerbated endocrine disorder in spite of the clinical remission of hemorrhagic fever [30–32]. Several hypotheses on how the Hantavirus infection causes hypopituitarism are as follows:

1. Hypotension or shock → pituitary gland ischemia → pituitary gland necrosis: This theory was supported by the study of Steer et al., which found pituitary gland damage in most of the HFRS patients who died during shock or oliguria [27], which is a common complication of Hantavirus Infection [33].
2. Depleted platelet → pituitary gland hemorrhage → pituitary gland damage: This theory was supported by the study of Valtonen et al., which found the hemorrhage foci in the pituitary gland in Hantavirus infected patients [29]. Besides, Stojanovic et al. found a correlation between Hantavirus infection and thrombocytopenia [34].

3. Inflammation of the pituitary gland → pituitary gland dysfunction: This theory was supported by the study of Hautala et al. as they isolated Hantavirus from stromal cells and vascular endothelial cells of the pituitary gland [35]. There is also evidence that the pituitary gland may undergo an auto-immune reaction after Hantavirus infection [36].

There are many other causes of hypopituitarism like empty sella syndrome, pituitary adenoma irradiation therapy, pituitary tumor or inflammation, etc. Clinicians should be aware of these possibilities and screen pituitary hormones if hypopituitarism is suspected.

## 20.2 Diseases of the Thyroid Gland

The thyroid gland is one of the largest endocrine organs. It uptakes dietary iodine, and then produces thyroid hormone through the following steps:

1. Transfer of iodide in the plasma into the thyroid cell through the sodium-iodide symporter (NIS),
2. Iodide oxidation into mono-iodotyrosine (MIT) and di-iodotyrosine (DIT) (i.e., organification), which is catalyzed by the hemecontaining protein, thyroid peroxidase (TPO),
3. Synthesis of iodothyronine from MIT and DIT, and linked to thyroglobulin (Tg),
4. Storage and release of thyroid hormone.

The thyroid gland is regulated by the feedback control loop including hypothalamus (which secretes thyrotropin-releasing hormone, TRH) and pituitary (which secretes thyrotropin, TSH). TSH is the key regulator of the morphology and function of the thyroid gland. The normal serum TSH level is between 0.4 and 4.2 mU/L, which is increased during primary hypothyroidism and reduced during thyrotoxicosis (hyperthyroidism) or secondary hypothyroidism. Either severe hypo or hyper thyroidism may cause a life-threatening condition.

### 20.2.1 Thyrotoxicosis

Thyrotoxicosis describes the effect of excessive thyroid hormones in various systems of the body in all cases. Thyrotoxicosis may be caused by primary hyperthyroidism, which means hyperfunction of the thyroid gland, most commonly seen in Graves' disease. Thyroiditis, which is usually caused by an autoimmune reaction or viral infection, can also cause thyrotoxicosis. Although thyrotoxicosis itself is a "benign" situation, excessive thyroid hormones may cause a severe medical condition like "thyrotoxic crisis"by exerting their influence on other systems of the body.

#### 20.2.1.1 Cardiovascular System

Excessive thyroid hormones directly increase sympathetic tone and decrease vagal tone, which causes tachycardia [37]. They also increase nitric oxide production and thus result in an increased systolic pressure, a decreased diastolic pressure, and an increased pulse pressure; this is frequently felt by patients themselves as a sense of palpitation [38–40]. In addition, thyrotoxicosis increases the metabolic rate, which needs an increased cardiac output [41]. As a result, this leads to complications of the heart including cardiac arrhythmias (e.g., atrial fibrillation and ventricular fibrillation), cardiac failure, cardiac ischemia or thrombosis, etc.

Cardiac arrhythmias are common in thyrotoxicosis patients; between 2% and 20% of them have atrial fibrillation, and about 15% of patients with unexplained atrial fibrillation are found to be thyrotoxic [41]. Atrial fibrillation decreases the efficiency of the heart, and when this happens with a patient with preexisting heart disease, cardiac failure or lethal arrhythmias may occur. Ohshima et al. reported an autopsy case of a 45-year-old woman with diffuse hyperplastic goiter (possibly Graves' disease) and thyroid crisis. They found hemosiderin-laden macrophages in the lungs, centrilobular necrosis, microscopic bleeding, fibrosis, and nodular regenerative hyperplasia of the liver, which indicated persistant heart failure [42]. Terndrup et al. reported a 22-year-old female with cardiopulmonary arrest. After basic life support (BLS) and advanced cardiac life support (ACLS) for 51 min, the patient still demonstrated apnea, pulselessness, and unresponsiveness, and resuscitative efforts were discontinued. Postmortem findings found nodular thyromegaly, elevated serum levels of T3 and decreased TSH, which indicated thyrotoxicosis [43]. Shirani et al. reported sudden death of two GD patients with enlarged hearts (420 and 425 g), dilated cardiac ventricles and ventricular walls free of the foci of fibrosis and necrosis [44]. Wei et al. reported a 30-year-old Chinese woman with GD who suddenly died after having a physical altercation. They found cardiomegaly with left ventricular hypertrophy in the postmortem examination [45]. Korte et al. reported an 18-year-old man who suffered a sudden cardiac arrest with ventricular fibrillation and was successfully resuscitated [46]. He had neither a medical nor family history of cardiac disease or sudden death, but was known to have Graves' disease. The blood test showed markedly elevated thyroid hormone levels, i.e., "thyroid storm" [47], which is sometimes caused by amiodarone or iodine contrast. Zhang et al. reported six cases of sudden death due to hyperthyroid heart disease between 2001 and 2016 in the Forensic Medicine School of China Medical University. They found an increase of cardiac weight, dilatation of cardiac chambers, myocardial hypertrophy, and focal necrosis [48]. These cases indicate thyrotoxicosis with preexisting heart enlargement as a potential cause of sudden death.

#### 20.2.1.2 Muscle

Thyrotoxic myopathy is more commonly seen in men than in women. Graves' disease occurs in about 3–5% of patients with myasthenia gravis, and about 1% of patients with Graves' disease develop myasthenia gravis. In most cases, myasthenia is aggravated during the thyrotoxic state and improves after the normal metabolic state is restored. Acute hypokalemic paralysis is a rare cause of acute weakness. Morbidity and mortality associated with unrecognized disease can occur and may include respiratory failure, lethal cardiac arrhythmias, and possibly death.

Thyrotoxic periodic paralysis (TPP), which has a particularly higher incidence in Asian and Latino men, is characterized by the sudden onset of hypokalemia and paralysis that primarily affect the lower extremities [49]. It can be triggered by extreme exercise, meals high in sodium or carbohydrate content [50, 51] etc. The underlying mechanism is thought to be skeletal muscle ion channel defects [52], as the $Na^+/K^+$-ATPase activity is higher in TPP than in other thyrotoxic subjects. Besides, TPP is found to be related with a high level of insulin [53] and an elevated serum testosterone level [54–56]. Recent research by Ryan et al. revealed the pathogenic gene mutation on *KCNJ18* that is responsible for TPP, which encodes an inwardly rectifying potassium channel, Kir2.6 [57]. Kir2.6 are primarily expressed in the skeletal muscle and probably contribute to cell membrane excitability. Furthermore, KCNJ18 has a thyroid hormone response cis element (TRE) within its promoter, which might up-regulate the expression of Kir2.6 to protect against membrane potential instability. Genetic analysis revealed mutations in Kir2.6 in multiple TPP patients. However, how these mutations cause predisposition for TPP remains a topic of further research.

#### 20.2.1.3 Other Systems

Thyrotoxicosis has variable effects on several other systems of the body. For energy metabolism, it increases the basal metabolic rate (BMR) and appetite, while also causing weight loss and muscle wasting. For the alimentary system, thyrotoxicosis increases the bowel movement and causes hepatic dysfunction in severe patients. These changes are unlikely to cause sudden unexpected death and are not discussed in this review.

Traditionally, there are three effective and relatively safe treatment options for Graves' disease: anti-thyroid agents (ATD), surgery (thyroidectomy), and radioiodine therapy (RAI). However, each kind of therapy has significant side effects and none is ideal [58]. Anti-thyroid drugs include thionamides (most commonly methimazole and propylthiouracil; act by inhibiting the oxidation and organic binding of iodide, impairing the conversion of thyroxine to triiodothyronine by type 1 deiodinase, and inhibiting the thyroid immune response) [59–61], iodine-containing agents (the Wolff–Chaikoff effect; inhibit hormone release and inhibit peripheral thyroxine conversion to triiodothyronine) [62, 63], β-blockers (blockage of the response to catecholamines) [64, 65], dexamethasone (inhibition of the peripheral conversion of thyroxine to triiodothyronine and suppression of the autoimmune reaction) [66, 67], lithium agents (temporary control of thyrotoxicosis in those who are sensitive to thiocarbamide and iodide) [68], etc. For surgery, the common complications include hypothyroidism, hypoparathyroidism and recurrent laryngeal nerve damage. The most serious postoperative complication is asphyxia caused by intratracheal hemorrhage and it should be treated immediately, or it may cause sudden death. Radioiodine therapy has been the favorite therapy but in recent years more physicians tend to prefer ATDs to RAI. In fact, according to the 2016 ATA guidelines for thyrotoxicosis, patients receiving one of the three treatment options were found to have the same long-term quality of life (QoL) [69].

### 20.2.2 Hypothyroidism

Hypothyroidism refers to the clinical condition featured by the reduced production of thyroid hormone, which affects about 4–10% of the population [70]. Hypothyroidism can be divided into primary and secondary. Primary hypothyroidism is usually caused by autoimmune destruction of the thyroid (i.e., autoimmune thyroid disease, AITD). Radioiodine therapy can also induce hypothyroidism occasionally. Secondary (or central) hypothyroidism is caused by disease of the hypothalamus or pituitary, which leads to insufficient secretion of thyrotropin-releasing hormone (TRH) or thyroid-stimulating hormone (TSH).

Hypothyroidism can affect almost all systems of the body. For example, hypotension, decreased pulse pressure, multiple serous cavity effusion, myxedematous tissue, stiffness and aching of muscles, impaired renal excretion of water, anemia, decreased energy metabolism and heat production, decreased intellectual functions, and changes in a variety of hypothalamus and pituitary hormones. Hypothyroidism is associated with decreased cardiac output due to the impaired relaxation of the vascular smooth muscle and decreased availability of endothelial nitric oxide; besides, thyroid hormones also impact the renin-angiotensin-aldosterone system and the beta-adrenergic system. As for molecular mechanisms, thyroid hormones regulate pacemaker-related genes in cardiomyocytes at the level of transcription [70]. Electrocardiograph usually shows bradycardia, flattened T waves, low voltage, bundle branch blocks, complete heart blocks, or even prolonged QT intervals leading to "torsades de pointes."

Myxedema coma is the most severe stage of hypothyroidism with a mortality rate of 20% or higher [71]. The pathogenic mechanism of myxedema coma is still not clear. The predisposing factors that contribute to its development include iodine insufficiency, hypothermia, hypoxemia, hypoglycemia, infection, trauma, the use of depressants or anesthetics, etc. The common clinical manifestations include severe myxedema, bradycardia, severe hypotension, delayed deep tendon reflexes, etc. The factors associated with higher mortality include advanced age, female, cardiac arrhythmias, persistent hypothermia, reduced consciousness, sepsis, and delay in therapy [72–74].

Treating myxedema coma is a multisystem challenge. Identification and treatment of the precipitating factor is essential. Aspiration and airway obstruction could occur due to the altered mental status and the myxedema of the larynx, which may lead to sudden death. Thus most patients will require assisted ventilation and controlled oxygen administration. Also, assessment of any pneumonia with imaging is needed to ensure the treatment of the possible underlying causes. Fluid resuscitation is needed while monitoring sodium and slow re-warming to avoid further hypotension. If hypotension is refractory to fluid resuscitation, then vasopressors should be initiated until levothyroxine has time to act. Hypotonic fluids should be avoided as low sodium can precipitate the altered mental status. Prompt initiation of thyroid hormone replacement therapy is of paramount importance when myxedema coma is highly suspected, even before having thyroid hormone results back. A delay could increase the mortality and morbidity of the patient [75]. Hydrocortisone is recommended to be administered prior to thyroid hormone replacement therapy, especially if the patient is hypotensive, to avoid adrenal crises, since levothyroxine will accelerate cortisol metabolism, and hypothyroidism may mask an underlying adrenal insufficiency [76, 77]. The administration of intravenous levothyroxine should follow. According to the recent ATA guidelines, the recommended initial dose is 200–400 mg IV once. TSH, FT4, and FT3 should be measured every 24–48 h until the patient's mental status starts to improve. One case report in 2017 suggests split high-dose oral LT4 as a therapeutic option in myxedema coma [74]. Another case report in 2019 indicates that treatment of a patient with a combination of levothyroxine 200 mg and liothyronine 50 mg for 5 days showed a successful improvement in the patient's condition; therefore, some reports recommended starting with 200–300 mg of levothyroxine and 10–25 mg of liothyronine as an alternative initial treatment [78]. This needs more cases to be confirmed.

## 20.3 Diseases of the Adrenal Gland

The adrenal gland is a pyramidal structure that lies above the kidneys. It is composed of cortex and medulla. The cortex can be further divided into Zona reticularis, Zona fasciculate, and Zona glomerulosa, from the inner to the outer. The adrenal cortex mainly produces three types of hormones—*glucocorticoids* (cortisol and corticosterone), *mineralocorticoids* (aldosterone and deoxycorticosterone), and *sex steroids* (mainly androgens). The adrenal medulla produces catecholamine, including epinephrine, norepinephrine, dopamine, etc.

Glucocorticoids affect many parts of the body. They increase blood glucose concentrations through glycogen (via glucogenesis and gluconeogenesis), protein (via proteolysis), and lipid (via lipolysis) metabolism. Glucocorticoids lead to sodium retention and potassium loss, which can cause hypernatremia and hypokalemia. They also induce negative calcium balance, resulting in osteopenia and osteoporosis. As for the immune system, glucocorticoids suppress the immunologic function in many ways, and thus they are used to treat a variety of autoimmune and inflammatory diseases.

The pituitary derived ACTH is the key hormone that controls adrenal glucocorticoid biosynthesis and secretion. It is regulated by CRH and arginine vasopressin (AVP) from the hypothalamus. The zona glomerulosa secretes aldosterone under the control of angiotensin II and potassium through the regulation of CYP11B2 transcription [79]. The adrenal hormones exert their effects by binding to their intracellular receptors: cortisol binds to the glucocorticoid receptor (GR, encoded by NR3C1) and aldosterone binds to the mineralocorticoid receptor (MR, encoded by NR3C2) [80–82].

Catecholamines regulate various cardiovascular and metabolic processes through the three main kinds of α, β, and dopaminergic receptors.

The adrenergic receptor α1 is a postsynaptic receptor that mediates vascular and smooth muscle contraction. It causes vasoconstriction and increases the blood pressure.

The adrenergic receptor α2 is a presynaptic receptor. It inhibits the release of norepinephrine, leading to down regulation of the central sympathetic outflow and blood pressure.

The adrenergic receptor β1 is located on the heart. It mediates positive inotropic and chronotropic effects on the heart, as well as increases renin secretion in the kidneys.

The adrenergic receptor β2 mediates bronchial, vascular, and uterine smooth muscle relaxation. It causes dilatation of these muscles. Besides, it also increases nor-epinephrine release from sympathetic nerve terminals.

The adrenergic receptor β3 regulates energy expenditure and lipolysis.

The adrenergic receptor D1 is located on the cerebral cortex and coronary, mesenteric, and renal vasculatures. It causes vasodilation of these vascular beds.

The adrenergic receptor D2 is a presynaptic receptor. It inhibits the release of norepinephrine at the sympathetic nerve endings, inhibits ganglionic transmission at the sympathetic ganglia, inhibits prolactin release in the hypophysis, and promotes catecholamine secretion at the adrenal medullary [83].

## 20.4 Pheochromocytoma and Paraganglioma

Catecholamine-secreting tumors are derived from the chromaffin cells of the adrenal medulla (pheochromocytoma, PCC, which mostly releases epinephrine) and the sympathetic ganglia (paraganglioma, PGL, which mostly releases both catecholamines).

The typical clinical manifestations of these tumors are headaches, palpitations, and diaphoresis. The other symptoms and signs may include paroxysmal hypertension, orthostatic hypotension, anxiety and fear of dying, headache, dyspnea, chest pain, nausea and vomiting, etc. Since these symptoms are also commonly seen in the general population, the identification of pheochromocytoma or paraganglioma from the simple symptoms and signs is a real challenge for clinicians. The diagnosis of PCCs and PGLs is based on (a) the detection of excessive production of catecholamines and (b) anatomical documentation of the tumor. Measurement of plasma and urinary fractionated catecholamines (epinephrine, norepinephrine, and dopamine) has been used for biochemical diagnosis of PCCs and PGLs in the past and the clearly elevated values (>2 times the upper limit of the normal range) are interpreted as positive [84, 85]. Besides, plasma fractionated metanephrines (metanephrine and normetanephrine) have shown a better accuracy with a mean sensitivity of

97% and a specificity of 93% across 15 studies [86]. A variety of medications such as tricyclic antidepressants, antipsychotics, L-dopa, amphetamines, cocaine, heroin, and even ethanol may cause elevations in catecholamines, and thus should be discontinued at least 2 weeks before assessments. For medical imaging of PCCs and PGLs, contrastenhanced CT or T2weighted MRI should be considered. PPGLs are highly heritable, as nearly 40% of these cases are associated with mutations in 15 well-established pathogenic genes [87–90].

### 20.4.1 Takotsubo Syndrome

First described in the 1990s by Sato et al., Takotsubo syndrome is characterized by symptoms similar to acute myocardial infarction without coronary artery obstruction, as well as acute severe left ventricular dysfunction which is mostly reversible with almost complete resolution in hours to weeks [91–94]. Takotsubo syndrome may also show typical electrocardiographic (ECG) changes of acute coronary syndrome (ACS) and myocardial infarction biomarker elevation [95, 96]. The ECG frequently shows a ST-segment elevation, but ST-segment depression and abnormal Q waves are relatively rare [97, 98]. For biomarkers, minor elevation of cardiac troponin and creatine kinase-MB is usually seen. Occasionally, these markers can be elevated significantly, which probably reflects more severe myocardial damage such as ST-segment elevation myocardial infarction [96]. Serum brain natriuretic peptide and N-terminal pro-B-type natriuretic peptide are usually increased in Takotsubo syndrome, which is related to ventricular stretching [99, 100].

A typical takotsubo syndrome patient has a unique circumferential left (bi-) ventricular contraction abnormality profile that extends beyond a coronary artery supply territory and appears to follow the anatomical cardiac sympathetic innervation [101]. The left ventricular wall motion abnormality is most commonly localized to the apical segments of the left ventricle [102]. There are several mechanisms for the development of Takotsubo syndrome: myocardial ischemia [96, 103], left ventricular outflow tract obstruction [104], myocardial toxicity of catecholamine [105, 106], sympathetic nervous system hyperactivation with autonomic nervous system dysfunction [107, 108], etc.

McGonigle et al. [109] reported a patient with "recurrent myocardial infarction" with pheochromocytoma. The patient had reversible tombstone-like ST segment elevation. Left ventricular angiography revealed discrete left ventricular apical "aneurysm" with a clot in the aneurysmal sac, with normal coronary arteries. With the current knowledge, this case is thought to be recurrent Takotsubo syndrome triggered by a pheochromocytoma [101]. Jessurun et al. reported a 30-year-old pregnant woman with pheochromocytoma who suffered acute anterior myocardial infarction with non-Q reinfarction [110]. Echocardiography showed mild hypokinesis of the mid and distal septum with moderate concentric left ventricular hypertrophy with a depressed left ventricular ejection fraction of 45%. This patient is now thought to be with Takotsubo syndrome. There were also several cases of "reversible pheochromocytoma induced cardiomyopathy," which can be remarkably improved by alpha receptor blockers [111–113]. Shams Y-Hassan reviewed 80 cases of PCCs and PGLs and found that pheochromocytoma-induced Takotsubo syndrome is characterized by a dramatic clinical presentation with a high complication rate and a relatively high recurrence rate [114]. Batisse-Lignier et al. reviewed 145 cases of PCCs and PGLs and found a higher rate of LV function in Takotsubo cardiomyopathy than other chronic catecholaminergic cardiomyopathies [115]. Rong Zhang et al. reviewed 163 cases of pheochromocytoma and cardiomyopathy. Their study highlighted the importance of early diagnosis of pheochromocytoma in cases of idiopathic heart failure to prevent progression to irreversible myocardial remodeling and death [116].

## 20.5 Diabetes Mellitus and its Complications

### 20.5.1 Diabetes Mellitus

Diabetes mellitus is a metabolic disease caused by insufficient insulin production by the beta cells in the pancreas. Deficiency of insulin can be either absolute or relative. Type 1 diabetes mellitus (T1DM) is caused by the destruction of the beta cells in the pancreas, usually secondary to autoimmunity, and its etiology is linked to the major histocompatibility complex and the human leukocyte antigen [117]. Type 2 diabetes mellitus (T2DM) is caused by insulin resistance, which is attributable to impaired glucose transport and increased fat breakdown due to excess fatty acids and proinflammatory cytokines. Like many other endocrine diseases, the etiology of T2DM includes both genetic predisposition and exposure to a series of environmental factors (e.g., sex, age, obesity, and ethnic background). Other types of diabetes include maturity-onset diabetes of the young (MODY), gestational diabetes, neonatal diabetes, and secondary diabetes due to a variety of causes. Chronic hyperglycemia induces nonenzymatic glycation of proteins and lipids, which can be measured by glycation hemoglobin (HbA1c). Glycation leads to damage in small blood vessels, resulting in diabetic retinopathy, nephropathy, and neuropathy [86].

Diagnosis of diabetes mellitus is made based on the following criteria: [118].

1. Fasting glucose level greater than 126 mg/dL (7.0 mmol/L).
2. A 2-h plasma glucose level greater than 200 mg/dL (11.1 mmol/L) during a 75-g OGTT.
3. A random plasma glucose greater than 200 mg/dL (11.1 mmol/L) with typical symptoms (polyuria, polydipsia, polyphagia, weight loss, etc.) or hyperglycemic crisis.
4. A HbA1c level greater than 6.5%.

Treatments of diabetes mellitus are complex and different for T1DM and T2DM. For T1DM, the cornerstone is intensive insulin treatment. For T2DM, treatments include diet, exercise, drugs, and finally, insulin. Drugs include:

1. Metformin.
2. Sulfonylurea.

3. Meglitinide.
4. Thiazolidinedione.
5. α-glucosidase inhibitor,
6. Glucagon-like-peptide-1 agonist (GLP-1).
7. Dipeptidyl peptidase IV inhibitor (DPP-4).
8. Sodium-glucose transporter-2-inhibitor (SGLT-2).

There are several acute complications of DM, including diabetic ketoacidosis, hyperosmolar hyperglycemic syndrome, and hypoglycemia.

## 20.6 Diabetic Ketoacidosis (DKA)

DKA is most commonly seen in T1DM; it can also occur in patients with T2DM that are suffering from stress like trauma, serious infections, and cardiovascular emergencies. In this condition, tissues cannot obtain glucose from the plasma due to insulin insufficiency, and severe hyperglycemia occurs. Then lipids undergo lipolysis into ketones (acetone, β-hydroxybutyrate, and acetoacetate) as a compensation for energy support.

In addition to the increased overproduction of ketone bodies, their clearance is decreased in DKA [119, 120]. There are also some other conditions that can cause acidosis or ketosis. For example, lactic acidosis [121, 122], uremic acidosis [123, 124], alcoholic ketoacidosis, [125–127] and starvation ketosis. These can be distinguished from DKA in many aspects. The characteristics of DKA include:

1. Hyperglycemia, ketonemia, and systemic acidosis: high anion-gap metabolic acidosis. Serum $HCO_3^-$ concentrations are usually less than 10 mg/dL.
2. Kussmaul respirations: deep, slow, hyperventilation, fruity odor of acetone.
3. Nausea, vomiting, and abdominal pain: may be associated with prostaglandin production by adipose tissue [128], and it usually resolves quickly with treatment of DKA in those without an underlying abdominal pathology.
4. Dehydration and electrolyte imbalance: diuresis and vomiting can cause severe loss of water and electrolytes, which results in dehydration and electrolyte abnormalities. This can cause sudden death by inducing cardiac arrhythmias, cerebral edema, shock, etc.

The treatments of DKA include:

1. Resolution of hyperglycemia. Insulin treatment is the cornerstone of DKA management. A low dose of insulin (beginning at 0.1 U/kg/h) should be given intravenously, or by infusion pump [129], as the subcutaneous route is probably ineffective because of tissue hypoperfusion and slower absorption in patients with shock or other critical conditions. The best route of insulin administration during DKA is still under debate. Frequent subcutaneous or IM injection has also been recommended, since patients who are treated with IV insulin therapy

have a more rapid fall in plasma glucose, particularly in the first hour [130, 131]. A study of Umpierrez GE et al. suggested that intravenous regular insulin can be replaced by subcutaneously administered insulin in the treatment of mild–moderate DKA [132]. Besides, some studies found that the time by which BG was brought to below 250 mg/dL in patients with DKA and DK was approximately 4–5 h, which is similar whether the administration was by the IV or IM route [133, 134].

2. Restoration of the circulatory volume and tissue perfusion. Patients with DKA usually suffer from a water deficit of 5–10 L. Hydration reduces hyperglycemia by decreased counter-regulatory hormones, enhanced renal glucose clearance, and augmented insulin sensitivity [135–137]. Repletion of fluids by administration of saline will recover renal perfusion, which in turn increases clearance of glucose and organic/inorganic acids. The general treatment is to administer 1000–1500 mL of normal saline over the first hour to restore the cardiovascular stability, and 200–500 mL/h until fluid depletion is corrected. When the serum glucose level is brought down to 250 mg/dL (13.9 mmol/L), saline should be replaced by 5% glucose and the aim of the therapy is to maintain the serum glucose concentration in that range for approximately 24 h to allow slow formation of osmotic equilibration across cell membranes as taking down serum osmolality too fast may result in cerebral edema [138]. This may be induced by an increased brain cell volume (caused by intracellular osmole retention) or an increased brain ECF volume (caused by an increased hydrostatic pressure or a decreased osmotic pressure in capillaries at the BBB) [139]. However, several other studies did not find a causal relationship between fluid administration and cerebral edema [140–142]. One possible mechanism depends on activation of the sodium/hydrogen ion exchanger 1 (NHE1) [143]. Insulin can activate NHE1 directly; besides, increased intracellular hydrogen ion, which is derived from dissociated β-hydroxybutyric acid and acetoacetic acid during DKA, also activates NHE1 [144]. Activation of NHE1 causes a sodium ion influx and a hydrogen ion efflux. Since hydrogen ions are bound to ICF proteins and thus can no longer be effective osmoles, NHE1 activation will result in an increased amount of effective osmoles in brain cells. Selective inhibitors of NHE1 like analogues of amiloride may be a possible medication for cerebral edema [143, 145]. Kuppermann et al. found no difference in the neurologic outcomes between pediatric DKA patients receiving sodium chloride of different concentrations (0.45% or 0.9%), or administered at different rates [142]. Shafi et al. compared vital clinical parameters, time for the correction of hyperglycemia and acidosis, and incidence of cerebral edema between 3% saline and 0.9% saline solutions on DKA and found no significant difference [146]. This suggests a fluid independent mechanism for the development of cerebral edema [140, 147, 148]. There are also other theories on the cause of cerebral edema, for example, the hypoxia-ischemia theory [141]. The symptoms of cerebral edema may include headache, recurrent vomiting, irritability, altered consciousness, incontinence, abnormal respiration pattern, a delayed rise in serum sodium after repletion, or cranial nerve dysfunction [149]. Mannitol administration is recommended as

soon as cerebral edema is suspected, which should not be delayed while waiting for the results of cerebral CT or MR [150].

3. Correction of electrolyte imbalance and acidosis. The most common ion disorder in DKA should be disturbance of potassium. Patients with DKA usually undergo a shift of potassium from the intracellular space to the extracellular fluid during DKA development. This is mainly caused by acidosis and osmotic diuresis. As a matter of fact, hyperkalemia occurs in most patients with DKA. Low plasma potassium levels indicate severe potassium depletion. According to the American Diabetes Association and the Canadian Diabetes Association, insulin administration should be delayed in DKA patients who have an initial plasma potassium level lower than 3 mmol/L [151, 152].Therefore, potassium should be supported to those without hyperkalemia or renal failure. The serum potassium level should be measured frequently as either hypo- or hyperkalemia can cause various life-threatening cardiac arrhythmias. These may include sinus bradycardia [153], ventricular tachycardia [153, 154], Brugada syndrome [155–157], cardiac arrest [158], etc. Among these, atrial fibrillation may be the most common arrhythmia, and it is associated with higher in-hospital mortality rates and complications including septic shock, pulmonary failure, mechanical ventilation, neurological failure, cerebral edema, acute kidney injury, acute hematologic failure, and cardiac arrest [159]. Replacement of bicarbonate is not recommended in DKA patients with a pH of 6.9 or higher [160].
4. Treat the correctable underlying cause. For example, insulin omission, sepsis, cerebrovascular disease, trauma, and myocardial infarction. Drugs like glucocorticoids, diuretics, antipsychotics, and alcohol can also induce DKA and HHS [161, 162].

## 20.7 Hyperosmolar Hyperglycemic State (HHS)

HHS occurs most commonly in elderly patients, and its mortality can be 5–16%, which is higher than DKA [161, 163]. Unlike DKA, HHS typically has a more severe degree of hyperglycemia (>30–33.3 mmol/L) and dehydration caused by osmotic diuresis, but without excessive ketones since insulin produced by the pancreatic beta cells still meets the need [151, 164, 165]. The distinguishing diagnostic factor of HHS from DKA is that the pH is greater than 7.3 and the bicarbonate level is greater than 20 mmol/L (ADA guidelines) or 15 mmol/L (UK guidelines). Besides, the serum osmolality is usually greater than 320 mOsm/kg. Osmolality = [2 × Na (meQ/L) + glucose (mg/dL)/18 + blood urea nitrogen (mg/dL)/2.8] or = [2 × Na (mmol/L) + glucose(mmol/L) + urea (mmol/L)]. Patients with HHS have higher concentrations of circulating hepatic insulin [166] and lower concentrations of hormones that can raise the blood glucose level (cortisol, growth hormone, and glucagon) than those with diabetic ketoacidosis [161]. The Joint British Diabetes Societies for Inpatient Care have particular guidelines for HHS separate from DKA [164]. Treatments of HHS have a lot of aspects that are similar to DKA and are not discussed in this review.

## References


1. Vance NF, Brittenham M. Hypopituitarism. NEJM. 1994;330:1651–62.
2. Schneider HJ, Aimaretti G, Kreitschmann-Andermahr I, et al. Hypopituitarism. Lancet. 2007;369:1461–70.
3. Nguyen R, Kirsten MF, et al. The international incidence of traumatic brain injury: a systematic review and meta-analysis. Can J Neurol Sci. 2016;43(6):774–85.
4. Schneider HJ, Kreitschmann-Andermahr I, Ghigo E, et al. Hypothalamopituitary dysfunction following traumatic brain injury and aneurysmal subarachnoid hemorrhage: a systematic review. JAMA. 2007;298(12):1429–38.
5. Benvenga S, Campenni A, Ruggeri RM, et al. Clinical review 113: hypopituitarism secondary to head trauma. J Clin Endocrinol Metab. 2000;85(4):1353–61.
6. Schneider M, Schneider HJ, Stalla GK. Anterior pituitary hormone abnormalities following traumatic brain injury. J Neurotrauma. 2005;22(9):937–46.
7. Caputo M, Mele C, Prodam F, et al. Clinical picture and the treatment of TBI-induced hypopituitarism. Pituitary. 2019;22(3):261–9.
8. Tanriverdi F, Taheri S, Ulutabanca H, et al. Apolipoprotein E3/E3 genotype decreases the risk of pituitary dysfunction after traumatic brain injury due to various causes: preliminary data. J Neurotrauma. 2008;25(9):1071–7.
9. Tanriverdi F, De Bellis A, Bizzarro A, et al. Antipituitary antibodies after traumatic brain injury: is head trauma-induced pituitary dysfunction associated with autoimmunity. Eur J Endocrinol. 2008;159(1):7–13.
10. Karaca Z, Tanrıverdi F, Ünlühızarcı K, et al. GH and pituitary hormone alterations after traumatic brain injury. Prog Mol Biol Transl Sci. 2016;138:167–91.
11. Karamouzis I, Pagano L, Prodam F, et al. Clinical and diagnostic approach to patients with hypopituitarism due to traumatic brain injury (TBI), subarachnoid hemorrhage (SAH), and ischemic stroke (IS). Endocrine. 2016;52(3):441–50.
12. Klose M, Juul A, Struck J, et al. Acute and long-term pituitary insufficiency in traumatic brain injury: a prospective single-centre study. Clin Endocrinol (Oxf). 2007;67(4):598–606.
13. Tanriverdi F, Agha A, Aimaretti G, et al. Manifesto for the current understanding and management of traumatic brain injury-induced hypopituitarism. J Endocrinol Invest. 2011;34(7):541–3.
14. Defense Centers of Excellence (DCoE) for psychological health and traumatic brain injury. 2017. https://dvbic.dcoe.mil/files/resources/DCoE_TBI_NED_Clnical_Recommendations.pdf. Accessed Sept 17.
15. Ghigo E, Masel B, Aimaretti G, et al. Consensus guidelines on screening for hypopituitarism following traumatic brain injury. Brain Inj. 2005;19(9):711–24.
16. Silva PP, Bhatnagar S, Herman SD, et al. Predictors of hypopituitarism in patients with traumatic brain injury. J Neurotrauma. 2015;32(22):1789–95.
17. Schneider M, Schneider HJ, Yassouridis A, et al. Predictors of anterior pituitary insufficiency after traumatic brain injury. Clin Endocrinol. 2008;68(2):206–12.
18. Kreitschmann-Andermahr I, Poll EM, Reineke A, et al. Growth hormone deficient patients after traumatic brain injury—baseline characteristics and benefits after growth hormone replacement—an analysis of the German KIMS database. Growth Horm IGF Res. 2008;18(6):472–8.
19. High WM Jr, Briones-Galang M, Clark JA, et al. Effect of growth hormone replacement therapy on cognition after traumatic brain injury. J Neurotrauma. 2010;27(9):1565–75.
20. Agha A, Phillips J, O'Kelly P, et al. The natural history of post-traumatic hypopituitarism: implications for assessment and treatment. Am J Med. 2005;118(12):1416.
21. Reifschneider K, Auble BA, Rose SR. Update of endocrine dysfunction following pediatric traumatic brain injury. J Clin Med. 2015;4(8):1536–60.
22. Rosario ER, Aqeel R, Brown MA, et al. Hypothalamic-pituitary dysfunction following traumatic brain injury affects functional improvement during acute inpatient rehabilitation. J Head Trauma Rehabil. 2013;28(5):390–6.

23. Popovic V, Aimaretti G, Casanueva FF, et al. Hypopituitarism following traumatic brain injury. In: JOL J, Christiansen JS, editors. Growth hormone deficiency in adults, vol. 33. Basel: Karger; 2005. p. 33–44.
24. Zaben M, El Ghoul W, Belli A. Post-traumatic head injury pituitary dysfunction. Disabil Rehabil. 2013;35(6):522–5.
25. Bhoelan S, Langerak T, Noack D, et al. Hypopituitarism after orthohantavirus infection: what is currently known? Viruses. 2019;11(4):340.
26. Steer A. Pathology of hemorrhagic fever: A comparison of the findings—1951 and 1952. Am J Pathol. 1955;31(2):201–21.
27. Lukes RJ. The pathology of thirty-nine fatal cases of epidemic hemorrhagic fever. Am J Med. 1954;16(5):639–50.
28. Lim TH, Chang KH, Han MC, et al. Pituitary atrophy in Korean (epidemic) hemorrhagic fever: CT correlation with pituitary function and visual field. AJNR Am J Neuroradiol. 1986;7(4):633–7.
29. Valtonen M, Kauppila M, Kotilainen P, et al. Four fatal cases of nephropathia epidemica. Scand J Infect Dis. 1995;27(5):515–7.
30. Sarıgüzel N, Hofmann J, Canpolat AT, et al. Dobrava orthohantavirus infection complicated by panhypopituitarism, Istanbul, Turkey, 2010. Emerg Infect Dis. 2012;18(7):1180–3.
31. Suh DC, Park JS, Park SK, et al. Pituitary hemorrhage as a complication of hantaviral disease. AJNR Am J Neuroradiol. 1995;16(1):175–8.
32. Jost C, Krause R, Graninger W, et al. Transient hypopituitarism in a patient with nephropathia epidemica. BMJ Case Rep. 2009;2009:pii: bcr02.2009.1538.
33. Pekic S, Cvijovic G, Stojanovic M, et al. Hypopituitarism as a late complication of hemorrhagic fever. Endocrine. 2005;26(2):79–82.
34. Stojanovic M, Pekic S, Cvijovic G, et al. High risk of hypopituitarism in patientswho recovered from hemorrhagic fever with renal syndrome. J Clin Endocrinol Metab. 2008;93(7):2722–8.
35. Hautala T, Sironen T, Vapalahti O, et al. Hypophyseal hemorrhage and panhypopituitarism during Puumala virus infection: magnetic resonance imaging and detection of viral antigen in the hypophysis. Clin Infect Dis. 2002;35(1):96–101.
36. Tarvainen M, Mäkelä S, Mustonen JE. Autoimmune polyendocrinopathy and hypophysitis after Puumala orthohantavirus infection. Endocrinol Diabetes Metab Case Rep. 2016;2016:16-0084.
37. Burggraaf J, Tulen JH, Lalezari S, et al. Sympathovagal imbalance in hyperthyroidism. Am J Physiol Endocrinol Metab. 2001;281(1):E190–5.
38. Kahaly GJ, Wagner S, Nieswandt J, et al. Stress echocardiography in hyperthyroidism. J Clin Endocrinol Metab. 1999;84(7):2308–13.
39. Fazio S, Palmieri EA, Lombardi G, et al. Effects of thyroid hormone on the cardiovascular system. Recent Prog Horm Res. 2004;59:31–50.
40. Napoli R, Biondi B, Guardasole V, et al. Impact of hyperthyroidism and its correction on vascular reactivity in humans. Circulation. 2001;104(25):3076–80.
41. Kahaly GJ, Dillmann WH. Thyroid hormone action in the heart. Endocr Rev. 2005;26(5):704–28.
42. Ohshima T, Maeda H, Takayasu T, et al. An autopsy case of sudden death due to hyperthyroidism. Nihon Hoigaku Zasshi. 1990;44(4):365–70.
43. Terndrup TE, Heisig DG, Garceau JP. Sudden death associated with undiagnosed Graves' disease. J Emerg Med. 1990;8(5):553–5.
44. Shirani J, Barron MM, Pierre-Louis ML, et al. Congestive heart failure, dilated cardiac ventricles, and sudden death in hyperthyroidism. Am J Cardiol. 1993;72(3):365–8.
45. Wei D, Yuan X, Yang T, et al. Sudden unexpected death due to Graves' disease during physical altercation. J Forensic Sci. 2013;58(5):1374–7.
46. Korte AKM, Derde L, van Wijk J, et al. Sudden cardiac arrest as a presentation of Brugada syndrome unmasked by thyroid storm. BMJ Case Rep. 2015;2015:bcr2015212351.
47. Nayak B, Burman K. Thyrotoxicosis and thyroid storm. Endocrinol Metab Clin North Am. 2006;35(4):663–86.

48. Zhang MZ, Li BX, Zhao R, et al. Forensic analysis of 6 cases of sudden death due to hyperthyroid heart disease. Fa Yi Xue Za Zhi. 2017;33(5):482–5.
49. Meseeha M, Parsamehr B, Kissell K, et al. Thyrotoxic periodic paralysis: a case study and review of the literature. J Commun Hosp Intern Med Perspect. 2017;7(2):103–6.
50. Klubo-Gwiezdzinska J, Wartofsky L. Thyroid emergencies. Med Clin North Am. 2012;96(2):385–403.
51. Vijayakumar A, Ashwath G, Thimmappa D. Thyrotoxic periodic paralysis: clinical challenges. J Thyroid Res. 2014;2014:649502.
52. Chan A, Shinde R, Chow CC, et al. In vivo and in vitro sodium pump activity in subjects with thyrotoxic periodic paralysis. BMJ. 1991;303(6810):1096–9.
53. Soonthornpun S, Setasuban W, Thamprasit A. Insulin resistance in subjects with a history of thyrotoxic periodic paralysis (TPP). Clin Endocrinol (Oxf). 2009;70(5):794–7.
54. Yao Y, Fan L, Zhang X, et al. Episodes of paralysis in Chinese men with thyrotoxic periodic paralysis are associated with elevated serum testosterone. Thyroid. 2013;23(4):420–7.
55. Biering H, Bauditz J, Pirlich M, et al. Manifestation of thyrotoxic periodic paralysis in two patients with adrenal adenomas and hyperandrogenaemia. Horm Res. 2003;59(6):301–4.
56. Guerra M, Rodriguez del Castillo A, Battaner E, et al. Androgens stimulate preoptic area Na+,K+-ATPase activity in male rats. Neurosci Lett. 1987;78(1):97–100.
57. Ryan DP, Da Silva MR, Soong TW, et al. Mutations ion potassium channel Kir2.6 cause susceptibility to thyrotoxic hypokalemic periodic paralysis. Cell. 2010;140(1):88–98.
58. Singer PA, Cooper DS, Levy E, et al. Treatment guidelines for patients with hyperthyroidism and hypothyroidism. JAMA. 1995;273(10):808–12.
59. Cooper DS. Antithyroid drugs. N Engl J Med. 2005;352(9):905–17.
60. Abuid J, Larsen PR. Triiodothyronine and thyroxine in hyperthyroidism: comparison of the acute changes during therapy with antithyroid agents. J Clin Invest. 1974;54(1):201–8.
61. Laurberg P, Vestergaard H, Nielsen S, et al. Sources of circulating 3,5,3′-triiodothyronine in hyperthyroidism estimated after blocking of type 1 and type 2 iodothyronine deiodinases. J Clin Endocrinol Metab. 2007;92(6):2149–56.
62. Emerson CH, Anderson AJ, Howard WJ, et al. Serum thyroxine and triiodothyronine concentrations during iodide treatment of hyperthyroidism. J Clin Endocrinol Metab. 1975;40(1):33–6.
63. Braga M, Cooper DS. Clinical review 129. Oral cholecystographic agents and the thyroid. J Clin Endocrinol Metab. 2001;86(5):1853–60.
64. Carvalho-Bianco SD, Kim B, Harney JW, et al. Chronic cardiac-specific thyrotoxicosis increases myocardial beta-adrenergic responsiveness. Mol Endocrinol. 2004;18(7):1840–9.
65. Hellstrom L, Wahrenberg H, Reynisdottir S, et al. Catecholamine-induced adipocyte lipolysis in human hyperthyroidism. J Clin Endocrinol Metab. 1997;82(1):159–66.
66. Vigneri R, Pezzino V, Filetti S, et al. Effect of dexamethasone on thyroid hormone response to TSH. Metabolism. 1975;24(11):1209–13.
67. Mechanick JI, Davies TF. Medical management of hyperthyroidism: theoretical and practical aspects. In: Falk SA, editor. Thyroid disease: endocrinolgy, surgery, nuclear medicine and tadiotherapy. 2nd ed. New York, NY: Lippincott-Raven; 1997. p. 253–96.
68. Lazarus JH, Richards AR, Addison GM, et al. Treatment of thyrotoxicosis with lithium carbonate. Lancet. 1974;2(7890):1160–3.
69. Ross DS, Burch HB, Cooper DS, et al. 2016 American thyroid association guidelines for diagnosis and management of hyperthyroidism and other causes of thyrotoxicosis. Thyroid. 2016;26(10):1343–421.
70. Udovcic M, Pena RH, Patham B, et al. Hypothyroidism and the Heart. Methodist Debakey Cardiovasc J. 2017;13(2):55–9.
71. Elshimy G, Correa R. Myxedema. StatPearls [Internet]. Treasure Island, FL: StatPearls Publishing; 2020.
72. Paull AM, Phillips RW. Primary myxedema with secondary adrenocortical failure. J Clin Endocrinol Metab. 1954;14(5):554–60.

73. Peterson RE, Wyngaarden JB, Guerra SL, et al. The physiological disposition and metabolic fate of hydrocortisone in man. J Clin Invest. 1955;34(12):1779–94.
74. Charoensri S, Sriphrapradang C, Nimitphong H. Split high-dose oral levothyroxine treatment as a successful therapy option in myxedema coma. Clin Case Rep. 2017;5(10):1706–11.
75. Roberts CG, Ladenson PW. Hypothyroidism. Lancet. 2004;363(9411):793–803.
76. Ilias I, Tzanela M, Mavrou I, et al. Thyroid function changes and cytokine alterations following major surgery. Neuroimmunomodulation. 2007;14(5):243–7.
77. Bajwa SJ, Sehgal V. Anesthesia and thyroid surgery: the never ending challenges. Indian J Endocrinol Metab. 2013;17(2):228–34.
78. Ueda K, Kiyota A, Tsuchida M, et al. Successful treatment of myxedema coma with a combination of levothyroxine and liothyronine. Endocr J. 2019;66(5):469–74.
79. Rainey WE. Adrenal zonation: clues from 11β-hydroxylase and aldosterone synthase. Mol Cell Endocrinol. 1999;151(1–2):151–60.
80. Weinberger C, Hollenberg SM, Rosenfeld MG, et al. Domain structure of human glucocorticoid receptor and its relationship to the v-erb-A oncogene product. Nature. 1986;318(6047):670–2.
81. Arriza JL, Weinberger C, Cerelli G, et al. Cloning of human mineralo-corticoid receptor complementary DNA: structural and functional kinship with the glucocorticoid receptor. Science. 1987;237:268–75.
82. Gustafsson JA, Carlstedt-Duke J, Poellinger L, et al. Biochemistry, molecular biology, and physiology of the glucocorticoid receptor. Endocr Rev. 1987;8(2):185–234.
83. Melmed S, Polonsky KS, Reed Larsen P, Kronenberg HM. Williams textbook of endocrinology. 13th ed. Holand: Elsevier; 2016.
84. Sawka AM, Jaeschke R, Singh RJ, et al. A comparison of biochemical tests for pheochromocytoma: measurement of fractionated plasma metanephrines compared with the combination of 24hour urinary metanephrines and catecholamines. J Clin Endocrinol Metab. 2003;88(2):553–8.
85. Neumann H, Berger DP, Sigmund G, et al. Pheochromocytomas, multiple endocrine neoplasia type 2, and von HippelLindau disease. N Engl J Med. 1993;329(21):1531–8.
86. Lenders JW, Pacak K, Walther MM, et al. Biochemical diagnosis of pheochromocytoma: which test is best? JAMA. 2002;287(11):1427–34.
87. Kantorovich V, Pacak K. New insights on the pathogenesis of paraganglioma and pheochromocytoma. F1000Res. 2018;7:F1000 Faculty Rev-1500.
88. Dahia PL. Pheochromocytoma and paraganglioma pathogenesis: learning from genetic heterogeneity. Nat Rev Cancer. 2014;14(2):108–19.
89. Fishbein L, Leshchiner I, Walter V, et al. Comprehensive molecular characterization of pheochromocytoma and paraganglioma. Cancer Cell. 2017;31(2):181–93.
90. Favier J, Amar L, Gimenez-Roqueplo AP. Paraganglioma and phaeochromocytoma: from genetics to personalized medicine. Nat Rev Endocrinol. 2015;11(2):101–11.
91. Sato TH, Uchida T, Dote K, Ishihara M. Tako-tsubo-like left ventricu-lar dysfunction due to multivessel coronary spasm. In: Kodama K, Haze K, Hori M, editors. Clinical aspect of myocardial injury: from ischemia to heart failure. Tokyo: Kagakuhyoronsha; 1990. p. 56–64.
92. Y-Hassan S, Falhammar H. Pheochromocytoma- and paraganglioma-triggered Takotsubo syndrome. Endocrine. 2019;65(3):483–93.
93. Y-Hassan S, Yamasaki K. History of takotsubo syndrome: is the syndrome really described as a disease entity first in 1990? Some inaccuracies. Int J Cardiol. 2013;166(3):736–7.
94. Dote K, Sato H, Tateishi H, et al. Myocardial stunning due to simultaneous multivessel coronary spasms: a review of 5 cases. J Cardiol. 1991;21(2):203–14.
95. Ghadri JR, Wittstein IS, Prasad A, et al. International expert consensus document on takotsubo syndrome (part I): clinical characteristics, diagnostic criteria, and pathophysiology. Eur Heart J. 2018;39(22):2032–46.
96. Akashi YJ, Nef HM, Lyon AR. Epidemiology and pathophysiology of Takotsubo syndrome. Nat Rev Cardiol. 2015;12(7):387–97.

97. Kurisu S, Inoue I, Kawagoe T, et al. Time course of electrocardiographic changes in patients with Tako-tsubo syndrome: comparison with acute myocardial infarction with minimal enzymatic release. Circ J. 2004;68(1):77–81.
98. Kosuge M, Ebina T, Hibi K, et al. Simple and accurate electrocardiographic criteria to differentiate Takotsubo cardiomyopathy from anterior acute myocardial infarction. J Am Coll Cardiol. 2010;55(22):2514–6.
99. Fröhlich GM, Schoch B, Schmid F, et al. Takotsubo cardiomyopathy has a unique cardiac biomarker profile: NT-proBNP/myoglobin and NT-proBNP/troponin T ratios for the differential diagnosis of acute coronary syndromes and stress induced cardiomyopathy. Int J Cardiol. 2012;154(3):328–32.
100. Omland T, Persson A, Ng L, et al. N-terminal pro-B-type natriuretic peptide and long-term mortality in acute coronary syndromes. Circulation. 2002;106(23):2913–8.
101. Y-Hassan S, Tornvall P. Epidemiology, pathogenesis, and management of takotsubo syndrome. Clin Auton Res. 2018;28(1):53–65.
102. Y-Hassan S, De Palma R. Contemporary review on the pathogenesis of takotsubo syndrome: the heart shedding tears: norepinephrine churn and foam at the cardiac sympathetic nerve terminals. Int J Cardiol. 2017;228:528–36.
103. Vitale C, Rosano GM, Kaski JC. Role of coronary microvascular dysfunction in takotsubo cardiomyopathy. Circ J. 2016;80(2):299–305.
104. El Mahmoud R, Mansencal N, Pilliére R, et al. Prevalence and characteristics of left ventricular outflow tract obstruction in Tako-Tsubo syndrome. Am Heart J. 2008;156(3):543–8.
105. Sharkey SW, Windenburg DC, Lesser JR, et al. Natural history and expansive clinical profile of stress (tako-tsubo) cardiomyopathy. J Am Coll Cardiol. 2010;55(4):333–41.
106. Wittstein IS, Thiemann DR, Lima JA, et al. Neurohumoral features of myocardial stunning due to sudden emotional stress. N Engl J Med. 2005;352(6):539–48.
107. Y-Hassan S. The pathogenesis of reversible T-wave inversions or large upright peaked T-waves: sympathetic T-waves. Int J Cardiol. 2015;191:237–43.
108. Y-Hassan S. Insights into the pathogenesis of takotsubo syndrome, which with persuasive reasons should be regarded as an acute cardiac sympathetic disease entity. ISRN Cardiol. 2012;2012:593735.
109. McGonigle P, Webb SW, Adgey AA. Phaeochromocytoma: an unusual cause of chest pain. Br Med J. 1983;286(6376):1477–8.
110. Jessurun CR, Adam K, Moise KJ Jr, et al. Pheochromocytoma-induced myocardial infarction in pregnancy. A case report and literature review. Tex Heart Inst J. 1993;20(2):120–2.
111. Wiswell JG, Crago RM. Reversible cardiomyopathy with pheochromocytoma. Trans Am Clin Climatol Assoc. 1969;80:185–95.
112. Sode J, Getzen LC, Osborne DP. Cardiac arrhythmias and cardiomyopathy associated with pheochromocytomas. Report of three cases. Am J Surg. 1967;114(6):927–31.
113. Case records of the Massachusetts General Hospital. Weekly clinicopathological exercises. Case 15–1988. A 26-year-old woman with cardiomyopathy, multiple strokes, and an adrenal mass. N Engl J Med. 1988;318(15):970–81.
114. Y-Hassan S. Clinical features and outcome of pheochromocytoma-induced takotsubo syndrome: analysis of 80 published cases. Am J Cardiol. 2016;117(11):1836–44.
115. Batisse-Lignier M, Pereira B, Motreff P, et al. Acute and chronic pheochromocytoma-induced cardiomyopathies: different prognoses? A systematic analytical review. Medicine (Baltimore). 2015;94(50):e2198.
116. Zhang R, Gupta D, Albert SG. Pheochromocytoma as a reversible cause of cardiomyopathy: analysis and review of the literature. Int J Cardiol. 2017;249:319–23.
117. Unger RH, Orci L. Paracrinology of islets and the paracrinopathy of diabetes. Proc Natl Acad Sci USA. 2010;107(37):16009–12.
118. American Diabetes Association. Diagnosis and classification of diabetes mellitus. Diabetes Care. 2010;33 Suppl 1:S62–9.

119. Nyenwe EA, Kitabchi AE. The evolution of diabetic ketoacidosis: an update of its etiology, pathogenesis and management. Metabolism. 2016;65:507–21. https://doi.org/10.1016/j.metabol.2015.12.007.
120. Dhatariya K. Blood ketones: measurement, interpretation, limitations, and utility in the management of diabetic ketoacidosis. Rev Diabet Stud. 2016;13:217–25. https://doi.org/10.1900/RDS.2016.13.217.
121. Madias NE. Lactic acidosis. Kidney Int. 1986;29(3):752–74.
122. Kamel KS, Oh MS, Halperin ML. L-lactic acidosis: pathophysiology, classification, and causes; emphasis on biochemical and metabolic basis. Kidney Int. 2020;97(1):75–88.
123. Moller-Petersen J, Andersen PT, Hjorne N, et al. Nontraumatic rhabdomyolysis during diabetic ketoacidosis. Diabetologia. 1986;29(4):229–34.
124. Brown D, Melamed ML. New frontiers in treating uremic metabolic acidosis. Clin J Am Soc Nephrol. 2018;13(1):4–5.
125. Fulop M. Alcoholism, ketoacidosis, and lactic acidosis. Diabetes Metab Rev. 1989;5:365–78.
126. Duffens K, Marx JA. Alcoholic ketoacidosis: a review. J Emerg Med. 1987;5(5):399–406.
127. Robert DH, Bokhari SRA. Alcoholic ketoacidosis. StatPearls [Internet]. Treasure Island, FL: StatPearls Publishing; 2019.
128. Chatzipanteli K, Head C, Megerman J, et al. The relationship between plasma insulin level, prostaglandin production by adipose tissue, and blood pressure in normal rats and rats with diabetes mellitus and diabetic ketoacidosis. Metabolism. 1996;45(6):691–8.
129. Trachtenbarg DE. Diabetic ketoacidosis. Am Fam Physician. 2005;71(9):1705–14.
130. Fisher JN, Shahshahani MN, Kitabchi AE. Diabetic ketoacidosis: low-dose insulin therapy by various routes. N Engl J Med. 1977;297(5):238–41.
131. Soler NG, FitzGerald MG, Wright AD, et al. Comparative study of different insulin regimens in management of diabetic ketoacidosis. Lancet. 1975;2(7947):1221–4.
132. Umpierrez GE, Guervo R, Karabell A, et al. Treatment of diabetic ketoacidosis with subcutaneous insulin aspart. Diabetes Care. 2004;27(8):1873–8.
133. Ehusani-Anumah FO, Ohwovoriole AE. Plasma glucose response to insulin in hyperglycaemic crisis. Int J Diabetes Metabol. 2007;15:17–21.
134. Basetty S, Yeshvanth Kumar GS, Shalini M, et al. Management of diabetic ketosis and ketoacidosis with intramuscular regular insulin in a low-resource family medicine setting. J Family Med Prim Care. 2017;6(1):25–8.
135. Wolfsdorf J, Craig ME, Daneman D, et al. Diabetic ketoacidosis in children and adolescents with diabetes. Pediatr Diabetes. 2009;10(Suppl 12):118–33.
136. Inward CD, Chambers TL. Fluid management in diabetic ketoacidosis. Arch Dis Child. 2002;86(6):443–4.
137. Jayashree M, Williams V, Iyer R. Fluid therapy for pediatric patients with diabetic ketoacidosis: current perspectives. Diabetes Metab Syndr Obes. 2019;12:2355–61.
138. Glaser N, Barnett P, McCaslin I, et al. Risk factors for cerebral edema in children with diabetic ketoacidosis. N Engl J Med. 2001;344(4):264–9.
139. Halperin ML, Maccari C, Kamel KS, et al. Strategies to diminish the danger of cerebral edema in a pediatric patient presenting with diabetic ketoacidosis. Pediatr Diabetes. 2006;7(4):191–5.
140. Hsia DS, Tarai SG, Alimi A, et al. Fluid management in pediatric patients with DKA and rates of suspected clinical cerebral edema. Pediatr Diabetes. 2015;16(5):338–44.
141. Long B, Koyfman A. Emergency medicine myths: cerebral edema in pediatric diabetic ketoacidosis and intravenous fluids. J Emerg Med. 2017;53(2):212–21.
142. Kuppermann N, Ghetti S, Schunk JE, et al. Clinical trial of fluid infusion rates for pediatric diabetic ketoacidosis. N Engl J Med. 2018;378(24):2275–87.
143. Van der Meulen JA, Klip A, Grinstein S. Possible mechanism for cerebral oedema in diabetic ketoacidosis. Lancet. 1987;2(8554):306–8.
144. Kamel KS, Schreiber M, Carlotti AP, et al. Approach to the treatment of diabetic ketoacidosis. Am J Kidney Dis. 2016;68(6):967–72.

145. Wu D, Kraut JA. Role of NHE1 in the cellular dysfunction of acute metabolic acidosis. Am J Nephrol. 2014;40(1):36–42.
146. Shafi O, Kumar V. Initial fluid therapy in pediatric diabetic ketoacidosis: a comparison of hypertonic saline solution and normal saline solution. Pediatr Endocrinol Diabetes Metab. 2018;24(2):56–64.
147. Felner EI, White PC. Improving management of diabetic ketoacidosis in children. Pediatrics. 2001;108(3):735–40.
148. Brown TB. Cerebral oedema in childhood diabetic ketoacidosis: is treatment a factor? Emerg Med J. 2004;21(2):141–4.
149. Karslioglu French E, Donihi AC, Korytkowski MT. Diabetic ketoacidosis and hyperosmolar hyperglycemic syndrome: review of acute decompensated diabetes in adult patients. BMJ. 2019;365:l1114.
150. Wolfsdorf JI, Glaser N, Agus M, et al. ISPAD clinical practice consensus guidelines 2018: diabetic ketoacidosis and the hyperglycemic hyperosmolar state. Pediatr Diabetes. 2018;19(Suppl 27):155–77.
151. Kitabchi AE, Umpierrez GE, Miles JM, et al. Hyperglycemic crises in adult patients with diabetes. Diabetes Care. 2009;32(7):1335–43.
152. Goguen J, Gilbert J, Canadian Diabetes Association Clinical Practice Guidelines Expert Committee. Hyperglycemic emergencies in adults. Can J Diabetes. 2013;37(suppl 1):S72–6.
153. McGreevy M, Beerman L, Arora G. Ventricular tachycardia in a child with diabetic ketoacidosis without heart disease. Cardiol Young. 2016;26(1):206–8.
154. Gapp J, Krishnan M, Ratnaraj F, et al. Cardiac arrhythmias resulting from a peripherally inserted central catheter: two cases and a review of the literature. Cureus. 2017;9(6):e1308.
155. Postema PG, Vlaar AP, DeVries JH, et al. Familial Brugada syndrome uncovered by hyperkalaemic diabetic ketoacidosis. Europace. 2011;13(10):1509–10.
156. Abrahim C, Maharaj S. DKA-induced Brugada phenocopy mimicking STEMI. Heart Asia. 2018;10:e011027. https://doi.org/10.1136/heartasia-2018-011027.
157. Haseeb S, Kariyanna PT, Jayarangaiah A, et al. Brugada pattern in diabetic ketoacidosis: a case report and scoping study. Am J Med Case Rep. 2018;6(9):173–9.
158. Abdulaziz S, Dabbagh O, Al Daker MO, et al. Hypokalaemia and refractory asystole complicating diabetic ketoacidosis, lessons for prevention. BMJ Case Rep. 2012;2012:pii: bcr-2012-007312.
159. Yang Y, Liu B, He J, et al. Impact of atrial fibrillation on in-hospital outcomes in patients with diabetic ketoacidosis. Am J Med Sci. 2019;358(5):350–6.
160. Chua HR, Schneider A, Bellomo R. Bicarbonate in diabetic ketoacidosis—a systematic review. Ann Intensive Care. 2011;1(1):23.
161. Fadini GP, de Kreutzenberg SV, Rigato M, et al. Characteristics and outcomes of the hyperglycemic hyperosmolar non-ketotic syndrome in a cohort of 51 consecutive cases at a single center. Diabetes Res Clin Pract. 2011;94(2):172–9.
162. Ananth J, Parameswaran S, Gunatilake S. Side effects of atypical antipsychotic drugs. Curr Pharm Des. 2004;10(18):2219–29.
163. Pinies JA, Cairo G, Gaztambide S, et al. Course and prognosis of 132 patients with diabetic non ketotic hyperosmolar state. Diabete Metab. 1994;20:43–8.
164. Scott AR. Joint British Diabetes Societies (JBDS) for Inpatient Care JBDS hyperosmolar hyperglycaemic guidelines group. Management of hyperosmolar hyperglycaemic state in adults with diabetes. Diabet Med. 2015;32(6):714–24.
165. Umpierrez G, Korytkowski M. Diabetic emergencies—ketoacidosis, hyperglycaemic hyperosmolar state and hypoglycaemia. Nat Rev Endocrinol. 2016;12(4):222–32.
166. Pasquel FJ, Umpierrez GE. Hyperosmolar hyperglycemic state: a historic review of the clinical presentation, diagnosis, and treatment. Diabetes Care. 2014;37(11):3124–31.

# Infectious Diseases 21

Shu-Bin Guo, Jun-Yu Wang, Xiao-Mei Zhu, Di Zhu, Rui-Qi Li, and Tian-Tian Wan

**Abstract**

The causes of sudden noncardiac deaths (SNCDs) are numerous and involve almost every systemic disease. A substantial number of sudden and unexpected deaths are caused by infections. Sudden death due to infectious disease may be classified by organ system involvement (e.g., cardiac—myocarditis; nervous system—meningitis and encephalitis) or according to the etiological agent (e.g., viral, chlamydial, bacterial, fungal, protozoal, or helminthic). This chapter provides an in-depth introduction to the causes of SNCDs by different pathogens and organ systems.

**Keywords**

Sudden noncardiac death · Infectious cause · Etiological agents

The world health organization defines sudden death as death within 24 hours of onset of various diseases. It is generally believed that sudden death occurs within 1, 6 and 12 hours of the disease. The National Heart, Lung and Blood Institute recently defined sudden cardiac death (SCD) as a sudden, unexpected, pulseless event with no obvious noncardiac cause, but the definition of sudden cardiac death is unclear and there is little research. In recent years, researchers have used different methods to investigate the incidence and causes of sudden death. Several studies have performed autopsies on patients who died of various causes, and based on the results of the autopsies, the causes of these sudden deaths can be divided into two categories: (1) actual SCD death and (2) sudden noncardiac deaths (SNCDs). However, since autopsy rates are low in most countries and it is difficult to determine the specific

S.-B. Guo (✉) · J.-Y. Wang · X.-M. Zhu · D. Zhu · R.-Q. Li · T.-T. Wan
Emergency Department, Beijing Chao-Yang Hospital, Capital Medical University, Beijing, China



H. Zhu (ed.), *Sudden Death*, https://doi.org/10.1007/978-981-15-7002-5_21

cause of sudden death by clinical examination and other evaluation methods, it is not possible to exclude that these deaths are caused by noncardiogenic diseases.

Currently, there are few studies on the incidence of sudden death from noncardiogenic diseases. However, the clarity of incidence, risk factors, and causes of SNCD may help guide clinicians in determining whether the cause of death is due to heart disease or nonheart disease. In an Australian study, the most common causes of noncardiac sudden death were epilepsy (23.8%), intracranial hemorrhage (23.8%), asthma (16.1%), and pulmonary embolism (12.5%) [1]. A national cohort study in Denmark concluded that, according to autopsy results [2], 28% of sudden death in young people was due to primary heart disease. The rate of sudden cardiac death was no more than 50% in patients aged 1 to 5 years, and dropped to 25% in patients aged 10 to 14 years and remained stable. Current studies suggest that age, female sex, location of hospitalization, and history of heart disease are independent risk factors for noncardiogenic sudden death. Identifying risk factors for sudden, noncardiac death could help in the early identification and prevention of those at risk in the future.

There are many causes of noncardiac sudden death, almost involving all systemic diseases. Some studies believe that infection, cerebrovascular disease, and nervous system disease are the main causes of SNCDs [3]. Sudden death from infectious diseases can be classified according to the system of affected organs (e.g., cardiovascular system—myocarditis; nervous system—meningitis and encephalitis), or by disease origin (e.g., virus, chlamydia, bacteria, fungi, protozoa, or worm infections). Lung infection is the most common cause of SNCD [3].

The spectrum of causes of sudden death is broad and varied. Many cases of sudden death are potentially preventable with correct diagnosis, and risk stratification and management being paramount. Despite advances in the diagnosis and treatment of infectious diseases, a large number of patients still die suddenly from infectious diseases. Sudden death due to infection may be directly caused by the factor of infection, or it may be caused by complications such as immunosuppression caused by infection or adverse reactions to drug treatment.

## 21.1 Viral Causes of Sudden Death

Viral infections in many systems in the body can cause sudden death, such as the respiratory system, cardiovascular system, and central nervous system. Virus infection needs our attention. At present, clinical diagnosis and treatment are very limited, so we need to make efforts to overcome these difficulties.

### 21.1.1 Viral Infections of Cardiovascular System

Viral myocarditis is a type of circulatory virus infection. A very important cause of sudden death is viral myocarditis [1]. In people under the age of 40, 12% of sudden deaths are caused by viral myocarditis [4]. Viral infections commonly cause myocarditis in developed countries [5]. In the later stages of the disease, viral myocarditis might develop into cardiomyopathy and heart failure [5]. And these patients finally develop life-threatening acute viral myocarditis [4]. The human enteroviruses, especially the coxsackie B viruses, predominate among viruses as the cause of myocarditis [4]. Coxsackie B virus easily attacks the human body during warm seasons [6].Viral infection and its inflammatory reaction is an important aspect of the pathophysiology of viral myocarditis [7]. An autoimmune mechanism is involved in the pathogenesis of viral myocarditis [7]. In addition, genetic variation can also cause viral myocarditis [8]. Currently, a lot of clinical treatments have been undertaken, but the results have been minimal. Studies have shown that IL-27 may be a new target for the treatment of viral myocarditis [9]. Heart transplantation is the only way once the disease results in chronic and dilated cardiomyopathy [4]. Viral myocarditis needs further study.

### 21.1.2 Viral Infections of Respiratory System

Lower respiratory infections (LRI) have made an important contribution to the cause of mortality and morbidity worldwide [10]. The cause of LRI is bacterial and viral, but the latter needs considerable attention. Viruses implicated include respiratory syncytial virus [11], influenza A [12, 13], and influenza B [14]. LRI is a preventable disease, and continued efforts to improve environmental pollution, improve childhood nutrition, and scale up more effective vaccines and vaccination programs will be important in reducing the morbidity of LRI [15].

### 21.1.3 Viral Infections of Central Nervous System

Viral encephalitis may cause rapid onset of neuroinflammation and eventually lead to death [16]. *Toxoplasma gondii* invasion of the human central nervous system is an important factor in brain mass lesions in patients with human immunodeficiency virus infections [17].This is a significant cause of sudden death [18]. Herpes simplex type 1 virus (HSV-1) can also cause fatal encephalitis [19].

The real-time polymerase chain reaction (PCR) of cerebrospinal fluid (CSF) is a very useful technique for diagnosing central nervous system infections. However, this technique is not common in China for the diagnosis of CNS infections [20]. Acyclovir can be used to treat HSV infections, and we should guard against the emergence of drug resistance [21]. So, we should make rational use of drugs and develop new drugs.

Viral infections causing sudden death usually involve the cardiac, respiratory, or the central nervous system. They are problems worthy of our concern. At present, clinical treatment and the ways of diseases diagnosed are limited. We should try harder to overcome these difficulties.

## 21.2 Bacterial Causes of Sudden Death

Bacterial infections are responsible for sudden death both in adults and children. Some studies have reported acute death from severe bacterial infections in adults, with most cases showing a sudden onset of septic shock. Bacterial infections of the respiratory, central nervous, and gastrointestinal systems account for the majority of cases of sudden unexpected death in the pediatric population. There are also many types of pathogenic bacteria.

Because sudden death from infection is difficult to diagnosis, many cases are confirmed from autopsy results. Combined with the literature and autopsy reports, we summarized some causes of sudden death caused by infectious diseases.

### 21.2.1 Bacterial Infections in the Cardiovascular System

*Borrelia burgdorferi*, *Corynebacterium diphtheria*, and *Neisseria meningitidis* may all be causative factors of myocarditis. In *B. burgdorferi*, cardiac involvement occurs in 1–8% of cases, and death may occur due to conduction disturbances. Myocardial damage is caused by the release of toxins in diphtheritic myocarditis. *Bartonella*-induced silent myocarditis has been considered as a cause of sudden death in athletes. Granulomatous myocarditis may also lead to sudden unexpected death. In fact, the pathogenic factors causing myocardial infectious diseases are not only limited to bacteria but also include viruses, spirochetes, etc. However, viral myocarditis is usually more common, but we cannot ignore bacterial infections. The mechanism of death caused by myocarditis includes arrhythmias, heart rupture, coronary artery occlusion, obstruction to pulmonary blood flow leading to fatal hemorrhage, and impaired myocardial contractility. The clinical manifestations of explosive myocarditis develop rapidly and the disease is critical, which directly endangers life. Explosive myocarditis is an inflammatory disease of the myocardium with sudden onset and severe hemodynamic disturbance.

Sudden death in infective endocarditis is caused by free-wall myocardial abscess perforation or rupture of a valve leaflet. Acute infective endocarditis occurs mostly in the normal heart. Pathogens are usually highly virulent bacteria such as *Staphylococcus aureus*. *Staphylococcus aureus* accounts for 10–20% of cases and is the main cause of endocarditis in intravenous drug abusers. Other bacterial causes include *Haemophilus*, *Actinobacillus*, *Cardiobacterium*, *Eikenella*, and *Kingella* (HACEK group). Positive blood bacterial culture is an important basis for the diagnosis of infective endocarditis. The most common sites of infection are the aortic and mitral valves, with the exception of intravenous drug users whose right-sided valves are primarily affected. Acute infective endocarditis often starts suddenly, accompanied by high fever, chills, and obvious symptoms of systemic toxemia. It is often part of a serious infection of the whole body. The course of the disease is acute and dangerous, and it is easy to cover up the clinical symptoms of acute infective endocarditis.

Syphilitic cardiomyopathy is an infectious disease caused by *Treponema pallidum*. Due to the lack of complete cure after syphilis, syphilitic heart disease often occurs 10–20 years after suffering from syphilis while aortitis caused by tertiary syphilis may cause sudden death due to rupture of aortic aneurysms with aortic dissection. The mechanism of death is either blood loss as a result of hypovolemic shock or a fatal cardiac tamponade caused by intrapericardial rupture.

### 21.2.2 Bacterial Infections in the Respiratory System

Acute epiglottitis is a clinical emergency which occurs suddenly and rapidly. The main clinical features are severe pharyngeal pain, dysphagia, dysphagia, and dyspnea caused by high epiglottis edema, which eventually leads to suffocation and respiratory cardiac arrest. The sudden death from acute epiglottitis occurs from respiratory obstruction as a result of swelling of the epiglottic folds, uvula, and vocal cords. In developing countries, the most common cause of acute epiglottitis is *Haemophilus influenzae* type B. In countries that have established immunization programs, the incidence of *H. influenzae* epiglottitis has decreased, while other bacteria, such as streptococcus, staphylococcus, and pneumococcus, have been considered as possible causes. Postmortem blood cultures are positive in 50–75% of cases. A particular type of epiglottitis is acute allergic epiglottitis, which usually develops within half an hour of medication or 2–3 h of eating. Gastro-esophageal reflux may be responsible for the onset of acute recurrent laryngeal dyspnea. So there is reason to think that changing body position may have an impact on allergic acute epiglottitis.

The most frequent causes of sudden death from acute bacterial infectious lung disease are lobar pneumonia and confluent bronchopneumonia. Some 90–95% of lobar pneumonia is due to *Streptococcus pneumoniae* type 3. Bronchopneumonia is mostly caused by staphylococci, streptococci, *H. influenzae*, *Pseudomonas aeruginosa*, and coliform bacteria. Although it is common, it should be taken seriously because it's often hard to find a specific pathogen clinically.

Diphtheria is an acute respiratory infection caused by *Corynebacterium diphtheriae*. It produces a gray pseudomembrane from the pharynx to the larynx, which may lead to respiratory obstruction and sudden death. Symptoms of systemic poisoning in severe cases are associated with myocarditis and peripheral nerve paralysis.

Legionnaire's disease is a clinical syndrome caused by *Legionella pneumophila*, a facultative intracellular organism, which is associated with outbreaks of sudden death. It causes severe pneumonia in the elderly, in smokers, and in immunocompromised patients. The organisms are usually found to transmit via droplet spread from contaminated air-conditioning units and water coolers. *Legionella pneumophila* can be demonstrated by a modified silver stain (Dieterle stain) or by immunofluorescence and culture.

There are a variety of bacteria that can cause infections in the lungs or respiratory system. Most of the time, doctors cannot quickly determine which bacteria (or multiple pathogens) are causing the disease. Doctors will confirm using blood, secretion, and imaging tests or tracheoscopy.

### 21.2.3 Bacterial Infections in the Central Nervous System

Bacterial infections of the central nervous system are a neurological emergency. Pyogenic meningitis may cause sudden unexpected death. The most common pathogens of acute bacterial meningitis are *Meningococcus*, *Pneumococci* and *Haemophilus influenzae*. The most common means of entry is blood transmission while other routes of infection include extension of local infection, such as paranasal sinusitis, osteomyelitis, direct implantation, and via the peripheral nervous system. Diffuse bacterial meningitis can follow rupture of a brain abscess, which may also lead to sudden death. These microorganisms may be demonstrated by microbiological culture of the cerebrospinal fluid (CSF) and examination of Gram staining of the CSF and brain tissue.

### 21.2.4 Bacterial Infections in the Urogenital Tract

Fulminant acute bacterial pyelonephritis may lead to sepsis, causing sudden death. An autopsy revealed renal tubular necrosis with interstitial suppurative inflammation. Renal papillary necrosis may also occur. There are two ways of infection. Bacteria enter the renal pelvis from the ureter and invade the renal parenchyma. 70% of acute pyelonephritis is caused from this pathway. The remaining cases of acute pyelonephritis are bacteria that invade the renal pelvis from the bloodstream into the renal tubules, mostly staphylococcal infections. Urinary tract obstruction and urinary stasis are the most common causes of acute pyelonephritis.

### 21.2.5 Bacterial Infections in the Gastrointestinal Tract

Severe bacterial enterocolitis can cause sudden death, especially among young people. *Vibrio cholerae* and *Clostridium perfringens* cause diarrhea due to ingestion of a preformed toxin present in contaminated foods. Intestinal invasive organisms such as *Salmonella*, *Shigella*, and enteroinvasive *Escherichia coli* invade and destroy mucosal epithelial cells. Dehydration and electrolyte imbalance are causes of sudden death.

Fulminant bacterial peritonitis often secondary to acute appendicitis, ruptured peptic ulcer, strangulated bowel, cholecystitis, acute salpingitis, and diverticulitis can lead to sudden death. Primary peritonitis may occur postsplenectomy and in patients with splenic hypoplasia. Patients with sickle cell disease may have functional or anatomical splenic insufficiency. The former is due to defects in opsonization of encapsulated bacteria. The latter is due to repeated bouts of infarction resulting in auto-splenectomy. In one study from Japan [22], the authors analyzed nine cases of sudden death from infection and found that despite the different types of bacteria, the onset of fulminant bacterial infection depended upon depressed bacterial phagocytosis in the liver or spleen. Underlying chronic illnesses should be identified as a predisposing common risk factor. It is important to understand the relations between underlying chronic illness and the onset of fulminant infection.

Actually, the cause of death in many cases is circulatory collapse caused by fulminant infection. Bacterial infection may not be identified at first histologic assessment. Also, the initial focus of bacteria may be unknown probably due to the very early entry of bacteria into the circulation. Once infection occurs, it produces endotoxins derived from lipopolysaccharide caused by bacteria or large amounts of cytokines caused by the host-immune response to the toxic superantigen, leading to acute volume loss. The onset of fulminant infection depends on the bacteria and the sensitivity of the host. In addition, trauma and some surgical procedures can cause explosive bacterial infections that can lead to sudden death. A general physician should always keep the possibility of fulminant bacterial infection in mind when examining patients with shock symptoms. Because acute bacterial infections can cause life and death within hours, correct diagnosis and emergency treatment must be made early.

## 21.3 Fungal Causes of Sudden Death

Sudden, noncardiac death from fungal infection is more likely to occur in immunocompromised hosts, such as AIDS patients. Pathogens include cryptococcus (meningitis or blood-borne disease) and *Pneumocystis carinii* (pneumonia). AIDS patients who inject drugs through the vein are susceptible to endocarditis caused by fungal infection, the most common pathogen is candida. These patients are prone to fungal thromboembolism, which can lead to sudden death. Sudden fungal death may also be due to complications of fungal diseases, such as fatal subarachnoid hemorrhage from meningitis caused by actinomycete infection or fatal frontal hemoptysis caused by fungal infection of the lung mucosa.

In recent years, with the increasing number of hospitals, the level of diagnosis and treatment has been increasing, and immunosuppressive agents, broad-spectrum antibacterial drugs, and various invasive diagnostic techniques have been widely used, leading to an increase in infections caused by conditional pathogenic fungi [23]. The hospital infection rate caused by fungi in developed countries in Europe and America is 0.19–2.62‰ [23–25]. Compared with developed countries, the incidence of hospital infections in China is higher, which is 3.8–29.3‰ [26].

The clinically common fungi are divided into yeast-like fungi, mold, and biphasic fungi according to different forms; pathogenic fungi and conditional pathogens are classified according to pathogenicity. The former includes histoplasma and coccidioides, coccidioides, dermatitis buds, coloring fungi, foot mycobacteria, spores, etc., and Candida, Cryptococcus, Aspergillus, Mucor, actinomycetes, Nocardia, etc., are conditional pathogens that can cause opportunistic infections in people with low immune function. The most common yeast-like fungi are mainly Candida (mainly *Candida albicans*, *Candida tropicalis*, *Candida glabrata*, *Candida parapsilosis*, etc.) and Cryptococcus; filamentous fungi mainly include Aspergillus, Mucor. The most common invasive fungal infections in clinical practice include Candida infection, Aspergillus infection and Cryptococcus infection, and the fourth place is occupied by Pneumocystis infection. According to China's invasive yeast-like fungal surveillance network (CHIFNET), the most common of the 3603 strains isolated in 2016 were Candida, of which 41.4% were *Candida albicans* and 15.8% were *candida parapsilosis*. *Candida glabrata* account for 9.0% and cryptococcal bacteria account for 10.5%. *Candida albicans* accounted for 30.9% of blood samples, and *Candida albicans* accounted for 23.1%, more common in catheter-related infections. 74.4% of cerebrospinal fluid specimens were *Cryptococcus neoformans* [27].

Different invasive fungal diseases often have different risk factors, for example, AIDS patients have risk factors due to CD4+ T lymphocyte reduction, clinical common oral candida infection, and cryptococcal meningitis; and blood disease patients with granulocytosis after chemotherapy, aspergillosis infection. Commonly, patients after transplantation are also susceptible to Aspergillus infection [28]. There are also certain regional differences in the distribution of different fungi. For example, Marnifi's yeast infection is more common in southern China such as Guangxi, Guangdong, Fujian, and Yunnan. People who are in close contact with a large number of flowers and soil in the work environment should also be alert to the inhalation of Cryptococcus, Aspergillus, etc., causing fungal infections.

Candida is widely colonized in the cavities of the upper respiratory tract, gastrointestinal tract, and genitourinary tract. Once the normal barrier is broken, the immune function is impaired or local flora is imbalanced, the candida colonized in these areas can grow and multiply, and can cause candidiasis, catheter-related bloodstream infection, etc., and easily through blood, involving other organs of the body. Therefore, for the isolation of Candida in sputum and urine specimens, it must be carefully identified whether it is due to colonization or infection. Once a positive culture of Candida bloodstream infection is obtained, it is highly valued and treated as soon as possible [29].

Unlike Candida infection, Aspergillus infection can be divided into acute invasive infection and chronic aspergillosis according to the patient's immune status. The former is more common in patients with neutropenia or posttransplantation immunocompromise, and the lung is most often affected. Lungs are most often involved, performance for cough, hemoptysis or sputum with blood, a lot of patients as a result of aspergillus sensitization performance for asthmatic hold back, breathing difficulties. Allergic bronchopulmonary aspergillosis (ABPA) has typical asthmatic manifestations, positive Aspergillus fumigatus skin test, or elevated serum-specific antibodies, which can assist in the diagnosis. Intracranial Aspergillus infections are often caused by sinusitis [30].

Another common clinical pathogenic fungus is Cryptococcus. Mostly inhalation infections can lead to simple pulmonary cryptococcosis or cryptococcal meningitis. Pulmonary cryptococcosis is not specific, and fever and respiratory symptoms are often not prominent. In clinical judgment, it is necessary to pay attention to the high-risk factors of patients and to identify them by the quantitative detection of cryptococcal capsular antigen. Patients with cryptococcal meningitis have typical fever, headache, nausea, vomiting, etc. Clinically, lumbar puncture, cerebrospinal fluid examination, positive ink staining, and positive cryptococcal culture can be diagnosed. Cryptococcal meningitis patients with typical fever, headache, nausea, vomiting and other manifestations, clinical need for lumbar puncture, do cerebrospinal fluid examination, positive ink staning and positive cryptococcal culture can be diagnosed, cryptococcal capsular antigen sensitivity and specificity can be up to 95%, conductive to diagnosis. The clinical manifestations of cryptococcal meningitis and tuberculous meningitis are similar and need to be distinguished by cerebrospinal fluid pathogen examination.

Liver failure is severe liver function damage caused by a variety of causes, and the mortality rate is extremely high. Due to the presence of severe immune paralysis, it is easy to have fungal infections. Clinically, widely used immunosuppressive agents and broad-spectrum antibacterial drugs have significantly increased fungal infections in patients with liver failure. The clinical symptoms of patients with liver failure and fungal infection are often atypical, and the diagnosis lacks effective means. At the same time, due to the decompensation of liver function and the existence of related complications, the choice of antifungal drugs and treatment timing have become a difficult problem in clinical practice.

In recent years, scholars in various countries have continuously explored the definition of liver failure. The Liver Failure and Artificial Liver Group of the Chinese Medical Association Infectious Diseases Section and the Hepatology Branch of the Chinese Medical Association, the Liver Failure Guideline (2018 Edition). Based on medical history, onset characteristics, and progression rate, liver failure is divided into four categories: acute liver failure (ALF), subacute liver failure (SALF), slow plus acute (subacute) liver failure (acute-on-chronic liver failure, ACLF or SACLF), and chronic liver failure (CLF). The incidence of liver failure combined with fungal infection is increasing year by year, and the clinical manifestations are concealed. There is still a lack of rapid and accurate diagnosis methods, and patients with liver failure have poor tolerance to antifungal drugs, difficult treatment, and high mortality. The main fungi involved in liver failure are *Candida albicans* and Aspergillus.

Common bacteria causing purulent meningitis include *Staphylococcus aureus*, *Streptococcus pneumoniae*, *Haemophilus influenzae*, *Escherichia coli*, and *Cryptococcus neoformans*, but it is rare to isolate *Actinobacillus urtica* from cerebrospinal fluid. *Actinobacillus urinae* is a rare bacterium, which is gram-negative and non-acid resistant filamentous bacteria. It needs 5% blood or 10% serum for growth. It grows well in 5% $CO_2$ environment. Yihong Meilan AGAR plate does not grow.

Controlling infection is also critical to reducing patient mortality and disability. Patients with comatose SAH have a higher risk of ventilator-associated pneumonia. In addition to respiratory infections, patients are also prone to urinary tract infections, the incidence of which is second only to the respiratory system. Therefore, patients should be prevented from developing infections such as catheter-related infections, ventilator-associated pneumonia, and blood infections during hospitalization. For patients undergoing external ventricular drainage, antibiotics can be used prophylactically.

A variety of complications often occur for SAH patients, including anemia, hypertension, arrhythmia, fever, and electrolyte abnormalities. The proportion of deaths due to complications is comparable to that from vasospasm and rebleeding. The study found that the most common complications in patients with severe SAH were fever, anemia, and hyperglycemia, and three complications were independent risk factors for clinical outcomes in SAH patients.

Malignant hematologic tumors require long-term chemoradiotherapy, which requires long-term use of broad-spectrum antibiotics and is prone to invasive fungal infections. Patients develop rapidly deep fungal infections and have a high mortality rate, which is the main cause of death in patients with malignant hematological tumors. Therefore, it is very necessary to select appropriate and effective drugs to prevent and treat fungal infections of malignant hematological tumors.

In addition, protozoans and helminths can also cause sudden death, which is not explained here because it is an uncommon manifestation. Despite advances in the diagnosis and treatment of infectious diseases, a large number of patients still die suddenly from infectious diseases. Sudden death due to infection may be directly caused by the factor of infection, or it may be caused by complications such as immunosuppression caused by infection or adverse reactions to drug treatment.

## References


1. Puranik R, Chow CK, Duflou JA, Kilborn MJ, McGuire MA. Sudden death in the young. Heart Rhythm. 2005;2(12):1277–82.
2. Risgaard B, Lynge TH, Wissenberg M, et al. Risk factors and causes of sudden noncardiac death: a nationwide cohort study in Denmark. Heart Rhythm. 2015;12(5):968–74.
3. Corsten MF, Heggermont W, Papageorgiou AP, et al. The microRNA-221/-222 cluster balances the antiviral and inflammatory response in viral myocarditis. Eur Heart J. 2015;36(42)
4. Daba TM, Zhao Y, Pan Z. Advancement of mechanisms of coxsackie virus B3-induced myocarditis pathogenesis and the potential therapeutic targets. Curr Drug Targets. 2019;20(14):1461–73.
5. Sagar S, Liu PP, Cooper LT Jr. Myocard Lancet. 2012;379(9817):738–47.
6. Druyts-Voets E, Van Renterghem L, Gerniers S. Coxsackie B virus epidemiology and neonatal infection in Belgium. J Infect. 1993;27(3):311–6.
7. Triantafilou K, Orthopoulos G, Vakakis E, et al. Human cardiac inflammatory responses triggered by Coxsackie B viruses are mainly Toll-like receptor (TLR) 8-dependent. Cell Microbiol. 2005;7(8):1117–26.
8. Zhu H, Lou C, Liu P. Interleukin-27 ameliorates coxsackievirus-B3-induced viral myocarditis by inhibiting Th17 cells. Virol J. 2015;12:189.
9. Liao Y, Chen KH, Dong XM, et al. A role of pre-mir-10a coding region variant in host susceptibility to coxsackie virus-induced myocarditis. Eur Rev Med Pharmacol Sci. 2015;19(18):3500–7.
10. GBD 2016 Lower Respiratory Infections Collaborators. Estimates of the global, regional, and national morbidity, mortality, and aetiologies of lower respiratory infections in 195 countries, 1990-2016: a systematic analysis for the Global Burden of Disease Study 2016. Lancet Infect Dis. 2018;18(11):1191–210.
11. Nam HH, Ison MG. Respiratory syncytial virus infection in adults. BMJ. 2019;366:l5021.
12. Wang X, Jiang H, Wu P, et al. Epidemiology of avian influenza A H7N9 virus in human beings across five epidemics in mainland China, 2013-17: an epidemiological study of laboratory-confirmed case series. Lancet Infect Dis. 2017;17(8):822–32.
13. Perez-Padilla R, de la Rosa-Zamboni D, Ponce-de-Leon S, et al. Pneumonia and respiratory failure from swine-origin influenza A (H1N1) in Mexico. N Engl J Med. 2009;361(7):680–9.
14. Thompson WW, Shay DK, Weintraub E, et al. Mortality associated with influenza and respiratory syncytial virus in the United States. JAMA. 2003;289(2):179–86.
15. GBD 2015 LRI Collaborators. Estimates of the global, regional, and national morbidity, mortality, and aetiologies of lower respiratory tract infections in 195 countries: a systematic analysis for the Global Burden of Disease Study 2015. Lancet Infect Dis. 2017;17(11):1133–61.
16. Furr SR, Chauhan VS, Moerdyk-Schauwecker MJ, Marriott I. A role for DNA-dependent activator of interferon regulatory factor in the recognition of herpes simplex virus type 1 by glial cells. J Neuroinflammation. 2011;8:99.
17. Marra CM. Central nervous system infection with *Toxoplasma gondii*. Handb Clin Neurol. 2018;152:117–22.

18. Gonzales Zamora JA. Dual infection of the central nervous system caused by Cryptococcus and Toxoplasma in a patient with AIDS: a case report and literature review. Acta Clin Belg. 2018;73(6):448–52.
19. da Cunha Sousa LF, Rachid MA, Lima GK, et al. Suppressor of cytokine signaling 2 (SOCS2) contributes to encephalitis in a model of Herpes infection in mice. Brain Res Bull. 2016;127:164–70.
20. Yang R, Zhang H, Xiong Y, et al. Molecular diagnosis of central nervous system opportunistic infections and mortality in HIV-infected adults in Central China. AIDS Res Ther. 2017;14:24.
21. Hou J, Zhang Z, Huang Q, et al. Antiviral activity of PHA767491 against human herpes simplex virus in vitro and in vivo. BMC Infect Dis. 2017;17(1):217.
22. Tajiri T, Tate G, Miura K, et al. Sudden death caused by fulminant bacterial infection: background and pathogenesis of Japanese adult cases. Intern Med. 2008;47(17):1499–504.
23. Wu GX, Khojabekyan M, Wang J, et al. Survival following lung resection in immunocompromised patients with pulmonary invasive fungal infection. Eur J Cardio-Thorac Surg. 2016;49:314–20.
24. Nur Y. Epidemiology and risk factors for invasive candidiasis. Therap Clin Risk Manage. 2014:95.
25. Lockhart SR, Naureen I, Cleveland AA, et al. Species identification and antifungal susceptibility testing of Candida bloodstream isolates from population-based surveillance studies in two U.S. cities from 2008 to 2011. J Clin Microbiol. 2012;50(11):3435.
26. Wang H, Xu YC, Hsueh PR. Epidemiology of candidemia and antifungal susceptibility in invasive *Candida* species in the Asia-Pacific region. Future Microbiol. 2016;11:1461–77.
27. Xiao M, Sun ZY, Kang M, et al. Five-year national surveillance of invasive candidiasis: species distribution and azole susceptibility from the China Hospital Invasive Fungal Surveillance Net (CHIF.NET) study. J Clin Microbiol. 2018;56(7):e00577-18. https://doi.org/10.1128/JCM.00577-18.
28. Sun Y, Meng F, Han M, et al. Epidemiology, management, and outcome of invasive fungal disease in patients undergoing hematopoietic stem cell transplantation in China: a multicenter prospective observational study. Biol Blood Marrow Transplant. 2015;21(6):1117–26.
29. Pappas PG, Kauffman CA, Andes DR. Clinical practice guideline for the management of Candidiasis: 2016 update by the Infectious Diseases Society of America. Clin Infect Dis. 2015;62(4):409.
30. Patterson TF, Thompson GR 3rd, Denning DW, et al. Practice guidelines for the diagnosis and management of aspergillosis: 2016 update by the Infectious Diseases Society of America. Clin Infect Dis. 2016;63(4):el–e60. https://doi.org/10.1093/cid/ciw326.

# Sudden Noncardiac Deaths Caused by Poisoning

22

Xiaobo Peng and Zewu Qiu

**Abstract**

Toxic diseases are currently on the rise, especially among adolescents and youth groups. Poisoning-induced death also constitutes the main cause of death. We mainly discuss the causes of toxic sudden noncardiac death. As can be seen, injuries to multiple systems such as the respiratory system, nervous system, digestive system, endocrine system, and immune system and electrolyte imbalance caused by poisoning can lead to sudden death. If a toxic disease is discovered in time, diagnosed, and given proper disposition, sudden death can be avoided. It is important that clinicians caring for poisoning patients need to be familiar with the characteristics of toxic diseases for accurate diagnosis and centralized management.

**Keywords**

Poisoning · Sudden death · Noncardiac death · Risk factors

## 22.1 Introduction

There are many kinds of poisons in the world, which are large in quantity. When you inhale, swallow, or touch the poison that makes you sick, poisoning will occur. Poisoning is a major cause of disease morbidity and mortality worldwide [1–3]. The number of drug poisonings has seen a rapid increase in the United States, especially among adolescents and youths [4–6]. According to a report of the American Association of Poison Control Centers (AAPCC), there were more than 2.1 million calls for poisoning in the United States in 2016. Moreover, deaths from toxic

X. Peng · Z. Qiu (✉)
Poisoning Treatment Department, The Fifth Medical Center of Chinese PLA General Hospital, Beijing, China



H. Zhu (ed.), *Sudden Death*, https://doi.org/10.1007/978-981-15-7002-5_22

diseases and poisoning have shown a rising tendency in many countries [7–9]. Between 1982 and 2013, poisoning was considered to be the second leading cause of accidental injury and death in the United States [10].

Poisoning can injure various organs of the body quickly and directly, resulting in damage to multiple organs. Large amounts of poison entering the human body, strong toxicity, and delayed disposition will lead to rapid deterioration of multiple vital organs, and even sudden death. On the basis of the International Classification of Diseases-10 (ICD-10) of the World Health Organization, sudden death refers to the death that occurs within 24 h after onset of symptoms, is nonviolent, and free of other explanation [11]. However, most of these deaths occur within 1 h or even less after the onset of symptoms [12, 13]. Sudden death is not necessarily accidental, unexpected death is not necessarily sudden, but they often coexist in combination of both [14]. Toxic diseases are a high risk factor for sudden death. In the presence of ambulance first-aid personnel, in addition to heart disease, drug poisoning and suicide are the most common causes of sudden death outside the hospital [15]. Mehtap Gurger reported that the most common nontraumatic sudden death poisoning patients in the emergency department accounted for 15.2% [16]. Poisoning-induced sudden noncardiac death (SNCD) is caused by poisoning-induced injuries to important organs other than the cardiovascular system, including the respiratory system, nervous system, digestive system, endocrine system, and immune system diseases and electrolyte disorders. In case of sudden death, respiration or heart beat will first stop, and then other functions will cease. This differs from the first stop of the heart in sudden cardiac death (SCD). The following illustrates the characteristics of sudden noncardiac death caused by poisoning.

## 22.2 Sudden Death Caused by Poisoning-Induced Respiratory Damage

Gas poisoning such as carbon monoxide and methane can directly give rise to asphyxiation, which causes death, especially in enclosed spaces [17, 18]. Poisoning for inhalation of toxic gases and irritating gases can directly damage the respiratory system, cause acute damage such as airway obstruction, pulmonary edema, and respiratory depression, and lead to sudden death due to acute respiratory failure. Other nongaseous forms of poisons can invade and be absorbed through the skin, digestive tract, injection, etc., causing damage to the upper respiratory tract, lungs, and respiratory center, leading to central respiratory depression, even pulmonary embolism, and bring about rapid death in severe cases.

### 22.2.1 Acute Airway Obstruction

Irritant gases and fumes such as ammonia, nitrogen dioxide, sulfur dioxide, metal fume, mercury, cadmium, etc., produce damage to the mouth, nose, throat, trachea, and bronchus through local stimulation, causing acute toxic pharyngitis and bronchitis. Acute airway obstruction and/or laryngospasm are caused, and mechanical obstruction of the throat can also be resulted from bronchial mucosal necrosis and defulvium. Acute laryngeal obstruction is manifested as inspiratory dyspnea, irritability, cyanosis, weak pulse and quick pulse, coma, and sudden death. When certain poisons and asphyxiating gases (hydride, organophosphorus, hydrogen sulfide, nitrogen, methane, barn gas, etc.) give rise to poisoning, the secretion of bronchial glands increases, and the trachea and bronchial smooth muscle spasm occurs, causing a large amount of secretions to block the bronchus, resulting in ventilation dysfunction or suffocation due to reflex edema of the throat, leading to "flash death."

Poisoning patients are often accompanied by unconsciousness and weakened oropharyngeal reflexes. For example, patients with acute alcoholism have a large amount of food in their stomachs. When vomiting is conducted, stomach contents easily enter the airway, resulting in suffocation and aspiration pneumonia. In severe cases, sudden death can occur due to asphyxia. Most of the patients with sudden death from acute alcoholism die from suffocation [19]. In the emergency treatment, it is often found that for some drunken patients who have already stopped heartbeat before coming to the hospital, a lot of aspirating vomit is often sucked out from the trachea during cardiopulmonary resuscitation [20–22]. Asphyxia, reflex cardiac arrest, or a combination of the two is considered to be the primary mechanism of death from acute alcoholism. Coma patients poisoned by sedative drugs and narcotics may also experience sudden death due to airway obstruction or pulmonary infection arising from aspiration caused by weakened laryngeal reflexes. Therefore, for poisoning-induced coma patients, preventing aspiration is a "top priority." The patient must not be in a supine position, and the head must be biased to one side to prevent vomit from entering the trachea. Inserting a stomach tube for gastric lavage is performed according to the situation, and the stomach contents are emptied with a view to prevent aspiration.

### 22.2.2 Acute Pulmonary Edema

Acute pulmonary edema is the most common symptom of respiratory tract poisoning. For example, acute irritating gas poisoning arising from chlorine, phosgene, hydrogen sulfide, ammonia, and nickel carbonyl can cause acute pulmonary edema. Poisoning in other routes can also cause acute pulmonary edema, such as organophosphorus poisoning, paraquat poisoning, diquat poisoning, etc. [23]. It is absorbed through the digestive tract, skin, and respiratory tract. The toxicity involves multiple organs in the body, and in severe cases, can cause multiple organ dysfunction syndrome (MODS). The lung is the main target organ, which is characterized by acute lung injury (ALI) or acute respiratory distress syndrome (ARDS). Sudden death may be caused in severe cases.

Methamphetamine poisoning is directly toxic to the lungs. It can be absorbed into the body through the mouth, lung, nose, intramuscularly, intravenously, and rectal and vaginal channels. There have been reports on poisoning in patients hiding drugs in their bodies [24–26]. It has been found that methamphetamine can cause acute pulmonary edema [27] and pulmonary hypertension [28, 29]. There was also pulmonary fever caused by inhalation of methamphetamine crack. Other pulmonary complications include pneumothorax, pneumomediastinum, pneumonia, acute lung injury, and pulmonary hemorrhage. Similar injuries also appeared after taking heroin and sucking cocaine crack [30].

### 22.2.3 Respiratory Muscle Paralysis

Some poisons act on the motor nerve or respiratory muscles, causing a decrease in respiratory muscle tension and paralysis. In the case of organophosphate poisoning, excessive acetylcholine excites neuromuscular conduction, causing muscle fibers to tremble and even paralyze, leading to paralysis of the respiratory muscles. The nicotinic action of organophosphorus pesticides can also cause the paralysis of respiratory muscle, and patients may suddenly develop respiratory failure.

Animal and plant poisoning tend to generate neurotoxin, which causes positioning. For example, animal toxins such as snake venom, scorpion venom, and bee venom are endotoxic or destructive to nerve tissue, which can cause fatty change to the peripheral nerve myelin, brain, spinal cord, and other tissues. With basket whelk poisoning, the paralytic shellfish poison contained in the basket whelk can block the sodium ions required for nerve impulse conduction from entering the nerve and skeletal muscle cells, thereby blocking nerve impulse conduction and depolarization of the muscle cells, producing strong muscle paralysis and leading to peripheral respiratory failure and respiratory arrest. Botulinum toxin can cause muscle relaxation, and respiratory muscle paralysis caused by these poisons may impede pulmonary ventilation and exchange seriously. If not treated in time, it may lead to respiratory failure and sudden death. Pesticides such as carbamates can also give rise to respiratory muscle paralysis.

Poisonous plants such as aconitums (monkshood, radix aconite agrestis, aconite, short-spedicel aconite root, etc.) may generate aconitine, which, with its severe toxicity, can cause rapid death if large doses are swallowed. Aconitine can excite and then inhibit the central nervous system and peripheral nerves, blocking the conduction of neuromuscular junctions. Severe poisoning patients suffer respiratory depression and blood pressure drops due to medullary respiration and vasomotor center paralysis, and finally die of respiratory and circulatory failure. Strychnos, Vietnamese sophora root, red fennel, *Gelsmium elegans*, thorn apple, henbane, coffee senna, ginkgo, etc., can also cause damage to the nervous system, which is mainly manifested as first excitement and then inhibition in the central nervous system. The patients suffer dizziness, headache, irritability, ataxia, muscle rigidity, convulsion, epileptic seizures, eclampsia, lethargy, high fever, blurred mind, and coma, and large doses of poisoning can cause death due to respiratory failure and circulatory failure.

For animal and plant toxin poisoning, special antidote should be applied as soon as possible. The special antidote for snake venom is antivenom, and that for botulism is anticreotoxin serum [31, 32]. Symptomatic and supportive treatment is applied, including smooth breathing, respiratory support, fluid replacement, prevention and treatment of shock, renal failure, and respiratory failure, and tetanus antitoxin and antibiotics are given to prevent wound infection.

### 22.2.4 Respiratory Center Suppression

Sedative hypnotics, anesthetics, central stimulants, and opioids can inhibit respiratory arrest caused by the medullary respiratory center in the event of poisoning. When organophosphorus pesticides and asphyxiating gases give rise to poisoning, the poisons enter the body in large quantities and go into the central nervous system through the blood-brain barrier and can directly inhibit the medullary respiratory center. For example, organophosphorus inhibits cholinesterase to accumulate acetylcholine in the brain, directly affecting the impulse conduction between synapses in the central nervous cells, causing central nervous system and respiratory dysfunction, and medullary respiratory center paralysis, leading to respiratory arrest. Respiratory depression due to diazepam-induced organophosphorus pesticide poisoning has been described in many human and animal studies although diazepam can treat epilepsy caused by organophosphorus pesticide poisoning [33]. Therefore, it should be noted that the application of sedative hypnotics during the treatment of organophosphate poisoning may result in respiratory depression [34]. Hydrogen sulfide poisoning inhibits cytochrome oxidase, causes it to lose the ability to transfer electron, blocks biooxidation, and leads to tissue hypoxia. High concentration of hydrogen sulfide poisoning (>1000 mg/m$^3$) can cause reflex respiratory central paralysis, and the poisoned person can immediately get stunned and suffer respiratory arrest.

After potassium cyanide, sodium cyanide, or other cyanide poisoning, cyanide ions can be released in the body and can rapidly combine with ferric iron in oxidized cytochrome oxidase to form oxidized ferric cytochrome oxidase, causing the pigment to lose the ability to transmit electrons, bringing about intracellular asphyxia, and resulting in poisoning due to tissue hypoxia. Oral administration of high-dose cyanide, such as sodium cyanide (50–200 mg), can cause extremely rapid death. Within 10–60 s, the patient will suffer sudden faint, difficulty breathing, and tonic spasm. After 2–3 min, the breathing stops, and then the patient dies after the heartbeat stops. In this case, there is almost no remedy. The toxicology of sodium azide is basically the same as that of sodium cyanide, and the symptoms are similar.

Severe poisoning by opium, heroin, fentanyl, and other narcotics causes deep coma, decreased blood pressure, and deep respiratory suppression. Severe hypoxia induced by acute respiratory dysfunction is the most common cause of sudden death. Morphine, barbiturates, hydrogen sulfide, cyanide, etc., can also directly inhibit the respiratory center, causing central respiratory failure, which is mainly manifested as moderate breathing, apathia, decreased blood pressure, coma, and even respiratory arrest.

### 22.2.5 Pulmonary Embolism

In a study of the reason for sudden noncardiac death in the 5–35-year-old population in Australia, pulmonary embolism is the fourth most common reason, second only to epilepsy, intracranial hemorrhage, and asthma [35]. Poisoning can cause pulmonary embolism. For instance, acute organophosphorus poisoning may bring about pulmonary thrombosis [36], and treatment of acute organophosphate poisoning by atropine may induce pulmonary embolism. In patients with a history of comorbidities, the probability of pulmonary thromboembolism (PTE) after acute organophosphorus poisoning is significantly higher [37]. A case report showed that deep venous thrombosis (DVT) in the upper extremity was caused by complications of acute organophosphorus poisoning [38], and mural thrombosis of severe organophosphorus poisoning was found at autopsy [39]. Infarction and gangrene requiring amputation are described as complications of acute organophosphorus poisoning in patients with primary vascular disease [40]. Atropine, as a therapeutic drug, may also cause pulmonary vasoconstriction by increasing serotonin levels [41].

## 22.3 Sudden Death Caused by Poisoning-Induced Acute Nervous System Damage

Acute neurological damage caused by poisoning includes cerebral hemorrhage, cerebral edema, epilepsy, and other acute symptoms. The common mechanism of sudden death caused by subarachnoid hemorrhage, brain stem hemorrhage, or large area cerebral hemorrhage is the formation of cerebral palsy caused by high intracranial pressure, direct compression of the brain stem, and interruption of blood supply, resulting in central respiratory failure or respiratory arrest, causing pulseless electrical activity (PEA), and leading to sudden death.

### 22.3.1 Cerebral Bleeding

Anticoagulant rodenticides, the most widely used rodenticides in most countries, including diphacinone, brodifacoum, bromadiolone, etc., and anticoagulant drugs such as warfarin can cause coagulation disorders, leading to stasis skin ecchymosis, gum bleeding, hematuria, and other multiple organ bleeding [42, 43]. In case of delayed diagnosis and treatment, sudden death may occur due to cerebral hemorrhage. Aspirin, dipyridamole, and other drugs can cause thrombocytopenia, dysfunction, and abnormal blood coagulation, leading to cerebral hemorrhage. Alcoholism, sympathetic drug poisoning, and drug poisoning such as amphetamine, cocaine, and norephedrine can also give rise to cerebral hemorrhage. Based on a prospective case-control study of forensic autopsy, Lucena et al. found that the incidence of cocaine-related sudden death was 14.0% [44]. Takayama reported a sudden death caused by subarachnoid hemorrhage in a cocaine abuser [45]. Cocaine is related with a high incidence of symptomatic vasospasm [46, 47]. Some mechanisms by which cocaine causes vasospasm include norepinephrine-induced vasoconstriction, influx of calcium into smooth muscle, and activation of endothelin-1 [47, 48].

### 22.3.2 Brain Edema

Many chemical poisons have a direct impact on the cellular metabolism of central nervous tissues. For example, acute triethyltin poisoning is considered to be a typical poison leading to cytotoxic cerebral edema. It inhibits the adenosine triphosphatase normally present in astrocyte processes and axons, thereby affecting the normal function of the sodium-potassium pump, and retaining astrocyte sodium and water selectively. After conversion of the tetraethyl lead into triethyl lead by the liver, severe intracellular edema can be caused by inhibition of the metabolism of glucose in the brain and reduction of the synthesis of high-energy phosphate bonds. Fluoroacetamide enters the body and forms fluoroacetic acid, which interferes with the normal tricarboxylic acid cycle, leading to adenosine triphosphate synthesis disorder and citric acid accumulation, causing cytotoxic cerebral edema. Organophosphate insecticides deactivate cholinesterase and hinder hydrolysis of acetylcholine, leading to the accumulation of acetylcholine. The accumulation of acetylcholine interferes with the impulse conduction between nerve cell synapses and impairs the function of brain cells. Moreover, some liposoluble poisons can change the permeability of nerve cells and inhibit the activity of enzymes and the oxidative phosphorylation process of cells, leading to edema due to damage to nerve cells. Cerebral edema can cause cerebral ischemia, hypoxia, and reduction of sodium in brain cells, giving rise to convulsions. Cerebral ischemia, hypoxia, and low sodium caused by poisons can result in or aggravate brain edema.

### 22.3.3 Epilepsy

Epilepsy can cause sudden unexpected death in epilepsy (SUDEP), the most common noncardiac factor in sudden death, nontraumatic cerebral hemorrhage, and acute asthma [35]. Some toxic diseases can cause severe epilepsy, such as the hypertoxic rat poisons tetramine [49, 50], fluoroacetamide, and sodium fluoroacetate [51], steroidal poisons including isoniazid and unsymmetrical dimethylhydrazine, organochlorine pesticides, pyrethrum vinegar, nereistoxin pesticides, phosphine, and other acute poisoning. The convulsions may take place intermittently, and the patients often have clear state of consciousness during the diapause and even suffer disturbance of consciousness in severe cases. Poisoning by fluoroacetamide and tetramine often manifests as systemic tonic spasm. Patients with severe cerebral edema often have epileptic seizures and convulsions. Some psychotic drug and narcotics poisoning also produces excitatory effects on the spinal cord, which can lead to convulsions. Sustained status of epilepsy can lead to respiratory disorders. Ventilatory failure with hypoxemia and hypercapnia in epileptic seizures caused by central nervous-mediated apnea may also be the cause of sudden death in some cases, and sudden death caused by clear apnea and respiratory failure can be observed sometimes [52–54]. For poisoning that can cause epilepsy, note to carry out timely sedative and antispasmodic treatment, keep the airway open, and protect the patients to prevent the patients from accidentally injuring themselves.

## 22.4 Sudden Death Caused by Poisoning-Induced Digestive Tract Injury

After poisoning by corrosive chemical poisons such as strong acids, strong bases, dichromic acids, and mercury salts by the digestive tract, the corrosive action can directly act on the digestive tract, causing tissue damage to bring about acute gastrointestinal bleeding and even perforation of the digestive tract. The bleeding occurs mainly in the upper digestive tract such as the esophagus and the stomach. A large amount of bleeding in a short time can cause circulatory failure, leading to sudden death due to hemorrhagic shock.

## 22.5 Sudden Death Caused by Endocrine System Lesion Due to Poisoning

With the exception of intramuscular insulin, oral hypoglycemic drugs can cause hypoglycemia. Since 1980s, there have been clinical reports and animal models that opioids (mainly methadone) are associated with glucose dysregulation, and hypoglycemia and sudden death during treatment with methadone and treatment with opioids have been reported [55]. In 2013, Faskowitz et al. found that methadone reduced blood glucose levels in a dose-dependent manner in a mouse model [56]. Hypoglycemia can cause changes in the electrical system of the heart, including extending QT interval, prolonging repolarization, and giving rise to ST wave changes. These ECG changes are attributed to hypokalemia, which results from the release of catecholamines caused by hypoglycemia [57]. Severe hypoglycemia, if not replenished in time to correct glucose, can cause necrosis and softening of brain tissue, and can lead to decorticate syndrome and gives rise to sudden death in severe cases.. Alcoholism and salicylic acid poisoning can also produce hypoglycemia [58].

## 22.6 Sudden Death Caused by Poisoning-Induced Electrolyte Imbalance

Acute barium salt, trimethyltin, and phenol poisoning can give rise to hypokalemia. Poisoning-induced acute renal failure and toxic hemolysis can result in hyperkalemia. Some drugs, such as digitalis, can inhibit the action of cell membrane sodium-potassium-ATPase, promote the outward transfer of potassium in cells, and also bring about hyperkalemia. Patients with hypokalemia and hyperkalemia can suffer various types of arrhythmia and even refractory arrhythmia . Failure to dispose of it in a timely manner can lead to sudden death.

## 22.7 Sudden Death Caused by Poisoning-Induced Immune Factors

As for biotoxin poisoning such as snake bites and wasp stings, in addition to the toxicity of the toxin itself, allergies are also an important cause of sudden death. In a study in the United Kingdom, allergic deaths caused by biotoxins accounted for a quarter. Relative to food, it is more likely to cause airway obstruction, and biotoxins more easily result in shock [59].

Overall, any poison can cause sudden death when bringing about direct or indirect serious damage to vital organs or electrolyte imbalance. Sudden death can be avoided if most of the toxic diseases are diagnosed in time and given proper treatment. Correct diagnosis, risk stratification, and management are paramount. With regard to toxic diseases, therefore, attention should be paid to the disposition of the causes and complications of acute poisoning, timely and correct use of special detoxification drugs, timely processing and prevention of various complications and delayed effects caused by poison damage, and protection of vital organs.

## References

1. Gallagher LM, Kappatos D, Tisch C, et al. Suicide by poisoning in New Zealand—a toxicological analysis. N Z Med J. 2012;125:15.
2. Gjersing L, Jonassen KV, Biong S, et al. Diversity in causes and characteristics of drug-induced deaths in an urban setting. Scand J Public Health. 2013;41:119.
3. Sinyor M, Howlett A, Cheung AH, et al. Substances used in completed suicide by overdose in Toronto: an observational study of coroner's data. Can J Psychiatr. 2012;57:184.
4. Manchikanti L, Helm S, Fellows B, et al. Opioid epidemic in the United States. Pain Physician. 2012;15:ES9–ES38.
5. Khan SQ, Berrington de Gonzalez A, Best AF, et al. Infant and youth mortality trends by race/ethnicity and cause of death in the United States. JAMA Pediatr. 2018;172(12):e183317.
6. Curtin SC, Tejada-Vera B, Warmer M. Drug overdose deaths among adolescents aged 15-19 in the United States: 1999-2015. NCHS Data Brief. 2017;(282):1–8.
7. Ren Y, Zhang M, Luo X, et al. Secular trend of the leading causes of death in China from 2003 to 2013. Afr Health Sci. 2017;17(2):532–7.
8. Wang SY, Li YH, Chi GB, et al. Injury-related fatalities in China: an under-recognised public-health problem. Lancet. 2008;372(9651):1765–73.
9. Kim KS, Kim SD, Lee SH. Trend of mortality rate and injury burden of transport accidents, suicides, and falls. J Prev Med Public Health. 2012;45(1):8–13.
10. Manini AF, Nelson LS, Olsen D, et al. Medical examiner and medical toxicologist agreement on cause of death. Forensic Sci Int. 2011;206(1–3):71–6.
11. World Health Organisation. International classification of diseases (ICD-10). version 2016. 2010. https://icd.who.int/browse10/2016/en. Accessed Jan 2019.
12. Jouven XDM, Guerot C, Ducimetière P. Predicting sudden death in the population, the Paris prospective study I. Circulation. 1999;99:1978–93.
13. Zipes DP, Wellens HJ. Sudden cardiac death. Circulation. 1998;98(21):2334–51.

14. Knight B. Simpson's forensic medicine, vol. 14. 11th ed. London: Hodder Headline Group; 1997. p. 105–12.
15. Marelsson S, Thornorgeirsson G. Sudden noncardiac arrest out-of-hospital in the Reykjavík area 1987-1999. Laeknabladid. 2001;87(12):973–8.
16. Gurger M, Turkoglu A, Atescelik M, et al. Sudden suspected death in emergency department: autopsy results. Turk J Emerg Med. 2014;14(3):115–20.
17. Hampson NB. U.S. mortality due to carbon monoxide poisoning, 1999-2014. Accidental and intentional deaths. Ann Am Thorac Soc. 2016;13:1768.
18. Hampson NB, Hauff NM. Risk factors for short-term mortality from carbon monoxide poisoning treated with hyperbaric oxygen. Crit Care Med. 2008;36:2523.
19. Blaas V, Manhart J, Port A, Keil W, Büttner A. An autopsy approach on bolus deaths. J Forensic Legal Med. 2016;42:82–7.
20. Brinkmann B. Ersticken. In: Brinkmann B, Madea B, editors. Handbuch gerichtliche Medizin. Band 1. 1st ed. Berlin: Springer; 2003. p. 785–6.
21. Dettmeyer R, Schütz H, Verhoff M. Rechtsmedizin. 2nd ed. Heidelberg: Springer; 2014.
22. Penning R. Rechtsmedizin systematisch. 2nd ed. UniMed Verlag: Bremen; 2006.
23. Wang Y, Gao D, Zuojun G, et al. Radiomics nomogram analyses for differentiating pneumonia and acute paraquat lung injury. Sci Rep. 2019;9(1):15029.
24. Hendrickson RG, Horowitz BZ, Norton RL, Notenboom H. "Parachuting" meth: a novel delivery method for methamphetamine and delayed-onset toxicity from "body stuffing". Clin Toxicol (Phila). 2006;44:379.
25. Cantrell FL, Breckenridge HM, Jost P. Transrectal methamphetamine use: a novel route of exposure. Ann Intern Med. 2006;145:78.
26. Kashani J, Ruha AM. Methamphetamine toxicity secondary to intravaginal body stuffing. J Toxicol Clin Toxicol. 2004;42:987.
27. Nestor TA, Tamamoto WI, Kam TH, et al. Crystal methamphetamine-induced acute pulmonary edema: a case report. Hawaii Med J. 1989;48:457.
28. Schaiberger PH, Kennedy TC, Miller FC, et al. Pulmonary hypertension associated with long-term inhalation of "crank" methamphetamine. Chest. 1993;104:614.
29. Chin KM, Channick RN, Rubin LJ. Is methamphetamine use associated with idiopathic pulmonary arterial hypertension? Chest. 2006;130:1657.
30. Gotway MB, Marder SR, Hanks DK, et al. Thoracic complications of illicit drug use: an organ system approach. Radiographics. 2002; 22 Spec no:S119.
31. O'Horo JC, Harper EP, El Rafei A, et al. Efficacy of antitoxin therapy in treating patients with foodborne botulism: a systematic review and meta-analysis of cases, 1923-2016. Clin Infect Dis. 2017;66:S43.
32. Bai L, Peng X, Liu Y, et al. Clinical analysis of 86 botulism cases caused by cosmetic injection of botulinum toxin (BoNT). Medicine. 2018;97(34):e10659.
33. McDonough JH Jr, Zoeffel LD, McMonagle J, et al. Anticonvulsant treatment of nerve agent seizures: anticholinergics versus diazepam in soman-intoxicated guinea pigs. Epilepsy Res. 2000;38:1.
34. Marrs TC. Diazepam in the treatment of organophosphorus ester pesticide poisoning. Toxicol Rev. 2003;22:75–81.
35. Puranik R, Chow CK, Duflou JA, et al. Sudden death in the young. Heart Rhythm. 2005;2(12):1277–82. Accessed 10 Mar 2019.
36. Pereska Z, Chaparoska D, Bekarovski N, et al. Pulmonary thrombosis in acute organophosphate poisoning—case report and literature overview of prothrombotic preconditioning in organophosphate toxicity. Toxicol Rep. 2019;6:550–5.
37. Lim Y-P, Lin C-L, Hung D-Z, et al. Increased risk of deep vein thrombosis and pulmonary thromboembolism in patients with organophosphate intoxication. Medicine. 2015;94:e341.
38. Naik M, Bhat T, Mir M, et al. Organophosphorus poisoning: a rare case of upper extremity deep vein thrombosis. Indian J Health Sci Care. 2016;9:339.
39. Anand S, Singh S, Saikia UN, et al. Cardiac abnormalities in acute organophosphate poisoning. Clin Toxicol. 2009;47:230–5.

40. Buckley NA, Dawson AH, Whyte IM. Organophosphate poisoning: peripheral vascular resistance–a measure of adequate atropinization. J Toxicol Clin Toxicol. 1994;32:61–8. Accessed 10 Mar 2019
41. Fritts HW, Harris P, Clauss RH, et al. The effect of acetylcholine on the human pulmonary circulation under normal and hypoxic conditions. J Clin Invest. 1958;37:99–110.
42. Dawson A, Garthwaite D. Rodenticide usage by local authorities in Great Britain. In: Department for Environment, Food & Rural Affairs, editor. Pesticide usage survey report 185. York: Department for Environment, Food & Rural Affairs; 2001.
43. Long J, Peng X, Luo Y, et al. Treatment of a long-acting anticoagulant rodenticide poisoning cohort with vitamin K1 during the maintenance period. Medicine. 2016;95(51):e5461.
44. Lucena J, Blanco M, Jurado C, et al. Cocaine-related sudden death: a prospective investigation in south-west Spain. Eur Heart J. 2010;31:318–29.
45. Takayama M, Waters B, Fujii H, et al. Subarachnoid hemorrhage in a Japanese cocaine abuser: cocaine-related sudden death. Legal Med. 2018;32:43–7.
46. Conway JE, Tamargo RJ. Cocaine use is an independent risk factor for cerebral vasospasm after aneurysmal subarachnoid hemorrhage. Stroke. 2001;32:2338–43.
47. Chang Y, Liu YP, Liu CF. The effect on serotonin and MDA levels in depressed patients with insomnia when far-infrared rays are applied to acupoints. Am J Chin Med. 2009;37:837–42.
48. Lange RA, Cigarroa RG, Yancy CW, et al. Cocaine-induced coronary-artery vasoconstriction. N Engl J Med. 1989;321:1557–62.
49. Whitlow KS, Belson M, Barrueto F, et al. Tetramethylenedisulfotetramine: old agent and new terror. Ann Emerg Med. 2005;45:609.
50. Deng X, Li G, Mei R, et al. Long term effects of tetramine poisoning: an observational study. Clin Toxicol (Phila). 2012;50:172.
51. Proudfoot AT, Bradberry SM, Vale JA. Sodium fluoroacetate poisoning. Toxicol Rev. 2006;25:213.
52. Tezer FI, Rémi J, Noachtar S. Ictal apnea of epileptic origin. Neurology. 2009;72:855.
53. Blum AS, Ives JR, Goldberger AL, et al. Oxygen desaturations triggered by partial seizures: implications for cardiopulmonary instability in epilepsy. Epilepsia. 2000;41:536.
54. Bateman LM, Li CS, Seyal M. Ictal hypoxemia in localization-related epilepsy: analysis of incidence, severity and risk factors. Brain. 2008;131:3239.
55. Plescia CJ, Manu P. Hypoglycemia and sudden death during treatment with methadone for opiate detoxification. Am J Ther. 2018;25(2):e267–9.
56. Faskowitz AJ, Kramskiy VN, Pasternak GW. Methadone-induced hypoglycemia. Cell Mol Neurobiol. 2013;33:537–42.
57. Snell-Bergeon JK, Wadwa RP. Hypoglycemia, diabetes, and cardiovascular disease. Diabetes Technol Ther. 2012;14(suppl 1):S51–8.
58. Lang JE, Pflaumer A, Davis AM. Causes of sudden death in the young—cardiac and non-cardiac. Prog Pediatric Cardiol. 2017;45:2–13.
59. Pumphrey RSH. Lessons for management of anaphylaxis from a study of fatal reactions. Clin Exp Allergy. 2000;30:1144–50.

# Digestive System Disease and Sudden Death

# 23

Shirui Qi, Zhongyin Wu, Heyue Jia, Bo Jin, Hui Li, Chuntao Liu, Shangqing Chang, Haiyan Zhu, Yating Zhu, Zheng Lu, Peng Li, Haibin Su, Jiang Xiong, Yu Wang, Wei Guo, and Gang Sun

S. Qi · Y. Wang
Emergency Department, Tianjin First Center Hospital, Tianjin, China

Z. Wu
Department of Vascular Surgery, Affiliated Hospital of Chengde Medical College, Hebei, China

H. Jia · Y. Zhu · J. Xiong · W. Guo
Department of Vascular Surgery, Chinese People's Liberation Army General Hospital, Beijing, China

B. Jin · Z. Lu
Liver Cirrhosis Diagnosis and Treatment Center, The Fifth Medical Center of Chinese PLA General Hospital, Beijing, China

H. Li · H. Su
Liver Failure Treatment and Research Center, The Fifth Medical Center of Chinese PLA General Hospital, Beijing, China

C. Liu · P. Li
Department of Gastroenterology, National Clinical Research Center for Digestive Diseases, Beijing Digestive Disease Center, Beijing Friendship Hospital, Capital Medical University, Beijing, China
e-mail: lipeng@ccmu.edu.cn

S. Chang
Emergency Department, The First Medical Center of Chinese PLA General Hospital, Beijing, China

H. Zhu
Emergency Department, The First Medical Center of Chinese PLA General Hospital, Beijing, China

Emergency Department, Hainan Hospital of Chinese PLA General Hospital, Haitangwan Bay, Sanya City, Hainan Province, China

G. Sun (✉)
Department of Gastroenterology and Hepatology, Chinese PLA General Hospital, Beijing, China


H. Zhu (ed.), *Sudden Death*, https://doi.org/10.1007/978-981-15-7002-5_23

**Abstract**

Although sudden death caused by digestive system diseases, accounting for about 7% of sudden death diseases, is not common compared with other diseases such as cardiovascular disease, it is also worthy of attention. Among them, sudden death caused by acute pancreatitis is the most common, accounting for 0.2%-0.5% of natural sudden death, and is one of the important causes of non-cardiac sudden death. This chapter mainly focuses on a series of sudden death related digestive system diseases, including ischemic bowel disease, variceal upper gastrointestinal bleeding in cirrhotic portal hypertension, hepatic encephalopathy, liver failure, acute suppurative cholangitis and acute pancreatitis. This type of disease is characterized by a rapid onset, a rapid progress, and a high mortality rate. Combining typical cases, this chapter describes the pathogenesis, diagnosis and treatment progress of the above-mentioned diseases that may cause sudden death.

**Keywords**

Digestive system disease · Sudden death · Pathogenesis · Clinical characteristics Diagnosis and treatment progress

## 23.1 Ischemia Bowel Disease

### 23.1.1 Introduction

IBD is defined as intestinal ischemic damage caused by insufficient blood supply. It can damage the small intestine, large intestine, or all segments of the intestine. IBD can be divided into chronic mesenteric ischemia (CMI), acute mesenteric ischemia (AMI), and ischemic colitis (IC) [1]. CMI is defined as chronic or persistent hypoperfusion of the bowel due to stenosis or occlusion of the mesenteric artery, also known as intestinal colic [2]. AMI is defined as acute hypoperfusion of the intestine due to obstruction or nonobstructive factors in the mesentery, including mesenteric venous thrombosis, arterial thrombosis, arterial embolism, and nonobstructive ischemia [3]. AMI and CMI are collectively called mesenteric ischemia (MI). IC is also known as colonic ischemia (CI) and defined as reversible or irreversible ischemic damage to the intestinal tract due to decreased colon blood supply. Reversible ischemic damage includes colitis and colon lesions (subepithelial edema or hemorrhage). Colitis usually recovers slowly, and the course of the disease lasts for several months. Colon lesions generally recover within 3 days. Irreversible ischemic damage includes colonic stenosis, gangrene, and fulminant colitis [4]. AMI is extremely susceptible to sudden death and is difficult to diagnose.

### 23.1.2 Case and Method

A death case occurred in August 2019. We analyzed the death process by reviewing the clinical symptoms, physical examination results, biochemical test results, and clinical treatment medications at the time of death.

A 59-year-old man was admitted to the hospital mainly because of "abdominal pain accompanied by melena for 25 h" with no previous medical history. PE: T 36.8 °C, P 66 cpm, R 22 cpm, BP 121/mmHg, $SPO_2$ 97%, clear consciousness, both lungs have rough breathing sounds, no dry or wet rales, HR 78 cmp, irregular S, soft abdomen, total abdominal tenderness, and suspicious rebound pain. CBC: Hb 163 g/L, HCT 0.476 L/L, WBC 13.54 × 109 g/L, PLT 121 × 109 g/L. CFT: APTT 39.7S, PT 21.5S, TT 12.0S, FIB 7.23 g/L, INR 1.99, D-dimer 6539 ng/mL. BBT: ALT 22.9 U/L, AST 68.1 U/L, TP 57.1 g/L, ALB 28.5 g/L, UREA 11.6 umol/L, CRE 142umol/L. SIM: CRP 27.40 mg/dl and PCT 59.50 ng/mL. This patient was administered hemostatic drugs; gastric acid inhibitors, drugs that inhibit digestive enzymes; antibiotics; and fluid infusion. After 12 h, CTA showed intestinal, colon, and rectal wall thickening, and abnormal lumen of superior mesenteric artery and inferior mesenteric artery. CTA diagnose report showed ischemic bowel disease. Two hours later, the patient was dead because his autonomic heart rate and blood pressure stopped.

### 23.1.3 Review and Treatment

#### 23.1.3.1 Etiology and Inducement

The essential pathological basis for this disease was local vascular damage, insufficient blood supply, or hypercoagulability. The major pathological process was intestinal ischemia, hypoxia, and reperfusion. The main pathological feature was a submucosal layer with a large number of hemosiderin cells and fibrous thrombosis. The cause of IBD was unknown; however, it may be related to the following four points: arterial thrombosis, arterial embolism, mesenteric venous thrombosis, and nonocclusive factors. Arterial thrombosis and arterial embolization are called occlusive factors. Previous studies have shown that the risk factors for IBD can be divided into five categories: demographic characteristics, behavioral characteristics, clinical complications, drugs. and iatrogenic factors [5]. Demographic characteristics include elderly and female. Behavioral characteristics include smoking, drinking, and strenuous exercise. IBD Patients are usually accompanied by heart failure, arrhythmia, atherosclerosis, diabetes, hypertension, dyslipidemia, irritable bowel syndrome, constipation, chronic obstructive pulmonary disease, and various other symptoms such as shock, arterial thrombosis, mechanical intestinal obstruction, and so on. Iatrogenic factors include aneurysm resection, gynecological surgery, bowel resection, coronary artery bypass surgery, barium enema, colonoscopy, and so on. Drugs commonly used in clinical practice include constipation-causing drugs, narcotic drugs, immunomodulators, nonsteroidal anti-inflammatory drugs, boosters, statins, chemotherapeutics, antibiotics, diuretics, steroid hormones, antipsychotics, cathartic drugs, and so on. Constipation-causing drugs include opioids, alosetron, tricyclic antidepressants, and antidiarrheals. Narcotic drugs include cocaine and amphetamine. Immunomodulators include interferons and tumor necrosis factor inhibitors. Yadav et al. [6] showed that age (>40), gender (male > female), and chronic obstructive pulmonary disease are related to death in patients with CI.

#### 23.1.3.2 Clinical Symptoms

Patients with IBD lack specific clinical signs and symptoms. Their symptoms and signs are not consistent.

Acute mesenteric ischia (AMI) has a rapid onset, a higher mortality, and no specific manifestation at an early stage. The AMI triad is defined as severe upper abdominal pain or umbilical pain without corresponding signs, organic heart disease with atrial fibrillation, and gastrointestinal emptying disorder [7]. The main symptoms of AMI are sudden and severe abdominal pain with frequent vomiting and diarrhea. It has been found that 15–25% of patients with AMI have no symptoms of abdominal pain. They only have unexplained abdominal distension and gastrointestinal bleeding. About 75% of patients have positive fecal occult blood. Bloody stools may occur in 15% of patients. Some patients may have intestinal obstruction. When the patient has severe intestinal ischemia, ulcers and perforations may occur, followed by fever, nausea, vomiting, and signs of peritonitis and sepsis. These factors eventually lead to septic shock.

#### 23.1.3.3 Biochemical Indicators and Imaging Characteristics

##### Biochemical Indicators

The peripheral white blood cells (WBCs) of patients with IBD are increased. About 75% of patients have WBC >15 × 109 g/L. However, this indicator lacks specificity, and IBD also occurs in patients with normal WBC [8]. It is worth noting that occult blood is often positive in these patients. Alkaline phosphatase (ALP), lactate dehydrogenase (LDH), and creatine kinase (CK) were elevated in patients with IBD. However, the determination of serum enzymes and biochemical indicators also lacks specificity for the diagnosis of AMI. Previous studies have shown that D-lactic acid, L-lactic acid, and intestinal fatty acid binding protein (I-FABP) can increase during intestinal ischemia [9]. D-Lactic acid is an isomer of L-lactic. It is one of the main fermentation products of intestinal bacteria. Normally, D-Lactic acid cannot be absorbed into the blood through the intestinal mucosal barrier. Tissues cannot produce D-lactic acid in the human body. Changes in blood D-lactic acid levels are closely related to intestinal permeability, which can reflect the intestinal barrier function, and are positively related to the degree of intestinal ischemic damage. D-Lactic acid can be used as an early indicator of intestinal ischemia detection, because it has higher specificity than other indicators [10]. Previous animal experiments have found that I-FABP exists in the cytoplasm of cells at the tip of the intestinal villi. Normally, peripheral blood vessels do not contain I-FABP. When intestinal damage occurs, the permeability of intestinal epithelial cells increases, which causes the intestinal villi to release I-FABP into the blood and can be detected in peripheral blood vessels [11]. Kanda et al. [12] found that serum I-FABP levels in patients with IBD were between 20 ug/L and 1496 ug/L, which were significantly higher than normal (<65 ug/L). This indicates that I-FABP has good sensitivity for the diagnosis of IBD. However, due to its poor specificity, complicated detection methods, and high cost, I-FABP is rarely used in clinical practice. D-Dimer (D-D) is often used clinically as an exclusion test for venous thrombosis. It is an end product of fibrin degradation and an important indicator of thrombosis and embolic disease. Block et al. found that when D-D > 0.9 mg/L, the accuracy of IBD diagnosis is 69%, specificity is 92%, and sensitivity is 60%, and it has a suggestive effect on the progress of the disease. In addition, when D-D > 3.17 mg/L, its sensitivity and specificity can approach that of CT angiography [13].

In addition, interleukin (IL) is a group of soluble proteins with different structures and functions secreted by many types of cells, which participate in the exchange of information between cells. Currently, IL has been found to be of several types including LI-1 to IL-33. Previous studies have showed that IL-6 has a significant upward trend in patients with acute intestinal ischemia [14].

### Abdominal X-Ray Examination

Abdominal X-ray is the most basic examination of AMI. The most typical sign is the "finger indentation" sign, which can indicate intestinal submucosal edema and bleeding. It should be noted that X-ray examination should not be performed during the period of gastrointestinal bleeding. Barium enema can cause the intestinal spasm. As the disease progresses, the intestinal canal can become stiff like a fence due to submucosal edema and thickening of the folds. In addition, the barium in the intestinal cavity forms a fan-like edge [15]. Barium test can also aggravate intestinal ischemia, which can cause bowel perforation when the patient is seriously ill. Therefore, barium examination is contraindicated in patients with peritoneal irritation. X-ray examination cannot show mesenteric vascular disease, which limits its diagnostic value for MI. On the other hand, a negative result cannot exclude MI.

### Ultrasound Examination

Ultrasound is a noninvasive imaging examination, which is simple, rapid, and effective. Type-B ultrasonic examination can show mesenteric vascular stenosis and occlusion. The other main signs are as follows: gas accumulation under the diaphragm, thickening of the intestinal wall, gas accumulation in the portal vein and mesenteric vein, and ascites. Ultrasound can be used for screening and identification of IBD. However, it is easily affected by interference factors, such as obese patients, peritoneal effusion, abdominal surgery history, gas accumulation, etc.

### Computed Tomography (CT) Examination

CT is the best choice for most patients. The reason is that it can comprehensively show the location and extent of lesions and can help identify acute or chronic abdominal pain caused by other causes. By measuring the morphology and inner diameter of blood vessels, nonocclusive mesenteric ischemia can be diagnosed early [16]. Contrast-enhanced CT and CT angiography (CTA) can directly observe the anatomy of the mesenteric artery trunk and its secondary branches, but it is not reliable for assessing branches below the third level [17]. CTA is the preferred test method for diagnosing MI. The sensitivity and specificity for AMI diagnosis are

96% and 94%, respectively [18–20]. However, the disadvantage of CTA is that it is impossible to perform intravascular drug perfusion treatment like intravascular angiography, and it is less sensitive to patients with nonocclusive mesenteric ischemia.

#### MRI and MRA

MRI is similar to CT, but its sensitivity and specificity are low, and it is time-consuming. Therefore, it is generally not used as an emergency examination method. MRA can show mesenteric arterial and venous trunks and their main branches. Its sensitivity and specificity for CMI diagnosis are 100% and 95%, respectively [21]. However, there is a certain false positive rate in the judgment of vascular stenosis. Therefore, it cannot effectively evaluate nonocclusive mesenteric ischemia disease. Overall, MRI is of great value in distinguishing between new and old thrombosis and distinguishing between reversible and irreversible bowel ischemia.

#### Angiography

It is the gold standard for the diagnosis of IBD. In addition, intravascular drug perfusion treatment and interventional treatment can be performed directly during the examination. Studies have shown that the sensitivity of DSA is between 90% and 100%, and the specificity is 100%, which has a significant advantage in the diagnosis of nonocclusive mesenteric ischemia. Application of DSA for diagnosis and treatment can reduce the mortality by 18–53% [1]. Angiography has significant advantages in the diagnosis of nonocclusive mesenteric ischemia. It is therefore the only way to diagnose nonocclusive mesenteric ischemia caused by mesenteric arterial spasm. Patients with severe hypotension and hypovolemia should not use this test. In addition, angiography is not used as a routine test because it is an invasive test method, which is expensive and has related complications.

#### Isotope Examination

Previous studies have shown that scanning techniques for the isotope $^{99}$Tc and $^{111}$In can show the ischemic area of acute mesenteric occlusion, which can be used as an assisted diagnostic measure for ischemic bowel disease. In patients with ischemic colitis, a colonic scan of white blood cells labeled with the isotope $^{99}$Tc revealed radionuclide accumulation in the ischemic site of the sigmoid colon. The sigmoid colon formed by it can be used as a diagnostic basis [22]. In addition, research has reported that the albumin-cobalt binding test is a new useful diagnostic indicator for acute intestinal ischemia, with a sensitivity of 100% and a specificity of 85.7% [23].

### 23.1.3.4 Diagnosis

At present, there is no uniform method for the diagnosis of IBD. Clinical diagnosis of patients with IBD needs to be combined with the patient's medical history, risk factors, clinical manifestations, and auxiliary examinations. IBD needs to be distinguished from gastrointestinal perforation, ulcerative colitis, acute gastroenteritis, Crohn's disease, acute pancreatitis, and acute appendicitis. According to the standards established by Williams and others, IBD can be diagnosed if it meets the following six requirements and excludes ulcerative colitis: (1) the acute onset of abdominal pain and blood in the stool; (2) localization of the left colon outside the rectum; (3) no antibiotics; (4) histological biopsy of bacterial culture or fecal examination was negative; (5) colonoscopy manifestations: mucosal congestion, edema, bleeding, and longitudinal ulcer scar (narrow type) in the acute phase, and chronic mucosa to ulcer scar formation in the chronic phase; (6) X-ray examination: thumb indentation sign in the acute phase and transient or narrow ulcer scar in the chronic phase; (7) pathological biopsy: mucosal edema, hemorrhage, necrosis, and protein component exudation in the acute phase, and hemosiderin in the chronic phase. If conditions permit, MRA, angiography, or CTA can be performed in some patients to improve the diagnosis of IBD.

#### 23.1.3.5 Treatment

The treatment of AMI includes medical treatment, interventional treatment, and open surgery. The medical treatment of AMI is as follows: (1) fasting and gastrointestinal decompression if necessary; (2) intravenous nutrition support to correct water and electrolyte balance disorders; (3) correct hypotension, hypovolemia, and arrhythmia; (4) maintain stable blood flow to ensure adequate oxygen supply; (5) early use of broad-spectrum antibiotics to prevent intestinal ischemia from worsening. The antibacterial spectrum should cover aerobic and anaerobic bacteria. Metronidazole and quinolone are commonly used. The third-generation cephalosporins are used in severe infection departments [23, 24]; and (6) adrenal glucocorticoids are used with caution to prevent the spread of necrotic toxins. Once AMI is diagnosed, vasodilators can be applied, and antithrombotic therapy can be initiated early. Aspirin can be given at 200–300 mg/day or clopidogrel t 150–300 mg/day. Patients' clinical symptoms should be closely observed to prevent bleeding; when patients have mesenteric venous thrombosis, anticoagulation and thrombolytic therapy should be performed. For patients with acute mesenteric arterial thrombosis, early intervention can be used when conditions permit. Interventional treatment includes intra-arterial thrombus removal, implantation of endovascular protectors, percutaneous stent implantation, transcatheter arterial infusion of vasodilators, and thrombolysis. Open surgery includes emergency revascularization, assessment of bowel viability, and removal of necrotic bowel segments, and it is the main treatment for AMI.

### 23.1.4 Discussion

In the above case, the patient was a middle-aged male who lacked health awareness and could not find that he had atrial fibrillation. He could not accurately report his condition to the doctor, which led to the misleading judgment of gastrointestinal bleeding. Among his biochemical indicators, D-dimer was significantly elevated, suggesting thrombosis. In the case of such patients, combined with their abdominal signs and test results, the doctor usually needs to make a CTA examination in time to rule out the possibility of AMI.

### 23.1.5 Conclusion

As a type of IBD, AMI is often secondary to patients with atrial fibrillation, and the onset is hidden. It is one of the rarer cases of acute abdomen and is more likely to be missed clinically, so timely diagnosis has a significant impact on the prognosis.

## 23.2 Variceal Upper Gastrointestinal Bleeding in Cirrhotic Portal Hypertension

### 23.2.1 Introduction

Portal hypertension is a group clinical syndromes caused by increased portal vein pressure. The most common disease is liver cirrhosis caused by various reasons. The basic pathophysiological characteristics of portal hypertension are obstruction of the portal vein system and (or) increased blood flow, increased static pressure in the portal vein and its branches, and associated collateral circulation. Clinical manifestations are ascites, esophageal and gastric varices (GOV), esophageal and gastric varices rupture and bleeding (EVB), and hepatic encephalopathy [25–27]. EVB has a high mortality rate and is one of the most common digestive emergencies. This article discusses the mechanism and the diagnosis and treatment of sudden death caused by varicose upper gastrointestinal bleeding in cirrhosis through actual cases.

### 23.2.2 Case and Method

The death occurred in January 2020. We analyzed the death process by reviewing the clinical symptoms, test results, clinical treatment, and medications during the treatment. The sharing of this case has been reviewed by the hospital ethics committee.

Patient Du, male, 49 years old, was admitted to the hospital because of "vomiting blood for 4 h." He reported dizziness, sweating, fatigue, blurred vision, and other symptoms. He had a history of hepatitis B cirrhosis and diabetes for 6 years. Admission examination: T36.4 °C, P129 times/min, R20 times/min, BP75/45 mmHg, $SPO_2$98%. Consciousness, pale skin and mucous membranes, normal soft abdomen, tenderness in the upper abdomen, no rebound pain and muscle tension, and no moving dullness. Blood test routine showed Hb 106 g/L, WBC 6.84 × 109 g/L, PLT 60 × 109 g/L. Coagulation function showed APTT 32.5S, PT 18.9S, TT 20.7S, FIB 1.35 g/L, INR 1.74, D-dimer 800 ng/mL. Blood NH3 229.6 umol/L. Biochemical display: ALT 29.4 U/L, AST38.0 U/L, TP 52.8 g/L, ALB 26.9 g/L, GLU13.19 mmol/L, K + 3.35 mmol/L. Abdominal CT showed cirrhosis, splenomegaly, and esophageal and gastric varices. He was observed in the emergency room and immediately given symptomatic treatment such as blood transfusion, fluid replacement, acid production, enzyme inhibition, and so on. He still showed several vomiting symptoms while in hospital, and 7 h later he underwent emergency gastroscopy at the bedside to stop bleeding, but the effect was not good. The patient lost his life after 11 h.

### 23.2.3 Review and Treatment

#### 23.2.3.1 Etiology and Inducement

Cirrhosis is a common late-stage progression of liver disease with various etiologies. The causes of cirrhosis include viral, alcoholic, cholestatic, circulatory disorders, drug or chemical poisons, genetic and metabolic diseases, immune diseases, parasitic infections, and nutritional disorders [25–27]. Cirrhosis due to any reasons may cause portal hypertension and varicose upper gastrointestinal bleeding [28, 29]. The common predisposing factors include improper diet (eating hard, fried foods, and excessive drinking), emotional instability, fatigue, increased abdominal pressure, and inappropriate medication. Changes in weather and temperature may also be contributing factors.

The risk factors for GOV bleeding include GOV level, red sign, and Child-Pugh classification [26]. Patients without varicose veins or small varicose veins develop varicose veins or develop large varicose veins at a rate of 8% per year. The incidence of varicose vein bleeding is 5–15%, and the mortality rate is as high as 20% within 6 weeks [26, 30–33]. Gastric varices are found in 5–33% of patients with portal hypertension. The incidence of gastric varices bleeding is lower than that of esophageal varices, but the amount of bleeding is often large, the condition is more serious, and the mortality rate can be as high as 45% [34, 35]. Although duodenal varices are rare, varices due to cirrhosis can also occur in upper gastrointestinal bleeding.

#### 23.2.3.2 Lethal Mechanism

Sudden death from varicose veins of the upper gastrointestinal tract due to cirrhosis is related to the following factors:

##### Hypovolemic Shock

Hypovolemic shock caused by varices and upper gastrointestinal bleeding in cirrhosis is one of the causes of sudden death. The occurrence of hypovolemic shock is related to the amount and speed of blood or body fluid loss. The blood volume is abruptly lost in a short period of time, resulting in a decrease in the cardiac output, which in turn causes tissue cell ischemia, hypoxia, and metabolic disorders.

##### Septic Shock

Due to the weak intestinal barrier of patients with cirrhosis and portal hypertension, the intestinal flora easily enter the bloodstream and become infected. The peritoneal infection rate in patients with varicose veins and upper gastrointestinal bleeding is 25–65% [36]. Pulmonary infection and abdominal cavity, thoracic cavity, and urinary tract infections can all cause systemic inflammatory response syndrome (SIRS) and severe sepsis and toxic shock from infection.

##### Multiple Organ Failure (MOF)

Patients with decompensated liver cirrhosis are often accompanied by impairment of the liver, kidneys, heart, and lung function. With varicose upper gastrointestinal bleeding, due to insufficient effective circulating blood volume and reduced coagulation factors, patients can have renal failure, liver failure, and electrolyte and acid-base balance disorders in a short period of time, and then induce coagulation system and respiratory system and circulatory system failure. Multiple organ failure is undoubtedly one of the additional or contributing factors to sudden death.

#### Hepatic Encephalopathy

Upper gastrointestinal bleeding is one of the important causes of hepatic encephalopathy. In the case of varicose upper gastrointestinal bleeding, the number of ammonia-producing bacteria in the intestine increases, a large amount of bleeding constricts the renal blood vessels, renal urinary dysfunction occurs, urea diffuses into the intestinal cavity, and ammonia production increases. Major blood loss causes hypotension and shock, leading to ischemia and hypoxia in the brain tissue and increased blood–brain barrier permeability. These factors lead to increased blood ammonia. Infection, electrolyte and acid–base imbalance, and the use of sedative drugs can all induce and exacerbate hepatic encephalopathy.

### 23.2.3.3 Diagnosis

Endoscopy is the gold standard for the diagnosis of varicose veins in cirrhosis and their bleeding. Multiple guidelines recommend gastroduodenoscopy (EGD) examinations within 12–24 h of bleeding [25–27, 37, 38]. The diagnosis of esophageal and gastric varicose vein bleeding can be established when the endoscope shows one of the following conditions, such as active bleeding (bleeding and spurting) of varicose veins and no bleeding lesions but obvious veins in other parts. Based on varicose veins, a thrombus head was found, or the surface of varicose veins was covered with blood clots [26].

Laboratory and imaging studies can to some extent determine the presence and severity of esophageal varices. B-ultrasound, CT, MRI, and liver elasticity tests can be used to assist the diagnosis of clinical portal hypertension. Upper gastrointestinal angiography and enhanced CT can also show the presence of gastroesophageal varices [39, 40]. But none of these methods can replace the upper gastrointestinal endoscopy.

The following manifestations suggest that EVB is not controlled: (1) vomiting fresh blood or nasal gastrointestinal aspiration of more than 100 mL of fresh blood ≥2 h after drug or endoscopic treatment and (2) hemorrhagic shock; in the case of no blood transfusion, hemoglobin decreased by 30 g/L during any 24 h period (hematocrit decreased by about 9%). The recurrent clinically significant active bleeding events after bleeding control include vomiting, melena, or blood in the stool; decreased systolic blood pressure > 20 mmHg or increased heart rate > 20 beats/min; and decreased hemoglobin >30 g/L without blood transfusion [38].

### 23.2.3.4 Treatment

The prevention and treatment of EVB includes: (1) prevention of first EVB (primary prevention), (2) control of acute EVB, (3) prevention of secondary EVB (secondary prevention), and (4) improvement of the liver function reserve [34, 35, 38–41]. Here mainly we introduce the treatment of acute active bleeding.

### Resuscitation and Medication

1. Supplement blood volume: Resuscitation and maintain hemodynamic stability. Excessive blood transfusion and insuffcient blood transfusion can cause damage. Indications for blood volume replenishment: (a) the systolic blood pressure is stable at 90–120 mmHg; (b) pulse <100 beats/min; (c) the urine volume > 40 mL/h and the blood Na+ concentration < 140 mmol/L; and (d) consciousness or improvement, with no obvious signs of dehydration.
2. Use of drugs that reduce the portal pressure: Drug therapy is the preferred treatment. Use vasoconstrictor as early as possible, such as vasopressin or somatostatin, until bleeding is controlled, or continuously use for 5 days. Beta-blockers are contraindicated during acute bleeding. (a) Somatostatin and its analogs including tetradecapeptide (cyclic 14 amino acid peptide, Stannin) and octapeptide (octreotide, Shanning). (b) Vasopressin: it is the strongest visceral vasoconstrictor, which can reduce the blood flow of all internal organs, leading to a decrease in the portal venous blood and a reduction in the portal pressure, but due to higher cardiac and cerebrovascular complications, it is less commonly used. Terlipressin is a synthetic vasopressin analog, which can effectively reduce hepatic venous pressure gradient (HVPG), reduce the portal vein blood flow, and has little effect on systemic hemodynamics.
3. Application of antibiotics: Studies have shown that early re-bleeding and mortality are related to uncontrolled bacterial infections. Antibiotics are recommended to prevent infection.
4. The role of proton pump inhibitors in the treatment of acute varices bleeding is controversial. They are recommended for use with peptic ulcers and can be used as adjuvant treatment after gastric mucosal lesions or endoscopic treatment.

### Endoscopic Treatment

Endoscopy is recommended within 12–24 h of bleeding. Patients with severe acute upper gastrointestinal bleeding and unstable disease are advised to undergo endoscopy immediately after resuscitation. Endoscopic treatment is designed to effectively control varicose vein rupture and bleeding, and to minimize or reduce varicose veins to prevent re-bleeding. Preoperative emergency endoscopy preparation for bleeding patients includes routine blood preparation, usually performed in the awake state; patients can be performed on with airway protection (tracheal intubation). Other conditions are similar to those of patients without bleeding. The contraindications of endoscopic treatment: with any contraindication of routine upper gastrointestinal endoscopy.

Endoscopic treatment includes endoscopic variceal ligation (EVL), endoscopic injection sclerostherapy (EIS), and tissue adhesive embolization, with reliable results [38, 42]. Therefore, esophageal and gastric fundus variceal ruptures should be treated with drugs and endoscopic ligation for acute bleeding. The combination of the two is more effective and has fewer complications. (1) EVL and EIS. (a) Indications: acute esophageal varices bleeding, recurrence of esophageal varices after surgery, moderate and severe esophageal varices without bleeding but with a significant risk of bleeding, and a past history of esophageal varices rupture and bleeding. (b) Contraindications: those who have contraindications for upper gastrointestinal endoscopy, hemorrhagic shock is not corrected, hepatic encephalopathy ≥ stage II, and excessively large or small varicose veins. (c) Course of treatment: the second ligation treatment is feasible for 10–14 days after the first EVL; the interval between each EIS is 1 week, and it usually takes 3–5 times. The best goal for both treatments is until the varicose veins disappear or almost disappear. (d) Follow-up: it is recommended to review the gastroscopy 1 month after the end of the course of treatment, and then to review the gastroscopy every 6–12 months thereafter. (2) Tissue adhesive treatment. (a) Indications: acute gastric varices bleeding and gastric varices with red signs or surface erosion and a history of bleeding. (b) Method: "Sandwich" method. The total amount is estimated based on the size of the gastric varicose veins, and it is best to occlude the varicose veins once.

After the treatment with drugs or conventional endoscopic ligation or sclerosis, 15–20% of patients still have repeated bleeding or active bleeding that cannot be effectively controlled, and other rescue treatments (such as TIPSS, Surgery) are unable performed, when the patient's life is seriously threatened, endoscopic esophageal metal stent rescue treatment shows a certain effect.

### Sengstaken-Blakemore Tube

If bleeding is difficult to control, a Sengstaken-Blakemore tube could be used to stop bleeding until endoscopic treatment, TIPSS, or surgery. It is an important treatment for severe bleeding. Balloon compression can effectively control bleeding, but the re-bleeding rate is high, and it needs to be used in combination with drugs and endoscopic treatment. The complications must be taken seriously, such as aspiration pneumonia, tracheal and esophagus obstruction, gastric mucosa compression, necrosis, and bleeding. The balloon should be deflated once every 8–12 h according to the condition. The extubation timing should follow the principle of the first deflation and then extubation. After the balloon is deflated and left unobserved for 24 h, extubation can be performed.

#### Interventional Therapy

Transjugular intrahepatic portosystem stent shunt (TIPSS) can quickly reduce the portal vein pressure, with an effective hemostatic rate of more than 90%. It has the characteristics of small trauma and low incidence of complications. It is recommended for the "final" treatment of esophageal and gastric fundus varices bleeding, HVPG >20 mmHg and liver function Child-Pugh grade B and C patients with high-risk re-bleeding, and can significantly improve survival [38, 43, 44]. (1) Indications: patients with esophageal and gastric varices rupture and bleeding who were not treated well with drugs and endoscopy, those with varicose veins rupturing and bleeding after surgery, and those with varicose veins rupturing and bleeding while waiting for liver transplantation. (2) Contraindications: Child-Pugh score of liver function >12 points, MELD score > 18 points, PACHE II >20 points, and irreversible shock status; right heart failure, central venous pressure > 15 mmHg; uncontrollable hepatic encephalopathy; carcinoma located in the first and second hepatic hilum; and intrahepatic and systemic infectious diseases. (3) Others: retrograde varicose vein occlusion under balloon obstruction, splenic artery embolization, percutaneous transhepatic varicose vein embolization, etc.

Surgical Treatment

In about 20% patients, re-bleeding within 24 h after the successfully stopping bleeding. Those who have failed standard medical treatment should be treated with surgery, and portal vein shunt surgery or shunt surgery can be considered [45].

In summary, it is recommended that patients with varicose veins of upper gastrointestinal bleeding in cirrhosis should immediately perform the following treatments: (1) fluid replacement and blood transfusion to correct patients' hypovolemic shock and stabilize the vital signs; (2) prevent bacterial infection, liver failure, and complications such as renal failure; prevention and treatment of hepatic encephalopathy; (3) pay attention to maintaining airway patency and tracheal intubation if necessary; (4) vasoactive drugs such as somatostatin that reduce varicose vein pressure should be applied immediately, and its analogues like vasopressin; (5) emergency upper gastrointestinal endoscopy and treatment should be performed as soon as possible under the condition of stable vital signs; (6) the treatment method for esophageal varices bleeding is EIS or EVL; EVL For the preferred option; patients with bleeding from varicose veins are preferred to endoscopic tissue adhesive injections. After failure of endoscopic hemostasis treatment, it is recommended to choose: (1) Sengstaken-Blakemore tube; (2) re-endoscopic treatment; (3) transjugular intrahepatic portosystemic stent shunt; and (4) surgery.

### 23.2.4 Discussion

An important cause of sudden death from upper gastrointestinal bleeding is hemorrhagic shock. In the above case, the patient's hospital was a teaching hospital and had a complete treatment for upper gastrointestinal bleeding. Patients have typical symptoms of acute blood loss, only 15 h from the onset to death. Except for interventional treatment and surgical treatment, the current treatment schemes for the treatment of upper gastrointestinal bleeding have been implemented, but they have not saved the lives of patients. The main reason for failing to perform interventional treatment is that the patient's condition has progressed rapidly, and abdominal enhanced CT cannot be performed for preoperative evaluation. Rapid blood loss makes conventional drug hemostasis ineffective, and a large amount of blood entering the intestine breakdown often leading to increased blood ammonia and hepatic encephalopathy. The inability to perform adequate preoperative evaluation is also an important cause of patients' death. Insufficient blood products and inadequate protection are also one of the reasons.

### 23.2.5 Conclusion

Sudden death due to upper gastrointestinal bleeding often occurs due to heavy bleeding and delayed treatment. Targeted treatment on the basis of understanding the pathogenesis principle will often achieve more results with less effort. Clinically, cases of upper gastrointestinal bleeding are very common, but cases of sudden death caused by major bleeding are not uncommon and often occur in the emergency room. By understanding the relevant knowledge and principles of upper gastrointestinal bleeding, and choosing a treatment method, we believe that better treatment results will be achieved.

## 23.3 Hepatic Encephalopathy

### 23.3.1 Introduction

Hepatic encephalopathy (HE) is a kind of central nervous system dysfunction caused by liver dysfunction and (or) portosystemic stent shunt (PSS), which is based on metabolic disorder. It is manifested as a broad-spectrum neurological or psychological abnormality from reversible subclinical changes to irreversible coma and even death, and other known encephalopathy are excluded. Hepatic encephalopathy is one of the main causes of death in patients with end-stage liver disease, with a mortality rate of more than 50% and poor prognosis. The North American Association for End-Stage Liver Disease Research (NACSELD) has confirmed that HE has an independent correlation with the death of patients with liver cirrhosis. The incidence rate of liver cirrhosis patients complicated with HE is 30–45%, and 40% have mild hepatic encephalopathy (MHE); 30–45% liver cirrhosis patients and 10–50% patients have dominant hepatic encephalopathy (OHE) after transjugular intrahepatic portosystemic shunt (TIPS). In the advanced stage of the disease (liver failure), the incidence and mortality rate of HE gradually increase with the increase of the child Pugh level [46]. This article discusses the mechanism of sudden death caused due to hepatic encephalopathy and its diagnosis and treatment through practical cases.

### 23.3.2 Case and Method

The death occurred in August 2019. We analyzed the death process by reviewing the clinical symptoms, examination results, test results, and clinical treatment of the death case. The case sharing has been reviewed by the Hospital Ethics Committee.

Patient Deng, a 50-year-old male patient, was hospitalized from 120 because of "defecation of black stool for 8 h and 6 h of sudden disturbance of consciousness." There was no previous physical examination history, with more than 20 years of drinking history, 250 mL/day. Admission examination: T 36.8 °C, P 170 times/min, R 33 times/min, BP 66/59 mmHg, $SPO_2$ 92%. Light coma, unable to cooperate with physical examination, pale skin and mucosa. Blood routine test showed HB 109 g/L, HCT 0.328 L/L, WBC 5.35 × 109 g/L, PLT 73 × 109 g/L. Coagulation function: APTT 36.7 s, PT 21.3 s, TT 20.9 s, FIB 1.61 g/L, INR 1.93, D-Dimer 1210 ng/mL. Blood ammonia 536.4 umol/L. Biochemical indicators: ALT 63.8 U/L, AST 82.0 U/L, TP 61.8 g/L, ALB 25.2 g/L, GLU 9.51 mmol/L, TBIL 59.4 umol/L, DBIL 34.4 umol/L, GGT 108 U/L, UREA 13.0 umol/L, CRE 97 umol/L. Abdominal ultrasound showed cirrhosis, splenomegaly and thickening of the gall bladder wall. The patients were intubated immediately after admission. Immediately endotracheal intubation, ventilator-assisted respiration, and symptomatic treatment such as reducing blood ammonia, boosting blood pressure, stopping bleeding, inhibiting acid, inhibiting enzyme, anti-infection, fluid replacement, etc., were given. After 10 h, the patient's heart rate and blood pressure could not be maintained and he lost his life.

### 23.3.3 Review and Treatment

#### 23.3.3.1 Etiology and Inducement

The main causes of hepatic encephalopathy are liver cirrhosis, abnormal portosystemic shunt, and other metabolic abnormalities caused by chronic liver disease. The causes of cirrhosis include chronic hepatitis B and C, alcoholic liver disease, drug-induced liver disease, autoimmune liver disease, and schistosomiasis; portosystemic shunt mainly includes hepatic vascular lesions such as Budd–Chiari syndrome, idiopathic portal hypertension, and portal hypertension after TIPS; metabolic abnormalities often include chronic liver damage caused by copper metabolism, iron metabolism, porphyrin metabolism disorders, and congenital urea circulation disorders. Other causes include severe hepatitis, fulminant liver failure, primary liver cancer, biliary tract diseases, acute fatty liver in pregnancy, etc. Common inducing factors include application of infection, gastrointestinal hemorrhage, ascite discharge, electrolyte disturbance, massive potassium drainage diuresis, high protein diet, constipation, hypnosis and sedation, anesthetics, uremia, surgery, proton pump inhibitors, etc. Among them, infection is the most common inducing factor, including abdominal cavity, intestinal tract, respiratory tract, and urinary tract infection, and abdominal infection is the most important. The occurrence of MHE has no obvious correlation with the etiology, but its incidence and mortality increase with the aggravation of the decompensation degree of liver cirrhosis.

#### 23.3.3.2 Pathogenesis and Lethal Mechanism

The pathogenesis and death mechanism of hepatic encephalopathy are not completely defined. Brain edema and astrocyte changes are the main pathological features. At present, there is no single theory that can explain the occurrence and death of HE, which may be related to the following theories and mechanisms [47–49]:

Ammonia intoxication hypothesis is the main pathogenesis of hepatic encephalopathy. The basis of the ammonia intoxication theory is that impaired astrocyte participates in the occurrence and development of hepatic encephalopathy. (1)

Inadequate ammonia clearance: in cirrhosis with portal hypertension, the detoxification function of liver cell dysfunction to ammonia and other toxic substances is reduced, the circulation of ornithine is blocked, and the process of ammonia to urea is disturbed. (2) Increased ammonia production: portal-integrated circulation shunting enables a large amount of toxic substances such as ammonia being absorbed into the blood by the intestinal tract to directly flow into human circulation through portal vein. Intestinal dysfunction increases the retention of nonabsorbed protein components in the intestinal tract. Active intestinal bacteria can release amino acid oxidase and urease, increasing ammonia production, especially during gastrointestinal hemorrhage and intestinal infection. Increased intestinal permeability can lead to the increase of ammonia in the portal vein. When kidney involvement alkalosis occurs, the hydrogen ion excretion in the renal tubules is reduced, the generation of ammonia ions decreases, and ammonia increases. In patients with hepatic encephalopathy, restlessness and muscle tremor increase adenylate decomposition, and cause an increase in ammonia production. (3) Toxic effects of ammonia on the brain: increased permeability of the blood–brain barrier; blood ammonia entering the brain tissue increases glutamine synthesis by astrocytes, leading to degeneration, swelling, and degeneration of astrocytes and neuron cells. As a result, brain edema and acute neurocognitive dysfunction are formed. Ammonia directly leads to imbalance of excitatory and inhibitory neurotransmitters, reduction of excitatory neurotransmitters such as acetylcholine, and enhancement of inhibitory neuron activity. The enhancement of inhibitory neuron activity increases inhibitory neurotransmitters such as glutamine and GABA, which impair the automatic regulation of intracranial blood flow. The increased ammonia interferes with the tricarboxylic acid cycle of the brain cell energy metabolism and affect the function of the nerve cell membranes, thus causing disorder in the excitatory activity of the central nervous system. In addition, ammonia can directly damage the electrical activity of nerves. In summary, the damage to the central nervous system caused by the increase of ammonia can cause the disease to rapidly progress into irreversible coma and death [50–52].

#### Damage of Inflammatory Mediators

The interaction between hyperammonemia and inflammatory mediators promotes the occurrence and development of HE. Inflammatory mediators can lead to the destruction of the blood–brain barrier, thus allowing toxic substances such as ammonia and inflammatory cytokines to enter the brain tissue, causing changes in brain parenchyma and brain dysfunction. Hyperammonemia can induce neutrophil dysfunction to release reactive oxygen species, which promote the body to produce oxidative stress and inflammatory response. Cytokines produced in the process of the inflammatory reaction in turn aggravate liver injury and increase HE. This forms a vicious circle.

#### Enterogenous Endotoxemia and Flora Disorder

Endotoxin level in patients with severe liver diseases are significantly increased, which is parallel to the degree of liver damage and reciprocal cause and effect each other with liver damage. Clinical observation shows that endotoxin in liver disease patients is correlated with the occurrence of hepatic encephalopathy, renal failure, hemorrhagic nephritis, and DIC. The mechanism of enterogenous endotoxemia [53]: (1) increased absorption of endotoxin—disturbance of intestinal flora, abnormal increase of bacteria, destruction or increase of the permeability of intestinal mucosa and vascular integrity, weakening of the intestinal mucosal barrier function, bilirubin and bile acid inhibiting phagocytosis of Kupffer cells caused by intrahepatic cholestasis, decrease of intestinal liner salt when bile excretion is blocked, etc. can lead to increase in the absorption of intestinal endotoxins; (2) dysfunction of endotoxin clearance: intestinal endotoxemia caused by dysfunction of Kupffer cells plays a decisive role in the induction of severe liver disease. When the liver function is incomplete, with the damage of hepatocytes, Kupffer cells and their peripheral cells change from the activated state to failure and their function is seriously damaged, and the scavenging effect of endotoxin is obviously weakened. Some studies have shown that the endotoxin level in patients with hepatic encephalopathy is significantly increased, and is positively correlated with the severity of hepatic encephalopathy, but the specific pathological mechanism has not been clearly explained.

#### Dysfunction of the Brainstem Reticular System

Neuronal activity of the brainstem reticular system and the nigrostriatal system in patients with severe cirrhosis is damaged to varying degrees, leading to the occurrence of HE, flapping wing-like tremor, and changes in muscle tone. In addition, the increase of pseudoneurotransmitters makes the wake-up function of the ascending activation system of the brainstem reticular structure unable to be maintained, resulting in coma. The damage degree of the brainstem reticular system is consistent with the severity of HE [54].

#### Manganese Poisoning Theory

In liver diseases, the manganese that is out of control enters the nerve cell, and generates low-valence manganese ions to be oxidized into high-valence manganese ions, which accumulate in the mitochondria through the specific affinity of manganese to the mitochondria and directly damage the brain tissue. At the same time, manganese ions generate a large number of free radicals during the valence state transition process, which leads to decreased activity of key enzymes in the respiratory chain of the mitochondria in the brain substantia nigra and striatum. Manganese can also affect the functions of 5-HT, norepinephrine, GABA, and other neurotransmitters, causing astrocyte dysfunction [55].

#### Amino Acid Imbalance, Inhibitory Neurotransmitter, and Pseudoneurotransmitter Theory

When liver function is damaged, the ability to degrade aromatic amino acids is reduced, and phenylalanine and tyrosine in the blood are increased, thus inhibiting the production of normal neurotransmitters. Increased levels of phenylalanine and tyrosine produce phenylethanolamine and hydroxyphenylethanolamine, known as pseudoneurotransmitters, which replace the normal neurotransmitter and lead to HE.

#### GABA (Gamma-Aminobutyric Acid)

It is a unique and main inhibitory neurotransmitter in the central nervous system. It exists in the form of compound receptors with benzodiazepine receptors in the brain. The content of GABA in the blood increases in HE, and the amount of GABA passing through the blood–brain barrier is increased, so that the level of endogenous benzodiazepine in the brain is increased.

#### Cerebral Edema and Stroke

All of the above mechanisms can lead to cerebral edema and neuroastrocytic lesions, which can cause irreversible damage to the nervous system, and even lead to sudden death due to cerebral hemorrhage, cerebral infarction, brain hernia, and other stroke [54].

*Other lethal mechanisms*: Infection and septic shock, respiratory failure, malignant arrhythmia, and hepatic encephalopathy are the leading causes of death in severe liver disease. Infection can induce hepatic encephalopathy, which aggravates primary liver disease. In addition, patients with hepatic encephalopathy are bedridden for a long time and have low immunity, which is extremely easy to promote exacerbation of infection and even septic shock. End-stage liver disease itself can cause hepatopulmonary syndrome and respiratory system damage; when complicated with hepatic encephalopathy, central nervous system involvement also affects the respiratory function, both of which aggravate respiratory system damage and eventually lead to respiratory failure. Various electrolyte disorders (hyponatremia) and acid–base imbalance complicated with hepatic encephalopathy can lead to malignant arrhythmia and even sudden cardiac death.

### 23.3.3.3 Diagnosis

Compared with other metabolic encephalopathy, the clinical manifestations of hepatic encephalopathy are not specific. It emphasizes clinical diagnosis based on severe liver disease or (and) portosystemic shunt and underlying diseases with related inducements, combined with clinical and related auxiliary examinations.

Clinical manifestations of HE are mainly the dysfunction of the higher nerve center (personality change, mental decline, abnormal behavior, and disturbance of consciousness) and abnormal movement and reflex (such as flapping-wing tremor, myoclonus, hyperreflexia and pathological reflex). At present, the West-Haven classification standard is mostly adopted to divide hepatic encephalopathy into five stages [56]:

- Stage 0(incubation period): That is, minimal hepatic encephalopathy, no abnormal behavior and personality, no neurological and pathological signs, and normal electroencephalogram, but only the psychological test or intelligence test shows a slight abnormality.
- Stage 1 (prodromal period): Mild personality changes and mental abnormalities, such as anxiety, euphoric excitement, apathy, sleep inversion, amnesia, etc., may have flapping-wing tremor; EEG is mostly normal. The clinical manifestations at this stage are not obvious and are easy to be ignored.
- Stage 2 (pre coma period): Sleepiness, abnormal behavior, slurred speech, dysgraphia, and disorientation. Neurological signs such as hypertonia, hyperreflexia,

ankle clonus, and Babinski sign are positive; flapping-wing tremor is positive, and electroencephalogram shows characteristic abnormalities.

- Stage 3 (lethargy period): Sleepiness but wakefulness, response when awake, unconsciousness or hallucination, continuous or aggravating of various neurological signs, positive flapping-wing tremor, increased muscular tension, and hyperreflexia of tendon reflex. Pyramidal sign often is positive, and electroencephalogram has abnormal waveform.
- Stage 4 (coma period): Coma and unable to wake up. Cannot cooperate with physical examination, and cannot lead to flapping wing tremor. In shallow coma, tendon reflex and muscle tension are still hypertonic. In deep coma, all kinds of reflexes disappear and muscle tension decreases. The electroencephalogram is obviously abnormal.

**Auxiliary Examination**

*Laboratory examination*: Elevated blood ammonia is of high value in the diagnosis of HE, especially in patients of HE with portal-systemic shunting, most of whose blood ammonia is increased. The elevated level of blood ammonia is not completely consistent with the severity of the disease, and sometimes patients with normal blood ammonia cannot be excluded from HE. Biochemical indexes such as bilirubin, alanine aminotransferase (ALT), aspartate aminotransferase (AST), albumin, prothrombin activity, renal function, and blood routine test were all used as routine laboratory indicators when HE was suspected. Other laboratory indicators: serum chitinase-3 like protein l (CHI3L1), a member of the glycosylase hydrolase family, is a protein secreted in the extracellular matrix by the liver. Its expression is significantly increased during cirrhosis and liver fibrosis, and the expression level of CHI3Ll reflects the degree of cirrhosis and liver fibrosis. Golgi protein 73 (GP73) is a transmembrane glycoprotein located in the Golgi body. In advanced liver disease caused by various causes, the expression level of GP73 in liver cells is increased.

*Neuropsychological test*: (1) Traditional paper–pen neuropsychological test includes the digital connection test (NCTA and B), the digit-symbol test (DST), the line-tracing test (LTT), and the serial dotting test (SDT); five subtests of the series dotting test. NCT and DST are simple and easy to operate, with strong operability, and are suitable for epidemiological investigation of MHE. MHE can be diagnosed if both NCT-A and DST are positive, or if any two of the five subtests are abnormal. (2) Critical flicker frequency (CFF): CFF is the minimum stimulus frequency that can cause flash fusion sensation, and it reflects brain nerve conduction dysfunction. It has moderate sensitivity and high specificity. CFF is an auxiliary inspection means, which is easy to interpret when used for diagnosing MHE. (3) New neuropsychological testing methods: animal naming test (ANT), gesture control and stability test, multi-sensory integration test, etc. (4) Others: repeatable battery for the assessment of neuropsychologic status (RBANS): it is one of the two neuropsychological examination tools recommended by ISHEN's guidelines, including Stroop and Encephal APP test, inhibitory control test (ICT), SCAN test, etc.

*Neurophysiological test*: The abnormality of electroencephalogram is mainly manifested by slow rhythm, which is not a specific change of HE, and typical electroencephalogram changes can only be detected in patients with severe HE, so it is only clinically used for auxiliary diagnosis of HE in children. Evoked potential detection, includes visual evoked potential, auditory evoked potential, and somatic evoked potential, among which endogenous time-related evoked potential P300 has the best sensitivity. And the MHE patients can show prolonged latency and reduced amplitude. The advantage of neurophysiological examination is that the result is relatively specific and there is no learning effect. Its shortcomings are poor sensitivity, the need for professional equipment and personnel, and poor consistency with neuropsychological test results.

*Imaging examination*: CT scan of the liver and brain can determine whether there is obvious portosystemic shunt, find brain edema, and exclude cerebrovascular accidents and intracranial tumors. MRI showed normal white matter area in patients with liver cirrhosis complicated with HE, but the mean diffusivity degree (MD) could still be significantly increased, which was related to HE staging, blood ammonia, neurophysiology, and neuropsychological changes. Functional magnetic resonance imaging (fMRI): resting fMRI analyzed by ReHo analysis can be used as a noninvasive examination method, which has an important value in revealing the cognitive changes of patients with cirrhosis [52].

#### 23.3.3.4 Classification of Hepatic Encephalopathy

*Classification according to the basic liver disease*: Hepatic encephalopathy was classified as type A, type B, and type C at the 11th Vienna WCOG in 1998 (Table 23.1). Type A develops rapidly on the basis of acute liver failure, and its pathophysiological characteristics are cerebral edema and intracranial hypertension. Type B is caused by portosystemic shunt without obvious liver dysfunction, and liver histopathological examination (liver biopsy) indicates a normal liver histologic structure. Type C is hepatic encephalopathy associated with liver cirrhosis, accompanied by portosystemic venous shunting, with manifestations of chronic liver injury, liver cirrhosis, and other liver-based diseases. Clinically, HE caused by liver cirrhosis is the most common type, that is, type C. At the same time, hepatic

**Table 23.1** Classification of hepatic encephalopathy recommended by the 11th World Congress of Gastroenterology (Vienna, 1998)

| Type of hepatic encephalopathy | Definition | Subclass | Subtype |
|---|---|---|---|
| Type A | Associated with acute liver failure | No | No |
| Type B | Portal-systemic shunt related | No | No |
| Type C | Associated with liver cirrhosis complicated with portal hypertension or portal-systemic shunt | Episodic | Precipitated |
| | | | Spontaneous |
| | | | Recurrent |
| | | Persistent | Mild |
| | | | Severe |
| | | | Treatment dependent |
| | | Minimal | No |

encephalopathy of type C can be further divided into paroxysmal type, persistent type, and mild type [57, 58].

*Classification by severity*: ISHEN established a grading standard called SONIC according to the severity of hepatic encephalopathy. Hepatic encephalopathy of grade 1 in MHE and West-Haven grades is classified as Covert HE (CHE), in which minimal hepatic encephalopathy (MHE) refers to hepatic encephalopathy that is usually found only through neuropsychological tests without obvious clinical symptoms. Overt hepatic encephalopathy(OHE) is a type of hepatic encephalopathy diagnosed by clinical standards, including hepatic encephalopathy of grade 2 and above [59].

#### 23.3.3.5 Diagnostic Criteria

*OHE*: According to clinical manifestations and signs and West—Haven grading standards, OHE diagnosis is not difficult, and neuropsychological, neurophysiological, and imaging examinations are generally not required. Key points of diagnosis: (1) there are basic diseases that cause HE, such as severe liver diseases and/or extensive portosystemic collateral circulation shunts; (2) clinically identifiable neuropsychiatric symptoms and signs; (3) excluding other diseases causing neuropsychiatric abnormalities, such as metabolic encephalopathy, toxic encephalopathy, neurological diseases (such as intracranial hemorrhage, intracranial infection, and intracranial space occupying), psychiatric diseases, etc.; (4) paying special attention to find out the inducement of HE (type C and type B), such as infection, upper gastrointestinal hemorrhage, massive ascites, etc.; and (5) blood ammonia increase.

*MHE*: Because patients have no obvious abnormal cognitive function, special examination is often needed to make a definite diagnosis, which is the focus of clinical attention. MHE can be diagnosed if it meets any one or more of the following main diagnosis points (1), (2), and (3–6). Main diagnostic points: (1) there are basic diseases causing HE, that is severe liver disease and/or extensive portosystemic collateral circulation shunt. (2) At least two abnormalities in traditional neuropsychological test indicators. (3) In the new neuropsychological test method (ANT, posture control and stability test, and multi-sensory integration test), there should be at least one abnormality; (4) abnormal CFF detection; (5) abnormal EEG, visual evoked potential (VEP), and brainstem auditory evoked potential (BAEP); and (6) fMRI abnormality.

#### 23.3.3.6 Differential Diagnosis

HE should be distinguished from the following diseases: (1) mental disorders; (2) intracranial lesions; (3) other metabolic encephalopathy, including ketoacidosis, hypoglycemia, hyponatremia, renal encephalopathy, pulmonary encephalopathy, etc.; (4) Wernicke encephalopathy; (5) toxic encephalopathy, including alcoholic encephalopathy, acute poisoning, withdrawal syndrome, heavy metal (mercury, manganese, etc.) encephalopathy, and toxic reactions of psychotropic drugs or salicylate drugs, etc.; (6) Parkinson's disease related to cirrhosis; (7) hepatic myelopathy; and (8) acquired liver and brain degeneration, etc.

#### 23.3.3.7 Treatment

*Treatment principles*: Clearing the inducement in time, treating the primary liver disease actively, maintaining the balance of liver function, promoting the clearance of ammonia metabolism, regulating neurotransmitters, restoring the acute neuropsychiatric disorder to the baseline state as soon as possible, and primary prevention and secondary prevention.

##### Remove the Inducement of MHE/HE

(1) Preventing and controlling infection: Since infection is the most common inducing factor, we should actively search for the source of infection and start using empirical antibacterial drugs as early as possible: even if there is no clear infection site, there is also a potential inflammatory state due to intestinal bacterial translocation and increased endotoxin level, and antibacterial treatment can reduce this inflammatory state. (2) Hemostasis and removal of intestinal hematocele: gastrointestinal bleeding is also a common inducing factor of HE, so bleeding should be stopped as soon as possible, and hematocele in the gastrointestinal tract should be removed. Meanwhile, intestinal tract should be acidified and stool should be kept normally. (3) Correcting electrolyte disorders (hypokalemia or hyperkalemia, hyponatremia or hypernatremia): alkalosis and electrolyte disorders related to insufficient effective circulation volume caused by excessive diuresis can induce HE, and in this case, it is necessary to suspend diuretics and supplement liquid and albumin. Hypovolemic hyponatremia (especially sodium lower than 110 mmol/L) should be supplemented with normal saline intravenously, while selective vasopressin type 2 receptor (V2) antagonist can be used for hyponatremia patients with high or equal volume. For patients with HE in grade 3–4, cerebral edema should be actively controlled and 20% mannitol or furosemide should be given. (4) Use sedative drugs and liver injury drugs with caution: sedative, hypnotic, analgesic drugs, and anesthetics can induce hepatic encephalopathy and should be avoided as much as possible. Some studies have shown that propofol can control the manic symptoms of HE more safely and effectively.

##### Treatment of Primary Liver Disease

(1) Improving liver function: Strengthening liver protection, promoting liver metabolism, reducing liver inflammatory response, etc. (2) Interrupting portosystemic shunting. (3) Artificial liver: it can remove some inflammatory factors, endotoxin, blood ammonia, bilirubin, etc., to a certain extent. The artificial liver modes commonly used to improve hepatic encephalopathy include hemoperfusion, hemofiltration, plasma filtration dialysis, molecular adsorption recirculation system (MARS), dual plasma molecular adsorption system (DPMAS) or plasma exchange combined hemoperfusion, etc., especially to relieve liver failure and preparation for liver transplantation. (4) Liver transplantation.

Promote ammonia metabolism and reduce the generation and absorption of enterogenous toxins. Hyperammonemia is one of the important factors in the occurrence of hepatic encephalopathy, so it is very important to reduce the generation and absorption of ammonia [60]. The main drugs for reducing blood ammonia are: (1) Lactulose: mainly reduce ammonia absorption and promote ammonia excretion by reducing pH value in intestinal tract, retaining water in intestinal tract and increasing stool volume, stimulating colon peristalsis, defecating smoothly, catharsis, restoring physiological rhythm of colon, promoting growth of intestinal acidophilic bacteria (such as lactobacillus), inhibiting proteolytic bacteria, reducing translocation of intestinal bacteria, transforming ammonia into the ionic state, etc., to improve hepatic encephalopathy. Take 15–30 mL orally each time, 2–3 times/day (adjust the dose according to the patient's reaction), with soft stool 2–3 times a day is appropriate. If necessary, it can be combined with retention enema. (2) Lactitol: the recommended initial dose of lactitol is 0.6 g/kg, which is taken three meal times, and the dosage is increased or decreased according to the standard of defecation twice a day. The principles of action and effect are the same as lactulose, which has the advantages of a fast onset of action, low incidence of abdominal distension, and low sweetness, and can be applied to diabetic patients. (3) LOLA: the dosage is 10–40 g/d, intravenous drip. LOLA promotes the utilization of ammonia in the brain and kidneys by promoting the circulation of ornithine in the liver and the synthesis of glutamine, thus consuming ammonia to synthesize glutamic acid and glutamine. LOLA can also reduce fasting blood ammonia and postprandial blood ammonia and reduce cerebral edema. (4) Rifaximin [61]: the dosage is 800–1200 mg/day, and is taken orally for 3–4 times. Theoretically, rifaximin can reduce the absorption of ammonia in intestinal tract, but its clinical effect is not good, especially for type B hepatic encephalopathy. (5) Microecological preparations [62, 63]: including probiotics, prebiotics, synbiotics, etc. It alleviates intestinal endotoxemia by promoting the growth of intestinal probiotic strains, inhibiting the growth of harmful flora, improving the nutritional status of intestinal epithelial cells, reducing the permeability of intestinal mucosa, and reducing bacterial translocation. It can also reduce inflammation and oxidative stress of liver cells, thereby increasing ammonia clearance of the liver.

Regulating neurotransmitters like arginine, glutamine, and branched chain amino acids is used clinically to competitively inhibit aromatic amino acids from entering the brain and reduce the formation of pseudoneurotransmitters [64].

*Nutritional support therapy*: The recommended daily ideal energy intake is 35–40 kcal/kg (1 kcal = 4.184 kJ), less food and more meals, add meals before bed (including at least 50 g of compound carbohydrates), and the fasting time in day time should not exceed 3–6 h. (1) Protein: the European society for parenteral nutrition guidelines recommended that the daily protein intake is 1.2–1.5 g/kg to maintain nitrogen balance. Daily dietary protein intake of obese or overweight liver cirrhosis patients is maintained at 2 g/kg. Patients with recurrent/persistent HE should take 30–40 g vegetable protein daily. Protein supplementation for HE patients should follow the following principles: it is forbidden to supplement protein from intestinal tract for patients with HE grade 3–4. Patients with MHE and L to 2 grade HE should limit the amount of protein to 20 g/day in the first few days. With the improvement of symptoms, 10–20 g protein can be added every 2–3 days. Plant protein is superior to animal protein. It is safe to supplement albumin intravenously. For patients with chronic HE, it is encouraged to have more meals a day but less food at each, and gradually increase the total amount of protein. The protein intake should be individualized. (2) Branched chain amino acid (BCAA): patients with grade 3–4 HE should be supplemented with parenteral nutrition preparations rich in BCAA (valine, leucine, and isoleucine). (3) Other micronutrients: trace elements and water-soluble vitamins, especially thiamine and zinc element. A multivitamin or zinc supplement may be replenished.

#### 23.3.3.8 Prevention

*Primary prevention*: Treatment of primary liver diseases and nutritional intervention. Etiological treatment can reduce injury and liver fibrosis from liver inflammatory, reduce pressure of portal vein, and prevent liver cirrhosis from progressing or reversing liver cirrhosis, which is of great significance in preventing and controlling the occurrence of HE and other complications. The main treatment measures include active prevention and treatment of infection, gastrointestinal hemorrhage, electrolyte disturbance, acid-base imbalance, constipation, and other inducing factors of HE; avoiding excessive diuresis and releasing a large amount of ascites; having more meals a day but less food at each; and avoiding excessive high protein diet.

*Secondary prevention*: The emphasis is on health education for patients and their families, control of elevated blood ammonia, and regulation of intestinal microecology. The patient should adjust the diet structure reasonably according to the liver function injury under the guidance of the doctor, and avoid taking a large amount of high protein diet at one time during the attack of hepatic encephalopathy. Lactulose and lactitol can be used as preventive drugs. Gradually guide the patient's self-health management, and guide the patient's family members to pay attention to the patient's behavior and personality changes, and at the same time, closely inspect whether the patient has loss of attention, memory, and orientation so as to achieve early detection, early diagnosis, and early treatment of HE as much as possible.

#### 23.3.3.9 Prognosis

Patients with mild hepatic encephalopathy can be relieved after active treatment. It will quickly progress to coma or even death in hepatic encephalopathy with no obvious inducement caused by acute liver failure. The inducement of hepatic encephalopathy on the basis of decompensated cirrhosis is clear, and the disease can be recovered and improved by actively removing the inducement and treating the primary disease. Patients with better liver function, after shunt operation and definite inducement, usually have better prognosis. Patients with hepatic encephalopathy on the basis of the end stage of liver cirrhosis suffer from slow progress, repeated attacks, gradual progress, poor prognosis, and rapid death without liver transplantation. Hepatic encephalopathy caused by fulminant liver failure has the worst prognosis.

### 23.3.4 Discussion

In the above cases, the patient is a middle-aged male, has a long history of drinking alcohol, lacks health awareness, and is unaware of the progression of his disease to liver cirrhosis. The lethal mechanism of hepatic encephalopathy has not yet been determined by the medical community, and the classification of hepatic encephalopathy has also produced a variety of standards due to different diagnostic methods. In this case, hepatic encephalopathy is a secondary change of varicose upper gastrointestinal hemorrhage in liver cirrhosis, and the very high blood ammonia concentration of the patient is extremely significant for brain damage. Usually, during gastrointestinal hemorrhage, ammonia is usually separated from the blood in the digestive tract and absorbed into the blood through the intestinal tract, resulting in high blood ammonia.

Although modern medicine has studied many methods to reduce the concentration of blood ammonia, there is a lack of faster and better methods to reduce the concentration of blood ammonia due to the lack of a clear understanding of its pathogenesis.

### 23.3.5 Conclusion

Through specific cases, we understand the harm of hepatic encephalopathy to the human body and also understand the methods of treating hepatic encephalopathy. However, these are no means that can be used once and for all. Lack of treatment measures to rapidly reduce the blood ammonia concentration is one of the biggest problems in the treatment of hepatic encephalopathy. We hope to find better treatment methods and save more patients by summarizing the past experience and exploring new things.

## 23.4 Liver Failure

### 23.4.1 Introduction

Liver failure refers to severe liver damage caused by various factors (virus, alcohol, drugs, etc.), resulting in a large number of liver cell necrosis, leading to severe dysfunction or decompensation of liver metabolism, synthesis, detoxification, secretion, biotransformation, immune defense, and other functions, and then form a group of clinical syndromes with coagulation mechanism disorders, jaundice, hepatic encephalopathy, ascites, and other main manifestations. Liver and coagulation failure gradually progress to multiple organ failure which may include nervous, circulatory, respiratory, and renal system. Liver failure may cause short time death or even sudden death. The survival rate of patients with liver failure is only 20–40% who were treated with comprehensive treatment. The mortality rate is very high and increased with other organ injuries involved. This article discusses the mechanism of death caused by liver failure and the diagnosis and treatment through practical cases.

The death occurred in August 2019. We respectively collected the clinical symptoms, lab results, and treatment to analyze the course of death. Sharing this case was approved by the hospital ethics committee.

### 23.4.2 Case and Method

Patient Zheng, male, 49 years old, was admitted to the hospital mainly because of "liver occupation for 2 months, hematemesis and black stool for more than 10 h." Due to the large amount of ascites and the space occupation throughout the liver and portal vein, he failed to take an active anti-tumor treatment program. This patient has no previous physical examination history. He has a drinking history of more than 30 years, about 150 mL/day. Physical examination on admission: T 36.6 °C, P 72 times/min, R 24 times/min, BP 91/57 mmHg, $SPO_2$97%. Consciousness, with yellow skin and mucous membrane. Blood routine test showed Hb 103 g/L, HCT 281 L/L, WBC 8.78 × 109 g/L, PLT 152 × 109 g/L. Coagulation function: APTT 28.0 s, PT 16.3 s, TT 14.5 s, FIB 3.60 g/L, INR 1.51, D-Dimer 1529 ng/mL. Blood ammonia 44.8 umol/L. Biochemical results: ALT 40.6 U/L, AST 75.1 U/L, TP 58.2 g/L, ALB 30.7 g/L, TBIL 297.2 umol/L, DBIL 272.8 umol/L, GGT 276 U/L, UREA 10.6 umol/L, CRE 84 umol/L. Abdominal CT showed cirrhosis and ascites, hepatic portal space occupying, expansion of intrahepatic and extrahepatic bile ducts, portal vein thickened and filling defect which was suspected emboli. The patient was treated with symptomatic and supportive treatment. Three days later, the patient's heart rate and blood pressure could not be maintained and he died.

### 23.4.3 Review and Treatment

#### 23.4.3.1 Pathogeny

The etiology of liver failure includes hepatitis virus, drugs, hepatotoxic substances, acute fatty liver disease of pregnancy, pathogen infection, and autoimmune liver disease. In China, HBV infection is the main cause of liver failure, followed by drug and alcohol abuse. In Europe and the United States, alcohol abuse and drugs are the main causes of liver failure, especially caused by acetaminophen which accounts for 40%. The most common cause of liver failure in children is genetic and metabolic diseases. The precipitating factors of liver failure include HBV reactivation, overlapping infection of other hepatotropic or nonhepatotropic virus, bacterial infection, gastrointestinal bleeding, virus mutation, and nonstandard antiviral treatment [65–68] (Table 23.2).

**Table 23.2** Etiology of liver failure

| Pathogenesis | Common classification |
|---|---|
| Hepatitis virus | Hepatitis A, B, C, D, and E viruses (HAV, HBV, HCV, HDV, and HEV) |
| Other viruses | Cytomegalovirus (CMV), epstein-barr virus (EBV), enterovirus, herpes virus, yellow fever virus, etc. |
| Drugs | Acetaminophen, antituberculosis drugs, antitumor drugs, some Chinese herbal medicine, antirheumatic drugs, and antimetabolic drugs |
| Hepatotoxic substance | Alcohol, toadstools, poisonous chemicals, etc. |
| Bacteria and parasites | Severe or persistent infection (e.g., sepsis, schistosomiasis, etc.) |
| Other liver diseases | Liver tumor, liver surgery, acute fatty liver of pregnancy, autoimmune liver disease, liver transplantation, etc. |
| Biliary tract diseases | Congenital biliary atresia, cholestatic liver disease, etc. |
| Metabolic abnormalities | Hepatolenticular degeneration, hereditary disorder of glucose metabolism, etc. |
| Circulatory failure | Hypoxia, shock, congestive heart failure, etc. |
| Other | Trauma, heat stroke, etc. |
| Unknown reasons | |

#### 23.4.3.2 Pathophysiology and Lethal Mechanism

##### Pathogenesis

The etiology and pathogenesis of liver failure are various and complicated which involve many factors. Hepatocyte mass necrosis, inflammatory cell infiltration, and hepatic ischemic necrosis are the key problems. The main factors involved in the development of liver failure include direct damage of virus or drug, related immune response, and injury caused by precipitating factors. Cellular immunity which involved mainly CTL plays a key role in clearing cytotoxin and is also the main factor causing cell apoptosis or death. In the innate immune cells, macrophages and Kupffer cells proliferate and secrete a large number of cytokines, which induce cytokine storm and delayed hypersensitivity and mediate apoptosis or death of liver cells through death receptors. In addition, the retention and accumulation of endotoxin and metabolites can lead to liver cell injury and rapid deterioration [69].

##### Systemic Inflammatory Response Syndrome and Multiple Organ Failure

In liver failure, various pathogenic factors not only directly damage liver cells, but also activate inflammatory cells such as monocytes and macrophages, releasing a large amount of inflammatory mediators (TNF-α β, interleukin-10, interferon inducible protein 10, vitamin D receptor, human leukocyte antigen, NO, etc.) or cytokines, which in turn activate monocytes and macrophages to form "cytokine burst." A large number of cytokines, small-molecular weight toxins, and vasoactive substances cause a sharp increase in inflammatory mediators, forming a network system of inflammatory mediators, which eventually leads to immune dysfunction, uncontrolled body inflammatory response, and multiple organ failure [70].

### DIC

The pathogenesis of DIC in liver failure is mainly endotoxin theory. In liver failure, the reticuloendothelial system is not functional enough to remove various substances. Endotoxin can directly activate FXII, damage capillary endothelial cells, and activate the coagulation system. Viruses, antigen-antibody complexes, drugs, and a large amount of tissue thromboplastin-like substances released by hepatocyte necrosis can cause coagulation system activation, platelet activation, fibrin deposition, resulting in diffuse microthrombosis in microvessels, and coagulation factor and platelet reduction by consumption, which is accompanied by secondary hyperfibrinolysis and prompt DIC. DIC itself and shock, multiple organ failure which caused by DIC can lead to sudden death [70].

### Classification, Staging, and Diagnosis of Liver Failure

The classification and stages of liver failure are not uniform at present. Based on the medical history, onset characteristics, disease progression speed, and histopathological characteristics of liver failure, China's 2018 guidelines for the diagnosis and treatment of liver failure classified liver failure into four categories [65]: acute liver failure (ALF), subacute liver failure (SALF), acute-on-chronic (subacute) liver failure (ACLF or SACLF), and chronic liver failure (CLF). (1) Acute liver failure: acute onset, complicated with grade II or higher hepatic encephalopathy, within 2 weeks without underline liver disease; the histology includes necrosis that can be massive, submassive, or bridging, accompanied by severe degeneration of surviving liver cells, and with no collapse or no complete collapse in the hepatic sinus network scaffold. (2) Subacute liver failure: the onset of the disease is slower than ALF. The clinical manifestations occur within 2–26 weeks. The pathological features mainly include co-existence of previous and new submassive necrosis or bridging necrosis. Collapsed reticular fiber or collagen fiber deposition may exist in older necrotic areas; residual hepatocytes have varying degrees of regeneration; and small bile duct hyperplasia and cholestasis can be seen. (3) Acute-on-chronic (subacute) liver failure: acute or subacute deterioration of liver function without chronic liver diseases. The pathological features are as follows: new hepatocyte necrosis can be seen in the background of pathological damage caused by chronic liver diseases. (4) Chronic liver failure: in patients with liver cirrhosis, progressive deterioration and liver decompensation developed, accompanied with ascites and/or hepatic encephalopathy. The histology includes diffuse hepatic fibrosis and the formation of dysplastic nodules with unevenly distributed hepatocyte necrosis. The staging and diagnosis of each type of liver failure are shown in Table 23.3 [71].

**Table 23.3** Classification and diagnosis of liver failure

| Classification | Diagnosis |
|---|---|
| Acute hepatic failure | Acute onset, complicated with grade II or higher hepatic encephalopathy, within 2 weeks without underlying liver disease and has the following behavior: (1) extreme fatigue, accompanied by obvious anorexia, abdominal distension, nausea, vomiting, and severe gastrointestinal symptoms; (2) jaundice gradually deepened in a short period, and serum total bilirubin (TBil) $\geq$ 10× upper limit of normal value (ULN) or daily increase $\geq$17.1 mol/L; (3) bleeding tendency, prethrombin activity (PTA) $\leq$ 40%, or international standardized ratio (INR) $\geq$ 1.5, and other reasons were excluded; (4) progressive shrinkage of the liver |
| Subacute liver failure | The onset of the disease is slower than ALF and the following manifestations at 2–26 weeks: (1) extreme weakness and obvious gastrointestinal symptoms; (2) jaundice rapidly deepened, serum Tbil $\geq$10× ULN or daily increase $\geq$17.1 mol/L; (3) with or without hepatic encephalopathy; (4) those with bleeding, PTA $\leq$ 40% (or INR $\geq$ 1.5) and other reasons excluded |
| Acute-on-chronic (subacute) liver failure | Hepatorenal syndrome, hepatopulmonary syndrome and other complications, as well as extrahepatic organ failure in patients with chronic liver diseases. Patients with jaundice rapidly deepened, serum Tbil $\geq$10 × ULN or daily increase $\geq$17.1 mol/L; there was bleeding, PTA $\leq$ 40% (or INR $\geq$ 1.5). On the basis of different chronic liver diseases, it can be divided into three types. Type A: chronic noncirrhotic liver diseases with slow and acute liver failure; Type B: chronic plus acute liver failure on the basis of compensatory cirrhosis, usually within 4 weeks; and Type C: chronic plus acute liver failure on the basis of decompensated cirrhosis |
| Chronic liver failure | In patients with liver cirrhosis, progressive deterioration and liver decompensation developed: (1) serum TBil increased, often <10 × ULN; (2) albumin (Alb) decreased significantly; (3) platelets decreased significantly, PTA $\leq$ 40% (or INR $\geq$1.5), and other reasons were excluded; (4) refractory ascites or portal hypertension; (5) hepatic encephalopathy |

#### 23.4.3.3 Treatment

Principles of treatment include early detection, diagnosis, and treatment. Comprehensive medical treatment should be based on the etiology. Active prevention and treatment of complications, artificial liver, and liver transplantation are also very important.

##### General Symptomatic Supportive Treatment

(1) The removal of precipitating factors: identify overlap infection with other hepatotropic or nonhepatotropic virus and bacteria, gastrointestinal bleeding, various stress states, fatigue, alcohol consumption, incorrect treatment, etc. (2) Reduce liver burden: bed rest, reduce physical exertion, strengthen the supply of nutrition and energy, and avoid the application of drugs causing liver injury. (3) Improve the liver function: by inhibiting liver inflammation, removing reactive oxygen species, promoting biological transformation and detoxification, stabilizing the cell membrane, improving cell membrane fluidity and integrity, regulating energy metabolism, reducing liver tissue damage, promoting liver cell repair and regeneration, and

reducing intrahepatic cholestasis, so as to improve the liver function. Anti-inflammatory drugs (glycyrrhizin), liver membrane protectants, antidotes, and anti-cholinergic drugs are recommended. (4) Nutritional support: recommend enteral nutrition, including high-carbohydrate, low-fat, and moderate protein diet. Intravenous supplement of calories, fluids, vitamins, and trace elements are recommended in patients with poor food intake. Also, night snack is recommended. (5) To correct hypoproteinemia and maintain water and electrolyte balance, especially to correct low sodium, low chlorine, low magnesium, low potassium; supplement coagulation factors and improve liver circulation. (6) Closely detect the change of illness and strengthen nursing management [65].

**Etiological Treatment**

*Hepatitis virus infection*: Mainly targeted at liver failure patients affected by HBV and HCV infection. For HBVDNA-positive patients, early and rapid reduction of HBVDNA load is the key to treatment. It is recommended to use nucleoside (acid) drugs for antiviral treatment immediately. Fast and effective nucleoside (acid) drugs are recommended, such as entecavir and tenofovir. Direct-acting antiviral agents are preferred in patients who are HCV RNA positive. Individualized treatment is carried out according to HCV genotype and patient tolerance, but the protease inhibitor is contraindicated in decompensated cirrhosis, which can aggravate the progress of liver failure. In the clinic, there is no special and effective treatment for end-stage liver failure caused by HCV infection. Liver transplantation may be the best treatment. For patients with confirmed or suspected herpes virus or varicella-zoster virus infection resulting in acute liver failure should be treated with acyclovir (5–10 mg/kg, 1 time /8 h, intravenous drip) [65].

*Liver failure caused by drug-induced liver injury*: Stopping all suspicious drugs on time. For patients with acute liver failure caused by excessive acetaminophen (APAP), if the intake of APAP happens within 4 h, the active peptide should be taken orally before the administration of N-acetylcysteine (NAC). For patients with large intake of APAP, the elevation of the serum drug concentration or transaminase indicates that liver injury is imminent or has occurred. NAC should be given immediately and artificial liver therapy should be carried out if necessary. NAC can improve the prognosis of mild hepatic encephalopathy in patients with acute liver failure caused by nonAPAP, and should be applied as early as possible. Penicillin G and silymarin should be considered for patients with acute liver failure diagnosed or suspected of mushroom poisoning [72].

*Alcoholic liver failure*: Abstinence is the basis of treatment. Patients with severe alcoholic liver disease with Maddary score $\geq 32$ can be treated with corticosteroid, usually at a dose of prednisone of 40 mg/day for 1 month. Infection should be closely monitored before and during treatment. The response to hormone can be evaluated by Lille score when corticosteroid is used for 7 days. If the Lille score $\geq 0.56$ on day 7 after treatment, corticosteroid should be stopped in time. N-acetylcysteine can be used in combination with corticosteroid. Some studies have reported that combined treatment can reduce the occurrence of severe alcoholic liver disease infection and hepatorenal syndrome [73, 74].

*Autoimmune liver disease*: For liver failure caused by autoimmune hepatitis, early use of corticosteroid (methylprednisolone, 1.0–1.5 mg/kg/day) may be effective, and liver transplantation should be considered if the treatment fails for a week [75].

*Acute fatty liver/HELLP syndrome in pregnancy*: Termination of pregnancy immediately. If the disease continues to progress after termination of pregnancy, artificial liver and liver transplantation should be considered [65].

*Hepatolenticular degeneration*: It can be treated with penicillamine and other copper expelling drugs, but the general curative effect is not good for liver failure patients. Plasma exchange, albumin dialysis, hemofiltration, and artificial liver support therapy combined with various blood purification methods can be used. Liver transplantation should be considered as early as possible for patients with end-stage liver failure [76].

#### 23.4.3.4 Prevention and Treatment of Complications

*Brain edema*: Intracranial pressure should be reduced in time in patients with intracranial hypertension. Mannitol (0.5–1.0 g/kg) or hypertonic saline should be used as soon as possible, and alternately using loop diuretics such as furosemide and osmotic dehydrating agents, and supplement human blood albumin which can improve colloid osmotic pressure and relieve brain edema. Also, artificial liver support therapy can be used. Mild hypothermia therapy can be considered for acute liver failure patients with uncontrollable intracranial hypertension, and indomethacin can be given to control intracranial hypertension under the condition of high cerebral blood perfusion.

*Hepatic encephalopathy*: Remove the predisposing factors using lactulose and ornithine-aspartic acid to reduce blood ammonia. Timely find infection and give anti-infection treatment to reduce systemic inflammatory response.

*Infection*: Prophylactic use of anti-infection drugs is not recommended. Attention should be paid to monitoring. The most common sites of infection are abdominal cavity, lungs, urinary tract, and blood. Once infection is found, antibiotics should be used empirically and immediately, and adjusted in time according to culture results.

*Hyponatremia*: Dilute hyponatremia caused by water and sodium retention is most common. When blood sodium is lower than 125 mmol/L, water can be properly limited. Hypertonic saline can quickly correct hyponatremia, but it will cause more water and sodium retention. Therefore, hypertonic saline solution is generally not recommended to correct hyponatremia. If there is severe hyponatremia (blood sodium level < 110 mmol/L) or hyponatremia encephalopathy occurs, 50–100 mL of 3–5% NaCl solution can be appropriately added intravenously. Tolvaptan, an arginine vasopressin V2 receptor blocker, mainly promotes free water excretion and corrects hyponatremia by selectively blocking the V2 receptor of collecting duct main cells. During application, the urine volume, physical signs, and electrolyte of patients should be closely monitored, and the increasing rate of blood sodium within 24 h should not exceed 12 mmol/L.

*Refractory ascites*: Low salt diet, 4–6 g/day. Furosemide combined with spironolactone can be used. Tolvaptan can be used in patients with poor response. Vasoactive drugs, such as midodrine and terlipressin, can improve the patient's hyperdynamic circulatory state to a certain extent and increase the body's response to diuretics. Patients with severe ascites may undergo paracentesis to release ascites, which can quickly relieve abdominal distension symptoms. However, we should be alert to circulatory dysfunction after releasing ascites, and it can be prevented by giving albumin infusion or vasoactive drugs.

*Acute renal injury (AKI)*: AKI is one of the common complications of liver failure. Once AKI occurs, the prognosis is poor. Prerenal AKI is the most common form. Hepatorenal syndrome (HRS) is a special form of prerenal AKI. Once AKI occurs in patients with liver failure, possible renal injury drugs, vasodilators or nonsteroidal anti-inflammatory drugs, should be discontinued. Use albumin or crystal solution to expand the volume. If infection is suspected, the infection should be controlled as soon as possible. If AKI does not improve after volume expansion, HRS should be considered and vasoconstrictors (terlipressin or norepinephrine) combined with albumin can be used for treatment. If terlipressin (1 mg/4–6 h) combined with albumin (20–40 g/day) is applied, the serum creatinine decreases by <25% after 3 days, and terlipressin can be gradually increased to 2 mg/4 h. If effective, the course of treatment is for 7–14 days; If not, stop using terlipressin. Norepinephrine (0.5–3.0 mg/h) combined with albumin (10–20 g/L) is also effective on HRS, but its effect is currently reported to be not as good as that of terlipressin. AKI, which is ineffective with vasoconstrictive drugs and meets the criteria of renal replacement therapy, can be treated with renal replacement therapy.

*Artificial liver*: Its therapeutic mechanism is based on the strong regeneration ability of liver cells. Through an external mechanical, physical, chemical, and biological device, it removes various harmful substances, supplements necessary substances, improves internal environment, and temporarily replaces some functions of failing liver, to create conditions for liver cell regeneration and liver function recovery or to wait for an opportunity for liver transplantation. Artificial liver support system can be divided into three types: nonbiological, biological, and combined system. Nonbiological artificial liver has been widely used in the clinic and proved to have certain effect.

*Liver transplantation*: Liver transplantation is the best choice for patients who have failed to respond to aggressive medical treatment. The MELD score is the main reference for evaluating liver transplantation [77].

### 23.4.4 Discussion

In the above cases, the patient is a middle-aged male with a long history of alcohol consumption and lack of health awareness, and the liver tumor was found to be terminal. And one of the hallmarks of a liver tumor in its end stages is liver failure. In the course of liver tumor development, necrosis and abnormal liver cells inevitably occur until the normal liver function is completely lost. As a secondary change of advanced liver tumor, liver failure plays an important role in predicting prognosis. On the basis of clear treatment of primary disease, targeted treatment is an effective method to treat liver failure. Another problem is the economics of treating liver failure. Despite the availability of advanced treatments like artificial livers and liver transplants, recipients are small, and few families can afford such high costs without health insurance.

### 23.4.5 Conclusion

By sharing the death case of liver failure, we aim to understand the course of death from sudden death caused by liver failure and to find better treatments to save more patients. Although there are so many treatments available to intervene in liver failure, a large number of patients with liver failure still die each year without timely and effective treatment. So, we still have a long way to go.

## 23.5 Acute Suppurative Cholangitis

### 23.5.1 Introduction

Acute suppurative cholangitis refers to various causes of biliary stenosis, secondary cholestasis, and acute suppurative bile duct infection. In physiological condition, continuous bile secretion and immune barrier of the bile duct epithelium can keep the bile duct sterile. The benign and malignant causes (stones, tumors, etc.) of the bile duct lead to biliary stricture or obstruction, which elevates the pressure within the biliary system, destroys the normal immune barrier, flushes the bacteria and endotoxins from the infected bile into systemic circulation, and induces systemic inflammatory response syndrome. The mortality of acute suppurative cholangitis can reach as high as 50%, if biliary decompression and drainage are not provided immediately [78, 79]. Here we will discuss the mechanisms of death caused by acute suppurative cholangitis and the diagnosis and treatment strategy based on a clinical case.

### 23.5.2 Case and Method

The case occurred in October 2019. We analyzed the death process by reviewing the clinical symptoms, examination results, test results, and clinical treatment of the patient. The case sharing has been approved by the ethics committee of our hospital.

#### 23.5.2.1 Case Report

An 89-year-old male patient was admitted to our hospital complaining of "jaundice for 14 days, and fever accompanied by asthma for 5 days." Past history includes hypertension and coronary artery stent implantation. Vital signs: T 36.7 °C, P 82/min, R 31/min, BP 160/79 mmHg, $SPO_2$ 94%. Physical examination revealed jaundice and tenderness of the right upper abdomen, rebound pain, and muscle tension. Laboratory tests: Hb 95 g/L, HCT 0.252 L/L,WBC 19.01 × 109 g/L, PLT 102 × 109 g/L, APTT 28.6S, PT 12.8S, TT 13.0S, FIB 3.93 g/L, INR 1.19, D-dimer 2028 ng/mL, ALT 213.3 U/L, AST 126.2 U/L, TP 60.3 g/L, ALB 32.5 g/L, TBIL 158.2 umol/L, DBIL 132.6 umol/L, GGT 675 U/L, CRP 80 mg/dL, PCT 21.25 ng/mL. Abdominal ultrasound showed extrahepatic bile duct expansion and gallbladder wall thickening. The patient received anti-infection, rehydration, and other conservative treatment. The patient could not tolerate the invasive procedure of ERCP because of his old age, and finally died after 2 days of hospitalization.

### 23.5.3 Review and Management

#### 23.5.3.1 Etiology and Incentives

The occurrence of acute suppurative cholangitis mainly depends on two factors: biliary obstruction and bacterial growth in the bile duct. A variety of causes can lead to bile duct stenosis or obstruction, and then induce acute suppurative cholangitis. Cholelithiasis is the most common cause of benign biliary obstruction and cholangitis, accounting for about half of the cases of acute suppurative cholangitis [80]. Other causes of benign biliary obstruction include benign stricture, external compression, and autoimmune diseases. The causes of malignant biliary obstruction include cholangiocarcinoma, gallbladder cancer, pancreatic cancer, ampullary cancer, and duodenal cancer. Secondary malignant obstruction of the biliary tract accounts for 10–30% of acute suppurative cholangitis [81].

The main route for bacteria to enter the bile duct is through retrograde infection from the duodenum. In addition, the bile duct can also be infected through the portal vein system and the periportal lymphatic system [82]. The most common pathogens of acute suppurative cholangitis include *Escherichia coli*, *Klebsiella*, and *Enterococcus* [83]. However, anaerobes and a variety of microorganisms are often found in patients with a previous history of biliary tract operation, in patients with severe concomitant diseases, and the elderly [84].

#### 23.5.3.2 Lethal Mechanism

*Septic shock*: In acute suppurative cholangitis, the increased pressure within the bile duct disrupts the tight junctions between the epithelial cells of the bile duct, and flushes a large number of microorganisms and endotoxins from the infected bile into systemic circulation, leading to a systemic inflammatory cascade reaction and septic shock, which is one of the main causes of death in patients with acute suppurative cholangitis [85].

*Multiple organ dysfunction syndrome (MODS)*: MODS is another important cause of death in patients with acute suppurative cholangitis. Bacteremia and endotoxemia lead to the activation of inflammatory cells in the body, excessive release of many kinds of inflammatory cytokines such as tumor necrosis factor and interleukin-6 into the circulatory system, resulting in systemic inflammatory cascade reaction, and eventually lead to the occurrence of MODS. Multivariate analysis showed that bacterial infection producing extended spectrum β-lactamases, leukocyte >20,000 cells/μL, serum total bilirubin >10 mg/dL, and an elevated serum urea nitrogen level were the risk factors for MODS, while timely decompression and drainage of the biliary tract were protective factors [86, 87].

#### 23.5.3.3 Diagnosis

In the past, the diagnosis of acute suppurative cholangitis mainly depended on the clinical symptoms of patients. Typical patients may have fever, right upper abdominal pain and jaundice, namely, Charcot's triad, while severe patients may have shock and neurologic symptoms, namely, Reynolds pentad. However, the sensitivity of these two diagnostic criteria in the diagnosis of acute suppurative

**Table 23.4** Tokyo Guidelines 2018: diagnostic criteria for acute cholangitis

| | |
|---|---|
| A Systemic inflammation | |
| A-1. | Fever >38 °C and/or shaking chills |
| A-2. | Laboratory data: evidence of inflammatory response:WBC(X1000/UL) < 4 or >10, CRP(mg/dL) ≥ 1 |
| B Cholestasis. | |
| B-1. | Jaundice:T-Bil ≥ 2 (mg/dL) |
| B-2. | Laboratory data: abnormal liver function tests:ALP, GGT, AST, ALT >1.5× STD |
| C. Imaging. | |
| C-1. | Biliary dilatation |
| C-2. | Evidence of the etiology on imaging (stricture, stone, stent etc.) |
| | Suspected diagnosis: one item in A + one item in either B or C |
| | Definite diagnosis: one item in A, one item in B, and one item in C |

*ALP* alkaline phosphatase, *ALT* alanine aminotransferase, *AST* aspartate aminotransferase, *CRP* C-reactive protein, *GGT* r-glutamyltransferase, *WBC* white blood cell, and *STD* upper limit of normal value

cholangitis is low and therefore not applicable. Initially published in 2007, the Tokyo guidelines established a more comprehensive diagnostic standard based on the clinical signs and symptoms, laboratory examination, and diagnostic imaging of patients. After two evaluations and revisions in 2013 and 2018, it has become a commonly used clinical diagnostic criterion for acute cholangitis (Table 23.4) [88].

### Clinical Signs and Symptoms

Fever, right upper abdominal pain, and jaundice (Charcot's triad) are common clinical manifestations of acute suppurative cholangitis, which can be seen in 60–80% of patients. Although the specificity of Charcot's triad can reach as high as 95.9%, studies have reported its sensitivity to be only 21.2–26.4%. In the same way, Reynolds pentad was only found in 4–8% of the severe patients. Therefore, the clinical application of the diagnostic criteria which only depend on clinical symptoms is seriously limited. In 2007, the Tokyo guideline diagnostic criteria, based on the clinical manifestations, laboratory examination, and diagnostic imaging of patients, were updated in 2013, and the sensitivity for the diagnosis of acute suppurative cholangitis was 91.8%, while the specificity reached 77.7% [88, 89]. Therefore, the 2013 diagnostic criteria for acute cholangitis were adopted by Tokyo Guidelines 2018 and used as the standard criteria in the clinical setting.

### Laboratory Examination

Inflammatory reaction, cholestasis, and etiological evidence can be found in laboratory examination. Abnormal white blood cell counts (leukocyte (X1000/UL) < 4 or >10), increase of serum creatinine protein levels (C-reactive protein ≥1 mg/dL), and other changes indicate systemic inflammatory response. In addition, procalcitonin (PCT) has been considered as a sensitive indicator of severe bacterial infection and sepsis in recent years, which can be significantly increased in acute suppurative cholangitis. It can be used to assist in assessing the severity of the disease and whether emergency biliary decompression and drainage is needed [90, 91]. Elevated T-Bil, (≥2 mg/dL) ALP, GGT, AST, and ALT levels (>1.5 times the upper limit of normal) are the manifestations of cholestasis. Among them, an increase of ALP can be seen in 74–93% of patients with acute suppurative cholangitis, and ALP recovers faster than other laboratory tests (such as bilirubin) after biliary decompression and drainage. Hence, it can be used as an indicator for judging whether biliary drainage is sufficient [92]. Blood specimen should be sent for culture to identify the causative organisms of acute suppurative cholangitis, and to guide anti-infection treatment. However, positive rates of blood culture range from 21% to 71% for acute suppurative cholangitis, and the procedure is time-consuming, which highly limits its clinical application. Therefore, the Tokyo Guidelines and the American Society of surgical infection/infectious diseases guidelines do not recommend routine blood culture examination [93, 94]. Blood culture was recommended only in a small number of patients with immune deficiency or severe infection, when such results may be helpful to guide the selection and course of antibiotics.

#### Imaging Examination

Imaging examination includes abdominal ultrasound, computed tomography (CT), magnetic resonance imaging (MRI)/magnetic resonance cholangiopancreatography (MRCP), ERCP, and EUS. Based on the findings of these imaging examinations, we can identify the causes of biliary stenosis/blockage that can cause acute cholangitis (stenosis, stone, stent, etc.). Abdominal ultrasound is often used as the first choice because of its minimal invasiveness, wide availability, convenience, and low price. It can detect abnormal dilatation of the bile duct and identify its causes. However, due to the influence of factors such as intestinal gas accumulation, it is easy to miss the diagnosis of distal choledocholithiasis and malignant lesions of the bile duct. Thus, abdominal ultrasound has a low diagnostic sensitivity. A meta-analysis showed that abdominal ultrasound has a sensitivity of 42% (95% CI: 28 to 56%) and a specificity of 96% (95% CI: 94 to 98%) for dilated common bile duct and a sensitivity of 38% (95% CI: 27 to 49%) and a specificity of 100% (95% CI: 99 to 100%) for all bile duct stones. Abdominal enhanced CT can be used to identify the causes of biliary obstruction such as cholelithiasis, benign strictures, and malignancies [95]. However, due to the presence of X-ray negative stones, it has a low sensitivity of 42% for bile duct stones [96]. MRCP can clearly delineate the morphology of intrahepatic and extrahepatic bile duct and pancreatic duct without the use of a contrast agent, and identify bile duct stenosis, dilatation, and large stones in the common bile duct. However, MRCP has a low diagnostic accuracy when displaying stones less than 6 mm [97]. ERCP is an invasive diagnostic and therapeutic procedure. It is the gold standard for the diagnosis of acute suppurative cholangitis, when the pus overflow was seen at the duodenal papilla through a duodenoscope. ERCP cholangiography can also show the delineation of the whole biliary tree, and find the cause of cholangitis. With the wide accessibility of MRCP, ERCP is now rarely used only for diagnostic purpose. ERCP has been recommended as the first-line biliary drainage procedure for acute cholangitis because of its less invasiveness and lower risk of adverse events than other drainage techniques [98]. In recent years, EUS has been emerging as a novel technique which provides both diagnostic and therapeutic effects for acute cholangitis. It demonstrates a sensitivity of nearly 100% and a specificity of more than 90% to the diagnosis of cholelithiasis, which is significantly better than MRCP, especially for the detection of small stones that are not easy to be identified by other inspection measures. EUS is superior to ERCP in the detection of cholangiopancreatic tumors, tumor invasion, and lymph node metastasis. In addition, EUS guided biliary drainage has been developed and reported as a useful alternative drainage technique when ERCP intubation fails [99, 100].

### Severity Grading Criteria for Acute Cholangitis

Based on patients' clinical signs and symptoms and routine laboratory examinations and whether or not combined with organ dysfunction, acute cholangitis was divided into three grades: mild, moderate, and severe (grade I, II, III) in Tokyo Guidelines of 2013. This severity grading criteria can be used to predict the prognosis of patients with acute cholangitis and determine which patients need emergency biliary decompression and drainage. Four case series studies from Japan and Taiwan confirmed its prognostic value in clinical application, and two of them evaluated the severity grading criteria as an indicator for biliary drainage. In these studies, patients with a higher severity grading had significantly higher 30-day mortality. However, 30-day mortality was significantly lower in patients with Grade II acute cholangitis who were treated with early or urgent biliary drainage. These findings suggest that the severity grading criteria in the Tokyo Guidelines of 2013 can be used to identify Grade II patients whose prognoses may be improved through urgent biliary drainage. Thus, this severity grading criteria were adopted in the Tokyo Guidelines of 2018 and used as the standard in the clinical setting (Table 23.5) [88].

**Table 23.5** Severity grading criteria for acute cholangitis in the Tokyo Guidelines of 2018

| |
|---|
| Grade III (severe) acute cholangitis |
| "Grade III" acute cholangitis is defined as acute cholangitis that is associated with the onset of dysfunction at least in any one of the following organs/systems: |
| 1. Cardiovascular dysfunction: hypotension requiring dopamine ≥5 μg/kg/min, or any dose of norepinephrine |
| 2. Neurological dysfunction: disturbance of consciousness |
| 3. Respiratory dysfunction: $PaO_2/FiO_2$ ratio $< 300$ |
| 4. Renal dysfunction: oliguria, serum creatinine >2.0 mg/dL |
| 5. Hepatic dysfunction: PT-INR > 1.5 |
| 6. Hematological dysfunction: platelet count $<100{,}000/mm^3$ |
| Grade II (moderate) acute cholangitis |
| "Grade II" acute cholangitis is associated with any two of the following conditions: |
| 1. Abnormal WBC count ($>12{,}000/mm^3$, $<4000/mm^3$) |
| 2. High fever (≥39 °C) |
| 3. Age (≥75 years old) |
| 4. Hyperbilirubinemia (total bilirubin ≥5 mg/dL) |
| 5. Hypoalbuminemia ($<$STD[a] × 0.7) |
| Grade I (mild) acute cholangitis |
| "Grade I" acute cholangitis does not meet the criteria of "Grade III (severe)" or "Grade II (moderate)" acute cholangitis at initial diagnosis. |

[a]STD: lower limit of normal value

#### 23.5.3.4 Management

**Initial Management**

Initial medical treatment includes the infusion of sufficient fluids and electrolytes, as well as analgesic administration and other symptomatic treatment. Empirical anti-infection therapy should be started as soon as a definitive diagnosis of acute cholangitis has been reached. Severity should be assessed according to the severity grading criteria for acute cholangitis. Moderate and severe patients should be fasting to enable immediate emergency drainage. At the same time, vital signs including blood pressure, heart rate, respiration rate, temperature, urine volume, oxygen saturation ($SPO_2$), and the patient's general status should be evaluated and closely monitored.

**Management Based on the Severity Grading of Acute Cholangitis**

Acute cholangitis should be managed in accordance with its severity. Alongside the initial treatment, severity assessment should be carried out using the severity grading criteria for acute cholecystitis in the Tokyo Guidelines of 2018. Timing treatment should be provided for patients based on the severity grading of acute cholangitis (Fig. 23.1) [100]. And the patient's general status and severity of disease should be reassessed within 24 h, 24–48 h after the start of treatment.

*Grade I (mild acute cholangitis)*: After initial treatment including antibiotics and general supportive care, most of the patients with mild acute cholangitis will get better without biliary drainage. However, if the patient's condition does not improve within 24 h after initial treatment, biliary drainage should be considered. For patients with choledocholithiasis, choledocholithotomy may be performed at the same time as biliary drainage.

*Grade II (moderate acute cholangitis)*: In addition to the initial treatment including antibiotics and general supportive care, patients with moderate acute cholangitis should consider early biliary drainage, including ERCP, PTBD, and EUS-BD. Treatment for the underlying etiology (bile duct stones, tumor, etc.) should

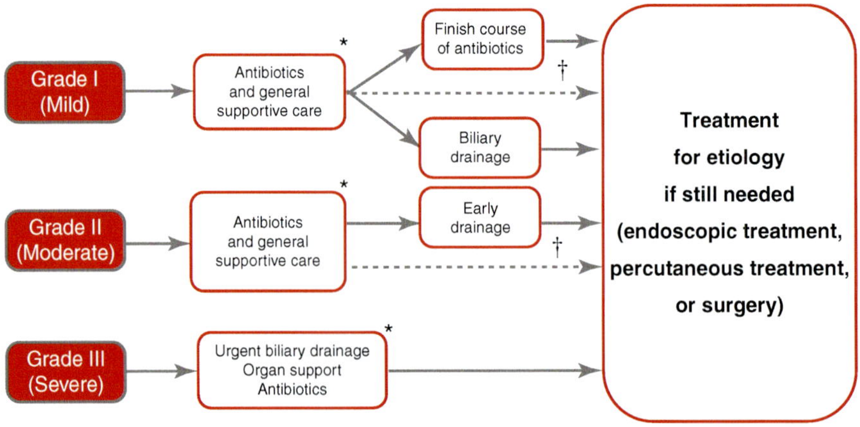


**Fig. 23.1** Flowchart for the management of acute cholangitis in the Tokyo Guidelines of 2018

not be provided until the patient's general condition has improved after early biliary drainage.

*Grade III (severe acute cholangitis)*: Severe acute cholangitis is characterized by sepsis-induced organ dysfunction. The condition of patients with severe cholangitis may deteriorate rapidly. In addition to the initial treatment, organ function support should be given immediately, including noninvasive/invasive mechanical ventilation (tracheal intubation followed by artificial ventilation) and vasoactive drugs. Urgent biliary drainage, including ERCP, PTBD, and EUS-BD, should be performed immediately after the patient's vital signs are stable. If the hospital is unable to perform such operations, the patient should be transferred to a hospital that can perform biliary drainage. The treatment of biliary obstruction should be delayed until the patient's condition is stable.

### Antimicrobial Recommendations for Acute Cholangitis

The primary goal of antimicrobial treatment for patients with acute suppurative cholangitis is to control sepsis and local inflammation of the bile duct and prevent the formation of intrahepatic abscess. Therefore, once suspected of acute suppurative cholangitis, empirical antimicrobial treatment should be provided immediately.

The common pathogens of acute suppurative cholangitis include *Escherichia coli*, *Klebsiella*, *Pseudomonas*, *Enterobacter*, *Acinetobacter*, etc. The selection of empiric antibiotics mainly depends on the type of strains prevalent in the area and the data of antimicrobial susceptibility. Common antibiotics include penicillins, cephalosporins, carbapenems, fluoroquinolones, etc. The resistance of *Enterobacteriaceae* strains has been widely reported, especially the gram-negative bacilli producing β-lactamase (ESBL) and carbapenemase, which have significantly affected the empirical antibacterial treatment of acute cholangitis. The Tokyo Guidelines of 2018 recommended that bile samples should be taken for bacterial culture and antimicrobial susceptibility test during biliary drainage. Once causative microorganisms and the susceptibility testing results are available, the application of antimicrobial therapy should be adjusted to specific antimicrobial agents targeting the organisms [94]. The guideline also recommends drug selection of empirical antibacterial treatment for community-acquired biliary tract infection and iatrogenic biliary tract infection; see Table 23.6 for details [94].

### Choice of Biliary Drainage

Patients with moderate or severe acute cholangitis should be treated with early/urgent biliary drainage. Drainage methods include endoscopic transpapillary drainage, percutaneous transhepatic drainage, and surgical drainage.

### ERCP

ERCP has become the first-line of therapy for acute cholangitis because of its less invasiveness and lower risk of adverse events compared to other drainage techniques. Endoscopic transpapillary biliary drainage methods include external drainage via nasobiliary catheters and internal drainage via biliary stents. Both methods were equally effective for patients with acute suppurative cholangitis. There is no significant difference in the success rate, effectiveness, and complications between the two procedures. The advantages of nasobiliary catheters over internal stents are the ability to obtain noninvasive cholangiograms and cholecystograms; to monitor

**Table 23.6** Antimicrobial recommendations for acute cholangitis in the Tokyo Guidelines of 2018

| | Community-acquired biliary infections | | | Healthcare-associated biliary infections[a] |
|---|---|---|---|---|
| Severity | Grade I | Grade II | Grade III[a] | |
| Antimicrobial agents | Cholangitis and cholecystitis | Cholangitis and cholecystitis | Cholangitis and cholecystitis | Healthcare-associated cholangitis and cholecystitis |
| Penicillin-based therapy | Ampicillin/sulbactam[b] is not recommended if >20% resistance rate. | Piperacillin/tazobactam | Piperacillin/tazobactam | Piperacillin/tazobactam |
| Cephalosporin-based therapy | Cefazolin,[c]<br>or Cefotiam,[c]<br>or Cefuroxime,[c]<br>or Ceftriaxone,<br>or Cefotaxime<br>± Metronidazole[d]<br>Cefmetazole,[c]<br>Cefoxitin,[c]<br>Flomoxef,[c]<br>Cefoperazone/sulbactam | Ceftriaxone,<br>or Cefotaxime,<br>or Cefepime,<br>or Cefozopran,<br>or Ceftazidime<br>± Metronidazole[d]<br>Cefoperazone/sulbactam | Cefepime,<br>or Ceftazidime,<br>or Cefozopran<br>± Metronidazole[d] | Cefepime,<br>or Ceftazidime,<br>or Cefozopran<br>± Metronidazole[d] |
| Carbapenem-based therapy | Ertapenem | Ertapenem | Imipenem/cilastatin, meropenem, doripenem, ertapenem | Imipenem/cilastatin, meropenem, doripenem, ertapenem |
| Monobactam-based therapy | – | – | Aztreonam ± metronidazole[d] | Aztreonam ± metronidazole[d] |
| Fluoroquinolone-based therapy[e] | Ciprofloxacin, Levofloxacin, Pazufloxacin ± Metronidazole[d]<br>Moxifloxacin | Ciprofloxacin, Levofloxacin, Pazufloxacin ± Metronidazole[d]<br>Moxifloxacin | | |

[a]Vancomycin is recommended to cover Enterococcus spp. for grade III community-acquired acute cholangitis and cholecystitis, and healthcare-associated acute biliary infections. Linezolid or daptomycin is recommended if vancomycin-resistant Enterococcus (VRE) is known to be colonizing the patient, if previous treatment included vancomycin, and/or if the organism is common in the community

[b]Ampicillin/sulbactam has little activity left against Escherichia coli. It is removed from the North American guidelines

[c]Local antimicrobial susceptibility patterns (antibiogram) should be considered for use

[d]Anti-anaerobic therapy, including use of metronidazole, tinidazole, or clindamycin, is warranted if a biliary-enteric anastomosis is present. The carbapenems, piperacillin/tazobactam, ampicillin/ sulbactam, cefmetazole, cefoxitin, flomoxef, and cefoperazone/sulbactam have sufficient anti-anaerobic activity for this situation

[e]Fluoroquinolones use is recommended if the susceptibility of cultured isolates is known or for patients with b-lactam allergies. Many extended-spectrum b-lactamase (ESBL)-producing Gram-negative isolates are fluoroquinolone resistant

the drainage volume; and to provide irrigation for hemobilia, mucin, or debris. However, it suffers from the disadvantage of patient discomfort and risk for dislodgement. On the other hand, the internal stents are associated with less postprocedure discomfort and avoid the potential problems of inadvertent removal of the nasobiliary catheter. The major drawbacks of the internal stent are that its patency and adequacy of drainage cannot be monitored. Furthermore, it has been found with a higher rate of blockage and more frequent hyperamylasemia. Thus, the choice of endoscopic transpapillary drainage, nasobiliary catheters, or biliary stents depends on the preference of the operator and the specific circumstances of each patient [101].

#### EUS-BD

EUS-BD has become the first-line of alternate therapeutic modality for biliary obstruction in patients who fail ERCP. The indications for EUS-BD include failure of ERCP intubation, and cases of benign and malignant bile duct obstruction that cannot be intubated by conventional transpapillary biliary drainage methods. The latter includes anatomical abnormalities after surgery and obstruction of the gastroduodenal lumen. Relative contraindications to EUS-BD are ascites, recent surgery, and anticoagulation therapy. EUS-BD consists of two puncture routes: intrahepatic and extrahepatic. Under the guidance of EUS, the intrahepatic puncture route is from the stomach to the left intrahepatic bile duct, while the extrahepatic puncture route is from the duodenum to the common bile duct. Once the puncture is successful, different drainage methods can be selected according to the etiology and anatomy of the obstruction, mainly including EUS-guided rendezvous technique (EUS-RV), EUS-guided antegrade stenting (EUS-AS), and EUS-guided transmural stenting (EUS-TS), which includes EUS-guided gastrostomy (EUS-HGS) and EUS-guided choledochoduodenostomy (EUS-CDS) according to different puncture sites. Compared with PTBD, EUS-BD has a higher success rate, while the incidence of adverse events is lower. Moreover, EUS-BD provides internal drainage, which is more in line with physiological conditions. Therefore, at present, EUS-BD has basically replaced PTBD as the first alternative measure for patients with acute suppurative cholangitis when ERCP is not an option [102].

#### PTBD

PTBD is another alternative to biliary drainage in patients with ERCP intubation failure. The technical success rate of PTBD is more than 90% in patients with intrahepatic bile duct dilation. However, the incidence of adverse events can be as high as 40%, including postprocedure bile leak, bleeding, cholangitis, drainage stent blockage or displacement, etc. PTBD is currently mainly used in patients with failed EUS-BD procedures. In addition, PTBD remains an alternative biliary drainage after ERCP failure in hospitals where EUS-BD is unavailable [103].

#### Surgical Drainage

Open surgical drainage was used to treat biliary obstruction and cholangitis before the introduction of endoscopic drainage and PTBD. At present, surgical drainage is not the first choice for patients with acute cholangitis because of its high incidence of complications. It is only performed when endoscopic or other drainage procedures have failed, as well as for patients with acute suppurative cholangitis who need surgery because of the primary disease [104].

### 23.5.4 Discussion

In the above-mentioned case, the patient was an old man with a history of hypertension and coronary heart disease, so the risk of operation was very high. ERCP is the first choice for patients with acute suppurative cholangitis. However, the patient cannot tolerate the ERCP procedure due to his poor physical condition. For elderly patients with acute suppurative cholangitis, the risk of sudden death is very high due to uncorrectable septic shock and continuous deterioration of the liver function.

### 23.5.5 Conclusion

For patients with acute suppurative cholangitis, the probability of sudden death is very low as long as the diagnosis is timely. After the biliary obstruction was relieved, the infection was more easily controlled and the probability of MODS was greatly reduced. Based on the characteristics of this disease, we need to ensure timely diagnosis.

## 23.6 Acute Pancreatitis

### 23.6.1 Introduction

Acute pancreatitis (AP) is defined as an inflammatory response after abnormal trypsinogen activation due to a variety of causes, followed by autodigestion of pancreas [105]. In severe cases, systemic inflammatory response syndrome occurs, and it can be accompanied by other organ dysfunction diseases. The process of most patients is self-limiting. About 15% of patients progress to severe acute pancreatitis with an overall mortality rate of 5–10%. Patients with severe pancreatitis have a higher mortality rate of 34–55% [106, 107]. According to autopsy data statistics, sudden death caused by acute pancreatitis is one of the important causes of noncardiac sudden death, which accounts for 0.2–2.5% of natural sudden death [108]. We understand the dangers of acute pancreatitis through a case report.

### 23.6.2 Case and Method

This death occurred in August 2019. We analyzed the death process by reviewing the clinical symptoms, laboratory tests, imaging tests, and clinical treatment medications at the time of death. The case has been reviewed by the hospital ethics committee.

#### 23.6.2.1 Case Report

We present the case of a 49-year-old male patient who was admitted with an abdominal pain and bloating for 38 h after overeating. He had history of pancreatitis. Admission examination revealed that the patient did not have fever (36.7 °C, axillary), the pulse rate was 142 bmp, the respiratory rate was 22 bpm, the blood pressure was 134/94 mmHg, and the oxygen saturation was 97%. The left mid-upper abdominal part was tender, no rebound pain or muscle tension. The results of the laboratory tests were showed as follows: blood routine showed WBC 21.78 × 109 g/L, N 87%, Hb 144 g/L, PLT 68 × 109 g/L. Blood biochemical indicators showed AMS2379U/L, LPS 1866 U/L, ALT 30.1 U/L, AST 76.5 U/L, TBIL 48.5 umol/L, DBIL 47.2 umol/L, GGT 90 U/L, UREA 12.9 mmol/L, CRE 220 umol/L, GLU 26.15 mmol/L. Coagulation function showed APTT 31.3S, PT 17.6S, TT 13.1S, FIB 6.95 g/L, INR 1.63, D-dimer 4516 ng/mL. Inflammation indicators showed CRP 30.18 mg/dL and PCT 88.17 ng/mL. Abdominal CT demonstrated signs of acute pancreatitis. The patient was given symptomatic treatments such as acid inhibition, enzyme inhibition, anti-infection, fluid replacement, hypoglycemia, and continuous hemofiltration. Three hours after admission, the patient developed unconsciousness, pale face, and progressive decrease in blood pressure. He was given rescue treatment, but eventually he failed to recover.

### 23.6.3 Review and Treatment

#### 23.6.3.1 Etiology and Inducement

The common causes of acute pancreatitis are mainly gallstones and alcohol misuse. Other factors include hypertriglyceridemia or hypercalcemia, trauma, autoimmune diseases, endoscopic retrograde cholangiopancreatography (ERCP), steroids, drugs, and genetic factors [109–111]. Smoking is associated with nonbiliary acute pancreatitis [112]. Severe acute pancreatitis is associated with obesity and abdominal fat content. Abdominal obesity rather than systemic obesity is an independent risk factor for the development of acute pancreatitis [113]. Common precipitating factors for AP include alcoholism, overeating, excessive fatigue, emotional agitation, excessive stress, strenuous exercise, and consumption of cold and frozen drinks.

#### 23.6.3.2 Lethal Mechanism

The mechanism of sudden death caused by acute pancreatitis is unclear. Current reports indicate that it may be related to the following factors:

##### Shock

Hypovolemic shock from acute pancreatitis is one of the causes of sudden death [114]. The possible mechanism is that pancreatic hemorrhage and necrosis release bradykinin, histamine, and other vasoactive substances to damage the pulmonary microvascular endothelium. Capillary permeability is increased, which promotes the exudation of a large amount of body fluids into the abdominal cavity and retroperitoneal space. The medium dilates small blood vessels, which causes a rapid decrease in the blood volume, and eventually leads to hypovolemic shock.

### Acute Respiratory Distress Syndrome (ARDS)

Acute pancreatitis complicated by ARDS involves intricate mechanisms, including multiple levels of inflammatory waterfall, coagulation, and fibrinolytic system imbalance, and the activation of pancreatic enzymes. These levels are interconnected in a complex network. (1) The inflammatory mediators caused by pancreatic hemorrhage and necrosis can trigger a waterfall-like cascade through "trigger action." A large number of inflammatory factors promote the accumulation and activation of inflammatory cells in lung tissue, aggravate lung tissue damage, and cause ARDS [115, 116]. (2) Pulmonary vascular injury caused by active trypsin: normally, trypsin inhibitors can inhibit the activation process of proteolysis. With an increase of trypsin in the blood circulation, trypsin inhibitors decrease, which can cause active trypsin to activate the kallikrein system and damage the pulmonary blood vessels. Active trypsin initiates the intravascular coagulation process, which promotes fibrin microthrombosis, involving pulmonary microcirculation, leading to ARDS. Autopsy studies have shown that fibrinoid thrombosis can be seen in the blood vessels of the lung tissue of patients with acute pancreatitis [117]. (3) Alveolar collapse caused by phospholipase: pancreatic lecithin is elevated in the serum of patients with hemorrhagic necrotizing pancreatitis. Lecithin is a major component of alveolar surfactants and plays an important role in exercising normal lung function. Lecithinase can accelerate the degradation of lecithin, reduce the activity of alveolar surfactants, atrophy of alveoli, and ARDS appears. At the same time, ARDS can aggravate the process of acute pancreatitis, form a vicious circle, and can affect other organs, eventually leading to MODS.

### Arrhythmia

(1) Enzymes and toxic substances released by pancreatic hemorrhage and necrosis directly damage myocardial cells. (2) Insufficient myocardial perfusion due to low blood volume. (3) Electrolyte disorders, hypokalemia, hypocalcemia, hypomagnesemia, etc. can induce severe arrhythmias and ventricular fibrillation, leading to sudden death.

## 23.6.3.3 Diagnosis

Anyone with epigastric pain, inexplicable shock, or elevated hematuria amylase should consider the possibility of acute pancreatitis. According to the revised Atlanta Classification, the diagnostic criteria for acute pancreatitis are: (1) abdominal pain (acute onset of persistent and severe epigastric pain, often radiating to the back), (2) serum amylase (or lipase) at least three times the upper limit of normal, and (3) abdominal imaging examination (CT, MRI, and ultrasonography) is consistent with the imaging changes of acute pancreatitis. Acute pancreatitis can be diagnosed by having two of the above three criteria [109, 118].

### Clinical Manifestations

Abdominal pain is the main symptom of acute pancreatitis. It is located in the epigastrium and periumbilical regions and often radiates to the back. Most of them are abrupt onset and constant. Nausea, vomiting, and abdominal distention are also frequent complaints. Fever often results from SIRS, secondary bacterial or fungal infection of necrotic pancreatic tissue. Fever and jaundice are more common in biliary pancreatitis. The clinical manifestations of acute pancreatitis leading to sudden death are diverse, and can also be manifested as transient death, death during sleep, death after sudden screaming, and death after coma. Due to the short time from the onset to death, there is probably no typical severe abdominal pain of acute pancreatitis in the clinic. Cases of sudden death because of acute pancreatitis have been reported in the past where diagnosis could not be made until autopsy [119].

#### Imaging

Ultrasound examination within 24–48 h at the beginning of the onset can initially determine the morphological changes of the pancreas and contribute to identify the biliary tract disease [120]. However, gas accumulation in the gastrointestinal tract during acute pancreatitis decreases the accuracy. Contrast-enhanced CT (CECT) scan is recommended as the standard imaging method for diagnosing acute pancreatitis. CECT diagnosis about 1 week after the onset is more valuable and can effectively distinguish the range of fluid accumulation and necrosis. CECT is the gold standard for diagnostic imaging to help establish disease severity [121]. However, the predictive accuracy of CT scoring systems for severity of acute pancreatitis is similar to that of clinical scoring systems. Therefore, it is not recommended to only evaluate the degree of severity of acute pancreatitis during initial admission [122]. In addition, an early CT scan does not show an alternative diagnosis, help with the distinction of interstitial versus necrotizing pancreatitis, or provide evidence of an important complication. An early CT scan is recommended when there is a clinical doubt about the diagnosis of acute pancreatitis, and other life-threatening disorders have to be excluded. In addition, MRI can also assist in the diagnosis of acute pancreatitis.

#### Etiological Diagnosis

The etiology of acute pancreatitis should be determined using detailed personal (i.e., previous pancreatitis, known cholelithiasis, alcohol intake, medication and drug intake, known hyperlipidemia, trauma, and recent invasive procedures such as endoscopic retrograde cholangiopancreatography (ERCP)) and family history of pancreatic disease, physical examination (i.e., body mass index (BMI)), laboratory serum tests (i.e., liver enzymes, blood lipid, calcium, virus, autoimmune marker, and tumor marker (CEA, CA19-9)), and imaging (i.e., right upper quadrant ultrasonography, CECT, magnetic resonance cholangiopancreatography (MRCP), ERCP, ampulla papillary sphincter pressure measurement, and pancreatic exocrine function detection) [117].

#### Graded Diagnosis

The 2012 Revision of the Atlanta Classification Criteria divided AP into the following three categories: mild acute pancreatitis (MAP): not accompanied by organ failure or local or systemic complications; moderate severe acute pancreatitis (MSAP): accompanied by transient organ failure (<48 h) or local or systemic complications; and severe acute pancreatitis (SAP): accompanied by persistent organ failure (>48 h). The diagnostic criteria for organ failure are based on the modified Marshall scoring system. Any organ score ≥2 points can be defined as organ failure [125]. Several scoring systems, such as Rason score system, Bedside Index for Severity in Acute Pancreatitis (BISAP), and modified CT Severity Index (MCTSI) score, have been developed to evaluate the severity of AP and promote clinical decision [122]. MCTSI score uses CT findings to judge the severity of AP, but early CT study can underestimate the severity of the disease [123, 124]. Rason score has 11 indictors including clinical factors, laboratory testing, response to fluid resuscitation, etc. It is cumbersome and not routinely used. BISAP score has five indicators and can be used at any time within 48 h of admission, which is relatively simple and effective for clinician.

#### 23.6.3.4 Treatment

The current treatment model for AP is a combination of internal medicine and multidisciplinary treatment.

##### Fluid Resuscitation

Insufficient blood vessel content is the most prominent pathophysiological change in the early stage of acute pancreatitis. Fluid resuscitation is the cornerstone of early treatment. The 2018 AGA guidelines recommend the use of a target-oriented method for fluid management [126]. Targeted therapy is defined as the titration of intravenous fluids to specific detectable clinical and/or biochemical indicators, such as heart rate, mean arterial pressure, central venous pressure, urine output, BUN, HCT, etc. The types of infusions include lactated Ringer's solution, normal saline, and colloid. At present, there is no high-quality evidence to prove that the recovery effect of lactated Ringer's solution is better than that of normal saline. Expansion with hydroxyethyl starch is not recommended because it can increase kidney damage in patients with sepsis [127].

##### Organ Function Maintenance

(1) Treatment of acute lung injury or respiratory failure: in severe acute pancreatic pancreatitis, oxygen inhalation through nasal tube or mask should be given to maintain oxygen saturation above 95%. Patients' blood gas analysis results should be monitored dynamically. When the disease progressed to ARDS, treatment strategies include mechanical ventilation and the use of high-dose, short-range glucocorticoids, and bronchoalveolar lavage under conditions [128]. (2) Treatment of acute kidney injury or renal failure: the treatment of acute renal failure is mainly supportive treatment, stable hemodynamic parameters, and dialysis. The indication of continuous renal replacement therapy (CRRT) is associated with acute renal failure, or the urine output ≤0.5 mL/kg/h; early with two or more organ dysfunction; SIRS with tachycardia, shortness of breath, the effect is not obvious after general treatment; with severe water and electrolyte disorders; and with pancreatic encephalopathy (PE). Combined with continuous venous-venous hemofiltration (CVVH) and continuous plasma filtration adsorption (CPFA) can be chosen [129]. (3) For SAP patients, special attention should be paid to maintaining the intestinal function. Because the stabilization of the intestinal mucosal barrier has an important role in reducing systemic complications, it is necessary to closely observe abdominal signs and defecation, monitor changes in bowel sounds, and give early

intestinal motility drugs, including rhubarb, magnesium sulfate, lactulose, etc., and use glutamine preparations to protect the intestinal mucosal barrier. Where conditions permit, early diet or enteral nutrition is important to prevent intestinal failure. Probiotics can regulate intestinal immunity and correct intestinal flora imbalance, thereby restoring the intestinal microecological balance. However, it is still controversial whether patients with severe acute pancreatitis should be treated with probiotics.

#### Nutritional Support

AGA recommends oral feeding of patients with acute pancreatitis as early as possible (within 24 h of onset). And enteral nutrition rather than parenteral nutrition is recommended for patients who cannot eat orally [118]. Enteral tube feeding should be the primary therapy in patients with predicted severe acute pancreatitis who require nutritional support but cannot eat. Glutamine should be the supplement. For patients with hyperlipidemia, fat supplementation should be reduced. When performing enteral nutrition, you should pay attention to whether the symptoms and signs of pancreatitis such as abdominal pain, intestinal paralysis, and abdominal tenderness are aggravated, and regularly test the electrolytes, blood lipids, blood glucose, total bilirubin and albumin, blood routine, and renal function, in order to evaluate the body's metabolism and adjust the amount of enteral nutrition [109]. Short peptide preparations can be used first, and then gradually transition to whole protein preparations. The enteral nutrition solution should be selected according to the patient's blood lipid and blood glucose.

#### Drug Treatment

The drug treatment of acute pancreatitis includes the inhibition of pancreatic exocrine and pancreatin inhibitors, adequate analgesia, and the application of antibiotics. At present, there is no breakthrough in drug treatment.

#### Minimally Invasive Treatment

In recent years, minimally invasive technology has developed rapidly and has gradually become the preferred intervention method for complications such as pancreatic necrosis infection and pancreatic pseudocyst. Currently, minimally invasive step-up therapy is considered the standard treatment for infectious pancreatic necrosis (IPN) [130]. Minimally invasive step-up therapy can be divided into two categories: (1) percutaneous retroperitoneal minimally invasive step-up therapy; (2) minimally invasive step-up therapy by stomach and/or duodenum. A large-scale retrospective study in 2016 compared the clinical prognosis of percutaneous retroperitoneal minimally invasive debridement therapy with open necrotic tissue wound surgery. Percutaneous retroperitoneal minimally invasive step-up therapy can reduce complications and mortality.

#### Etiology Treatment

(1) Endoscopic treatment of biliary pancreatitis: At present, ERCP is the first method to relieve biliary obstruction in patients with acute biliary pancreatitis. The IAP/APA guidelines point out that patients with biliary pancreatitis and cholangitis need emergency ERCP within 24 h [14]. For those without common bile duct

obstruction and cholangitis, early ERCP is not beneficial. In recent years, EUS has been used for the examination of common bile duct stones, and it has received increasing attention in the diagnosis and treatment of biliary pancreatitis. It can find small bile duct stones that are difficult to diagnose by MRCP. The IAP/APA guidelines recommend cholecystectomy for patients with mild biliary pancreatitis during hospitalization [118]. Studies have shown that delaying cholecystectomy for several weeks increases the risk of recurrence (up to 30%). However, early cholecystectomy in patients with necrotizing pancreatitis will increase the incidence of infection, and surgery is required after pancreatitis has healed [105]. (2) The incidence of hypertriglyceridemia pancreatitis is gradually increasing. Because HTGP is prone to exacerbation, the triglyceride (TG) level is positively correlated with the severity of the disease at the time of onset. Therefore, early lipid-lowering treatment may reduce the severity of the disease and improve the prognosis of patients with hypertriglyceridemia. The current early lipid-lowering programs can be divided into two categories: noninvasive drug treatment (insulin, heparin, etc.) and invasive blood purification treatment (plasma replacement, hemofiltration, etc.) [130].

### 23.6.4 Discussion

Acute pancreatitis, requires prompt treatment. In the above case, the patient suffered from abdominal pain due to overeating 38 h ago, but failed to pay attention because of previous pancreatitis. He did not fast, and even used nonsteroidal anti-inflammatory drugs (NSAID) on his own during abdominal pain, directly delaying the diagnosis and treatment. At the time of his consultation, he already had MODS and shock. At last, he was prone to sudden death. Because many acute pancreatitis are diagnosed after autopsy, the clinical attention to pancreatitis is insufficient.

### 23.6.5 Conclusion

Acute pancreatitis is one of the most common causes of sudden death in the digestive system. It has rapid onset, many complications, and a high degree of severity. But it is often confused with surgical acute abdomen and other digestive diseases of internal medicine. Once doctors ignore it, it is prone to become severe and even causes sudden death. We share the death case to let everyone know about the danger of acute pancreatitis.

## References

1. Brandt LJ, Boley SJ. AGA technical review on intestinal ischemia. Gastroenterology. 2000;118(5):954–68.
2. Jaster A, Choudhery S, Ahn R, Sutphin P, Kalva S, Anderson M, et al. Anatomic and radiologic review of chronic mesenteric ischemia and its treatment. Clin Imaging. 2016;40(5):961–9.
3. Corcos O, Nuzzo A. Gastro-intestinal vascular emergencies. Best Pract Res Clin Gastroenterol. 2013;27(5):709–25.

4. Brandt LJ, Feuerstadt P, Longstreth GF, Boley SJ. ACG clinical guideline: epidemiology, risk factors, patterns of presentation, diagnosis, and management of colon ischemia (CI). Am J Gastroenterol. 2015;110(1):18–44.
5. Flynn AD, Valentine JF. Update on the diagnosis and management of colon ischemia. Curr Treat Option Gastroenterol. 2016;14(1):128–39.
6. Yadav S, Dave M, Edakkanambeth VJ, Harmsen WS, Tremaine WJ, Zinsmeister AR, et al. A population-based study of incidence, risk factors, clinical spectrum, and outcomes of ischemic colitis. Clin Gastroenterol Hepatol. 2015;13(4):731–8.
7. Brandt L, Boley S, Goldberg L, Mitsudo S, Berman A, et al. Colitis in the elderly. A reappraisal. Am J Gastroenterol. 1981;76(3):239–45.
8. Kozuch PL, Brant LJ. Review article: diagnosis and management of mesenteric ischemia with an emphasis on pharmacotherapy. Aliment Pharmacol Ther. 2005;21(3):201–15.
9. Van der Voort PH, Westra B, Wester JP, Bosman RJ, van Stijn I, Haagen IA, et al. Can serum L-lactate, D-lactate, creatine kinase and I-FABP be used as diagnostic markers incritically ill patients suspected for bowel ischemia. BMC Anesthesiol. 2014;14:111.
10. Assadian A, Assadian O, Senekowitsch C, Rotter R, Bahrami S, Furst W, et al. Plasma D-lactate as a potential early marker for colon ischaemia after open aortic reconstruction. Eur J Vasc Endovasc Surg. 2006;31(5):470–4.
11. Levy E, Menard D, Delvin E, Montoudis A, Beaulieu JF, Mailhot G, et al. Localization, function and regulation of the two intestinal fatty acid-binding protein types. Histochem Cell Biol. 2009;132(3):351–67.
12. Kanda T, Hujii H, Tani T, Murakami H, Suda T, Sakai Y, et al. Intestinal fatty acid-binding protein is a useful diagnostic marker for mesenteric infarction in humans. Gastroenterology. 1996;110(2):339–43.
13. Akyildiz H, Akcan A, Oztürk A, Sozuer E, Kucuk C, Karahan I. The correlation of the D-dimer test and biphasic computed tomography with mesenteric computed tomography angiography in the diagnosis of acute mesenteric ischemia. Am J Surg. 2009;197(4):429–33.
14. Sutherland F, Cunningham H, Pontikes L, Parsons L, Klassen J. Elevated serum interleukin-6 levels in patients with acute intestinal ischemia. Hepato-Gastroenterology. 2003;50(50):419–21.
15. Acosta S, Nilsson TK, Bjorck M. Preliminary study of D-dimer as a possible marker of acute bowel ischaemia. Br J Surg. 2001;88(3):385–8.
16. Woodhams R, Nishimaki H, Fujii K, Kakita S, Hayakawa K. Usefulness of multidetector-row CT (MDCT) for the diagnosis of non-occlusive mesenteric ischemia (NOMI): assessment of morphology and diameter of the superior mesenteric artery (SMA) on multi-planar reconstructed (MPR) images. Eur J Radiol. 2010;76(1):96–102.
17. Resch T, Lindh M, Dias N, Sonesson B, Uher P, Malina M, et al. Endovascular recanalisation in occlusive mesenteric ischemia feasibility and early results. Eur J Vasc Endovasc Surg. 2005;29(2):199–203.
18. Acosta S, Wadman M, Syk I, Elmstahl S, Ekberg O. Epidemiology and prognostic factors in acute superior mesenteric artery occlusion. J Gastrointest Surg. 2010;14(4):628–35.
19. Cangemi JR, Picco MF. Intestinal ischemia in the elderly. Gastroenterol Clin N Am. 2009;38(3):527–40.
20. Wadman M, Syk I, Elmståhl B, Ekberg O, Elmstahl S. Abdominal plain film findingsin acute ischemic bowel disease differ with age. Acta Radiol. 2006;47(3):238–43.
21. Laissy JP, Trillaud H, Douek P. MR angiography: noninvasive vascular imaging of the abdomen. Abdom Imaging. 2002;27(5):488–506.
22. Stathaki MI, Koutroubakis IE, Koukouraki SI, Kouroumalis EA, Karkavitsas NS. Is there a role for Tc-99m(V) DMSA scintigraphy in ischemic colitis? World J Gastroenterol. 2008;14(35):5432–5.
23. Polk JD, Rael LT, Craun ML, Mains CW, Davis-Merritt D, Bar-Or D. Clinical utility of the cobalt-albumin binding assay in the diagnosis of intestinal ischemia. J Trauma. 2008;64(1):42–5.
24. Theodoropoulou A, Koutroubakis IE. Ischemic colitis: clinical practice in diagnosis and treatment. World J Gastroenterol. 2008;14(48):7302–8.

25. Clinical Services and Standards Committee of the British Society of Gastroenterology. U.K. guidelines on the management of variceal haemorrhage in cirrhotic patients. Gut. 2015;64(11):1680–704.
26. De Franchis R, Baveno VI Faculty. Expanding consensus in portal hypertension: report of the Baveno VI Consensus workshop: stratifying risk and individualizing care for portal hypertension. J Hepatol. 2015;63(3):743–52.
27. European Association for the Study of the Liver. EASL clinical practice guidelines for the management of patients with decompensated cirrhosis. J Hepatol. 2018;69(2):406–60.
28. Acute upper gastrointestinal bleeding: management. 2012. NGC:009131 National Clinical Guideline Centre—National Government Agency [Non-U.S].
29. Esophageal varices. World Gastroenterology Organisation Global Guidelines. 2014.
30. Carbonell N, Pauwels A, Serfaty L, Fourdan O, Lévy VG, Poupon R. Improved survival after variceal bleeding in patients with cirrhosis over the past two decades. Hepatology. 2004;40(3):652–9.
31. Tripathi D, Stanley AJ, Hayes PC, Patch D, Millson C, Mehrzad H, et al. UK guidelines on the management of variceal haemorrhage in cirrhotic patients. Gut. 2015;64(11):1680–704.
32. Kim YD. Management of acute variceal bleeding. Clin Endosc. 2014;47(4):308–14.
33. Vorobioff JD, Groszmann RJ. Prevention of portal hypertension:from variceal development to clinical decompensation. Hepatology. 2015;61(1):375–81.
34. Li M, Xu X. Researches on the prevention and treatment of bleeding gastroesophageal varices secondary to portal hypertension in patients with cirrhosis. Zhonghua Gan Zang Bing Za Zhi. 2015;23(4):247–9. (in Chinese)
35. Kim DH, Park JY. Prevention and management of variceal hemorrhage. Int J Hepatol. 2013;2013:434609.
36. Lee YY, Tee HP, Mahadeva S. Role of prophylactic antibiotics in cirrhotic patients with variceal bleeding. World J Gastroenterol. 2014;20(7):1790–6.
37. Hwang JH, Shergill AK, Acosta RD, Chandrasekhara V, Chathadi KV, Decker GA, et al. The role of endoscopy in the management of variceal hemorrhage. Gastrointest Endosc. 2014;80(2):221–7.
38. Chinese Society of Hepatology, Chinese Medical Association; Chinese Society of Gastroenterology, Chinese Medical Association; Chinese Society of Endoscopy, Chinese Medical Association. Guidelines for the diagnosis and treatment of esophageal and gastric variceal bleeding in cirrhotic portal hypertension. J Chin Hepatol. 2016;32(2):203–19. (in Chinese)
39. Hearnshaw S, Logan R, Lowe D, Travis S, Murphy M, Palmer K. Acute upper gastrointestinal bleeding in the UK: patient characteristics, diagnoses and outcomes in the 2007 UK audit. Gut. 2007;60:1327–35.
40. Garcia-Tsao G, Bosch J. Management of varices and variceal haemorrhage in cirrhosis. N Engl J Med. 2010;362:823–32.
41. Garbuzenko DV. Contemporary concepts of the medical therapy of portal hypertension under liver cirrhosis. World J Gastroenterol. 2015;21(20):6117–26.
42. Sarin SK, Kumar A. Endoscopic treatment of gastric varices. Clin Liver Dis. 2014;18(4):809–27.
43. Huang L, Yu QS, Zhang Q, Liu JD, Wang Z. Transjugular intrahepatic portosystemic shunt versus surgical shunting in the management of portal hypertension. Chin Med J. 2015;128(6):826–34.
44. Orloff MJ, Hye RJ, Wheeler HO, Isenberg JI, Haynes KS, Vaida F, et al. Randomized trials of endoscopic therapy and transjugular intrahepatic portosystemic shunt versus portacaval shunt for emergency and elective treatment of bleeding gastric varices in cirrhosis. Surgery. 2015;157(6):1028–45.
45. Chinese Medical Association Surgery Branch, Department of Portal Hypertension. Expert agreement on diagnosis and treatment of esophageal and gastric varices bleeding in cirrhotic portal hypertension. J Pract Surg. 2015;23(10):1086–90. (in Chinese)

46. Hadjihambi A, Arias N, Sheikh M, Jalan R. Hepatic encephalopathy: a critical current review. Hepatol Int. 2018;12(61):135–47.
47. Tranah TH, Paolino A, Shawcross DL. Pathophysiological mechanisms of hepatic encephalopathy. Clin Liver Dis. 2015;5(3):59–63.
48. Elwir S, Rahimi RS. Hepatic encephalopathy: an update on the pathophysiology and therapeutic options. J Clin Transl Hepatol. 2017;5(2):142–51.
49. Ochoasanchez R, Rose CF. Pathogenesis of hepatic encephalopathy in chronic liver disease. J Clin Exp Hepatol. 2018;8(3):262–71.
50. Kenston SS, Song X, Li Z, Zhao J. Mechanistic insight, diagnosis, and treatment of ammonia-induced hepatic encephalopathy. J Gastroenterol Hepatol. 2019;34(1):31–9.
51. Jayakumar AR, Norenberg MD. Hyperammonemia in hepatic encephalopathy. J Clin Exp Hepatol. 2018;8(3):272–80.
52. Zwingmann C, Butterworth R. An update on the role of brain glutamine synthesis and its relation to cell-specific energy metabolism in the hyperammonemic brain: further studies using NMR spectroscopy. Neurochem Int. 2005;47:19–30.
53. Grover VP, Tognarelli JM, Massie N, Crossey MM, Cook NA, Taylorrobinson SD. The why and wherefore of hepatic encephalopathy. Int J General Med. 2015;8(1):381–90.
54. Felipo V. Hepatic encephalopathy: effects of liver failure on brain function. Nat Rev Neurosci. 2013;14(12):851–8.
55. Krieger D, Krieger S, Theilmann L, Jansen O, Gass P, Lichtnecker H. Manganese and chronic hepatic encephalopathy. Lancet. 1995;346(8970):270–4.
56. Chinese Society of Gastroenterology, Chinese Society of Hepatology, Chinese Medical Association. Consensus on the diagnosis and treatment of hepatic encephalopathy in China (Chongqing, 2013). Chin J Hepatol. 2013;21(9):641–51.
57. Amodio P. Hepatic encephalopathy: diagnosis and management. Liver Int. 2018;38(6):966–75.
58. Ferenci P, Lockwood A, Mullen K, et al. Hepatic encephalopatlly—definition, nomenclature, diagnosis ,and quantification: final report of the working party at the 11th World Congresses of Gastroenterology, Vienna. Hepatology. 2002;35(3):716–21.
59. Patidar KR, Bajaj JS. Covert and overt hepatic encephalopathy: diagnosis and management. Clin Gastroenterol Hepatol. 2015;13(12):2048–61.
60. Fischer JE, Rosen HM, Ebeid AM, James JH, Keane J, Soeters PB. The effect of normalization of plasma amino acids on hepatic encephalopathy in man. Surgery. 1976;80(1):77–91.
61. Coronel-Castillo CE, Contreras-Carmona J, Frati-Munari AC, Uribe M, Méndez-Sánchez N. Efficacy of rifaximin in the different clinical scenarios of hepatic encephalopathy. Rev Gastroenterol Mex. 2020;85(1):56–68.
62. Tilg H, Cani PD, Mayer EA. Gut microbiome and liver diseases. Gut. 2016;65(12):2035–44.
63. Schwenger KJ, Clermont-Dejean N, Allard JP. The role of the gut microbiome in chronic liver disease: the clinical evidence revised. JHEP Rep. 2019;1(3):214–26.
64. Dam G, Aamann L, Vistrup H, Gluud LL. The role of branched chain amino acids in the treatment of hepatic encephalopathy. J Clin Exp Hepatol. 2018;8(4):448–51.
65. Liver Failure and Artificial Liver Group, Chinese Society of Infectious Diseases, Chinese Medical Association et al. Guideline for diagnosis and treatment of liver failure. Chin J Hepatol. 2019;27(1):18–26.
66. Wendon J, Cordoba J, Dhawan A, Larsen FS, Manns M, Samuel D, et al. EASL clinical practical guidelines on the management of acute(fulminant)liver failure. J Hepatol. 2017;66(5):1047–81.
67. Flamm SL, Yang YX, Singh S, Falck-Ytter YT. American gastroenterological association institute guidelines for the diagnosis and management of acute liver failure. Gastroenterology. 2017;152(3):644–7.
68. Sarin SK, Choudhury A, Sharma MK, Maiwall R, Al Mahtab M, Rahman S, et al. Acute-on-chronic liver failure: consensus recommendations of the Asian Pacific association for the study of the liver (APASL): an update. Hepatol Int. 2019;13(4):353–90.
69. Shao J, Li S, Liu Y, Zheng M. Extracellular vesicles participate in macrophage-involved immune responses under liver diseases. Life Sci. 2020;240:117094.

70. Dong V, Nanchal R, Karvellas CJ. Pathophysiology of acute liver failure. Nutr Clin Pract. 2020;35(1):24–9.
71. Han T, Li LJ. Guideline for diagnosis and treatment of liver failure. J Clin Hepatol. 2018;35(1):38–44.
72. Tujios SR, Lee WM. Acute liver failure induced by idiosyncratic reaction to drugs: challenges in diagnosis and therapy. Liver Int. 2018;38(1):6–14.
73. Louvet A, Mathurin P. Alcoholic liver disease: mechanisms of injury and targeted treatment. Nat Rev Gastroenterol Hepatol. 2015;12(4):231–42.
74. Im GY. Acute alcoholic hepatitis. Clin Liver Dis. 2019;23(1):81–98.
75. Ishibashi H, Komori A, Shimoda S, Gershwin ME. Guidelines for therapy of autoimmune liver disease. Semin Liver Dis. 2007;27(2):214–26.
76. Yi LP, Zhang W, Wu Z, Duan WJ, Wang Y, Huang J, et al. Present status of diagnosis and treatment of hepatolenticular degeneration. Zhonghua Gan Zang Bing Za Zhi. 2019;27(3):161–5.
77. Emmanuel T, Audrey C, Silvio N, Josh L, Yaman T, Mark G, et al. International liver transplantation consensus statement on end-stage liver disease due to nonalcoholic steatohepatitis and liver transplantation. Transplantation. 2019;103(1):45–56.
78. Andrew DJ, Johnson SE. Acute suppurative cholangitis, a medical and surgical emergency. A review of ten years experience emphasizing early recognition. Am J Gastroenterol. 1970;54:141–54.
79. Shimada H, Nakagawara G, Kobayashi M, et al. Pathogenesis and clinical features of acute cholangitis accompanied by shock. Jpn J Surg. 1984;14:269–77.
80. Gigot JF, Leese T, Dereme T, et al. Acute cholangitis. Multivariate analysis of risk factors. Ann Surg. 1989;209:435–8.
81. Kimura Y, Takada T, Kawarada Y, et al. Definitions, pathophysiology, and epidemiology of acute cholangitis and cholecystitis: Tokyo Guidelines. J Hepato-Biliary-Pancreat Surg. 2007;14:15–26.
82. Attasaranya S, Fogel EL, Lehman GA. Choledocholithiasis, ascending cholangitis, and gallstone pancreatitis. Med Clin North Am. 2008;92:925–60.
83. van den Hazel SJ, Speelman P, Tytgat GN, et al. Role of antibiotics in the treatment and prevention of acute and recurrent cholangitis. Clin Infect Dis. 1994;19:279–86.
84. Tanaka A, Takada T, Kawarada Y, et al. Antimicrobial therapy for acute cholangitis: Tokyo Guidelines. J Hepato-Biliary-Pancreat Surg. 2007;14:59–67.
85. Navaneethan U, Jayanthi V, Mohan P. Pathogenesis of cholangitis in obstructive jaundice-revisited. Minerva Gastroenterol Dietol. 2011;57:97–104.
86. Schwed AC, Boggs MM, Pham XD, et al. Association of admission laboratory values and the timing of endoscopic retrograde cholangiopancreatography with clinical outcomes in acute cholangitis. JAMA Surg. 2016;151:1039–45.
87. Lee BS, Hwang JH, Lee SH, et al. Risk factors of organ failure in patients with bacteremic cholangitis. Dig Dis Sci. 2013;58:1091–9.
88. Yokoe M, Hata J, Takada T, et al. Tokyo Guidelines 2018: diagnostic criteria and severity grading of acute cholecystitis (with videos). J Hepatobiliary Pancreat Sci. 2018;25:41–54.
89. Sulzer JK, Ocuin LM. Cholangitis: causes, diagnosis, and management. Surg Clin North Am. 2019;99:175–84.
90. Umefune G, Kogure H, Hamada T, et al. Procalcitonin is a useful biomarker to predict severe acute cholangitis: a single-center prospective study. J Gastroenterol. 2017;52:734–45.
91. Shinya S, Sasaki T, Yamashita Y, et al. Procalcitonin as a useful biomarker for determining the need to perform emergency biliary drainage in cases of acute cholangitis. J Hepatobiliary Pancreat Sci. 2014;21:777–85.
92. Watanapa P. Recovery patterns of liver function after complete and partial surgical biliary decompression. Am J Surg. 1996;171:230–4.
93. Solomkin JS, Mazuski JE, Bradley JS, et al. Diagnosis and management of complicated intra-abdominal infection in adults and children: guidelines by the Surgical Infection Society and the Infectious Diseases Society of America. Clin Infect Dis. 2010;50:133–64.

94. Gomi H, Solomkin JS, Schlossberg D, et al. Tokyo Guidelines 2018: antimicrobial therapy for acute cholangitis and cholecystitis. J Hepatobiliary Pancreat Sci. 2018;25:3–16.
95. Abboud PA, Malet PF, Berlin JA, et al. Predictors of common bile duct stones prior to cholecystectomy: a meta-analysis. Gastrointest Endosc. 1996;44:450–5.
96. Buyukasik K, Toros AB, Bektas H, et al. Diagnostic and therapeutic value of ERCP in acute cholangitis. ISRN Gastroenterol. 2013;2013:191729.
97. Sun Z, Zhu Y, Zhu B, et al. Controversy and progress for treatment of acute cholangitis after Tokyo Guidelines (TG13). Biosci Trends. 2016;10:22–6.
98. Ramchandani M, Pal P, Reddy DN. Endoscopic management of acute cholangitis as a result of common bile duct stones . Dig Endosc. 2017;29 Suppl 2:78–87.
99. Boulay BR, Lo SK. Endoscopic ultrasound-guided biliary drainage. Gastrointest Endosc Clin N Am. 2018;28:171–85.
100. Miura F, Okamoto K, Takada T, et al. Tokyo Guidelines 2018: initial management of acute biliary infection and flowchart for acute cholangitis. J Hepatobiliary Pancreat Sci. 2018;25:31–40.
101. Liu C-T, Li P, Zhang S-T. ENBD. In: Mine T, Fujita R, editors. Advanced therapeutic endoscopy for pancreatico-biliary diseases. Tokyo: Springer Japan; 2019. p. 51–62.
102. Sharaiha RZ, Khan MA, Kamal F, et al. Efficacy and safety of EUS-guided biliary drainage in comparison with percutaneous biliary drainage when ERCP fails: a systematic review and meta-analysis. Gastrointest Endosc. 2017;85:904–14.
103. Nennstiel S, Weber A, Frick G, et al. Drainage-related complications in percutaneous transhepatic biliary drainage: an analysis over 10 years. J Clin Gastroenterol. 2015;49:764–70.
104. Lai EC, Mok FP, Tan ES, et al. Endoscopic biliary drainage for severe acute cholangitis. N Engl J Med. 1992;326:1582–6.
105. Portelli M, Jones CD. Severe acute pancreatitis: pathogenesis, diagnosis and surgical management. Hepatobiliary Pancreat Dis Int. 2017;16:155–9.
106. Roberts SE, Akbari A, Thorne K, Atkinson M, Evans PA. The incidence of acute pancreatitis: impact of social deprivation, alcohol consumption, seasonal and demographic factors. Aliment Pharmacol Ther. 2013;38:539–48.
107. Vege SS, Gardner TB, Chari ST, Munukuti P, Pearson RK, Clain JE, Petersen BT, Baron TH, Farnell MB, Sarr MG. Low mortality and high morbidity in severe acute pancreatitis without organ failure: a case for revising the Atlanta classification to include "moderately severe acute pancreatitis". Am J Gastroenterol. 2009;104:710–5.
108. Lankisch PG, Schirren CA, Kunze E. Undetected fatal acute pancreatitis: why is the disease so frequently overlooked? Am J Gastroenterol. 1991;86:322–6.
109. Forsmark CE, Vege SS, Wilcox CM. Acute pancreatitis. N Engl J Med. 2016;375:1972–81.
110. Lankisch PG, Apte M, Banks PA. Acute pancreatitis. Lancet. 2015;386:85–96.
111. Whitcomb DC. Genetic risk factors for pancreatic disorders. Gastroenterology. 2013;144:1292–302.
112. Sadr-Azodi O, Andren-Sandberg A, Orsini N, Wolk A. Cigarette smoking, smoking cessation and acute pancreatitis: a prospective population-based study. Gut. 2012;61:262–7.
113. Smeets X, Knoester I, Grooteman KV, Singh VK, Banks PA, Papachristou GI, Duarte-Rojo A, Robles-Diaz G, Kievit W, MGH B, Verdonk RC, Van Santvoort HC, JPH D, Belias M, EJM VG, Dutch Pancreatitis Study G. The association between obesity and outcomes in acute pancreatitis: an individual patient data meta-analysis. Eur J Gastroenterol Hepatol. 2019;31:316–22.
114. Di Paolo M, Marradi I. Haemorrhagic complication of acute necrotizing pancreatitis presenting with sudden death. J Clin Forensic Med. 2006;13:271–3.
115. Pastor CM, Matthay MA, Frossard JL. Pancreatitis-associated acute lung injury: new insights. Chest. 2003;124:2341–51.
116. Browne GW, Pitchumoni CS. Pathophysiology of pulmonary complications of acute pancreatitis. World J Gastroenterol. 2006;12:7087–96.

117. Zhao X, Andersson R, Wang X, Dib M, Wang X. Acute pancreatitis-associated lung injury: pathophysiological mechanisms and potential future therapies. Scand J Gastroenterol. 2002;37:1351–8.
118. IAP/APA evidence-based guidelines for the management of acute pancreatitis. Pancreatology 2013;13:e1–15.
119. Turner B. Acute pancreatitis: symptoms, diagnosis and management. Nurs Times. 2003;99:38–40.
120. Banks PA, Bollen TL, Dervenis C, Gooszen HG, Johnson CD, Sarr MG, Tsiotos GG, Vege SS. Classification of acute pancreatitis—2012: revision of the Atlanta classification and definitions by international consensus. Gut. 2013;62:102–11.
121. Karagoz A, Unluer EE, Oyar O, Topal FE, Topal F. The ability of emergency physicians to diagnose and score acute pancreatitis on computed tomography. Eur J Trauma Emerg Surg. 2017;43:287–92.
122. Bollen TL, Singh VK, Maurer R, Repas K, van Es HW, Banks PA, Mortele KJ. A comparative evaluation of radiologic and clinical scoring systems in the early prediction of severity in acute pancreatitis. Am J Gastroenterol. 2012;107:612–9.
123. Siregar GA, Siregar GP. Management of severe acute pancreatitis. Maced J Med Sci. 2019;7:3319–23. Open Access
124. Balthazar EJ, Ranson JH, Naidich DP, Megibow AJ, Caccavale R, Cooper MM. Acute pancreatitis: prognostic value of CT. Radiology. 1985;156:767–72.
125. King NK, Powell JJ, Redhead D, Siriwardena AK. A simplified method for computed tomographic estimation of prognosis in acute pancreatitis. Scand J Gastroenterol. 2003;38:433–6.
126. Crockett SD, Wani S, Gardner TB, Falck-Ytter Y, Barkun AN. American gastroenterological association institute guideline on initial management of acute pancreatitis. Gastroenterology. 2018;154:1096–101.
127. Zhao G, Zhang JG, Wu HS, Tao J, Qin Q, Deng SC, Liu Y, Liu L, Wang B, Tian K, Li X, Zhu S, Wang CY. Effects of different resuscitation fluid on severe acute pancreatitis. World J Gastroenterol. 2013;19:2044–52.
128. Bhadade RR, de Souza RA, Harde MJ, Khot A. Clinical characteristics and outcomes of patients with acute lung injury and ARDS. J Postgrad Med. 2011;57:286–90.
129. Sun B, Zhang C, Lin T, Liu S, Wang Z, Zhang J, Liu C. Effect of continuous renal replacement therapy during percutaneous drainage in severe acute pancreatitis patients: a retrospective cohort study. Zhonghua Wei Zhong Bing Ji Jiu Yi Xue. 2019;31:714–8.
130. Faghih M, Fan C, Singh VK. New advances in the treatment of acute pancreatitis. Curr Treat Option Gastroenterol. 2019;17:146–60.

# Part V

# Chinese Medicine to Prevent Sudden Death

# Prevention and Control of Sudden Death in Traditional Chinese Medicine

# 24

Xiaoyong Chen and Zengduo Wang

**Abstract**

This section introduces Chinese medicine from six aspects: "The Fundamental Theory of Traditional Chinese Medicine," "Characteristics of TCM in Disease Prevention and Treatment," "Chinese Medicine to Prevent Sudden Death," "Case Analysis," "Characteristics of Traditional Chinese Medicine," and "National Policy for the Development of Chinese Medicine." Theoretical research on the prevention and treatment of sudden death by medicine, the treatment methods, and the special diagnosis and treatment methods related to traditional Chinese medicine have greatly enriched the clinical treatment methods against sudden death. At the same time, Chinese medicine is also an important part of world medicine.

**Keywords**

Traditional Chinese medicine · Holistic concept · Cure for disease · Sudden death
Traditional Chinese medicine technology

## 24.1 The Fundamental Theory of Traditional Chinese Medicine

The fundamental theory of Traditional Chinese Medicine (TCM) is based on the philosophical view of harmony between man and nature. The core concepts of TCM are holism and treatment based on syndrome differentiation. The fundamental theory of TCM mainly includes the theory of Yin and Yang, visceral manifestation (heart, liver, spleen, lung, kidney system), five movements and six climates, essence, Qi and blood (Qi: information-energy-substance theory), constitution, etiology,

X. Chen (✉) · Z. Wang
University of Sanya, Sanya, Hainan, China



H. Zhu (ed.), *Sudden Death*, https://doi.org/10.1007/978-981-15-7002-5_24

pathogenesis, health preservation, and meridian theory. Visceral manifestation serves as the core concept and information-energy-material theory serves as the foundation. These theories expound the physiological and pathological phenomena in the human body and are used to guide clinical diagnosis and treatment. The following is a brief introduction to the theory of Yin and Yang, five elements, visceral manifestation, and Qi, blood essence, and fluid.

### 24.1.1 The Theory of Yin Yang and Five Elements

The theory of Yin Yang and five elements are based on the long-term medical practice of ancient Chinese medical scientists. Yin Yang and five elements are used in the medicine to illustrate the origin of human life, physiological phenomena, and pathological changes and also guide clinical diagnosis and prevention. As important parts of the TCM theory, they have profound impacts on the formation and development of the TCM theory. It can be said that TCM is the philosophy of ancient China, and it is how ancient Chinese understood the nature and the world. Many scholars believe that the ancient Chinese concept of nature, especially the Yin and Yang and the five elements theory hindered the progress of science. When explaining the phenomenon, Chinese natural philosophers often resort to this natural philosophy. For example, electricity is interpreted as "the Yin and Yang interact and form electricity"; the earthquake is considered to be that "Yang is unable to come out, and Yin cannot steam." Thus, the extreme forms of empiricism and mysticism run through the entire ancient Chinese scientific theory system.

### 24.1.2 The Visceral Manifestation Theory

*Questions (Su Wen) · Discussion on Six System and the Manifestations of the Viscera.* "Visceral" refers to the internal organs in the body; "manifestation" refers to the physiological and pathological phenomena that are manifested outside. The visceral manifestation refers to the signs of the physiological activities and pathological changes of the internal organs. For example, Zhang Jingyue wrote in the "Lei Jing (Classified Canon)": "Visceral manifestation means the signs of inner organs." Visceral manifestation theory is the study of the signs of the various organs of the body. The manifestation here includes three aspects, namely the physiological functions, pathological changes, and the interrelationships of various organs. It can be seen that it mainly studies the laws of visceral activities and their interrelationships by observing the signs outside the body.

### 24.1.3 The Theory of Qi, Blood, Essence, and Body Fluid

Qi, blood, essence, and body fluid are the material basis for the physiological activities of meridians and organs. They are the basic substances that constitute the human body and maintain human life activities. The formation of these substances and their metabolism in the body depend on the normal physiological activities of the body, organs, and meridians. Therefore, there is always a close relationship between these basic substances, organs, and meridians in both physiological and pathological conditions.

#### 24.1.3.1 Qi

Qi is a subtle and energetic substance, constantly running in the human body. It is one of the basic substances that constitute the human body and maintain human life activities. The Qi runs continuously, promotes and regulates the metabolism of the human body, and maintains the life of the human body. If Qi stops moving, the life ends.

#### 24.1.3.2 Blood

Blood is a kind of nutritious red liquid substance that travels through the vessels and is one of the basic substances that make up the human body and maintain human life. *Plain Questions:·Discussion on Regulation of Channels* emphasizes that "The Qi and blood constitute the body."

#### 24.1.3.3 Essence

Essence is formed by the combination of a vital material from parents and the acquired nutrition. It is the origin of human life and the basic substance that constitutes the human body and maintains human life activities. For example, as discussed in *Plain Questions:· Discussion on Important Ideas in the Golden Chamber,* "Essence is the foundation of the body." Essence is generally stored in or between the internal organs as a form of liquid. For example, Spiritual Pivot (*Lingshu)·Basic State of Spirit* said, "The five internal organs store essence." As discussed in *Plain Questions:· Special Discussion on Channels and Vessels*, "When food is taken into the stomach, Jing (nutrient substance) is transported to the liver to nourish the sinews."

#### 24.1.3.4 Body Fluid

Body fluid is a general term for all kind of normal water in the body, including the internal fluids of the organs and their normal secretions. Body fluid is one of the basic substances that constitute the human body and sustain life activities. The contents of the body fluid are very extensive. Except for the essence stored in the organs and the blood running in the vessel, all the other normal fluids belong to the body fluid. Therefore, body fluid is not only a basic substance that constitutes the human body, but also one of the basic substances for maintaining human life activities.

## 24.2 Characteristics of TCM in Disease Prevention and Treatment

The diseases prevention and treatment of TCM mainly includes the characteristics of holism, treatment based on syndrome differentiation, and preventive treatment of disease. It not only studies the stage of disease occurrence and development but also highlights the concept of disease prevention.

### 24.2.1 TCM's Concept of Holism

The concept of holism is the idea of unity and integrity. TCM attaches great importance to the unity and integrity of the human body and its relationship with the natural world. It believes that the human body is an organic whole, and the various components that make up the human body are structurally inseparable, functionally coordinated, and mutually supplementary. It also affects each other in pathological conditions. The human body and the natural world are also inseparable. The changes in the natural world affect the human body at any time. Human beings maintain normal life activities in the process of adapting to nature and transforming nature. The concept of holism is the embodiment of ancient Chinese materialism and dialectical; it is reflected in the physiology, pathology, diagnosis, syndrome differentiation, and treatment in TCM

The concept of holism is mainly reflected in the fact that the human body is an organic whole, the unity of human and external environment, the unity of human and natural environment, and the unity of human and social environment.

#### 24.2.1.1 TCM Believes that the Human Body Is an Organic Whole

The human body is made up of several organs and tissues. Each of the organs and tissues has its own unique physiological functions, and these different functions are an integral part of the human body, which determines the internal harmony of the human body. That is to say, the various components of the human body are structurally inseparable, physiologically interconnected, mutually supportive and restrictive, and also interact with each other in pathological conditions. This unity of the human body is centered on the five zang-organs, six fu-organs, and the meridian system. All organs of the human body can be included in the five zang-organs system, which is in the center of human body. The whole body is connected by the meridian system and unified through the functions of essence, Qi, blood, and body fluid.

Under the guidance of the holistic concept, TCM believes that the normal physiological activities of the human body rely on each of the organs to play their own functions. On the other hand, it also relies on the interaction between the organs to maintain their physiological balance. Each of the organs has its own functions but cooperates together, forming the unity of the human body.

In the understanding and analysis of the pathological condition of the disease, TCM also focuses on the overall pathological changes caused by local lesions and considers both the local pathological changes and overall pathological response. In general, the pathological changes in a certain part of the human body are often related to the condition of the organs, blood, Yin and Yang. Due to the physiological and pathological interactions and mutual influences of tissues and organs, it is possible to understand the internal disease through external changes such as complexion, tongue, and pulse and make a correct diagnosis and carry out appropriate treatment.

The human body is an organic whole. When treating local lesions, it is necessary to take appropriate measures from the whole. For example, the tongue is the orifice of the heart, there is an interior—exterior relationsihp between the heart and the small intestine, so the method of clearing the heart and the small intestine heat can be used to treat the erosion of the tongue. It is like "Draw Yang from Yin, draw Yin from Yang, needle the right side to treat the left and needle the left to treat the right" (*Plain Questions:· Major Discussion on the Theory of Yin and Yang and the Corresponding Relationships Among All the Things in Nature*); "If the disease is in the upper part of the body, acupoints located on the lower part of the body can be needled to treat it; if the disease is in the lower part, at the part of the acupoints can be needled" (Spiritual Pivot · Beginning and Ending). These are the principles of treatment under the guidance of the holistic view.

#### 24.2.1.2 TCM Believes that Human and the External Environment Are Unified

The holistic concept of TCM emphasizes the overall harmony of the human body's internal and external environment. It believes that the human body is an organic whole, emphasizing the unity of the internal and external environment of the human body. The so-called external environment refers to the natural and social environment on which human beings live. According to modern medical theory, life systems include eight levels, which are cells, organs, organisms, groups, organizations, communities, societies, and supranational systems. Numerous adjustments are being made to survive in the environment, based on changing material flows, energy flows, and information flows. The relationship between man and nature is the basic component of ancient Chinese philosophy. In ancient Chinese philosophy, the meaning of heaven can be roughly categorized into three types: one refers to the natural sky, the second refers to the heaven of domination, and the third refers to the heaven of righteousness; the meaning of human is roughly two: one refers to the subject of cognition and practice in real life and the second refers to the ideal personality in the sense of value. The relationship between man and heaven essentially includes the relationship between man and nature and society. The ancient Chinese philosophical monism believes that man and nature are unified and the whole universe is unified. Man and nature have material unity and follow the same laws. According to the simple materialism of "Nature and Man have the same Qi," Chinese medicine uses the natural science materials such as medicine, astronomy, and meteorology to demonstrate and enrich the theory of harmony between man and nature, and puts forward that "man and nature correspondence" (*Plain Questions: · Discussion on Cough*) emphasizes that "the man who understands nature can understand human condition" (*Plain Questions: · Discussion on Pain*), and the study of humans is put in the center of human-nature relations.

The external environment includes the natural environment. Man and nature have the same origin and attributes. People are born in nature, and the laws of human life are inevitably regulated and influenced by nature. The material unity of man and nature determines the unity of the laws of life and nature.

Human beings live in the natural world, which provides conditions for human beings to survive. Changes of nature can directly or indirectly affect the human body, and the body undergoes physiological and pathological changes accordingly. The theory "man and nature correspondence" shows that there are changes in the three Yin, three Yang, Six Qi, and five elements. The human body also has the Qi movement of three Yin, three Yang, six meridians, and five zang-organs. The movements of the five elements and the Yin and Yang of nature are in harmony with the movements of the human body. Therefore, the human body and the natural world are closely related. Human beings can not only adapt to nature actively but also actively change nature to maintain health and survive. This is the unity of the human body and the natural environment. It is embodied in the following aspects.

Humans live because of Qi of the nature: TCM believes that Qi is the origin of the world, which is the result of the interaction between Yin Qi and Yang Qi. Nature is the origin of life, and the Yin Qi and Yang Qi provide the most suitable environment for the beginning of life. Life is an inevitable outcome of natural development. Like all things in the nature, people are the product of the Yin and Yang and the result of the regular changes in the material nature. Human beings are born in nature, and nature provides the necessary conditions for the survival of mankind. Therefore, "the heavens feeds people with five Qi, and the earth feeds people with five flavors" (*Plain Questions: · Discussion on Six System and the Manifestations of the Viscera*). Metabolism is a fundamental feature of life and life is both an automatic system and an open system, so it must constantly exchange material, energy, and information with the external environment. Human body is a complex system. Qi is the basic substance that constitutes the human body and the material basis for life-sustaining activities. Lifting in and out is the basic form of Qi movement. In short, human beings are products of nature and survive in nature.

The influence of nature on the human body—the unity of man and nature, the common law of man and nature—is subject to the laws of the Yin and Yang five elements. The physiological activities of human beings change correspondingly with the movements of nature. If you violate the laws of nature, it will lead to adverse consequences.

#### 24.2.1.3 Chinese Medicine Emphasizes the Overall Unity of Human and Social Humanities Environment

TCM believes that the progress and development of humans should be in harmony with the social environment and productivity. One can live and develop better when adapting to the progress and development of the social environment.

### 24.2.2 Treatment Based on Syndrome Differentiation

TCM emphasizes treatment based on syndrome differentiation in all stages of disease development. It is the basic principle to understand and treat diseases and is a special research and treatment method. The commonly used syndrome differentiation methods in clinical practice are as follows: eight-class syndrome differentiation, syndrome differentiation of Qi and blood, syndrome differentiation of viscera, syndrome differentiation of six meridians, syndrome differentiation of

Wei-qi-ying-xue, syndrome differentiation of Sanjiao (Triple Energizer), and syndrome differentiation of meridians.

Syndrome differentiation is the process of understanding syndromes. The syndrome is a summary of the pathological reflection of the body at a certain stage of the disease, including the location, cause, and nature of disease. Thus, the syndrome reveals the nature of the disease more comprehensively, deeply, and correctly than the symptoms. Syndrome differentiation is based on the information collected by the four diagnostic methods. Distinguish and summarize the cause, nature, and location of the disease.

The treatment is based on the results of syndrome differentiation. Syndrome differentiation and treatment are two parts that are inseparable from each other in the process of diagnosis and treatment of diseases. Syndrome differentiation is the premise and basis for treatment. The correctness of the syndrome can be tested by the effect of the treatment. Syndrome differentiation is the process of understanding disease and solving disease. It is also the embodiment of the combination of theory and practice in TCM.

The term syndrome is a pathological summary of a certain disease stage. It is more comprehensive and accurate than the symptoms in revealing the nature of the disease because it includes the location, cause, and nature of the disease, reflecting the nature of the pathological changes at a certain stage of the disease.

"Syndrome differentiation" refers to the analysis of the data, symptoms, and signs collected by the four diagnostic methods (inspection, smelling and hearing, consultation, and pulse-taking). The treatment is based on the results of syndrome differentiation. Syndrome differentiation is the premise and basis, while treatment serves as the means and method.

The process of treatment based on syndrome differentiation is the process of understanding diseases and treating diseases. Syndrome differentiation and treatment are two aspects that are inseparable from each other in the process of diagnosis and treatment. It is a combination of theory and practice. Syndrome differentiation is to analyze, synthesize, and identify the causes, nature, symptoms, and signs (such as pulse and tongue) collected by the four diagnostic methods (inspection, smelling and listening, consultation, and pulse-taking).

TCM focuses not only on the similarities and differences of the "disease" but also on the difference between "syndromes" and further understanding of the disease through syndrome differentiation. For example, a cold may have symptoms such as aversion to cold, fever, and headache and body pain. However, due to the cause of the disease and the reactivity of the body, it is characterized by wind-cold, wind-heat, or summer heat-dampness. Only by discerning which type of syndrome the cold belongs to can we correctly choose different treatment principles and use appropriate treatment methods such as pungent-warm exterior relieving method, pungent-cool or summer-heat relieving method. The treatment based on syndrome differentiation is completely different from the symptomatic treatment of giving painkillers for headaches, giving antipyretics for fever, and taking specific measures for only one symptom. It is also different from the simple treatment of treating all patients with the same disease with the same prescription.

TCM believes that different syndromes can appear in different stages of one disease; different diseases may have the same syndrome. Therefore, in the treatment of diseases, the principle of "different treatment of the same disease" or "same disease with different treatment" can be adopted. "Different treatment of the same disease" means different treatments for different syndromes appearing at different stages of the same disease. For example, in the early stage of measles, when the rash is not appeared completely, the method of promoting rash eruption can be applied; in the middle of the measles, the lung heat is usually obvious, and the treatment must focus on clearing the lung heat; and in the later stage of the measles, the lung Yin and stomach Yin are often impaired so at this time treatment should be based on nourishing Yin and clearing heat. "Different diseases with the same treatment" means that different diseases have the same type of syndrome during the development process, so the same treatment can be used. For example, arrhythmia and amenorrhea are two completely different diseases, but both of them may have blood stasis syndrome. The treatment can be performed with Xuefu Zhuyu Decoction for blood circulation. This principle of solving different contradictions in the process of disease development with different methods is the embodiment of the essence of syndrome differentiation.

### 24.2.3 Preventive Treatment of Diseases

The idea of preventive treatment of diseases in TCM has important guiding significance in the prevention of modern diseases. With the development of society, people's desire for health is growing, and they gradually realize that the simple "treatment of diseases" is passive, and pay more attention to "preventive treatment of diseases." This idea is recognized as one of the most advanced preventive medical thought and has become a hot spot in modern medical research. The idea of "preventive treatment of diseases" has a long historical process, and it is the summarization and sublimation of the combination of practice and theory in the history of the past. It is based on the "Huang Di's Inner Classics" and "Classics on Difficulties" in the Spring and Autumn Period and the Warring States Period. It was developed in the Eastern Han Dynasty from "On Cold Damage," matured in the "On Febrile Disease" of the Qing Dynasty, and gradually became a system after the enrichment and improvement of the ancient doctors.

The theory of preventive treatment of disease is reflected in Huang Di's *Inner Classics* and according to *The Plain Question:·Major Discussion of Regulation of Spirit According to the Changes of the Four Seasons,* "The changes of Yin and Yang in the four seasons are the roots of all the things in nature. So the sages cultivate Yang in spring and summer while nourish Yin in autumn and winter in order to follow such roots. Violation of these roots means destruction of the primordial base and impairment of the body. Thus the changes of Yin and Yang in the four seasons are responsible for the growth, decline and death of all things. Violation of it brings about disasters. This is what to flow the Dao (law of nature) means. The Dao is followed by the sage, but violated by the foolish. Following the rules of Yin and Yang ensures life while violating them leads to death. Abidance by them brings about peace while violation of them results in disorders. If the violation is taken as abidance, disease known as inner conflict will be caused. Therefore, the sages usually pay less attention to the treatment of a disease but more to the prevention of it. To resort to treatment when a disease has already occurred and to resort to regulation when a disorder has already been caused is just like to dig a well when one feels thirsty and to make weapons when a war has already broken out. It is certainly late." This shows the four seasons and the change of the cold and the warm are the foundation of the growth and development of all things. Therefore, people who know how to live according to the laws of nature can maintain the Yang in their own body in spring and summer and maintain the Yin in their body in autumn and winter to obey the fundamental changes of natural cold and heat. If a person violates the fundamentals of Yin and Yang changes in the four seasons, it is damaging the true spirit of his own body. If it obeys it, there will be no stagnation, and this way of obedience to the Yin and Yang is knowing how to maintain health and how to live in accordance with the laws of nature, to obey at all times according to the laws of nature. People who live according to the laws of nature do not need treatment, because they have no disease. If the disease has already been formed, it is like to dig a well when one feels thirsty and to make weapons when a war has already broken out. It is certainly late.

As discussed in *Spiritual Pivot:· The Occurrence of All Diseases,* "Wind, rain, and heat, they cannot attack the body if there is no weakness in the body. If a person is suddenly attacked by strong wind and heavy rain but does not fall ill, it is due to the fact that there is no weakness in his body. Evil cannot attack people under normal condition. The occurrence of disease must be caused by weakness of the body complicated by attack of deficiency-evil. When abnormal changes of weather attack a person whose body is weak, it will damage the body and cause disease; when a person's body is strong and the weather changes are normal, no disease will be caused. The attack of the body by deficiency-evil is due to abnormal changes of weather and weakness of the body. The confrontation between the deficiency and excess gives rise to the occurrence of serious disease." Six evils will not harm the human body alone. Even if someone suddenly suffers from heavy storms and does not get sick, it is because of the Zheng-Qi of his body. But when the person's Zheng-Qi is weak, the evil will make people sick. Some people are sick because of the evil spirits. It is because they are weak when encountering evil spirits. *Plain Questions:* · As written in *Ancient Ideas on How to Preserve Natural Healthy Energy*, "When the sages in ancient times taught the people, they emphasized the importance of avoiding Deficiency-Evil and Thief-Wind in good time and keep the mind free from avarice. In this way Zheng-Qi in the body will be harmony, Essence-Spirit will remain inside, and disease have no way to occur." If the concept of preventive treatment of disease can be applied in people's daily diet, it can effectively prevent the occurrence of some diseases. It is especially important to apply the idea of preventive treatment of disease in critical illness like sudden death.

Sudden death is a natural, unexpected death. According to the standards set by the World Health Organization, it is defined as a noninvasive, unpredictable sudden death that occurs within 6 h. Most of them occur within 1 h of the onset of symptoms. It also defined as 1 h sudden death. Sudden death refers to the irreversible stopping of biological functions. TCM related to sudden death is called phlegm syndrome that includes cardiac arrest, shock, heart failure and coma. It is mainly divided into three categories: Yin collapse syndrome, Yang collapse syndrome and phlegm block syndrome.

## 24.2.4 The Concept of Chinese Medicine Dying

### 24.2.4.1 Reverse Pattern

The main clinical manifestation of reverse pattern is sudden fainting, unconsciousness and coldness of the extremities. If the condition is mild, the patient usually wakes up in a short period of time, but if the condition is serious, the fainting time is much longer, and in the worst conditions, it will lead to death. The causes of reverse pattern mainly include emotional internal injuries, physical fatigue, loss of blood, and abstemious diet. The pathological mechanism is the disorder of qi. It is considered that qi and blood, yin and yang are out of order. "Jingyue Quanshu, Reverse Flow": there are two kinds of reverse qi. One is deficient, the other is excessive. Those who suffer from qi deficiency will have their body and spirit lassitude. For instance, the complexion is pale, the body temperature is cold and the pulse is weak. Those who suffer from excessive qi, their expression looks like angry, the pulse feels like string and wire and the chest feels full. This is called desertion pattern. There are two types of blood desertion. Both the blood collapse and reverse can cause blood desertion. Blood collapse usually occurs while the giving birth, the qi will also be collapsed if the person loses the blood heavily. The blood reverse that is the blood and the qi upsurge to the body. Qi reverse, blood reverse and phlegm reverse are common to reversal patterns diseases. And the are very serious conditions should be treated as soon as possible. The treatment principle is resuscitation.

### 24.2.4.2 Desertion Pattern

Desertion pattern is a critical condition caused by sinister infestation, visceral collapse, qi and blood damage, and yin and yang separation. The main symptoms are sweating, eye-closing and mouth-opening, urine and stool incontinence and unconsciousness which are known as spirit dissipation and obnubilation. Its pathological mechanism is lack of vitality, dysentery, sinister poisoning, consumption of fluids, blood loss, desertion of qi and collapse of yang, damaging of the five internal organs. Because of the exhaustion, yin and yang can not nourish each other, the meridians networks are weakened. The main causes are external scorpion venom, insect venom, sharp injuries, The etiology of desertion pattern are emotional disorders, clinical misuse of sweating, vomiting and excreting. The clinical manifestations are mainly sudden dizziness or fainting, paralyzed limbs, cold sweats on the limbs, freezing cold of the body, incontinence, atrophic tongue, a dark purple tongue with the white sticky coating, a deep and slow pulse. The principle of treatment is to replenish qi, resuscitate yang and strengthen the weakness. The main application prescription is Shenfu Decoction. Desertion pattern is divided into yin and yang, up and down, "Leizhengzhicai, Tuo syndrome" records: discontinued wheeze, shortness of breath, heavy sweat, yang collapse, spirit chaos and dissipated soul. This is yin desertion. Up desertion, down desertion and up and down desertion...there is always yin and yang pivot which is not strong enough. The up desertion patient can not breathe smoothly and sweats heavily. This is so called yang collapse.

The down desertion patient, heavy bleeding, serious excretion, can cause yin desertion. The up and down desertion patient feels dizzy and has stroke, snoring, heavy sweat and incontinence. This is called yin and yang desertion. Ye Tianshi said in the "Clinical Guide Medical Case": the suffocation of internal organs is caused by internal blockage and external desertion. It is considered as the same disease but the blockage inside and the desertion outside.

#### 24.2.4.3 Block Pattern

Block pattern is based on evil and internal block, which is empirical and urgent to go evil. Because of its critical appearance during the coma, the poor prognosis has been transformed into disqualification, causing sudden death. The closed-end block is divided into "yang block," "yin block," "qi block," "heat block" and other blocks. Among them, the main causes of sudden death are "yang block," "yin block" and "qi block."

The Yang block syndrome is common in stroke and viscera. The pathogenesis of the disease is internal damage, excessive labor, unhealthy diet, emotional injury, qi deficiency and evil, always yin and yang disorders, qi and blood disorder. The main clinical manifestations are sudden fainting, unconsciousness, yellow greasy moss, and slippery pulse strings. Treatment should save the yin and return to the sun.

Yin block syndrome is common in strokes and viscera syndrome, which is empirical. The pathogenesis of the disease is caused by the clearing of evil inside. Clinically, the main manifestations are sudden fainting, unconsciousness, tightness of the jaws, lack of mouth opening, solidification of both hands, closeness of the stool, strong limbs, dark lips, restlessness, and limbs are not warm, flow of phlegm, the moss is greasy, and the pulse is slow and gentle. Treatment should be gentle and open, and phlegm and sorrow.

The air-sufficient syndrome refers to the evil spirits of wind, fire, sputum, and sputum, the turbulence of the air, the yin and yang, the occlusion of the sputum, and the stagnation of the nine sputum, the stunned, the jaws closed, the two hands hold, two It will not pass the syndrome of the main symptoms. The main causes of the disease and pathogenesis are the main reasons for the formation of air-sufficiency syndrome: strong mental stimulation, occlusion of the god machine; sandstone, insects, sputum and other obstruction of the veins, lumens, resulting in occlusion of the air machine; drowning, electric shock and other accidents, resulting in Heart and lungs are blocked. Clinically, sudden onset of sudden urgency, severe fainting, or visceral colic, or two occlusions, thick breathing, high sound, strong pulse and string is the main performance. The dialectical basis of the air-tightness syndrome is that it is mainly characterized by sudden fainting or cramping, occlusion of the second stool, thickening of the mass, and pulse. The main cause of sudden death caused by poor prognosis is sedation of air-blocked syndrome and stroke of air-tightness syndrome. Treatment is based on qi stagnation, phlegm and phlegm.

### 24.2.5 The Syndrome Differentiation and Treatment of Chinese Medicine Death

The phlegm syndrome is divided into sputum, blood stasis, and sputum. At the same time, syndrome differentiation of blood stasis and blood stasis must be divided into real and false.

#### 24.2.5.1 Syndrome Differentiation Treatment of Phlegm and Blood Stasis Syndrome

Certificate Name: Discouraged (positive) Symptoms: Sudden by emotional abnormalities, mental stimulation, sudden fainting, I do not know human factors, or cold limbs, breathing gas, mouth fists, thin white tongue, pulse or sinking string. Governing Law: Kailuan, Shuqi, Jieyu. Representative party: Tongguan Sanhe Wujian drinker addition and subtraction. Commonly used TCM: saponin, asarum, agarwood, black peony, betel nut, medlar, woody, sandalwood, clove, musk. Addition and subtraction: If the liver is hemiplegic, dizzy and painful, and the face is red and disturbed, it can be added to the vine, the stone cassia, the magnet, etc.; if there is heat, the disease will see the throat, For those who are suffocated, they can add biliary southern stars, fritillaria, orange red, bamboo leaching, etc.; if they wake up, they will be crying and laughing, and those who are not restful can add sacred gods, distant phoenix, sour jujube and so on.

Name of the certificate: suffocating (defective) Symptoms: There are obvious emotional factors such as emotional tension, fear, pain or standing too long before the onset. The vertigo is dizzy when the attack occurs, pale, weak breathing, sweating cold limbs, pale tongue, and subtle pulse. Governing Law: qi, back to Yang, wake up. Representative side: Shengmai injection, Shenfu injection, Siwei Huiyang drink. Commonly used TCM: ginseng, Ophiopogon japonicus, Schisandra, aconite, gun ginger, licorice. Addition and subtraction: sweating more, add jaundice, atractylodes, calcined keel, calcined oysters, strengthen the effect of Qi, more solid and antiperspirant; heart palpitations, plus Yuanzhi, Baiziren, sour jujube and so on, soothe the nerves; The valley is not fragrant, the appetite is weak, plus atractylodes, sputum, tangerine peel and stomach.

Name of the certificate: bloody (positive) symptoms: Many of them are irritated and angry, suddenly fainting, I don't know the personnel, the teeth are closed, the face is red and purple, the tongue is red, and the pulse string is powerful. Governing Law: Pinggan Qianyang, qi and qi. Representative party: Lingjiao hook vine soup or Tongfu frying addition and subtraction. Commonly used TCM: antelope horn (or goat horn), Uncaria, Angelica tail, safflower, hawthorn, black medicinal, green skin, woody, fragrant, and diarrhea. Addition and subtraction: If you are irritable, the liver is hot, add chrysanthemum, paeonol, gentian; if you see yin deficiency, vertigo headache, add raw land, sputum, mother of pearl.

Certificate Name: Bloody (Dummy Certificate) Symptoms: due to excessive blood loss, sudden fainting, pale, lips without brilliance, limbs tremor, spontaneous sweating, cold mouth, mouth suffocation, weak breathing, pale tongue, pulse or fine powerless. Governing Law: nourishing qi and blood. Representation: Urgent use of ginseng soup, followed by ginseng raising soup. Commonly used TCM: ginseng, astragalus, angelica, rehmannia, white peony, Schisandra, Atractylodes, Poria, Polygala, licorice, cinnamon, ginger, jujube, dried tangerine peel. Addition and subtraction: If the skin is cold, the breathing is weak, add aconite, dry ginger and warm yang; if the mouth is dry and less, add yogurt, jade bamboo, sand ginseng to nourish; heart sputum less sputum, add longan meat, jujube Peace of mind.

Certificate Name: Tan Jue Symptoms: Suffering from cough and phlegm, how wet and sputum, sudden fainting after irritating or severe coughing, throat snoring, or vomiting and sputum, breathing gas, greasy tongue coating, slippery pulse. Governing the law: tempering. Representative: Guided soup added and subtracted. Commonly used TCM: tangerine peel, medlar, pinellia, gallbladder, scorpion, scorpion, white mustard. Addition and subtraction: If the phlegm heat, dry mouth constipation, yellow greasy tongue coating, pulse slippery, add jaundice, medlar, bamboo ru, melon glutinous rice heat and reduce fire.

#### 24.2.5.2 External Treatment of Phlegm and Blood Stasis

1. Acupuncture therapy Main points: Shuigou, Zhongchong, Yongquan, Zusanli. Matching points: Deficiency of the sea, Guanyuan, Baihui; empirical cooperation with Valley, Taichong. Operation: the main point uses acupuncture, the deficiency syndrome uses the supplement method, and the empirical method uses the diarrhea method; the acupoints in the gas sea, Guanyuan, Baihui use moxibustion method; Hegu, Taichong use the diarrhea method.
2. Ear needles Choose Shenmen, adrenal gland, heart, subcortical, acupuncture, strong stimulation, each time 15–30 points.
3. Prevention of phlegm needs to strengthen daily exercise and nutrition, cultivate the sentiment and avoid the vicious spirit and the environmental stimulation.
4. For those who have already issued sputum, it is necessary to strengthen nursing, closely observe the development and changes of the disease, and take corresponding measures to treat.
5. After the patient wakes up, he should eliminate his nervousness and give different diets for different causes.
6. All patients with phlegm and blood stasis should refrain from smoking alcohol and spicy scented products to avoid heat and sputum and aggravate the condition.

#### 24.2.5.3 Disqualification

De-certification is mainly divided into three types: syndromes of gas, yin and yang.

##### Dialectical Treatment of Syndrome Differentiation

Name of the certificate: gas symptoms: pale, ambiguous, low-pitched, tired, tired, sweaty, and cold. Light tongue, white moss, weak pulse card machine: true qi deficiency Governing Law: Yiqi Gutuan Representative: Dushen Soup Commonly used

TCM: ginseng, can also be replaced by Dangshen addition and subtraction: If asthma, add schisandra; sweat leak, add calcined dragon, schisandra, scutellaria; two cannot help, add aconite, cinnamon.

Name of the certificate: Yin symptoms: sorrowful or irritated, flushed, hot and hot, dry mouth, drink, constipation, oliguria, dry skin and wrinkles, red tongue and dry, fine pulse. Card machine: true yin is exhausted Representative: Shengmai San commonly used TCM: ginseng, Ophiopogon japonicus, Schisandra addition and subtraction: imaginary sun rises and sees hot flashes, plus raw oysters, armor, schisandra to nourish yin and yang; dry mouth and throat dry plus stone sputum, pollen, scrophularia stagnation and stagnation; constipation plus Maren, Xuanshen, Shengdizeng liquid intestines.

Name of the certificate: Yangtuan symptoms: suddenly sweating is not only sweating, like sweat, sorrowful, flustered, shortness of breath, cold limbs, incontinence, tongue curling, and pulse. Card: true yang Governing Law: Returning to the Sun Representative party: Shenfu soup Commonly used TCM: ginseng, aconite Addition and subtraction: If sweat is not enough, add schisandra, calcined keel, calcined oysters; heart sputum chest tightness, add magnets, white sputum; limbs cold, add cassia twig, angelica; Qizhao plus Schisandra, jaundice.

#### Prevention of Syndrome

1. Active treatment of primary disease, such as tonifying spleen and qi, converging and stopping bleeding, regulating yin and yang, clearing heat and detoxification
2. Adjust the emotions, ventilator, avoid stagnation of liver qi and fire and damage of blood yin
3. Diet, avoid eating fat and spicy and spicy products, in order to prevent damage to the spleen, lack of the blood
4. Because of deficiency of kidney fire, the seniors, should avoid overwork and cold stimulation, because of too much labor and qi deficiency, the coldness is damaging the yang, and finally become the collapse of yang.

### 24.2.5.4 Closed

Closed card mainly introduces the positive closedness, yin closed and air-closed syndrome with poor prognosis or critical illness during coma.

1. Yangshuo certificate: Certificate Name: TanrefushiZheng Clinical manifestations: suffering from headache, dizziness, upset and irritability, sudden onset, hemiplegia, tongue slanting, strong tongue, unclear or faint, sturdy and sticky. The tongue is dark red, or has a freckle, and the pulse is slippery. Governing Law: venting heat all night, extinguishing wind and turning phlegm. Formula: Taoren Chengqi Decoction. Commonly used TCM: peach kernel, licorice, mirabilite, rhubarb. Acupuncture treatment often takes acupuncture treatments such as Twelve Wells, Shuigou, Taichong, Laogong, and Fenglong.

   Name of the certificate: TanhuoyuzhiZheng Clinical manifestations: symptoms of closed syndrome plus facial redness, bad breath, bad breath, and restlessness. The yellow moss is greasy, and the pulse string is slippery. Governing Law: Extinguish the wind and clear the fire. Prescription: Addition and subtraction of antelope hook and vine soup. Commonly used TCM: Antelope tablets, frost mulberry leaves, Jingchuan shell, fresh raw land, double hook vine, chrysanthemum, Fu wood, raw white shao, raw licorice.

2. Prevention of Yangshuo prevent: A light diet, regular living, and avoid overwork. After the illness, strengthen the care. In the coma, closely observe the changes in the condition, pay attention to changes in face, breath, sweating, etc., to prevent the conversion to the syndrome.
3. Yin closed certificate: The yin closed test is urgently treated with Su Hexiang Pills (or nasal feeding) to warm the aroma, followed by the decoction of the phlegm and phlegm. Commonly used Chinese medicines include Su Hexiang, benzoin, borneol, buffalo horn concentrate powder, artificial musk, sandalwood, agarwood, clove, fragrant, woody and so on.
4. Air tightness certificate: Name of the certificate: suffocation Symptoms: God is dizzy, his teeth are closed, his hands and feet are cautious, like a stroke but no mouth sputum, the sequelae of hemiplegia, the pulse is late. Etiology and pathogenesis: mood swings, anger is on the air, against the gas on the rush to clear the blind, blinded. Governing Law: Reversing qi, dispersing and opening and closing. Commonly used prescription: Bawei Shunqisan. Commonly used TCM: ginseng, atractylodes, medlar (peeling), green skin, dried tangerine peel (to white), white peony, black medicinal herbs, licorice.

   Name of the certificate: a gas-closed card stroke Clinical manifestations: stroke faint servant, unconscious, mouth and eyes skewed, half-length body, closed jaws, two hands holding solid, face red gas, snoring, restlessness, dry stool, yellow greasy moss, pulse string number. Etiology and pathogenesis: liver gas rises indefinitely, blood and blood reverse, and the folder is smoldering, clearing sputum occlusion. Governing Law: Open and close, open the wind and wind. Commonly used prescriptions: Zhibao Dan; Zhengan Xifeng Decoction. Commonly used TCM: Achyranthes bidentata, raw vermiculite (rolling fine), raw keel (mashed), raw oyster (mashed), raw turtle version (mashed), Sheng Hang, Scrophulariaceae, Asparagus, Chuanxiongzi (Crushed), raw malt, capillaris, licorice.
5. Prevention of air-tightness syndrome: After the illness, care should be strengthened. In the case of visceral coma, it is necessary to closely observe changes in the condition, pay attention to changes in facial appearance, breathing, sweating, etc., in order to prevent the transformation to occlusion. Strengthen oral care, promptly remove sputum, feed or nasal feeding Chinese medicine should be a small number of frequent service. During the recovery period, it is necessary to strengthen the passive activities of the limbs, perform various functional exercises, and cooperate with acupuncture, massage, physiotherapy, massage and so on. If the hemiplegia is severe, the affected limb will be prevented from being deformed due to pressure. Language disadvantaged, should strengthen language training. Long-term bedridden, protects local skin and prevents acne.

### 24.2.6 First Aid Methods for Sudden Death of Chinese Medicine

The first-aid methods of Chinese medicine for sudden death are mainly reflected in three aspects: external treatment of acupuncture, internal administration of Chinese patent medicine, and injection, which are introduced as follow:

#### 24.2.6.1 Acupuncture

**Body Needle**

1. Acupoints: Philtrum, Ten Xuan, Shaoshang, Neiguan, Baihui, Yongquan, Xinshu. Limb twitching plus Hegu, Taichong; snoring in the throat plus fenglong, sputum. Operation: Take a strong stimulation method, the above order is appropriate.
2. Philtrum, Feishu, Suliao, Ten Xuan, Quchi. Operation: Take a strong stimulation to disperse the lung Qi.

**Moxibustion Method**

1. Acupoints: Qihai, Guanyuan, Shenque, Baihui, Zusanli, Yongquan, Xinshu. Operation: Acupuncture and moxibustion can be used together for Zusanli and Neiguan. The technique should be gently applied. Moxibustion should be applied for the remaining points including Qihai, Shenque Guanyuan to achieve recovered pulse, arrested sweat and warm limb.
2. Philtrum, Danzhong, Baihui, Hegu, Zusanli. Operation: Burning rush moxibustion. Burning rush moxibustion is one of the moxibustion methods which refers to the moxibustion method of burning directly on the acupoints after ignition with the lamp grass vegetable oil. Also known as lamp grass moxibustion, lighting, quenching. When operating, apply an appropriate amount of oil and move quickly to prevent burns caused by fuel drops. When the flame is burning the skin of the acupoints, a slight "shoot" sound can be heard, and the light is extinguished, which is called a sputum. Each acupoint usually can only apply a moxibustion. After moxibustion, the area might be slightly red, and should be cleaned to avoid infection.

**Ear Acupuncture**

Acupoints: heart, brain point, subcortical, adrenal gland. Operation: Take all the upper points, choose one ear, strong stimulation, leaving the needle until the recovery of heartbeat and waking of the patient.

**Triangular Needle**

1. Acupoints: Shaoze, Ten xuan, Philtrum, Baihui. Operation: Use a triangular needle to puncture, squeeze a few drops of blood, to strengthen the heart and pulse, protect the brain and refresh the mind.
2. Acupoints: Philtrum, Feishu, Suliao, Ten Xuan, Quchi. Operation: puncture with a triangular needle, squeeze out a few drops of blood to disperse the lung and promote Qi.

## 24.3 Characteristic Chinese Medicine for Preventing Sudden Death

1. Angong Niuhuang Pill, Zhibao Dan, and Su Hexiang Pills were administered by nasal feeding to refresh the brain.
   (a) Formulation of Angong Niuhuang Pills: bezoar, buffalo horn concentrate, artificial musk, pearl, cinnabar, realgar, berberine, astragalus, medlar, turmeric, borneol.
   (b) Formulation of ZhiBao Dan: raw black rhinoceros (buffalo horn generation), raw oysters, amber, cinnabar, realgar, bezoar, borneol, musk, benzoin, gold foil, silver foil.
   (c) Formulation of Su Hexiang Pills: Su Hexiang, benzoin, borneol, buffalo horn concentrate, artificial musk, sandalwood, agarwood, clove, fragrant, woody, frankincense (system), medlar, atractylodes, medlar meat, cinnabar.
2. The Tongguan Powder is blown into the nose to induce sneeze to reveal the lungs.
3. Four flavors of Huiyang drink is used to recuperate depleted Yang and to treat collapse.

### 24.3.1 Injection

1. Shenfu injection is used to recuperate depleted Yang and to treat collapse;
2. Qingkailing injection, Xingnaojing injection, Xuesaitong injection is used to refresh the brain, and to strengthen heart and pulse.
3. Shenmai injection is used to replenish Qi and to save Yin.

## 24.4 Case Analysis

### 24.4.1 Ancient Chinese Case

The most famous case of Chinese medicine to prevent sudden death is probably the story of a famous doctor Bianque. There is a record in the "Historical Records of the Biography of Bianque and Canggong": Bianque was around the Guo Country, and the prince of Guo Country was dead. ...... Bianque said: "I come from Qi, Bohai, Qin Yue... I heard that the prince unfortunately died, I may be able to make him alive again... Bianque asked his student Ziyang to sharp the needles with a stone and to apply acupuncture on the points of Wai Sanyang Wuhui. After a while, the prince come alive..." This story told about that Bianque went to the Guo Country and heard that the prince of the Guo Country was dead for less than half a day and has not been put into a coffin. So he rushed to the palace gate to tell the minister, saying that he could bring the prince back to life. The Chinese minister thinks that what he said is a nonsense, and that there is a reason for resurrection. Bianque sighed and said: "If you don't believe me, try to see the Prince. You should be able to hear his tinnitus, his nose is swollen, and the warmth of the thighs and the genitals." the minister reported that to the King. The King was shocked and came out to meet Bianque.

Bianque said: The illness that the Prince received was the so-called "corpse." People accept the Qi of yin and yang between the heaven and the earth. Yang controls the upside and the outside, yin controls the downside and the inside, and the harmony of yin and yang means a good health. Now the yin and yang of the Prince are dysfunctional, while the inside and the outside are unreasonable and the up and down are unreasonable, causing the princes to have confused Qi and pulse, pale, no consciousness, and a dead silence. In fact, he is not dead. Bianque asked his student to give first aid with acupuncture, and stabbed the prince's Sanyang and Wuhui points. Soon the Prince really woke up. Bianque further adjusted the prescription, so that the prince can sit up. The decoction was used to regulate yin and yang. For more than 20 days, the illness of the prince was cured. After the incident came out, people said that Bianque had the stunt of make the dead come back to life.

In addition, the first emergency handbook of China "The Elbow Reserve Emergency" recorded 36 prescriptions for the treatment of sudden death in the use of external stimulation methods, such as "Scallions" "Nasal, male left, female right," "onion piercing ears," "sudden death and limbs do not receive, Yakita. Horse urine one liter, water three buckets, boils into two buckets to wash. Also take a cow hole a liter, Warm wine is poured into the mouth. The cave, the thin manure is also. The moxibustion each points 100 hundred times including 1 in. below the heart, 3 in. upward of the umbilicus, and 4 in. below the umbilical, to cure."

### 24.4.2 Modern Case

*Case 1*: Patient Ji, male, 43 years old. First diagnosed on May 15, 1967. Suddenly fainted in May last year, limbs cramps, no foaming. At the beginning, the illness happened every 1–2 months, and the frequency gradually increased to every 2–3 days. After treatment with Chinese and Western medicine, the effect was not obvious. At present, the patient feels weak, dizzy, and is easy to wake up at night, and the appetite is about 75 g. The tongue is greasy and the pulse is slippery. The symptom belongs to the sputum certificate—the wind and the sun are disturbed, the sputum is turbidity inside, and the plan is to flatten the liver and stagnate the yang.

30 g of mother-of-pearl, 60 g of raw iron, 9 g of white peony, 9 g of southern star, 9 g of sarcophagus, 30 g of night vine, 15 g of cassia seed, 3 g of medlar, 5 doses.

On the 20th of May, the second diagnosis: there is on fainting and convulsions in the past 5 days, and dizziness has been significantly improved, the appetite has also increased, the spirit is better than before. The greasy coating on the tongue is light, the pulse is slippery. The mother of pearl is removed from the original prescription and to administrate another ten doses. After treatment with the adjustment of prescription according to the symptom for 1 month, the illness was cured on June 22, and the patient returned to work. There was no recurrence after 4 years of follow-up. (Note: selected from Longhua Hospital affiliated to Shanghai College of Traditional

Chinese Medicine. Selected from Medical Cases. Shanghai People's Publishing Press. 1977)

*Case 2*: Patient He, female, 26 years old. Because of the loss of blood after the initial birth, she feel awkward. One day, she suddenly fainted, and become unconscious and pale, she wake up when she was moved and behave as normal. At the beginning, she thought it was accidental and did not keep in mind. After that, she had frequent episodes which occurred every two to three days for up to dozens of times. Multi-party treatment is not effective. The pulse is weak, the tongue is reddish and the moss is not covered, the complexion is opaque, there is no convulsions in the hands and feet, the eyes are skewed, and the sputum is up. It is not a stroke, but a bloody sputum. Expelling yin and yang, and using Baiwei Tang to taste.

Codonopsis 30 g, Angelica 24 g, Baiwei 10 g, Salvia miltiorrhiza 10 g, jujube kernel 12 g, licorice 10 g. The patient was cured after the administration of more than ten doses. No recurrence was seen in 3 years. (Note: selected from the Hunan Provincial Institute of Traditional Chinese Medicine. Hunan Province, the old Chinese medicine doctor case selection · Zeng Shaozhen. Hunan Science and Technology Press · 1981 medical case three)

## 24.5 Traditional Chinese Medicine

The characteristic technology of TCM mainly introduces the external treatment methods of TCM, including acupuncture, cupping, scraping and some external treatment methods of ethnic minorities.

### 24.5.1 Acupuncture

Acupuncture is a general term for acupuncture and moxibustion. Acupuncture consists of "needle" and "moxibustion" and is an important part of Oriental medicine. Its contents include acupuncture theory, acupoints, acupuncture techniques and related instruments. In the process of formation, application and development, it has a distinct Chinese national cultural and regional characteristics are a valuable legacy based on Chinese culture and scientific traditions. In 2006, the Chinese Academy of Traditional Chinese Medicine reported that acupuncture and moxibustion were listed in the first batch of national intangible cultural heritage by the State Council.

In ancient China, people accidentally bumped some parts of the body surface with some hard objects such as stones and thorns, and pain was alleviated unexpected. The ancients began to consciously use some sharp stones to puncture certain parts of the body or artificially puncture the body to bleed to relieve pain. People have mastered the techniques of excavation and grinding, and can produce some more sophisticated stone tools suitable for piercing the body to treat diseases. This stone is the oldest medical tool meteorite. People use the "meteorite" to penetrate a part of the body to treat the disease. At the time, meteorites were more commonly used for incision and drainage of surgical suppurative infections, so they were also called needle stones or stones. "Shan Hai Jing" said: "There are stones like jade, can be needles," which is an early record of stone needles. China has discovered meteorites in archaeology. It can be said that meteorite is the foundation and predecessor of the tool of the later generation.

Moxibustion is produced after the discovery and use of fire. In the process of using fire, people found that the pain in a certain part of the body was relieved or eliminated by the burning and baking of the fire, and then learned to use the animal skin or bark to wrap the hot stones and sand for local hot ironing which was further developed to ignite branches or hay to treat diseases. After a long period of exploration, the flammable Ai Ye, which has the function of Wentong meridian, was chosen as the main material for moxibustion treatment, and it is warmly stimulated on the surface of the body surface, so that moxibustion and acupuncture become an important method for disease prevention and treatment. Because it has the characteristics of easy burning, fragrant aroma, abundant resources, easy processing and storage, it has become the most important moxibustion raw material. "Broken and stabbed" gradually developed into acupuncture, "hot and ironed" gradually developed into moxibustion, which is the predecessor of acupuncture therapy.

Acupuncture therapy was first seen in the book The Yellow Emperor's Internal Classics, which was published in the Warring States Period. "The Yellow Emperor's Internal Classic" said: "Hidden cold is full of disease, and moxibustion is recommended for its treatment," it refers to moxibustion, which describes the shape of the nine needles in detail, and a large number of acupuncture theory and technology. The needle of the needle tool, the traditional needle, the word from gold to salt, the "gold" means "metal," such as gold, silver, bronze and other materials, "salty" means "sour," "gold" and "Salty" united to say: "an appliance that produces a sour feeling." It is not excluded that the ancients used fried bamboo needles as a disposable needle. The name of this bamboo needle is "Zhen," and the "salty" in its shape is still the meaning of "sour sputum."

The needle method refers to pierce the needle tool (usually refers to the needle) into the body of patient at a certain angle under the guidance of the theory of TCM, and using acupuncture methods such as twisting and lifting to stimulate specific parts of the body to achieve the purpose of treating diseases. The point of penetration is called the body acupoint, referred to as acupuncture points. According to the latest acupuncture textbook statistics, the human body has a total of 361 positive acupoints. The moxibustion method uses pre-made moxibustion or moxibustion grass to burn, smoke and iron on certain acupuncture points on the body surface, and uses heat stimulation to prevent and treat diseases. Usually Ay Tsao is most commonly used, so it is called moxibustion, and there are other methods such as moxibustion, wicker moxibustion, wick moxibustion, and mulberry moxibustion. And moxa moxibustion is most commonly used today.

### 24.5.2 Cupping

Cupping is therapy of action using cans as the tool to generate negative pressure by means of burning, pumping, etc., so that it is adsorbed on the body surface, causing local blood stasis, so as to achieve the passage of vitality, qi and blood circulation, swelling and pain relief, hurricane and cold, etc. Cupping therapy has a long history in China. As early as in the book of the Western Han Dynasty, the book "Fifty-two Diseases" has a record of "corner method." The corner method is similar to the cupping therapy of later generations. Cupping therapy had also been prevalent in ancient Greece and ancient Rome.

Initially cupping therapy was mainly used for surgical treatment of sores to absorb blood and drain. With the continuous deepening of medical practice, the tool materials and methods of operation have been improved and developed. Some experts believe that the mechanism of cupping therapy from the physiological physiology It belongs to an arterial congestion (medically referred to as fill-in-filled hyperemia), which is beneficial to the body and can increase the supply of oxygen and nutrients in the local blood circulation. The main manifestations are small arteries and telangiectasia, increased local blood content, mild swelling of organs or tissues, slightly increased volume, bright red color, and dark purple color in patients with severe or long disease, which may cause blood stasis for a long time. Functional activity is also enhanced due to local arteriole expansion, increased blood flow, enhanced material metabolism, and elevated temperature. This symptom can disappear quickly or after a while. Modern use of cupping is often in conjunction with acupuncture to gradually expand the scope of treatment including the illness of internal, external, maternal and pediatric.

There are many kinds of cupping tools. At present, glass jars, bamboo cans, gas cans, etc. are mainly used in clinical practice.

Cupping is relatively simple in clinical operation, easy to take, ignited with tweezers and alcohol cotton balls, and then pulled out in the cans; quickly cover the cans on the parts to be extracted and suck them.

### 24.5.3 Application Methods and Precautions of Cupping

The application of cupping is mainly divided into retained cupping, movable cupping, flash cupping, and a method of bloodletting treatment by acupuncture.

1. Retained cupping: After the can is adsorbed on the body surface, the can is sucked and removed and placed in the operation site, generally for 5–10 min; mostly used for cold and dampness, neck and shoulder pain.
2. Movable cupping: Apply the oil to the cans, hold the cans, hold the bottom of the cans, push and pull up and down several times, until the skin is flushed; for large areas, muscles, such as the back; multi-purpose In the case of colds, coughs and other diseases.

3. Flash cupping: Immediately after the jar is pulled out, it is repeatedly sucked up and down several times until the skin is flushed; it is mostly used for facial paralysis.
4. Pricking cupping: first use a plum blossom needle or a triangular needle in local spurs or puncture bleeding; then cupping to make the tank bleeding 3–5 ml; mostly used for skin diseases such as acnes.

When cupping, do not burn the opening of the can, otherwise it will burn the skin; the time of keeping the can should not exceed 20 min, otherwise it will damage the skin; the skin areas with allergies, ulcers, edema and heart, large blood vessels, lower abdomen, are not suitable for cupping.

### 24.5.4 Scraping

The scraping is guided by the theory of TCM meridians and acupoints. Through special scraping instruments and corresponding methods, a certain medium is taken, repeated scraping and rubbing on the body surface, until red miliary or dark red bleeding spots appear on the skin or "Out of the sputum" changes, in order to achieve the effect of promoted blood circulation. Because of its simplicity, convenience, low cost and efficiency, it has a wide range of clinical applications and is suitable for medical and family health care. Scraping can also be used in combination with acupuncture, cupping, puncture and bloodletting to strengthen the effect of promoting blood circulation, removing evil spirits and detoxifying.

### 24.5.5 Common Tools

#### 24.5.5.1 Types of Scraping Plates

Common tools for scraping mainly include scraping plates and scraping oil. The material of the scraping tool is not fixed and has various forms. Many daily utensils can be used as scraping tools, such as copper coins, silver yuan, porcelain spoons, tender bamboo boards, cotton yarns, clam shells, etc. Now there are modern materials such as resin and silica gel. The scraping tools made for clinical applications are mainly made from horns, jade and vermiculite, and each has its own characteristics.

1. Horn scraping board in the clinical use is mainly made from buffalo horn. Buffalo horny taste, salty, cold, Xin can divergence, qi and blood swelling; salty soft and firm; cold can clear away heat and detoxification, cool blood and shock. The texture is tough, smooth and durable, rich in raw materials and easy to process. The horn-shaped scraping board should avoid hot water for a long time soaking, roasting or electric baking; after scraping, the scraper should be dried immediately, coated with olive oil, and stored in the scraper sleeve.

2. Jade scraping board is more suitable for facial scraping, because its material jade texture is gentle and smooth, easy to hold, comfortable to touch, and has the functions of moisturizing and stimulating muscles, clearing away heat and detoxifying, calming and calming the nerves, and warding off evil and turbidity. It should be cleaned after use. Avoid collisions; avoid contact with chemical reagents.
3. Stone scraping board is made from the Suibin pumice stone. This stone contains a variety of trace elements. The infrared radiation band is extremely wide, which can dredge the meridians, clear away heat and detoxification, soften and firm the knot, and can warm the skin of the human body. The scraped vermiculite scraping plate has a thickness of less than 3 mm. Because vermiculite may contain harmful substances, it is necessary to carefully distinguish the authenticity when purchasing. It is necessary to purchase meteorites do not contain harmful substances that are tested by national authorities.

#### 24.5.5.2 Types of Scraping Oil

Scraping oil is mainly divided into liquids and creams.

1. Liquids mainly include cold boiled water, vegetable oil (such as sesame oil, tea seed oil, rapeseed oil, soybean oil, peanut oil, olive oil), medicated oil (such as safflower oil, bruise oil, rheumatoid oil), etc., not only prevent the scraping board scratches the skin and can also moisturize the skin, open pores, and promote blood circulation. In addition, it is also possible to use Chinese herbal medicines with the functions of clearing away heat and detoxifying, promoting blood circulation to remove blood stasis, relieving pain, that are boiled into a liquid medicine according to the symptom. Scraping oil should be used and store away from fire; skin allergies are banned for scrapping, and the areas with trauma, ulcers, scars, and malignant tumors are partially banned for scrapping.
2. Cream refers to the choice of fine texture of paste-like substances, such as vaseline, moisturizer, snake oil, Futalin cream. The TCM extract having the functions of promoting blood circulation, relieving pain, and aroma opening can also be used as a cream. Cream products should be stored in the dark, dry and cold place; appropriate scraping medium should be selected according to the needs of the disease, such as Futalin cream has analgesic and anti-inflammatory effects, and is effective for rheumatic joint disease.

### 24.5.6 Clinical Application

#### 24.5.6.1 Operation Key Points

When scraping, fully expose the scrapping area and evenly apply a medium such as scraping oil to the skin. The operator holds the scrapping board in the hand, firstly with light and slow techniques. After the patient adapts, the technique gradually increases and accelerates, so that the patient can tolerate it. When scraping, it should be unidirectional, follow the meridian wiping, focus on the pain points, acupuncture points, and wipe out the sputum. Generally, you can first wipe the back Du Meridian and the foot sun bladder through the back Shu point to follow the route, invigorate the yang, adjust the function of the viscera and enhance the disease resistance; then scrape the local Ashi or the acupoint according to the symptom, you can get better curative effect. After scraping, the patient should drink warm boiled water to help the body detoxify and exorcise.

#### 24.5.6.2 The Application of Scraping

Scraping has the functions of regulating blood circulation, promoting blood circulation, relieving collaterals, exorcism and detoxification, and has been widely used in the treatment of various diseases such as internal, external, maternal and pediatric, as well as beauty and health care. Especially suitable for painful diseases, bone and joint degenerative diseases such as cervical spondylosis, recovery of frozen shoulder; for cold, fever, cough and other respiratory diseases, scaping can be used in clinical combination with cupping; for acne, chloasma and other damage-causing diseases, it can be used in combination with acupuncture, puncture and bloodletting, etc.; it is also suitable for the prevention and treatment of sub-health, chronic fatigue syndrome and other diseases.

#### 24.5.6.3 Scraping Precautions

1. After scraping, 1–2 days, the occurrence of local mild pain, itching and other symptoms are normal; cold bath; in the summer should be avoid in 30 min after the sputum; the fan or air conditioner should not be blown straight; in winter, keep warm.
2. Scraping therapy has strict direction, time, technique, strength and indications, contraindications and other requirements. Improper operation can easily cause uncomfortable reaction, even the condition is aggravated, it should strictly follow the operating rules or follow the doctor's advice, and should not be operated randomly at home.
3. Patients with bleeding tendency, high extent of skin irritation, extreme weakness, and severe heart failure should be banned for scraping or carefully scraped.

### 24.5.7 Special Treatment Methods for Ethnic Minorities

#### 24.5.7.1 Line Moxibustion in Zhuang Medicine

Medicine line moxibustion is a folk therapy that has been passed down in Zhuang. It is ignited by Chinese medicinal herbs and ignited by TCM. It directly burns the specific acupuncture points or parts of the body surface of for moxibustion to achieve the purpose of treating diseases. It is the traditional natural therapy of Zhuang nationality in Guangxi, China. The material of the moxibustion therapy is a medicine line, which is made by ramie and processed by soaking in a precious drug solution. Each line of the medicine line is 30 cm long, and each ten pieces are tied into one bundle. The size is divided into three types: the diameter of the first drug line is 1 mm, which is suitable for acupuncture points in the thicker parts of the moxibustion for the treatment of sputum diseases, or for the use of moxibustion in winter; the diameter of the second medicine line is 0.7 mm, which is the most commonly used one. It is suitable for various diseases; the diameter of the third medicine line is 0.25 mm, which is suitable for acupuncture points where the skin of the moxibustion is thinner or the moxibustion treatment of children. The spare medicine line should be bottled, tightly covered, placed in a dark and dry place, not placed in a place with high temperature or near the stove, and should not be exposed to sunlight or strong light, and should be protected from moisture and mildew, so as not to affect the efficacy. Zhuang medicine sprouted in the primitive society. In the long-term labor and life practice, the Zhuang ancestors gradually recognized the nature and role of drugs and mastered simple methods of treatment. In fact, the so-called medicine line moxibustion therapy, mystery is hidden in the lines. These special lines are soaked in various herbs and heated by an alcohol lamp to point to a specific acupuncture point of the patient. TCM pays attention to meridians. Although the medicine line is only on the surface of the skin, because it is heated by fire, the drugs on the line will pass from the acupuncture points on the skin to the meridians of the human body through the warming effect, thereby achieving the purpose of treatment. The medicine line moxibustion therapy has a good effect on headache, rhinitis and skin diseases.

When performing moxibustion, the therapist first uses the end of the line with the food and the thumb, and exposes the thread 1–2 cm. At the second step of ignition, the exposed line ends are ignited on the kerosene lamp (alcohol lamp, candle, etc.). If there is a flame, you must extinguish it. You only need to have little fire on the thread. The therapist will apply the end of the line aligned on the acupuncture point, and the wrist and thumb will flex. The thumb (finger) will firmly and agile the Martian thread directly on the acupuncture point. As soon as the fire is extinguished, it is one strong. Generally, a moxibustion is one strong, and the moxibustion can have a slight burning sensation.

Medicine line moxibustion therapy emphasizes the timing of treatment, early treatment (timely treatment), treatment of small (small disease, early treatment of mild disease), treatment (complete treatment, not halfway). As for the course of treatment, it needs to be flexible according to different diseases. The course of acute disease should be short, the course of chronic disease should be long, and the interval between intractable chronic diseases should be shorter, usually 2–3 days. The condition continues to improve during the interval, which is called aftereffect, and the interval can be extended appropriately. Efficacy, especially in some chronic diseases, such as lobular hyperplasia of the breast, after the tumor disappears, it is necessary to continue treatment for a course of treatment to consolidate the effect.

### 24.5.8 Yao Doctor "Three Baths Postpartum"

#### 24.5.8.1 Yao Medicine

Yao medicine is an important part of the composition of Chinese national medicine. It is a unique theoretical system formed by the Yao people living in the southwest of China in the process of looking for ways to treat diseases. The Yao people live in deep forests in the mountains. The natural conditions are foggy and rainy. Different cockroaches can be seen everywhere. Therefore, they are vulnerable to diseases, and they are prone to many diseases such as postpartum diseases, rheumatism and skin diseases. The mountainous terrain is complex, with abundant rainfall and lush vegetation, and has a rich and diverse flora and fauna. Yao medicine has a long history of development. The ancient book "Nanzhong Jixing" mentioned "to live in the mountains, with the benefits of Amomum villosum L., lycium, nan, lacquer, skin, and vine." "Good knowledge of herbs, taking for treatment with good efficacy"; "Ling outside the answer" refers to "emergency drug arrow, eager to remove the meat with a sword, so is not dead" and so on. Yao Medicine Bath has been recognized and promoted in the accumulation of many years. When the medicated bath is used, it can be immersed in warm water and medicinal power to make the blood flow. In winter, it can also be used to resist the cold and make up for the shortage of clothing caused by poverty. With the accumulation of experience, the Yao people have created a decoction prescription for postpartum women on the basis of medicated baths for the prevention and treatment of postpartum diseases.

#### 24.5.8.2 Three Baths Postpartum

Yao folk women began medicinal bath within 1 h after childbirth, and they could work in the field 3 days postpartum. They benefited from Yao Medicine Bath's "three baths postpartum," also known as "three days to work." This is the post-natal care of Yao women for thousands of years. The main method is external treatment method with the characteristics of Yao medicine bath. This medicinal bath uses the natural native Yao medicine of Dayao Mountain. It is developed according to the ancient millennium of Yao people. It has the function of promoting postpartum uterine contraction, repairing the birth canal, reducing lochia, dredging meridians, relieving phlegm and relieving pain, removing saprophytic muscles, replenishing vital energy, and relieving Fatigue, enhance immunity, whitening and moisturizing, prolactin and other effects can effectively treat postpartum lochia, poor milk discharge, postpartum spasm and other diseases. Its usage is: use 40–50 kg of hot water with a temperature of about 80–90 °C every time, pour it into the bucket, soak the medicine for 25–30 min, then repeatedly squeeze the medicine to make the medicine cool naturally. Appropriate temperature (in principle, not lower than 45 °C), then enter the barrel and slowly wash, the bathing time is about 20 min, avoid putting head into the water, starting from the third day after birth, once a day for 3 consecutive days , the whole body can be washed (the women with cesarean section does not wash the incision). The first bath can remove odor and phlegm; the second bath can shrink the abdomen and repair the damaged birth canal; the third bath can quickly restore physical strength and improve immunity. The punk bucket used in the medicated bath is also called the yellow bucket, which is generally a wooden barrel made of fir of 1 m × 0.6 m × 0.7 m.

#### 24.5.8.3 The Treatment Mechanism of "Three Baths Postpartum"

The "three baths postpartum" is the best embodiment of the three treatment methods of "through the veins, Kaiguan Tongyu, and detoxification" in the Yao medical system. Through the method of postpartum medicated bath, the medicine is inserted into the vein, so as to achieve the purpose of detoxification, and elimination of disease and evil through sweating, promote postpartum repair and maintain break-even. In the Qing Dynasty, Wu Shangxian mentioned in the "Liang Li Wen": "The principle of external treatment, that is, the rule of internal treatment; the medicine for external treatment, that is, the medicine for internal treatment; The Yao medicinal bath belongs to the category of TCM external treatment and is a kind of transdermal drug delivery system. As the largest organ of the human body, the skin regulates blood circulation, absorption and secretion and excretion. Postpartum skin care is relatively open, and it can be quickly applied through skin administration. The human body is immersed in the syrup, plus the warming effect, the skin telangiectasia, the drug directly penetrates into the human body, promotes blood and lymph circulation, accelerates metabolism, avoids the first-pass effect of the liver and the damage of the drug to the gastrointestinal tract, through physical effects. It has a therapeutic effect with pharmacological effects. In addition, the medicated bath has the characteristics of warmth, can eliminate fatigue, regulate the body's qi, yin and yang, and also has a certain effect of disease prevention and health care.

## 24.6 National Policy for the Development of Chinese Medicine

As a unique health resource, huge potential economic resources, scientific and technological resources with original advantages, excellent cultural resources and important ecological resources, Chinese medicine plays an important role in economic and social development. With the in-depth development of Chinese new industrialization, informationization, urbanization, and agricultural modernization, the process of population aging is accelerating, and the health service industry is booming. With increasing demand for Chinese medicine services, there is an urgent need for inheritance, development, and utilization of TCM, aiming to fully play the role of Chinese medicine in deepening the reform of the medical and health system for the benefit of human health.

The development of Chinese medicine adheres to the people-oriented and service-oriented principle. To meet the health needs of Chinese people as a starting point and a foothold, we must persist that the development of Chinese medicine for the benefit of the people and Chinese medicine, the outcomes of Chinese medicine benefit the people, enhance people's health and well-being, and ensure that the people enjoy safe, effective and convenient Chinese medicine services. Insist on innovation and highlight characteristics. Inherit and innovate throughout the development of Chinese medicine, correctly grasp the relationship between inheritance and innovation, adhere to and carry forward the advantages of TCM, adhere to the original thinking of TCM, make full use of modern science, technology and methods, and promote the continuous development of Chinese medicine theory and practice. Advance the modernization of TCM, and constantly form new features and new advantages in innovation, and keep the Chinese medicine handed down. Insist on deepening reforms and inspiring vitality. Reform and improve the institutional mechanism for the development of Chinese medicine, fully play the decisive role of the market in resource allocation, stimulate investment and consumption, promote industrial restructuring, and fully play the role of the government in formulating plans, introducing policies, guiding investment, and regulating markets. Create a market environment of equal participation and fair competition, and constantly stimulate the potential and vitality of the development of Chinese medicine. Adhere to overall planning and coordinated development. Adhere to the mutual complementarity between Chinese medicine and Western medicine, fully utilize their respective advantages, promote the integration of Chinese and Western medicine, and develop Chinese medicine in opening. We will take into account all aspects of TCM development, focus on urban and rural, regional, domestic and international Chinese medicine development, promote the comprehensive development of Chinese medicine, health care, scientific research, education, industry and culture, promote the coordinated development of TCM, and continuously enhance the integrity and systematisms during the development of Chinese medicine.

The development of TCM first needs to improve the medical service capacity of Chinese medicine, push ahead the health care services for Chinese medicine, vigorously promote the inheritance and education of Chinese medicine, boost the innovation and development of Chinese medicine, enhance the development level of Chinese medicine industry, carry forward the culture of Chinese medicine, promote the Chinese medicine seat home and abroad, and contribute to the benefit of human health.

GPSR Compliance

*The European Union's (EU) General Product Safety Regulation (GPSR) is a set of rules that requires consumer products to be safe and our obligations to ensure this.*

*If you have any concerns about our products, you can contact us on ProductSafety@springernature.com*

In case Publisher is established outside the EU, the EU authorized representative is:

Springer Nature Customer Service Center GmbH
Europaplatz 3
69115 Heidelberg, Germany

**Batch number: 10756339**

Printed by Printforce, the Netherlands